Psychology for Nursing

Psychology for Nursing

BT Basavanthappa MSc (N) PhD

Professor & Principal (Rtd)
Govt College of Nursing, Bangalore
PhD Guide for Research Work

Member
Faculty of Nursing, RGUHS, Karnataka

Examiner
UG and PG, Courses on Nursing Various Universities

Ex-Programme Incharge
IGNOU, BSc Course, Karnataka and Goa

Life Member
Nursing Research Society of India, New Delhi

President
RGUHS, Nursing Teachers Association, Karnataka

Winner
Bharat Excellence Award and Gold Medal
Vikas Ratan Gold Award
UWA Life Time Achievement Award

Shree Veeranjaneya "Shrujanashri" Award

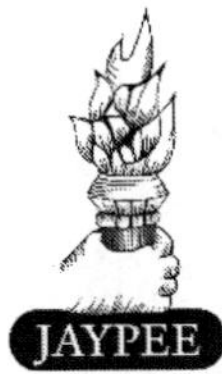

JAYPEE BROTHERS MEDICAL PUBLISHERS
The Health Sciences Publisher
New Delhi | London

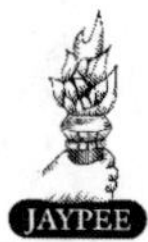

Jaypee Brothers Medical Publishers (P) Ltd

Headquarters
Jaypee Brothers Medical Publishers (P) Ltd
23/23-B, Ansari Road, Daryaganj
New Delhi 110 002, India
Phone: +91-11-23272143, +91-11-23272703
+91-11-23282021, +91-11-23245672
E-mail: jaypee@jaypeebrothers.com

Corporate Office
Jaypee Brothers Medical Publishers (P) Ltd.
4838/24, Ansari Road, Daryaganj
New Delhi 110 002, India
Phone: +91-11-43574357
Fax: +91-11-43574314
E-mail: jaypee@jaypeebrothers.com

Overseas Office
JP Medical Ltd
83 Victoria Street, London
SW1H 0HW (UK)
Phone: +44 20 3170 8910
E-mail: info@jpmedpub.com

EU GPSR Authorised Representative
Logos Europe, 9 rue Nicolas Poussin
17000, La Rochelle, France
Phone: +33 (0) 6 67 93 73 78
E-mail: Contact@logoseurope.eu

Website: www.jaypeebrothers.com
Website: www.jaypeedigital.com

Psychology for Nurses

First Edition: 2010, Reprint: 2026

ISBN: 978-93-5025-007-5

Printed at: Samrat Offset Pvt. Ltd.

To
my parents
and
my nursing profession
and
my dear students

Preface

It gives me immense pleasure and satisfaction to present this title "Psychology for Nursing" to nursing community. In offering this title, I remain grateful to readers who supported my all titles on Nursing and who have provided constructive feedback as well as encouraging comments.

This book is intended to provide an easily comprehensible, non-intimidating and concise text on the subject matter of psychology to the nursing students. It has been written in accordance with the needs of the present existing syllabus prescribed for the nursing course at degree level. The information provided is based on established knowledge and practice and also backed by scientific principles. Every attempt has been made to maintain simplicity and lucidity of language and style.

I hope, this book will continue to serve as good source not only for nursing students but also a source of reference and revision to the nurses who are in service and educational settings.

And I am aware of manifold reason, errors might erept in and shall feel oblige, if such errors are brought to my notice for proper action. Once again I sincerely welcome constructive criticism from readers that would help me to enrich my knowledge.

BT Basavanthappa

Acknowledgments

I owe a great deal of thanks to many who encouraged and supported me with their time and encouragement throughout.

- Shri G Basavannappa, Former Minister of Karnataka State for having initiated and supported me to take up this "Noble Nursing Profession" as my career.
- Dr (Mrs) Manjula K Vasundhra, Former Professor and HOD of Community Medicine, Bangalore Medical College, who continuously encouraged me to write texts in the field of Nursing since nursing is a major force in Medical and Health services.
- My father Shri Thukkappa, who continues to grace for the progress of my career and all-round development of my personality for the welfare of the community.
- My mother Smt Hanumanthamma who continues to be a bright spot in the lives of all who knew her and whose grace gave me strength to progress in my life.
- My wife Smt Lalitha, who gives meaning to my life in so many ways. She is the one whose encouragement keep me motivated, whose support gives me strength and whose gentleness gives me comfort.
- My lovely children BB Mahesh and BB Gaanashree, for all the joy they provided me and all the hope that they instill me and who bare with patient throughout my works of the nursing texts. They keep me young at heart.
- Finally, my warmest appreciation goes to M/s Jaypee Brothers Medical Publishers, New Delhi, for sharing my vision for this book and giving me the chance to turn vision into reality.

BT Basavanthappa

Contents

1

CHAPTER

Historical Development of Psychology

Psychology is apparently concerned with the search for laws that explain the various activities of the animals on the one hand while on the other it aspires to explain the behavior of saints, geniuses and spiritual leaders. The main function of psychology is to explain the states of experience and analyse the process of behavior in the conscious, unconscious, normal, abnormal, child, adolescence, young, old, animal and man, individual and groups. Ideas, concepts, postulates, methodology, theories and subject matter of every science observed to undergo changes and development and the beginning of every branch of knowledge is seen to be shrouded in confused, disordered and undeveloped thoughts. As new advances are made these same thoughts taken an order, clarity and organizations. Sometimes they are also replaced by new ideas than seem to be completely alien to existing thought and normally with time the old theories are discarded to replace the new. With the emergence of new ideas and theories the scope of a science tends to become more precise, sometimes more limited, at other times more extended. Generally, the science is the study of a well-defined and properly delimited subject and the definition applies to each and every science, but in fact the methods of study and scope take on precisions only after gradual development.

Ever since man woke to the mystery of thought and began to make some conjectures on the various changes took place in his mind and body during conditions of sleep, waking, dreaming, etc. he has been making a constant progress in the field of psychology, however silly and ridiculous such conjectures may appeared. The history of psychology coincides with the history of civilization but it cannot be traced any further than Greek times no records are available. In Greek times the various sciences were not distinct from philosophy, for it was the philosophers duty to cogitate upon the stars, earth, soul, mind, body, education, politics and every conceivable subjects. So that psychology emerged as a branch of philosophy.

Greek Philosophers' Views on Psychology

There is not much to be gained by a detailed account of the views of all Greek philosophers for few of them had anything enlightening to say on psychology. From our standpoint, only the views of Democritus, Plato and Aristotle are worth mentioning, for only these thinkers made an effort to elucidate the nature of knowledge and its process. The views of Democritus, Plato and Aristotle are as given below:

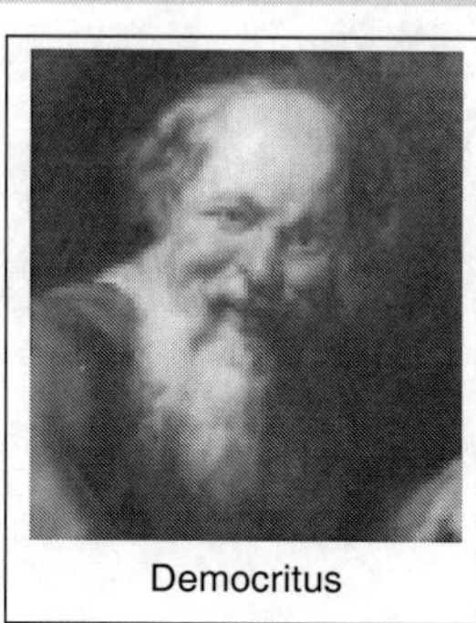
Democritus

1. Democritus's views—Democritus (460-370 BC) was influenced by the mechanistic explanations of natural phenomena, and he believed the world to be constituted of dynamic atoms or very small particles, atoms that are indivisible, imperceptible, ultimate and permanent. He further believed that they possessed the same qualities, but that they differed in respect of weight and number. Every object of the natural world, including the soul, was made up of these particles, and at death atoms were disorganized. And since both the body and soul were constituted of atoms nothing was left after death. In considers the world to be constituted of atoms, although an atomistic explanation of human psychology is a difficult task, indeed.

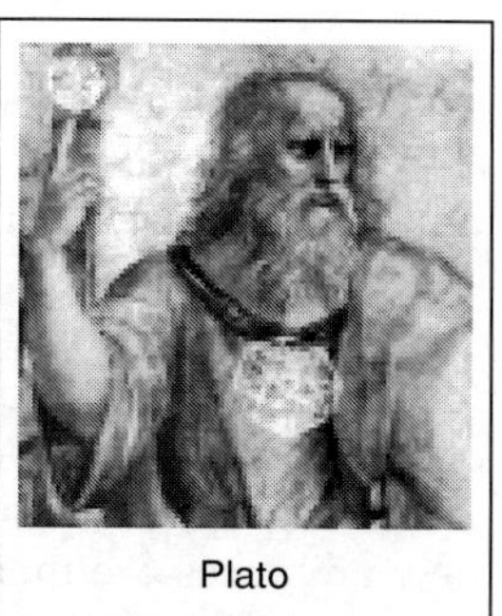
Plato

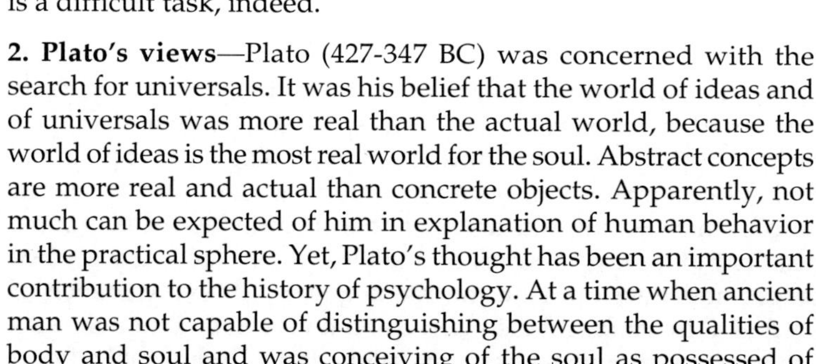

2. Plato's views—Plato (427-347 BC) was concerned with the search for universals. It was his belief that the world of ideas and of universals was more real than the actual world, because the world of ideas is the most real world for the soul. Abstract concepts are more real and actual than concrete objects. Apparently, not much can be expected of him in explanation of human behavior in the practical sphere. Yet, Plato's thought has been an important contribution to the history of psychology. At a time when ancient man was not capable of distinguishing between the qualities of body and soul and was conceiving of the soul as possessed of physical traits, Plato defined the quality of body and soul, pointing out their essential differences. In his opinion the soul is definitely not physical, and even after the body's destruction the soul continues to live. It, he believes, is capable of thinking upon abstract subjects, for it can rise above its physical environment to the world of pure ideas, a world that is far more real than the physical one. Knowledge is a function of the soul, and the soul alone can know beauty, good, the real and ultimate element.

Plato, the philosopher divided the soul into three parts located in different parts of the body.

- Appetitive represents peremptory desires, physical lusts and greed.
- Rational which was immortal and divine and located in the brain.
- Spirited affective.

According to him appetitive and rational are in conflict and the spirited affective can be enlisted on either side. Plato said 'health is the result of harmony between body and mind whereas disharmony between them results in *mania* or *gross ignorance*.' Plato distinguished two kinds of madness—one resulted from human ailments when the appetitive soul lost the domination of the rational and other was produced by time disturbances of the soul.

In addition to his opinions on the psychology of the human soul, Plato also made certain excursions into the field of interaction between society and the individual. It was a definite belief with Plato that man's behavior is the outcome of his social system, the system into which he has been born. He considers man's tendency to learn as the very basis of his behavior within society occur. Man's natural instincts, those with which he is born, are subject to radical change through the agency of education. An individual's personality is moulded according to the circumstances in which he finds himself or education which is given to him, and his behavior in his social environment is conditioned by it. Thus, it can be seen that if certain desired changes are to be introduced into society it is necessary that the system of education should be improved. In his famous work *Republic Plato* has upto forward an ideal system of education suited to his ideal state. Plato's thought is characterized by imbalance for he has placed the utmost stress on the importance of society, as much as to say that compared with society the individually of man is of no account.

3. Aristotle's views—Aristotle's (330-322 BC) was the most substantial contribution to Greek thought in the field of psychology. From the standpoint of history of psychology his contribution can be evaluated from the following aspects:

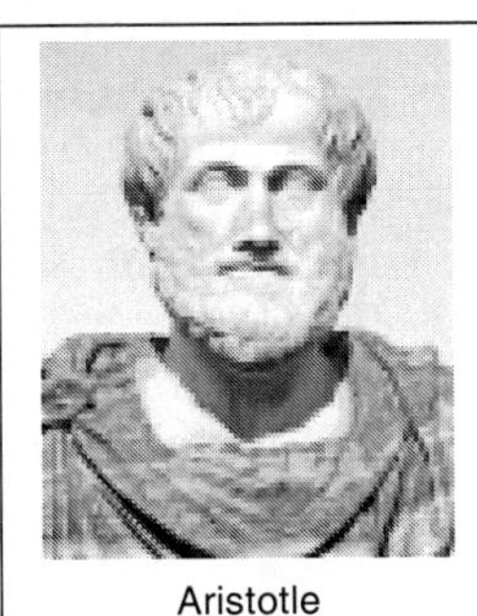

Aristotle

i. Establishment of relation between soul and body—Aristotle has constructed an edifice of knowledge that allows for a very intimate relationship between soul and the physical being, both on the practical and the intellectual level.

   Plato's pupil believed that the soul was the center of psychic life, located in the heart, and derived its energy from natural heat and that it was vulnerable to changes in temperature, black bile and the emotions.

   Cold black bile leads to apoplexy, numbness, fearfulness and becoming disheartened.

   Hot black bile produced cheerfulness, bursting into song, ecstasy and the eruption of sores.

   Music is the release of repressed emotions or passions, that is abreaction.

   Passion must be purged continuously to avoid violence.

   Theater is collective cathartic device. Aristotle first accurately described the affections of desire, anger, fear, courage, envy, joy, hatred and pity. 3

ii. Improvement of body and soul dualism—The dualistic view of the body and soul had been prevalent from ancient times to Plato, who had completely supported it, but now Aristotle improved upon it. He has given an explanation of the soul's nature that reduces body and soul to manifestations, one of the others, so that the functions of the body appear to be caused by the soul, and those of the soul by the living organism. But in improving upon this dualistic principle Aristotle did not have recourse to the atomism of Democritus, for he has explained the relationship on the basis of matter and form. What he says in effect is that matter and form are to be seen together everywhere. It is the matter of which an object is made that determines the uses to which the object will be put, and all that is latent in matter is manifested in real shape in form. For example, each and everyone of the body's parts physical, but their functions differ on account of their various shapes or forms. This form is the soul, and, accordingly, each and every organ of the body has its soul which finds expression in the organ's own specific functions. The soul of the eye, for example, lies in its ability to see, if there is no soul, the eye cannot see. This point is furnished illustrated by the fact that a statue has eyes but they do not see, for they do not have any soul. Soul, in this sense, always accompanies the eye; consequently the moment the eye is opened one can see.

iii. Analysis of human experience—Aristotle went further to the explanation of man's experiences in ordinary day-to-day life. A detailed account of the psychology of adolescence, old age, sleeping, waking and dreaming states. In explaining the nature of memory he places much emphasis upon the importance of proximity, similarity and contrast. When things are seen in close proximity to each other the thought of one results the other. Similarity and contrast both help memory, for perception of anything may help recollection of things similar or contrasted. Black reminds one of white no less than of black itself. It should be noticed that these views on the nature of memory are incorporated into the theory of association. Further, he made detailed investigation into the functions of sense organs, and besides memory he cogitated upon learning, emotion, imagination, argument, etc. his thinking is not confined to the activities and processes of the living or waking world; instead he tried to glance into the realm that borrows its importance from dreams or foretelling. In his work 'Ethics' he analyses the psychology of pleasure and tries to solve the problems of self-control. In Politics, another of his writings, he puts forward to numerous human problems, while in his De Oratore he has engagingly shown how an orator tries to arouse emotions in the audience.

iv. Interaction of society and individual—In the study of interaction between society and individual, for Aristotle has laid stress on the fundamental psychological principle that society and the individual, instead of being independent entities, are parts of an interacting system. Modern psychology believes the interaction between individual and environment to be the sole determinant of personality. The kind of interaction that the living being evinces with the environment is an expression of its nature. Similarly, the nature of the environment can be judged from the beings reaction to it. Aristotle's ideas on the social behavior of the individual are important. But subject are completely at variance with Plato's views. For, Plato believes that education is a must if human behavior is to be changed, but Aristotle holds the view that man's fundamental nature cannot be changed, even by education. He holds that the instincts are the causes and determinants of his social behavior and conduct. It is Plato's opinions that the individuals nature depends upon the nature of society, while Aristotle holds the contrary opinion, that is, that nature of society depends primarily upon the individuals nature. Society, according to Aristotle, is the outcome of human tendencies that are not subject to change, from which it follows that society, too, cannot be changed. Interpreted in this light it appears that Aristotle presents a negative or pessimistic outlook on human life.

Heraclitus (535-470 BC): A philosopher believed that mental health depended not only on the integrity of body parts but on an equilibrium between opposite psychological tendencies that existed in the soul. He recognized soma and psyche.

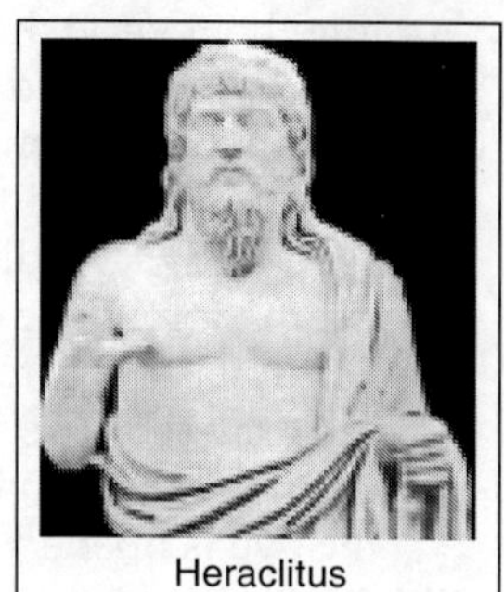
Heraclitus

Hippocrates (450-355 BC): The father of Medicine. He believed that the body contained four essential humors—blood, phlegm, yellow bile and black bile—which were secreted by different organs, possessed different qualities, and varied with the seasons. The brain was regarded as a seat of life, and its normal functioning required a harmony between the humors. Crasis is the appropriate interaction between internal and external forces while dyscrasis is the presence of excessive bodily humor which had to be removed by purging. The smaller excess of body humors produced choleric (black bile), melancholic (yellow bile), phlegmatic (phlegm) and sanguine (blood) personalities. The Hippocratic authors gave first rational classification to mental diseases, including epilepsy, mania, depression, paranoia (which today called mental deterioration), postpartum psychosis, organic toxic delirium, and phobias. They described some of the symptoms of "hysteria" and named it believing that it was confined to women and was caused by wandering uterus (Thus, marriage and intercourse were the recommended cure).

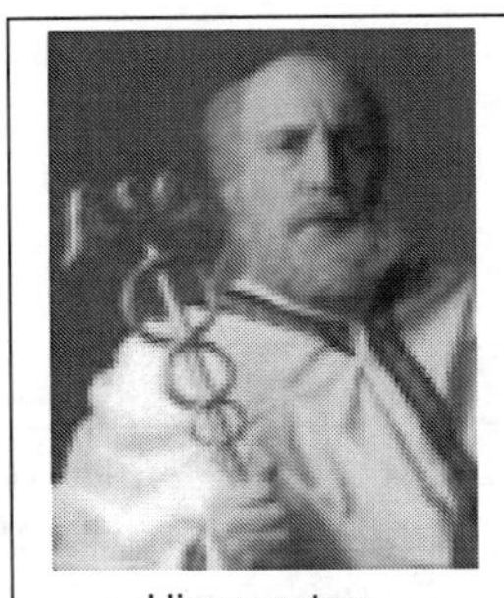
Hippocrates

Greek philosophers also advocated three psychological therapies for mental illnesses—the therapy of the world, induced sleep and dream divination. Words were used to alleviate illness in different ways—as prayers, magical incantations, cheering speeches, rhetorical speeches meant to persuade and Plato's verbal dialectics. In the 6th Century BC, the Greek philosophers of Ionia believed that human mind was composed of atoms in motions, and mental illness occurred when there were changes in the size and motions of the atoms, in the amount of humors and vital substances. They believed Mania and Lyssa are the dreaded Goddesses sent by angry God.

VIEWS OF EPICURUS (340-430 AD)

It was on the time of ruins of the Greek civilization that the philosophy of Hedonism took its stand. Tendencies of this age are reflected and succinctly engraved on the mental framework of Epicurus, who based his hedonism on the atomism of Democritus, a hedonism that differed from the Socratic theory of pleasure pain. It was a hedonistic philosophy characterized by rigidity, indifference and even an inaction. It was Epicurus view that this world is a vale of tears, and it is for man to make the best of it, to derive as much pleasure from it as is possible. This is the pleasure of a peaceable, calm and placid life. He stressed the fact that man differs from the animal, for he is self-conscious, intelligent, capable of looking into the future and the past. Man cannot, said Epicurus, crush his should for the sake of physical pleasures, he cannot sacrifices the past or the present to a few moments of pleasure, for his life is not merely one of sensual pleasures. Pleasures that he derives from them are pleasures for him, in fact, pleasure that are superior to pleasures of a purely sensual nature. Man does not, or would not, like to lead the meaningless, disorganized and violent life of the animal, he prefers placid and calm pleasures. His intelligence tells him that indiscriminate indulgence undermines health while control and limited indulgence give energy to the soul. Dissatisfaction can be avoided only when desires are few, because all our numerous wishes cannot be fulfilled. Epicurus had divided desired into the inevitable, unnecessary and meaningless, etc. He holds that only those desires should be fulfilled which help health and promote peace. Pleasures of inactivity are superior to a life of anxiety for it gives permanent peace.

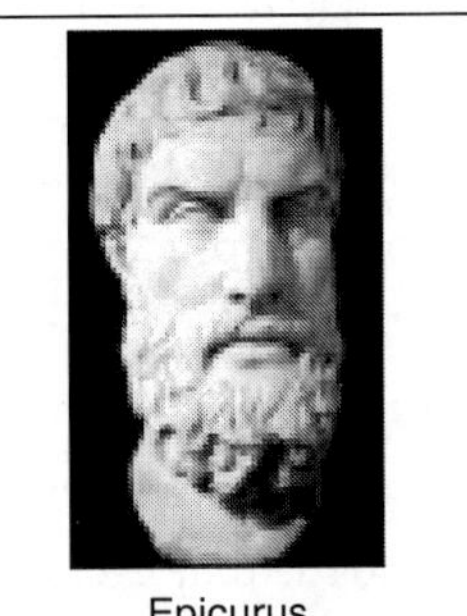
Epicurus

CHURCH FATHERS VIEWS

The Church Fathers philosophy chiefly finds expression in the views of Paul, Origen and Augustine, whose philosophical ideas were based primarily on the mind-body dualism of

Plato. As is apparent from every aspect of Christian religion, they expressed despair regarding the physical body and its values. Man is by nature animalistic, a concept to which is attached the moralistic prejudice of sin, crime and the desire to be rid of them. This Christian religion was aimed at slaves, soldiers, fisherman and the lowest level of artisans and farmers, but soon it permeated society in its entirety. Philosophical and religious idealogy of the Mediterranean world bears unmistakable marks of this Christian religion. There was a rediscovery of Aristotelian philosophy in the field of psychology after this phase of Epicurean hedonism and Church despair. This rediscovery led to an increasing interest in naturalism, due to which research in the field of science and medicine found encouragement. As a consequence, the human soul was considered in the same terms as the various objects of everyday life and experience. In the light of this reconsiderations of Aristotelian thought the philosophy of the Church Fathers lost ground or was reinterpreted in a more naturalistic direction. And hence it would be no exaggeration to remark that psychological thought during and immediately after the renaissance is colored by Aristotelian philosophy. Thomas Aquinas attempted a reconciliation between the humane naturalism of Aristotle on the one hand, and the mind-body dualism of Plato and the Church Fathers on the other. It was an unsuccessful attempt. The influence wielded by Aristotelian psychology was strong enough to turn the philosophy of Church Fathers towards naturalism. Saint Augustine (345-430 AD) wrote a book 'Confession' which was first book that centered on psychological introspection and on psychological autobiographical insights. It has been rated as "the earliest forerunner of psychoanalysis" "psychoanalysis without a psychoanalyst listening and interpreting the confessions".

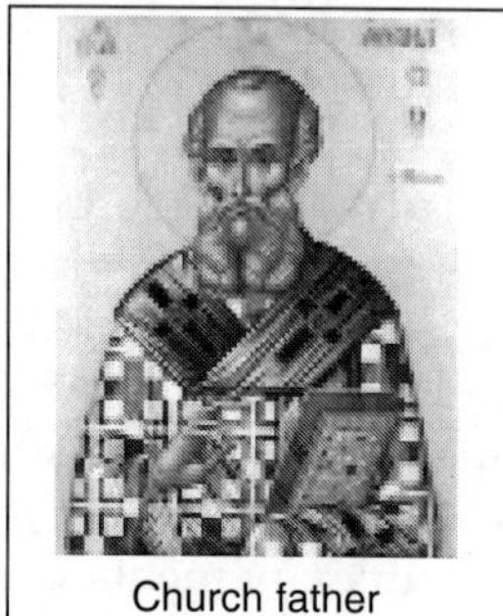
Church father

CONTRIBUTIONS OF INDIVIDUALS AND INSTITUTIONS IN THE PERIOD OF RENAISSANCE

While the majority of contributions in this renaissance came from individual effort, much valuable work was also done by institutions. In this connection much important work was done in France and more particularly in Paris during the latter half of the seventeenth century. In 1671 the Paris Academy of Sciences was given royal aid, and it is a matter of regret that while in France scientific progress was aided by the state, in England people of the genius of Newton had to toil on alone. And the royal society that Newton misnomer to call it aid. Much the same conditions existed in Spain and Portugal where people were engaged in geographical discoveries. Even these discoveries, as is evident from the history of Columbus, though some aid from the government was forthcoming. As Germany was divided into numerous small states at the time, scientific progress could not be financed by the state, even its scientists were scattered far and wide. In Italy the conditions were, if anything, worse, for there, even a genius like Galileo had continually to withstand much hostile criticism from the church and state. Only in the field of biological sciences did Italy contribute anything important during this period, and even here much of the credit for it must go to scientific methods. Harvey published his theory concerning the circulation of blood in 1628, but what was even more important was that he succeeded in demonstrating and proving his principle.

It is evident from the foregoing sketch of the development of psychology during the Greek period and renaissance that in this period there was a steady development of scientific methods, objective observation and empirical tests. The importance of the renaissance period for psychology lies not in developments of psychological concepts but in the advent of the scientific method. Observation and empirical tests gradually took the place of tradition and testimony during this period. And with this development of the scientific method a strong foundation for psychology was laid, which was responsible for the progress made in the centuries to come. Thus, even before the 17th century the foundations of psychology as a science had been laid, although the psychological laboratory came into existence much later.

Rene Descartes (1596-1650), a French thinker of great eminence, saw the light of day in the district of Touraine in 1956 and from his very infancy evinced a philosophic tendency. Descartes, who was once philosopher, now became a psychologist for he abandoned the abstractions of soul and mind for the actuality of consciousness. On the other hand, by accepting scientific suggestions in his thinking he supported the scientificity that was all the craze. He accepted this scientific process in order to explain psychological elements. Besides, even while he lived, the study of physiology and psychology were coming into close contact, and out of this combination was born determinism and reflexism. When the two sciences came very close together and threatened to merge emphasis was placed on the coordinated activity of mind and body. Again, Descartes made a definite contribution by placing so much reliance on scientific methodology, so that his insistence on determinism brought about requisite changes in the field of psychology. Physiology also left its impression upon psychology, so that psychology no longer remained the science of the soul. This constitutes, in its very precise form, the contribution that Descartes made to the development of psychology. A deductive rationalist. He introduced the concept of reflex are to explain all animal, and much human, behavior. "A sense organ is stimulated, there is a tug on the 'strings' leading to brain; animal spirits are released into hollow behaves. In the case of man, however, a 'dam' may be raised through the faculty of will". Believed that man had a thinking substance, the soul, which did not interact with the body, thus creating a misleading mind-body dichotomy which still haunts the study of man.

BARUCH SPINOZA

Baruch Spinoza (1632-1677): Portuguese/Dutch philosopher has been called as perhaps the greatest of pre-Freudian psychologists. Challenged Descartes' mind-body dualism and replaced it with a concept of psycho-physiological parallelism, supplying the epistemological foundation of psychosomatic medicine. He remarks that by emotion he understands those changes of mode in the body by means of which activity increases or decreases, is assisted or retarded, besides which he comprehends in emotion the visible forms of such changes. At another juncture Spinoza writes that emotion, which is considered the excitement or oppression of the soul, is an indistinct concept through which the mind announces the increase or decrease in the existence potential of its body or some part of it, and which, once it is accepted, determines the mind to cogitate upon one object instead of another.

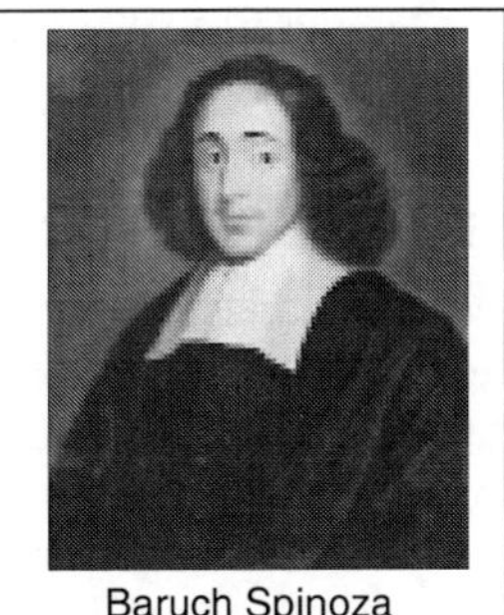

Baruch Spinoza

Spinoza contends that in life that every basis of motivation is self-preservation. Self-preservation is motivation. It is for this that man desires. Desire or proper volition is an essential part of motivation. Spinoza remarks that there can be no cogitation superior to the one concerning the tendency towards an effort to preserve oneself. He further remarks that desire is that object or project which is kept in mind while acting. And self-preservation is possible only when a person acts intelligently and with some desire. Objective performance of one's duty consists in acting on the basis of his own good, directed by his intelligence, in conducting one's life on his principle and in maintaining one's existence. In the opinion of Spinoza man is motivated by a strong desire to continue living, so he indulges in acts that bring him physical or mental satisfaction. It is in this way that the adjustment of life is attained.

According to Spinoza the different levels of knowledge are the following:

1. *Sensory knowledge:* The first source of our knowledge is the sense, with the help of which we know or become conscious of the external world. Spinoza accepts the dichotomy between mind and body, and the differences of form and mode in the bodies of different persons. For this reason it is feasible that all the various sensations that occur may be experienced differently by separate persons, just as the same object leads different individuals to different conclusions. A piece of rope appears a snake to one, a piece of rope to another. To summarize, Spinoza holds that sensory knowledge is individual and personal, and hence it cannot be universal.
2. *Intellectual knowledge:* As a general rule, the proper knowledge of any subject can occur only at the intellectual level. According to Spinoza, the origin and development of sciences and mathematical concepts depends upon the intelligence or brain. Knowledge gleaned by the brain has association, logicality, cogitation and conception. For this reason the facts of science and mathematics have universality or universal validity, and are free from self-contradiction.
3. *Intuition:* Both the former sources of knowledge yield information concerning the external world, but a third kind, intuition, depends upon dignity and majesty, it arises from sublimity. Eternal truths are grasped only by this level of knowledge. Knowledge of this kind is confined to saints, philosophers and other people with extraordinary powers. In fact, only the knowledge received from this third source, on this level, is true knowledge. According to Spinoza only this third kind of knowledge is real; he has also clarified how the ordinary mortal can attain to this level, after having achieved the two previous levels.

LEIBNITZ (1646-1716)

With regard to body-mind relation. Using the casual relationship as a basis Leibnitz demonstrated that just as physiological processes occur on account of specific laws and causes, so do mental functions happen due to certain specific laws and causes. Physiological and mental processes are not influenced by the functioning of the soul. Hence the body and mind function in their separate and individual capacities, there being no interaction between the two. In order to elucidate this principle Leibnitz made use of an example of two watches that are constructed to tell time. Both tell the same time, yet neither influences the other in any manner, their functioning is independent of the other. Mind and body function on similar lines, and the natural interaction that apparently exists between the two is on account of a pre-established harmony. We can understand the present variations in the mind only if we are aware of the variations that have taken place in the past. Similarly, the changes in the body can be understood only on the basis of changes that have occurred in the past within that body. This theory propagated by Leibnitz is called Parallelism.

Leibnitz has also reflected upon the nature of relations that exist between mental occurrences. Mental activity he has divided into two classes—vivid or conscious and amorphous or unconscious. From the viewpoint of vividity he has divided consciousness into four classes—self-conscious, conscious, subconscious, and unconscious. And, in fact, the Freudian psychoanalytic psychology has it basis in this division of consciousness. Freud has made use of no other than these words. Leibnitz has opined that thoughts which are indistinct remain in the unconscious and the subconscious, while experiences or thoughts that are distinct or vivid come to the conscious or self-conscious level. Monad is the center of consciousness; it is a very subtle element. All knowledge, in his opinion, is self-knowledge, and every monad sees only that which it possesses within itself. Perception is an internal condition that only lights up things or exhibits external things. Apperception is a conscious condition and is the reflected knowledge of an internal condition. Monad is the center of consciousness; it is a very subtle element. All knowledge, in his opinion, is self-knowledge, and every monad sees only that which it possesses within itself. Perception is an internal condition that only lights up things or exhibits external is an things. Appreciation is a conscious condition and is the reflected knowledge of an internal condition. Monad, according to this philosopher, is the basis of these forms or conditions of consciousness. And it is through the instrumentality of these monads that thoughts are present, to begin with, in man's mind. It is his contention that these monads are indivisible, eternal, subject to change due to no external influence but only to changes that occur within each individual monad. Leibnitz remarks that they have no window through which something can come out or go in because of impressions these monads are present at the very outset. Monads constitute the entire existence.

Descartes, Spinoza and Leibnitz, each of them is a rationalist. They believe that the basis of knowledge is thought. According to Descartes internal or innate thoughts are true and vivid. In this manner, in his opinion, some thoughts are innate, but according to Leibnitz all of them are so. Man does not receive anything from outside, all knowledge is present inside him in a potent condition, and along with gradual development it keeps on emerging.

GEORGE BERKELEY (1685-1753)

Berkeley agreed with the Locke that knowledge is possible only through sensation, but he also believed that the external object has no independent existence, it depends upon our own mind. The entire world is nothing more than imagination. He held that no distinction between primary and secondary quality. Berkeley hold that primary qualities reside not in the object but in the mind. Concepts also exists in mind, and apart from concepts no object has any distinct existence. No object has any existence if it is not experienced. This is subjective idealism, according to which the mind is the very basis of this universe. From sensations Berkeley passers on to perception, and opines that external objects are possible only when they produce direct knowledge. In the absence of such direct knowledge these external objects have no existence.

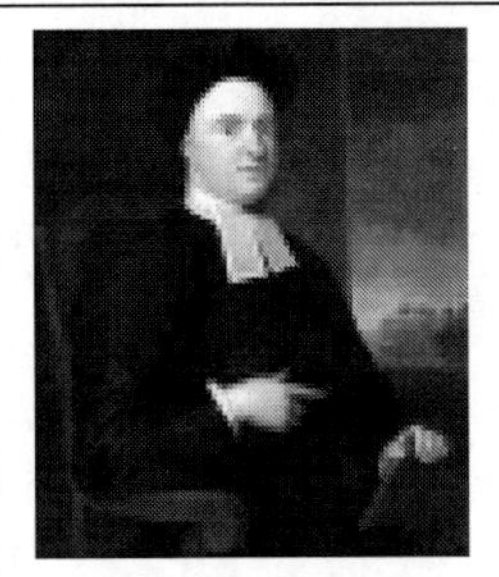
George Berkeley

Berkeley accepted the existence of soul and God, on account of which he can be called religious and theistic. In spite of his theory of visual space perception has its importance from the point of view of psychology. He holds that association can be made use of to explain the various experiences muddled up in perception. In explaining the functioning of the retina he has remarked that with its aid we view any object in only two dimensions—above, below, left or right. Knowledge of the third dimensions is derived from the sensation of touch which gives is knowledge of thickness, roundedness, roughness, smoothness but such knowledge is not the subject of visual perception.

Berkeley's contention concerning perception is subject to the following difficulties:
1. Berkeley's theory concerning direct or perceptual knowledge is not quite psychological, because his rejection of all objective existence precludes the possibility of perception. How can there be perception if there is no existent? He contends that an object has existence only because we perceive it, but what this implies is that perception is possible only if some object has existence.
2. In the opinion of Berkeley the only two elements that participate in perception are the object perceived and the preceptor while from the psychological standpoint such an activity demands three elements, namely, however, known and knowledge.
3. Berkeley holds that all that we perceive is either the thoughts or ideas of the mind or the sensations originating in the senses. Neo-realists hold, to the contrary, that the mind perceives an object directly and not through the medium of thoughts.
4. Berkeley argues that objects are complex ideas since they appear to be different when viewed by separate individuals. Yet the variability of perception does not reduce the objectivity of matter, for it can change in appearance when conditions change.

JOHN LOCKE (1632-1704)

British philosopher John Locke, the father of modern empiricism. Every aspect of psychology is considered in the various books written by John Locke, but the chief problem engage him was the means by which the human organism came into the possession of universal truth was complete to reflect upon the nature of human mind. Sensation, Locke believes, in the very cause of experiences of some object and reflection, which is a kind of mental process, the reaction that mind makes into the experience and thoughts. According to Locke reflection is considered an essential part of perception. Perception is of three kinds—external, internal and direct. Lockes' importance for the history of psychology lies in his contribution to the principle of association in its original form. He threw fresh light upon memory and association and how the two are related. Empiricism was explained beautifully by him. Generally speaking, the following objections can be raised against empiricism form the standpoint of modern psychology:

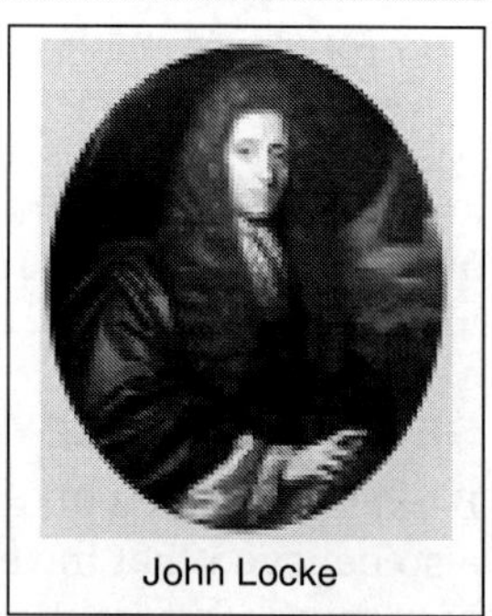

John Locke

- *Mind is not passive:* According to empiricists mind passively receives sensations. While on the other hand, as has been proved by modern psychological researches, mind selects in the reception of sensations. A man cannot equally attend to all the sensations and therefore he does not experience those sensations to which he does not pay any attention.
- *Mind is active in making ideas:* According to empiricists mind makes idea soon the basis of sensations received by it. Then how can it remain passive? Does it not become active in the process of making ideas.

- *Absence of distinction between knowledge and ideas:* While John Locke and David Hume have tried to distinguish between knowledge and ideas they could not explain the distinction properly because in fact both ideas and knowledge are two aspects of the same process.
- *Absence of explanation of the relation of ideas and objects:* According to empiricists the idea is different from the object. But they do not point out as to what is the nature of this object? It is different from the idea. And if so then how can we have knowledge of the object through the idea? The explanation advanced by empiricists in this connection is not satisfactory.
- *Opposed to Gestalt psychology:* According to empiricists the sensations reach the mind one by one. As against this the modern Gestalt psychologists believe that perception is not a putting together of different bits of sensations but it is a whole.
- *Empiricism culminates into skepticism:* According to the empiricists, the knowledge based on experiences is relative, indefinite and particular. It is clear that such a knowledge cannot solve philosophical problems. We cannot hope to arrive at universal empiricism in philosophy, therefore, is skepticism.
- *Absence of proper explanation of perceptions:* According to empiricists our sense organs are the medium through which the qualities of the external object reach the mind. According to modern psychology perception also depends on past experience, mental set, attention and interest besides sensations.

THOMAS HOBBES (1588-1679)

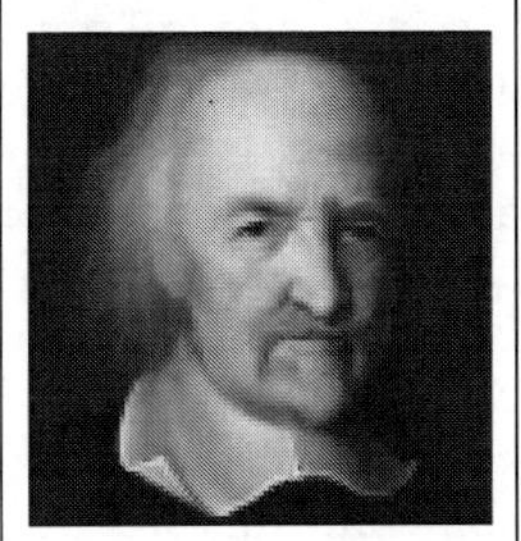
Thomas Hobbes

Thomas Hobbes who was responsible for an important changes in traditional thinking on psychology. He made a detailed study of the human mind. In this process, among the various mental characteristics that he studies the most important are his studies on sensory perception and perceptual knowledge. His standpoint is all the more interesting for it forms the part of the foundation of social psychology. He holds the view that innate elements of a human tendency are the very basis for social organization and social behavior. According him, social organization and social behavior are determine dialy by hunger, thirst, sex, fear, desire for honor, pleasure seeing and avoidance of pain. He placed much stress upon government and culture as elements in social control, organization and behavior. Laws of nature inspired him to analyse human behavior. Hobbes psychology in fact, is based upon an empirical viewpoint which contents that all knowledge is based on experience and believed only the experience acquired by our five senses—taste, smell, sound, touch and light constitutes truth.

This Hobbes, the empiricist, managed to give psychology a new turn by his scientific thinking. Sensory experiences and perceptual knowledge were considered the source of thought or experiences. Association is the other field to which Hobbes contributed. He laid the foundation of associations by explaining the relationship between experiences on the basis of independent and controlled associated thinking. Empiricism finds its first champion in Hobbes, in connection with which he plundered much from coffers of science. His views one particularly valuable from the psychological standpoint. He practically banished God and soul from the field of psychology both of which had been accredited by Descartes and other thinkers before him. Experience and perceptions were the most important in his opinion.

DAVID HUME (1711-1776)

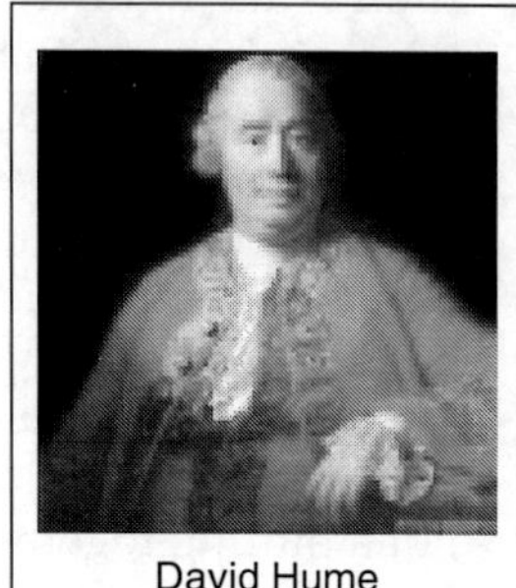
David Hume

David Hume was the British empiricist philosophy, attempted to storm the ultimate fortress of empiricism. He believed that perceptual knowledge is the basis of mental experience. Association of thought is the process which makes mental functioning possible. No divine force or concept is necessary for this purpose. Hume accepts three possible sources of knowledge—perception, inference and imagination. All our mental activities takes place on the basis of perceived knowledge. Hume laid emphasis only upon the unification of experience without accepting God or soul as a substance. Experience is all that is necessary for the process of thinking. And he made use of the principle of association in order to explain the unity of experience. His theory of association differs somewhat from the principles propounded by other empiricists. His chief contribution to psychology lies in his theory of association. According to him all objects take the form of experience and thought. It is only through the mutual relationship of concepts that we can know our dreams, memory and experience.

DAVID HARTLEY (1705-1757)

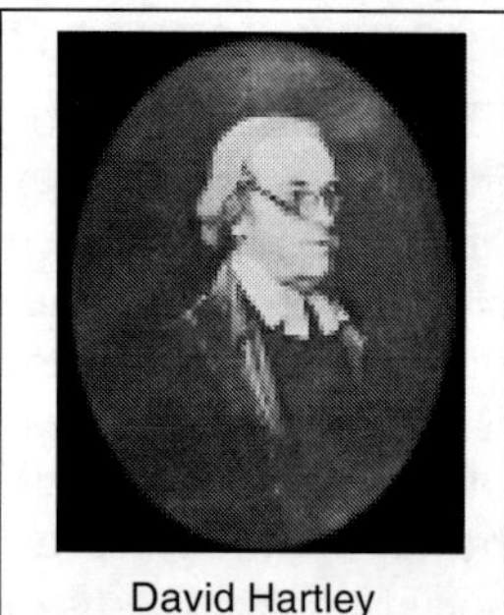
David Hartley

Hartley was a contemporary of Hume he was not influenced by the Latters views, instead, he explained all mental activity from the psychological standpoint. He has chosen to explain all mental activity on the basis of physiological mobility, and he established a similarity between motor habit and such a mental phenomenon as memory. In a motor habit there is an order or series of motor activities in which every activity activates or sets into motion of every other unit. In other words, one activity is followed by another in the motor habit. It is his contention that in mental activity there is an order the mind in a particular order. After sometime this order of experiences becomes organized and takes on the form of memory. He remarks that thought or idea is the name give to an organized form of ideas or thoughts through the process of association. In the manner he accepts the physiological basis for all mental activity. He has opined that all the mental activity depends upon nerve fiber. Sensation, images and ideas are all born out of nerve fiber, without it they cannot arise.

THOMAS REED (1710-1792)

Thomas Reed was responsible for establishing the Scottish School of Psychology. The history of psychology guided in the following respects from the efforts of Reed:

1. Reed's primary task was the refutation of Hume's philosophy of agnosticism. Hume had laid emphasis only upon conscious effort after denying the existence of the external world, but Reed pointed out the necessity of believing in the external world because, as he reasoned, the mind provides us knowledge of this same external world. His contention is that we know undoubtedly that there is a mind within us, a mind having the power of thinking. Besides, we can act in a rational manner and that we also have within us the capacity to perceive actual objects.

2. Another contribution of Reed to the history of psychology lies in the importance which he attached to sense organs in the functions of the mind. In his opinion it is these sense organs which provide the mind with the knowledge of the external world. And, in the form of common observation, he developed a new method upon which his whole system of psychology is based. It is on the basis of common observation that we believe credulity of the sense so that we are enabled contact with the external world.
3. The third contribution of Reed to psychology concerns intellectual powers and innate concepts. Associationists believed that the child's mind is bereft of all thoughts of feelings, but on the contrary, Reed believed in Descartes notion of innate ideas. Reed contends that we are sentient and intelligent beings born with some innate powers by means of which we try to solve our problems, to know the external world and to forecast what can possibly occur in future. Besides this the child is further equipped naturally for distinguishing between right and wrong. Every individual being is free to adopt what is either true or what is false. Reed's arguments indicate very clearly that he was opposed to associationism, and wanted instead to study psychology in the light of innate powers on the basis of common observation.

Brett, a historian of psychology, has written of Reed that he has elucidated the simple and complex mental activities in his system of psychology, if it can be called that. He examined consciousness and laid emphasis upon experience, and for this he accepted the importance of sense organs. Thoughts are formed from experiences received through the sense organs. From this it is further evident that Reed accepted the inductive method in which specific experiences lead to general experiences or laws. Although this viewpoint of Reed resembles associationism to a certain extent, yet he does not express any faith in the latter view point.

Concerning the contribution of the Scottish school to the development of psychology Gardner Murphy has stated explicitly that such contribution is more general than specific. In his words, "Because of its insistence upon the unity and coherence of mental life and because it pictured the individual as an active entity, not as a mere field in which ideas assembled and reassembled, the greatest contributions of the Scottish school were necessarily general rather than specific". If contributed little to the solution of specific problems until the school became blended to some extent with associationist movement. And the contribution of the Scottish school was not very productive in so far as the development of psychology is concerned because the progress in this field of science has been primarily based upon scientific thinking. In fact, by reinstating the soul Thomas Reed and his followers did not science a disservice by sending it back to the point of its departure. We will see later on that this same tendency took the form of faculty psychology and developed in Germany under the leadership of Wolff. Whateverelse may be the fact, there can be no denying that the influence of Reed and his followers was no longer limited to Scotland but had spread to France, England, American and other countries. His new theory became a subject which was debated by the general populations and it was in this form that it became famous as a school of psychology.

WOLFF (1679-1735)

Wolff has mentioned two faculties or powers of the mind, namely knowing and feeling. Under feeling he mentioned two important kinds pleasure and pain. He remarks that pain arises in a condition where something is lacking while pleasure arises under conditions of satisfaction or satiation. A sense of pleasure is not at all possible under any circumstances of want. The faculty of knowledge has been divided into various composite faculties by Wolff-sensation, perception, memory, imagination, argument, etc. According to him the knowledge received by sensation and perception is complemented and completed by the imagination. For memory he believe to be the power of recollecting older experiences. Further elements an the faculty of knowledge are understanding, judgment and general concept. In expanding upon argument he says that the power of argument gives is as definite conclusions based upon concepts. According to him the functioning of the mind and body are equally important for life. Just as the functioning of body depends upon the sensations created by stimuli belonging to the external world, mental functioning depends upon the thoughts that arise in it. Both work equally.

ETIENNE BONNETED CONDILLAC (1715-1780)

Condillac, the French Psychologist has attempted an explanation of psychological life on the basis of sensation. According to him sensation is sufficient for an explanation of mental life; the principle of association is not required for purpose. Man is naturally endowed with an innate power of receiving and absorbing sensate experience, and among the various sensations that smell is the most prominent, one owes the first and foremost knowledge of external world to the organ of smell. Similarly the other sense organ provides sensation of different kinds. He contents pleasure and pain are also comprehend in sensation, feeling of pleasure continually increased and also recollected but the feeling of pain as far as possible, is eliminated. He believes memory to be another form of sensation, for when sensation returns to the mind it constitutes memory.

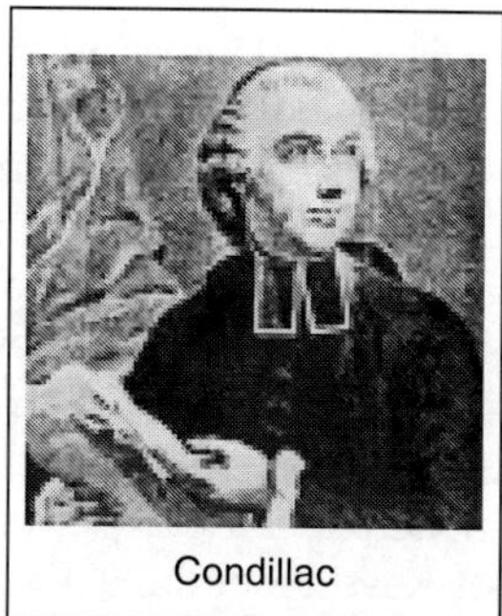

Condillac

PIERRE JEAN GEORGE CABANIS (1757-1808)

Pierre Jean George Cabanis was a very great surgeon and hence it was only national that he should take an appropriate interest in psychology. He made a study of the reflex activity on three different levels—spinal cord level; semiconscious level and thought and volition level. He stated that the first level of reflex activity concerned with the spinal cord, for the reflex activity within the spinal cord took place when some stimulus was present. Then, the reflex activity that takes place at the semiconscious level is not brought to the conscious notice of the individual. And at the highest level reflex activity is concerned with thought and volition. Another aspect of respect in which Cabanis exhibited his genius is in connection with his analysis of the 'modus operandi' of the brain. He pointed out that the mechanical principles applicable to reflex activity are also applicable to the functioning of the brain. He illustrated that brain diseases and mental diseases are related on the basis of statistics. He expressed his views on social psychology, i.e. he accepted social stimulation and the laws of individual behavior as the basis and also accepted the importance of ethical or moral assumption. It was in the manner Cabanis, starting with simple things like reflex activity penetrated to such a complex phenomenon on the moral aspect of human behavior.

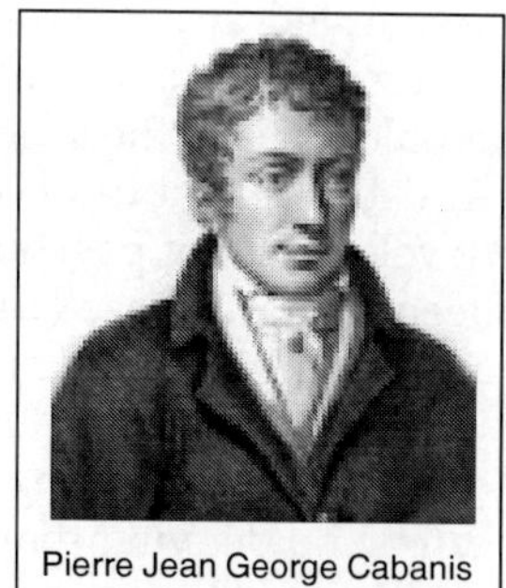

Pierre Jean George Cabanis

MARIE FRANÇOIS XAVIER BICHAT (1771-1802)

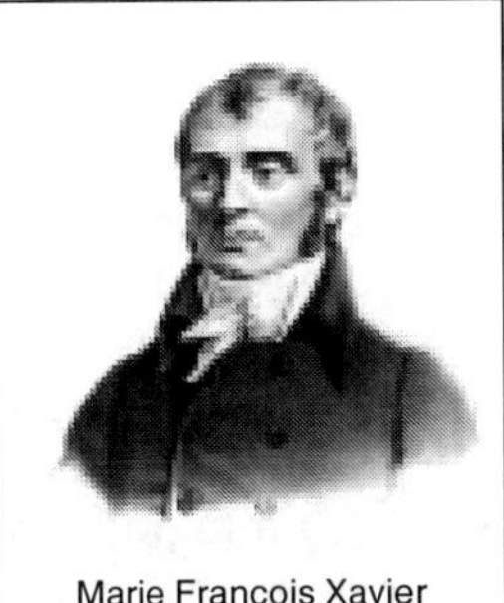
Marie François Xavier

Bichat a doctor scientist, who turned to psychology like Cabanis. Being a doctor he concentrated his attention on physiological psychology. He proceeded into the relationship between the nervous system and mental diseases. The body of human being is constructed upon some nerves. These nerve fibers take on different forms and organizations for the formation of different parts of the body such as muscles, glands, etc. He took the problem of neuropathology in which he also studied various mental deformities. In this way he studied the abnormal psychology.

PHILIPPE PINEL (1745-1826)

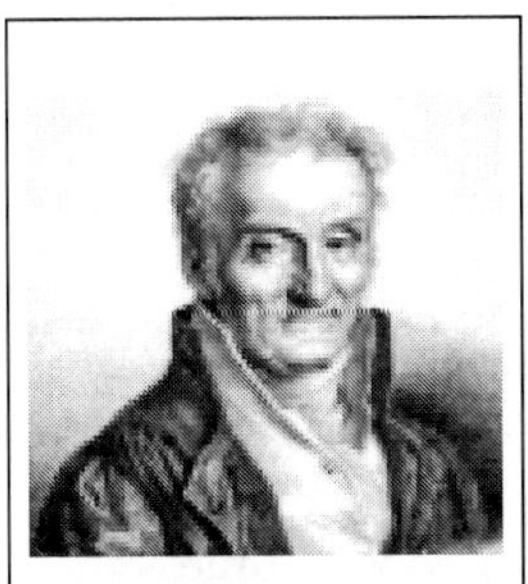
Philippe Pinel

Pinel was one of the scientists seriously interested in problem of mental diseases and he was one to bring almost fantastic changes in the field of pathology. A French physician, abolished forcible restraint in the management of mentally ill. Esquire was his pupil. Started moral states. Pinel propagated the notion that the insane should be treated with sympathy and not with instrument hatred and disgust. Pinel laid stress mainly on following three things with regard to abnormal psychology. These are—

- Aberration of the mind implies aberration in the personality
- Diseases should be classified and cured
- A humanistic movement should be initiated ensuring sympathetic behavior towards mentally insane.

CEASAR BECCARIA

Beccaria, the founder of the modern science criminology shows direct evidence of this humanist thought. He opposed any violent and strong punishment for the common trivial infringement of law and the cruelty to him quite unnecessary and over-strict. He also supported the principle of psychological hedonism in the field of criminologies. According to psychological hedonism man naturally hunts for pleasure object desired are not ends in themselves, they are the means to pleasure. Pleasure is the natural end of all our desires. On this basis he attempted to establish that man commits a crime only when his desire force him to do it, e.g. hungry man steals a bread.

JEREMY BENTHAM (1748-1832)

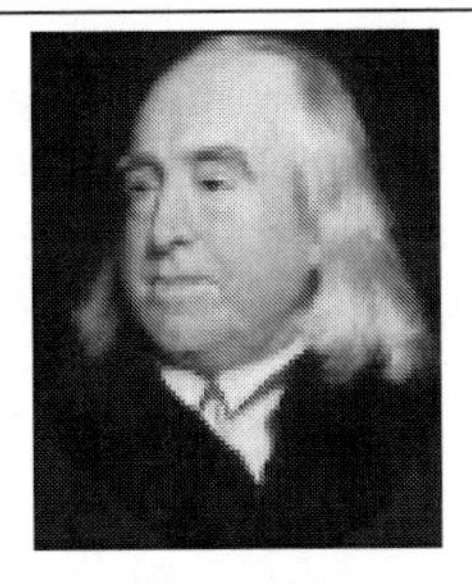
Jeremy Bentham

Bentham's hedonistic principle is utilitarian or practical. Man is by nature selfish, for he engages in work only when it affords him pleasure. Work is done for another only if it fulfils some or the other purpose but the note of hope marked out in this principle depends upon the fact that in spite of his innate selfishness he does desire the pleasure of another. The cause of this is that the object of every person is pleasure, and hence the good of society includes the good of every individual. For some such reason as this Bentham remarks that each should count for one and none for more than one. It is evident from this statement that every individual is entitled to an equal share or unit in the common good. Besides, the utilitarian principle of good is considered more important. Bentham holds that if some one form of good is shared by the majority of people then its universality or preponderance is more than for a good the use of which is confined to one individual. And it was on this basis that Bentham's fundamental principle, greatest good of the greatest number, took place. This theory of his not only explains human activity but also social organization. As a matter of fact, it is the duty of every politician should merge in the general or social good. Society and the individual should be integrated or identified to such an extent that the interests of the two should not be separate, they should depend upon each other.

A careful perusal of the humanitarian movement will show that this motivational theory of Bentham's which he is content to use for social welfare, resembles the humanitarian principle. And the influence of this Benthamite principle is in evidence even today in the field of economics. The Benthamite principle in fact blends utilitarianism, hedonism and humanitarianism.

Bentham takes it for granted that man is selfish by nature. According to him, "To obtain the greatest portion of happiness for himself is the object of every rational being. Every man is nearer to himself than he can be to any other man, and no other than can weigh for him his pleasures and pains". Even his benevolent acts only conceal some particular self-interest. Man indulges in acts of benevolence only when he is confident of gaining something by it. To quote Bentham, "Dream not that men will move their little finger to serve you, unless their own advantage in so doing be obvious to them. Men never did so and never will, while human nature is made by so doing they can serve themselves". In the opinion of Bentham, the root of every motivation among mankind is formed by the principle of self-preference. And the meaning of duty, law and good behavior can be understood only in terms of pleasure and pain.

Yet, in spite of all his belief in the selfishness of man, Bentham evinced faith in altruism as well, for he thought that the final moral idea is the "greatest number". Man's objective should be the search for the greatest good of his own kind. Social good or collective good is the ideal of life, not personal good. Collective good is the criterion of morality.

GERMAN PSYCHOLOGY

In the 19th century the important psychologists who contributed to the development of psychology in Germany were—Fries, Herbart, Gall, Weber, Fechner, Johannus Muller, Lotz and Helmholtz.

- **Freis** did research work on the functioning of mind. His viewpoint was experimental. Hence his views have become scientific. He took interest in anthropology hence he has viewed thinking as a function of the physiological structure. He has accepted the existence of three functions—knowledge, feeling and will-power and conceived of self of man as the center of these powers. He clarified the mutual relation between the three powers and light on the mind's method of working.
- **Herbart**—Contrary to Fries, Herbart does not accept the three powers to be separate. According to him in reality mind is a single unit and all the three powers are different aspects of this unit. Like Fries, Herbart too concentrated on the nature of mind. In his opinion, the newborn infant's mind is devoid of any impressions and concepts. New concepts start coming gradually into the mind when the child comes in contrast with

the environment. Relations are established among these concepts on the basis of similarity, dissimilarity or contrast. For example white becomes associated with black and red with yellow and hence our attention goes to black when hearing mention of white and to yellow when we hear of red. On the basis of this mutual relation between different concepts Herbart established the theory of Apperception which has an important place in modern education. In this way is the unity of all concepts. The nature of the soul is similar to the mind. It remains in the brain and governs the body. Herbart did not differentiate between soul and mind. He did not believe in any divine power in the soul. According to him mind or soul is like a stage on which different concepts come and go. Herbart classified mental activities and defined development in them. He accepted the following mental functions under knowledge, feeling and power:

1. Presentation	Higher—Understanding and judgment
	Lower—Imagination and memory
2. Feeling	Higher—Artistic and moral
	Lower—Pleasure and pain
3. Will	Higher—Rational will and passions
	Lower—Instincts and appetites

As has been mentioned earlier Herbart was an empiricist. Hence he has given special importance to sensation which in its basic form is indistinct and can be understood after it has combined with past experiences and acquired visible form. Man has sensation by different external and internal sense organs. Herbart has accepted both higher and lower types of knowledge, feelings and will which has already been given in the table. He also defines the Limen of consciousness. Clear concepts lie above this Limen and the indistinct ones within it. Herbart has also unsuccessfully tried to combine spiritual facts in Psychology. His main contribution can be said to be in child psychology and educational psychology. While analyzing mental functions he forgot their physical basis.

Gall—Frans Joseph Gall discussed Phrenology in his book published in 1810. The second part of this book was published in 1819. In the development of Phrenology his pupil Spurzheim was also with him but who left him later on. In reality Spurzheim gave more prominence to Phrenology than did Gall. Phrenology is based on the following three views:

1. On the external shape and construction of the skull depend the shape and construction of the brain
2. There are many faculties in the brain. Gall has accepted 37 faculties and Propensities of the mind
3. The various faculties and propensities are present in different parts of the brain. Hence Phrenology divides the brain into 37 parts and names every part on the basis of its mental faculty. In addition to Germany and England, Phrenology also got prominence in America. But its popularity started decreasing at the start of the 20th century. Gradually new facts related to the brain started emerging and phrenology was proved to be completely imaginary. Its importance lies only in that it encouraged scientific discoveries in both fields of mind and brain and established a relation between them.

Weber and Fechner—Among the famous psychologists of the 19th century, the names of Weber and Fechner have won great fame. Both of them together developed psychophysics and presented the famous Weber-Fechner law. In the field of scientific study of sensations they made some valuable contributions.

Beneke—German psychologist Beneke contributed to the development of lower **faculty psychology** though his views were different from other psychologists. Like Herbart, he too was an empiricist and believed psychology to be assisting and did not accept it as a part of it. On the subject of the faculties of mind he supported. Herbart's concepts of apperception mass. He reflected on the various faculties of the mind. His views were so similar to Herbart's that some people accused him of stealing Herbart's views.

Johannus Muller—Johannus Muller made important contributions to the development of German psychology in the 19th century. He defined the structure and working of the nervous system. He made important discoveries on the subject of sensations and reflected on the action of memory. He clarified the biological and physical basis of psychology.

Lotze—A German psychologist of the 19th Century Lotze defined space perception. He has accepted space perception to be based on many things, signs and symbols. In the beginning these depend on the experience of man but later on adopt mental form. Lotze also defined tactual and visual sensation in addition to space perception. In this connection he mentioned local sign without which space perception is not possible. Visual sensation also depends on local sign movement. By previous experience man can guess the direction by the help of local signs. In the history of psychology, Lotze's views on visual psychology and local signs and space perception have an important place.

Helmholtz—In the development of experimental psychology in Germany in addition to Fechner and Wundt, the contribution of Helmholtz is important. He psychologically defined the mental process connected with color vision. He believed red, blue and green to be the three primary colors. These colors are related to three different cones in the retina and by the excitation of a particular cone, that particular color is seen. The principle of Helmholtz cannot blindness. Herring's theory is more acceptable in this respect. In addition to visual sensation Helmholtz has also analyzed auditory sensation. In the context of sensation and perception, he also mentioned unconscious inference. Helmholtz laid special stress on experimental method. Hence his experiments helped the development of experimental psychology.

FRENCH PSYCHOLOGY

In the 19th century, in the development of psychology in France, four psychologists were prominent—Biran, Ampere, Comte and Cousin. In addition Pinel, Taine, Ribot and Binet too did important work. The psychology of this age was empiricist though the experimental tendency was not so developed here as it was in Germany. The contribution of French psychology in this century was in the field of abnormal psychology which had an important influence on development in the 20th century.

Biran—French psychologist Biran stressed the method of introspection and self-observation in psychological study. He defined self-observation in psychological study. He defined self and threw light on the development of self in individuals. The existence of self is not clear to the individual in the beginning. During the process of adapting to the environment, when an individual recognizes himself as different from other then gradually the development of the self takes place. By gaining the ability to control physical motions by will power the ego emerges in thin development. In this way Biran has traced the development of the ego in an individual, as a result of the process of adjustment.

Ampere—Ampere studied the immediate consciousness of man and tried to find out how sensations and ideas get related to each other. In this way he studied the process of involuntary association. Secondly, he tried to find out how to use the faculties of the mind for the scientific study of the world. In order to achieve these aims Ampere presented the doctrine of association of ideas and the theory of knowledge. He tried to clarify the mental functions and behavior. In this respect his principle of concretion is important. According to it when one kind of sensation mixes with another kind of resistance then their concertinos takes place in such a way that it is seen in the form of simple association. Ampere defined the principle of concertinos by the sensations occurring in different sense organs. For example while reading a song already heard, its tune automatically comes in the mind because by concretion a simple association between the two has been formed. Ampere also defined the sensations caused by different muscles and established a casual relation between these sensations and self-consciousness. He defined the immediate and general forms of consciousness. His views were greatly respected in the contemporary scientific society.

Cousin—In the study of psychology Cousin laid stress on observation and threw light on the principle of direct perception and consciousness. He was influenced by Reid, Biran and Ampere in this respect. The fact is that he lacked originality. He was only an eclectic.

Auguste Comte—Auguste Comte is in fact famous as the creator of Sociology, but in psychology, especially in the development of social psychology also he is known for his contributions. Comte was humanist and positivist. He traced the development of human society. In this development he believed the religious to be the first stage, philosophical the second and the scientific the third stage. In the present scientific stage efforts are made to understand the world by observation, reason and cogitation. In this way Comte imparted strength to the strength tendency in psychology and encouraged evolutionism.

Pinel—The contribution of French psychologist Pinel is in the field of abnormal psychology. He suggested kind and humane treatment of the insane and pointed out that the persons who have a defect the brain require sympathy and treatment. In this way he inspire psychologists for research in a new direction.

Taine—French psychologist Taine published an important book related to intelligence. He defined psychological actions on the basis of associationism. In this he threw light on the physical basis of mental actions. In the field of abnormal psychology, the studies of Taine on hypnotism, illusion and delusion are important.

Ribot—Ribot was a professor of experimental psychology. But his greatest contribution is in the psychology of attention on which he published a separate book in which he believes attention and consciousness to be based on physical motions and actions. In addition Ribot wrote a book on the psychology of feelings.

Binet—In 1903 French psychologist Alfred Binet published his famous book on the experimental study of intelligence. In 1905 he created the Binet-Simon test study of intelligence in association with Simon. Binet did detailed research on intelligence. He threw light on the nature of intelligence and he discovered three tendencies—definite order, desired adaptation and the tendency of self-criticism. In 1908 he amended the Binet-Simon standard and defined mental age. The last amendment of Binet-Simon standard was published in 1911.

BRITISH PSYCHOLOGY

In the development of British Psychology in the 19th century, the following three tendencies can be clearly seen:

1. Associationism
2. Hypnotism
3. Evolutionism.

1. *Associationism*—In the 19th Century most of the British psychologists defined different psychological processes on the basis of the principle of association. This tendency was most prominent in Britain in this period. The chief exponents of this theory were—James Mill, John Stuart Mill, Thomas Brown, Hamilton, Alexander Baine and Herbert Spencer. James Mill published a book on the analysis of human mind to be based on sensations and ideas. According to him mental function was equal to a mental compound. Contrary to this son John Stuart Mill believed mental work to be mental chemistry. James Mill has an important place in British associationism. He has defined the process of the development of concept or ideational association. He differentiated between the strength of associations on the basis of permanence, certainty and facility. His son JS Mill defined the different mental actions more minutely. Stuart Mill stressed similarity, contiguity and inseparability. He took frequency to be a part of contiguity. John Stuart Mill amended the principle of association presented by his father. Thomas Brown was the founder of the Scottish psychological community. He found the association principle to be useful in the form of suggestion in defining psychological actions. Brown believed association to be suggestion as he found some faults in the principle of association. He defined 9 laws of suggestions in which recency, frequency and liveliness were the main ones. Brown created the background to the modern doctrine of Gestalt, by defining relative suggestion. Sir William Hamilton presented the famous theory of Reintegration in the field of Psychology. According to it the organization found in the mind is not simple but rather complicated. Due to the tendency towards organic unification and re-integration man remembers all past experiences related to a present experience. In Hamilton's theory of reintegration we get the prototype of the modern doctrine of Gestalt. Alexander Baine threw light on the physiological bases of mental processes. He spoke of association in explaining intelligence and stressed the laws of continuity and similarity. He tried to create a synthesis between philosophical psychology and physiological psychology. In British associationism Herbert Spencer is famous for Evolutionary associationism. According to it there is evolutionary order in mental actions which evolve from simplicity to complexity. In this evolution, both heredity and environment are important. In elaborating upon the mutual relation between heredity and environment Spencer threw light on the mutual relation between Psychology and Zoology.
2. *Hypnotism*—In the 19th century, three doctors Elliotson, James Braid and James Esdaile threw light on the form of hypnotism. Elliotson treated some patients on the basis of theory of animal-magnetism. James Braid used the word Hypnotism for the first time because mesmerism or animal magnetism had fallen into disrepute. Braid used Hypnotism in the treatment of many persons and analyzed its form in half a dozen of his books and essays, due to which the opposition to it in England decreased. James Esdaile too started using Hypnotism in his treatments. Due to the efforts of these doctors Hypnotism was given an important place in abnormal psychology and mental treatment.

3. *Evolutionism*—In the British Psychology of 19th century, the tendency of Evolutionism is also as important as associationism. The credit of promoting it goes to Charles Darwin. By the revolutionary books of Darwin The Principle of Evolutionism won recognition in the scientific world. Therefore it also came into use in the field of psychology. By the research work of Darwin mental evolution in psychology was examined on the basis of Zoology. As a result of this research the fields of child psychology and animal psychology got encouragement.

So, in brief, in the 19th century special research work was undertaken in Associationism, Evolutionism, and Hypnotism by British Psychologists and important literature on these subjects came into existence.

FRANCIS GALTON (1822-1911)

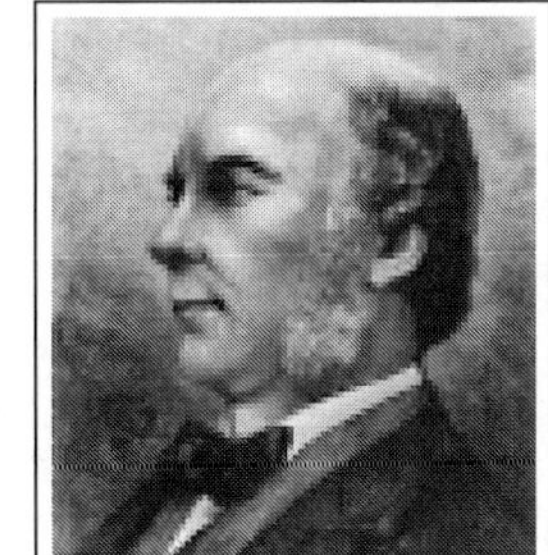
Francis Galton

A versatile English scientist. He has made great contributions to many branches of knowledge among which Psychology also is one. Galton has often been referred to as the pioneer in Differential Psychology, which studies individual differences. Some of his experiments with the study of imagery are very famous and are quoted often in the study of Psychology. He was also perhaps responsible for using statistics in understanding Psychological data.

WILHELM WUNDT (1832-1902)

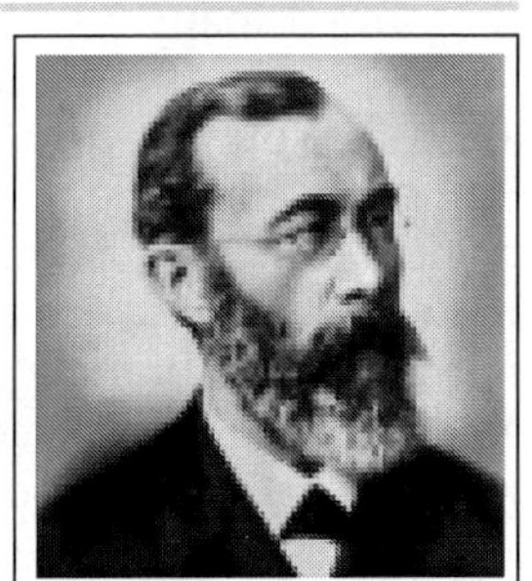
Wilhelm Wundt

Founder of the first Psychological Laboratory at Leipzig in 1879. One of the earliest scientists of Germany who were responsible for making Psychology into a separate science. Many of the early experimental psychologists were his students. He wrote a number of books on different aspects of Psychology.

Wundt has played an important role in the development of modern psychology in Germany. He established the first psychological laboratory of the world and encourages psychological experiments. He himself performed many experiments and it deserves special mention that all his experiments were of a scientific nature. He wrote books on psychology—physiological psychology and folk psychology. He made psychology systematic and in this way made it easy for the students to study psychology. Wundt analyzed and explained such mental processes as sensation, perception and concepts. The basis of this study was experimental. He explained the part that was played by the nervous system and sense organs in the development of sensation. He accepted sensation and feeling to be a necessary element of the mind and described intensity, quality and duration in defining sensation. He performed different psychophysical experiments concerned with intensity in sensations and defined them on this basis. While defining it he threw light on the simple form of sensation. He made direct perception the basis of extent and duration.

According to him there are three dimensions of feeling, i.e. pleasant or unpleasant, peace and excitement, rest and tension. To him, concept is related to direct perception, the nature of perception was combined from of feeling and memories, ideas and concepts emerge from direct perception. He classified ideas and concepts on the basis of their qualities. Accordingly three kinds of ideas which includes:

- Intensive ideas—Associated on the basis of consonance and resistance
- Space ideas—Connected with space
- Time ideas—Related to time.

He talked about apperception that it was related to the upper portion of the brain. The action of apperception occurs by the combination of the nerves. Association has an important role in the development of apperception. The awareness of association goes to the brain through the medium of nerves, where perception evolves. The sensation of individual acquire meaning on the basis of association. In the action of remembering there is the contribution of both apperception and association, ideas and concepts develop on the basis of association and the action of remembering takes place on this basis. Like this he found out many fact by experiments in the laboratory.

HERMAN VON HELMHOLTZ

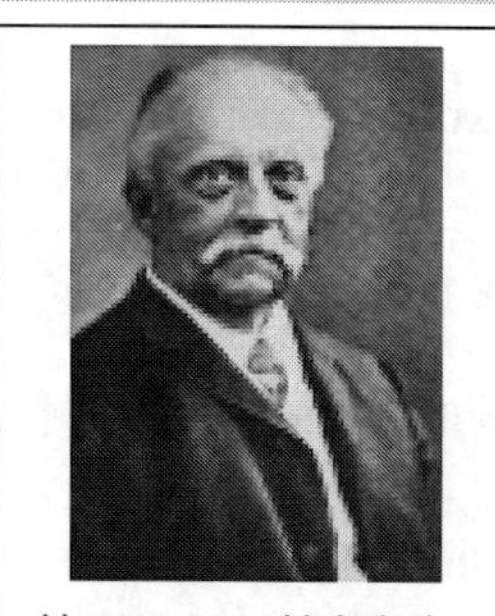
Herman von Helmholtz

Helmholtz was a German, interested in science, stared and studied physics, but it was not sufficient to study science for livelihood. Hence he also had to study science for livelihood. Hence he also had to study medicine. At the age of 24 he published an article on medicine in which he said that the cells of ganglia were attached one by one to different vein. This fact was welcomed in the field of medicine. When he was appointed as surgeon in the army, he performed many psychological experiments and made intense study of energy. He conducted experimental examination of Thomas Young's principle of color victim and found it to be defective and amended this principle as "Young-Helmholtz principle of color vision". He also studied auditory sensation and maintained that there are thousands of nerves in the inner membrane of the ears, mere nerves of membrane for the ear can be compared to stringed musical instrument. He has said defining unconscious that for direct knowledge an unconscious inference is most necessary. Every person indulges in unconscious inferences, and this action is natural. According to him direct knowledge is related with the stimulus and the specific sense organ. It is also related to with the preconception of man and his unconscious inference. In addition he also studied temperature and said that it can be measured. He accepted the relationship between psychology and human psychology.

J MCKEEN CATTEL (1860-1944)

Cattel was the American interested in experimental psychology. He did experiments concerning reaction and worked in the field of measurement of direct knowledge by using tachitoscope. He designed many necessary mental tests to measure individual difference. He experimented on individual differences, reaction time, association, direct knowledge and psychophysics, etc. He also used statistics in reaction time experiments. He established psychological laboratories and studied direct knowledge of children on the basis of experiment and presented important facts.

EH WEBER

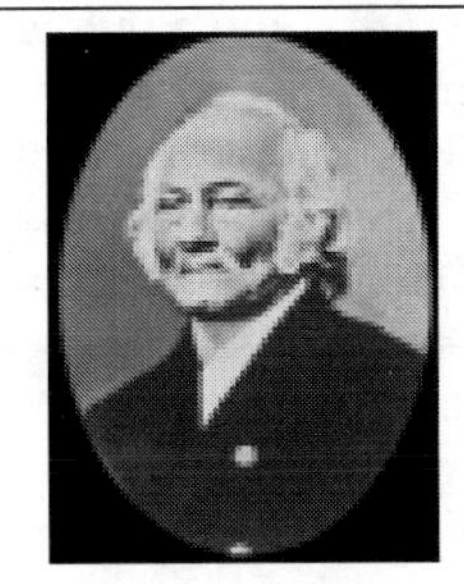

Ernst Weber

EH Weber of Germany can be accepted as the founder of experimental psychology. He was interested mainly in physical structure of sense organs. He did detailed experiments on the sensations of eye, nose, ears and skin. Many scientists of Germany and others countries had experimented widely in these fields but Weber for the first time found out new facts by the experimental method and from them arrived at psychological conclusions. From the view of history of psychology, the most important contribution of Weber is the principle which later on became famous as the "Weber-Fechner Law".

FECHNER (1801-1887)

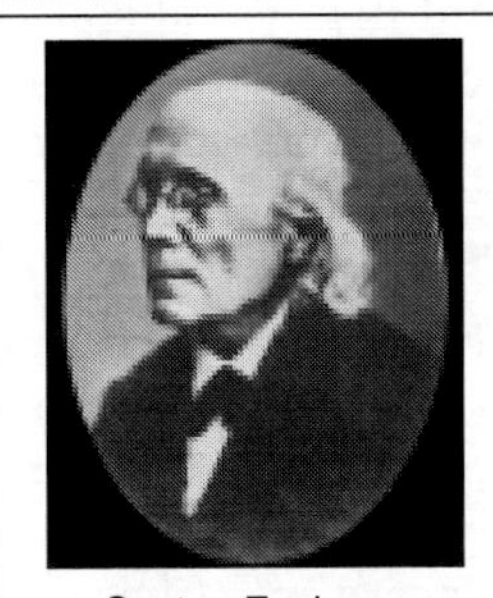

Gustav Fechner

Fechner published his book "Elements der Psycho Physic", this he defined psychophysics and determined into sphere. According to him psychophysics was a science studying the relations of interdependence between the mind and the body, as well as the functional relations sensations, perception, feelings, actions, attention, etc. come in its sphere. Fechner experimental for years with Weber law and found that when a uniform increase is affected in our stimulus, then there is a similar increase in the sensations resulting from them. Thus increase does not occur in simple ratio but is in comparison to increase in the excitement. Hence relation between excitement and sensation is shown by a curve. It is seen that this curve always bends down in the graph of stimuli and sensation on the basis of this he discovered a law that the sensations are in a ratio of the Log of stimuli responsible for them. If sensation in shown by 'S' stimulus by R and constant as C their Fechner's law can be expressed by this by "S = C Log R". This equation known as "Weber-Fechner Law".

JOHANNES MULLER

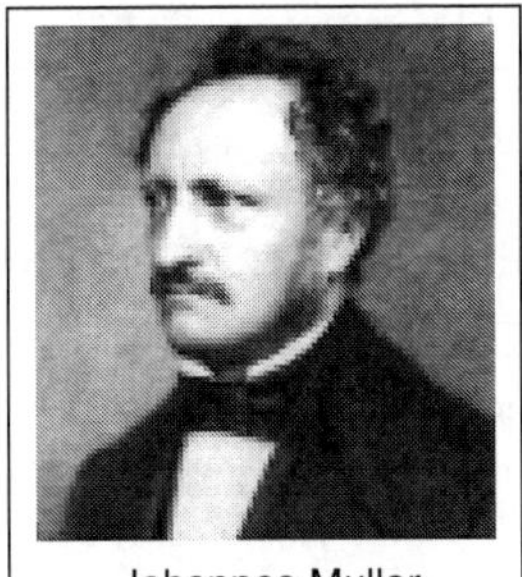

Johannes Muller

Muller was interested in physiology, generally in the actions related to sensation and he centered his study on optical sensation. Mostly his experiments were related to the action of the external organs of the eyes and space perception. He also threw light on reflex action. He has propounded a very important principle related to sensation which is known as the doctrine of "specific energies". Accordingly there is special kind of energy in the nerves of the body, when a nerve connected with a stimulus, then a unique reaction occurs, e.g. Optic nerve—vision.

WILLIAM JAMES (1842-1910)

Hailed by many as the father of modern psychology. James is undoubtedly one of the greatest names in psychology. He was an American and was one of the early scholars of psychology who were responsible for establishing the subject in America. His book the

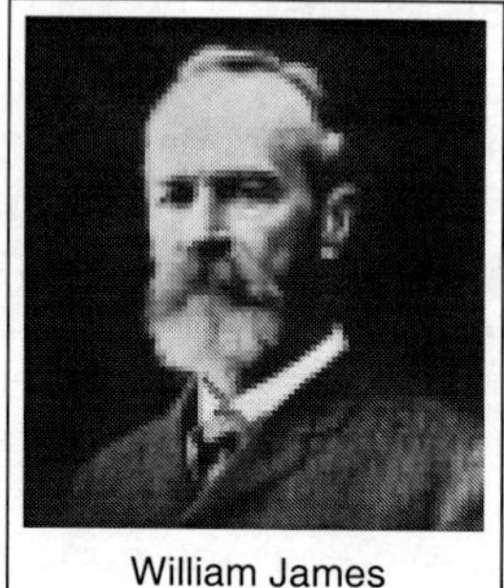
William James

"Principles of Psychology" is one of the best books even today, though some of his teachings are now out-moded. His theory of emotions also has attacted the attention of all psychologists belonging to different schools.

William James did detailed study and analysis of consciousness, self and intellectual process. According to him, the characteristics of consciousness is personal it is changing, it is continuous and is related to some objects. He has accepted mind to be the stream of consciousness. Awareness of consciousness is created by action. All mental actions are isolated from each other. This streams of actions is known as the mind. There is no association among thoughts. They never be similar.

William James described three forms of the soul—Material, social and spiritual. Material soul is physical soul kept in mind the relations between body and clothes. Social soul depends on the social relations of the individual, spiritual soul of the person in the part of him whose work is intellectual and emotional.

EL THORNDIKE (1874-1949)

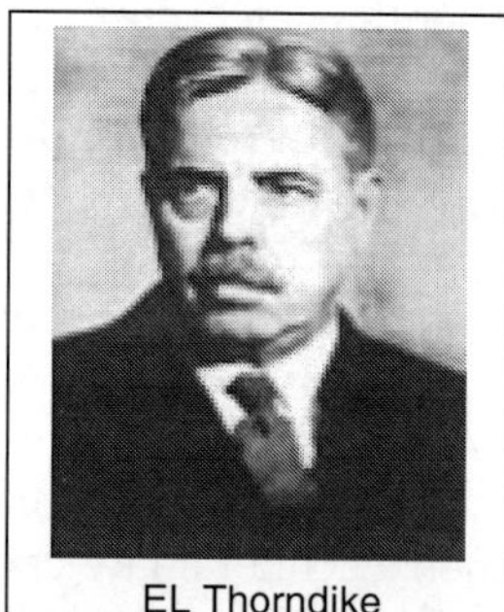
EL Thorndike

Thorndike was an American psychologist. His major interest was at first animal psychology. He did very valuable work concerning animal learning. Thorndike greatly emphasised, as a result of his experiments, the "trial and error method" in learning. Since his concern in earlier years was mostly with animal learning, he switched over in later years to the study of learning process in human beings and attained a very high position as an educational psychologist.

Thorndike first presented his theory in his book "Animal Learning" published in 1898. The clearest form of his theory seen in the three volume treatise on "Educational Psychology". His theory may be understood in a systematic way with the help of three major laws. (i) Law of readiness (ii) Law of Exercise and (iii) Law of effect. He has stressed the following five things, which assist in the progress of learning—(i) interest in the work (ii) interest in improvement (iii) significance (iv) problem attitude (v) attentiveness. Further he added another two which includes absence of irrelevant emotion and absence.

EDWARD B TITCHENER

There are two different ways in which behavior of living organism can be described, either according to structure or in terms of its functioning. Both points of view have been adopted in the history of psychology.

Titchener began the development of structuralism, a system of psychology which differed from associationism and faculty psychology. It is also called existentialist psychology. Titchener give it a psychological ground. Experience he analyzed with the help of the introspective method. Nervous system is believed to be the actual basis of experience and mind the sum total of mental experiences. It has the three mental elements—Sensation, image and affection, the qualities of which are quality, intensity, duration and clearness.

Mind and body have a parallel relationships. Attention is the pattern formed in consciousness. Structuralism stressed the need for the development of applied psychology.

JOHN DEWEY (1859-1952)

Dewey stressed the fact of utility and encouraged the study of psychology as it benefits the society and individual solving some problems. He brought to psychology a pragmatic approach. He pointed out that mental facts possess a continuity as well as a function. He stressed the fact of mental function is mental elements. According to him mental activity continues without any cessation or interpretation and there is no stages in which it is possible to accept the explanation that one activity has come to a stop and another has begun. He further pointed out that the continuity is also true of stimulus and reaction but accepting the existence of a functional relationships between a living being and his environment Dewey has opined that the individuals psychological efforts amount to nothing more than an effort to adjust to his environment. Every mental activity has some objective and functions, it is for this reason that stress is laid on mental functions.

JAMES ROWLAND ANGELL (1869)

Angell indicated that functionalism is related to process and hence he opposed to structuralism, which is related content. He noted that difference between functionalism and structuralism. The functional school stresses the importance of utility, and it believes that the study of psychology should not be made for its own sake but for the advantage it will bring. Psychology studied in order to improve the efficiency of the individual. Angell pointed out that the aim of functionalism is to find out has and why particular mental activity takes place and functionalism fills the gap left in the study of psychology by inquiring into the mechanics of mental actions.

HARVEY CARR

According to Harvey mental activity is a concept which symbolizes such diverse mental function as direct knowledge, memory, imagination, thinking, volition, decision, etc. On the subject he has written "mental activity is concerned with acquisition, fixation, retention, organization and evaluation of experiences and their subsequent utilization in the guidance of conduct. He believed all mental actions are based on mind and body. The term 'mental' refers to the both psychological as well as physiological aspect. The study of behavior required that both psychological and bodily basis of mental activity be observed and examined. He believes all mental activity to be directed towards the establishment of the most efficient adjustment. On the subject of environment, he pained out that circumstances of the environment also inspire the individual to activity, and that environment is found to contain differing conditions which gives rise to varying kinds of behavior.

In addition James Cattel, Edward Thorndike, Robert S, Wordwoth contributed substantially to progress of functionalism. In brief:

- Functionalism stressed the need for a study of complete personality
- Functionalism accepts the mind and body duality with skepticism choosing to believe both of them to be identical
- Functionalism placed much stress on adjustment and accepted the facts that an individual achieves a satisfaction adjustments between his life and environment
- Functionalism helped prefers in different branches of psychology, child psychology, education psychology, animal psychology.

JB WATSON (1878-1958)

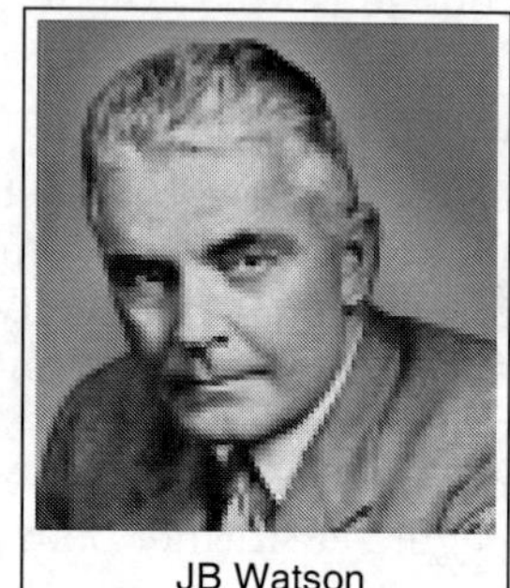
JB Watson

An American psychologist. He was particularly interested in animal psychology and child psychology. He was very zealous about making psychology a science and so, emphasised objective and experimental methods and also started a new school of psychology called "behaviorism." According to this school, the scope of psychology is limited only to objectively observable and measurable reactions. He objected to the usage of terms like mind, consciousness etc. Watson also believed that what we are, is mostly because of our environment. By having a proper environment he claimed that any child could be made into a scientist or a philosopher or a criminal.

John Broadus Watson believed to be the father of the behaviorist school. Taking the behaviorist standpoint Watson offered novel explanations of the different mental and other processes traditionally the subject matter of psychology. He also put forth numerous new ideas on the subject. A short account of them will clarify his contribution to psychology and the influence he had on its development. The main ideas of the man are the following:

1. *Explanation of behavior:* Watson attempted to explain all internal and external, acquired and instinctive, behavior of men and animals through stimulus-response or S-R. all behavior has its beginning in some stimulus, seeing by the eye when light reaches it, hearing by the ears when sound reaches them. A stimulus causes a response in the living organism, responses that are either internal or external, either acquired or instinctive. Many complex reactions or responses are developed in individuals on account of the learning that takes place during some of his activities.
2. *Sensation and perception:* In view of the fact that much of his research was confined to animal psychology it is not surprising to note that Watson did not put much faith in the verbal report method. Instead he used what he called verbal response. When a person sees yellow color and says that he sees yellow this saying so constitutes his verbal response. But in actual fact Watson could not prove how verbal report differs from verbal response. Watson did not believe in any sensation and perception apart from the response of the senses and the organism.
3. *Memory images:* According to Watson all behavior is the outcome of motion in the senses and muscles: he did not believe in the concept of memory images. He tried to illustrate or to establish that the so-called memory images are no other than the reaction of the senses and muscles. For example, reactions of the eye muscles and latent sound motions form part of any image formed by the eye.
4. *Feeling and emotion:* According to Watson feelings are also sensory motor activities. The feelings of pleasure, for example, is the outcome of various sensations received from the sense organs and the consequent motion in muscles. In explaining the phenomenon of emotion Watson resorts to purely physiological considerations and points out that it is the outcome of a definite and pronounced imbalance between the total organism and the visceral, along with the glandular organization and glandular activity during different emotional states. According to Watson, them, in an unusual state certain internal and external changes take place in the place in the organism. Through his research on the basic emotions like fear, anger and love, and their expression in children Watson tried to prove that the other emotions are all required. And that the principle of conditioned reflex works in the acquiring of these emotions.

5. *Learning:* In his explanation of the phenomenon of learning Watson enunciated the law of use, replacing the law of effect suggested by Thorndike. According to Watson in learning, the principles of recency and frequency work, both of which are comprehended under the law of exercise. In this way Watson believed that to begin with, all learning is done by trial and error, and consequently this is the method to which the grants recognition. Later on, he tried to explain all learning on the basis of conditioned reflex or response, a theory propagated by Pavlov the Russian physiologist. The truth of the matter is that Watson's parallels the older notion of associationism because he could not offer any satisfactory explanation of many elements, such as reinforcement, in Pavlov's theory.
6. *Thinking:* Thinking was also given a behaviorist explanation in terms of latent motor activity by Watson, for it was his belief that all behavior is sensory motor activated. It is often observed that some children and quite a few organ ups think aloud, but on the other hand, the majority of adult people think without talking aloud. It was Watson's view that the reason behind the change was that external activity was replaced by some internal behavior. According to this theory the vocal organs function during thinking but their movement is so subtle that it is not perceptible. One often sees movements of the tongue and face during thinking. One direct effect of this watsonian explanation was the immediate increase in experiments on this subject and it was found in many of them that some activity of the vocal organs is almost inevitable in thinking. But there is no way of finding out how this activity would differ with differing kinds of thinking. Besides, all experiments did not provide evidence of this activity.
7. *Environmentalism:* Watson placed greater stress on environment than on heredity as factors in the development of personality although this does not have much of a connection with behaviorism. Watson declared that if he were given the authority to condition a normal child's environment completely he could turn that child into anything, doctor, engineer, artist, scientist, advocate, businessman or any other kind of specialist. He could even turn him into a beggar or a thief, irrespective of the intelligence of its parents, their tendencies, abilities, business, race, etc.

Watsonian behaviorism arose as a reaction against the structural and functional psychologies in vogue. Watson defined psychology as the science of behavior and objectivity elaborated upon the nature of behavior. He effected a complete refutation of the concept of consciousness and the introspective methods. He emphasized the importance of animal psychology and analyzed behavior, sensation, perception, memory images, feeling and emotion, learning and thinking from the behaviorist standpoint. According to him the development of personality depends upon the environment. Behavior is guided by the senses and it can be explained in terms of stimulus and response. Watson's importance is not owing to his ideas on psychology but to his hopeful, realistic and progressive attitude. After Watson the work done by the early behaviorists and the later behaviorists deserves mention in the history of behaviorism. Max Meyer and AP Weiss are among the more important early behaviorists while the chief among the later behaviorists are Hunter, Tolman, Hull, Skinner and Karl S Lashley. Among them many not only modified the ideas originally propagated by Watson but even went to the length of contradicting them.

SIGMUND FREUD (1856-1939)

He was an Austrian psychiatrist, Founder of Psychoanalysis, concept of libido, regression, transference, sublimation, id, ego, superego, conscious, preconscious, Oedipus complex,

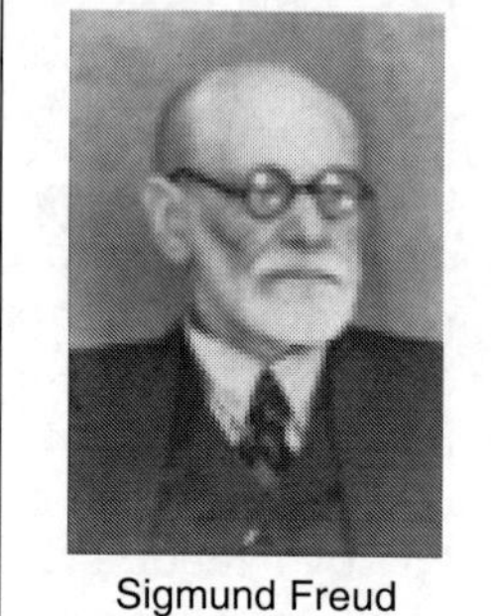
Sigmund Freud

psychopathology of dreams, topographical (regions of unconscious, preconscious) and structural (id, ego, superego) modes described properties of cocaine.

According to Freud, the field of our mental activities is of three kinds—Conscious, foreconscious, and unconscious. It is the Freudian theory of the unconscious that has much value for psychology, as psychoanalysis has analyzed the unconscious and thus contributed to psychological information.

According to Freud just as only 1/10th part of an iceberg remains above the water, while the 9/10th is concealed below the water, similarly the conscious level of the man's mind is a very small part of the unconscious. Thus according to Freud most of the human activities are motivated from the unconscious. Freud devised many methods to explore the unconscious. It was this technique which came to be known as psychoanalysis.

In his books Freud has very much emphasized the role of unconscious process in human behavior. According to Freud almost the entire mental life is directed from the unconscious forces. The conscious level is a very small part of the unconscious mind. The unconscious is the reservoir of the unfulfilled motives. It store repressed desires do not disappear but go to the unconscious of the man, and there await suitable chances for manifestation. Of these almost all the desires are sexual. It is the sexual desires which are the causes of much of the behavior of human beings. Freud calls the universal aspect of these sexual desires with the name libido. Libido is the motivating force in human life.

The Id: Thus, according to Freud man's unconscious is the storehouse of instinctive impulses, frustrated desires and repressed feelings. It is not in the contact of the environment. Freud calls it Id. In the Id there are the directing forces of the man. Earlier Freud conceived it to be directed by the pleasure principle alone, but later on he accepted the existence of death instinct as well. Thus in the Id there are impulses connected both with life and death. These impulses assume the form of particular desires which are directed towards the environment. Thus they very much influence the conscious life of a man. In the Id most of these desires are sexual.

The Ego: In the beginning Freud conceived Id as unconscious and the ego as conscious, and explained their conflict in terms of the conflict of the unconscious and conscious. Later on he modified his concept of the polarity of the conscious and the unconscious. Earlier he thought that the conscious level is the level of the ego and on this level the unwanted desires are repressed and sent to the unconscious. But later on Freud found that many of his patients who were analyzed, themselves did not know their resistances. Consciously they were presenting some sort of resistance while remembering their past experiences. This showed that the resistance and repression is unconscious. Thus Freud concluded that in resistance and repression the ego is unconscious. According to this modified view ego is partly conscious and partly unconscious. In the conscious aspect it is in the contact of the environment. This contact with the environment is through the muscles. The ego is also concerned with the inner mind of the man. This is the internal unconscious. The contact of the ego with this unconscious is proved through conscious pleasure and pain. According to Freud there is a constant conflict between this conscious and the unconscious level. The ego mediates between both these worlds because it is partly conscious and partly unconscious. In his famous book *"The ego and the Id"* Freud writes, "The ego tries to mediate between the world and the Id, to make the Id comply with the world's demand and, by means of muscular activity, to accommodate the world to the Id's desires". Thus id is always in search of pleasure. Id searches for pleasure blindly according to pleasure principle. But the Id must work through the Ego and the Ego follows the reality principle. In the beginning Ego is weak and undeveloped. Hence it has to face many difficulties to fulfill Id's desire. It runs after the objects which are not found in the environment. When the ego has to leave his favorite object, it keeps it's imagine in it and identifies itself with the object. Thus by adopting the characteristics of the rejected object, the Ego gradually develops. When successfully developed the Ego is systematic and well-organized and adjusted to the environment. The Id is always primitive and unorganized.

The Super Ego: Super Ego is called conscience to the ordinary sense. It is also known as ego ideal. In the analysis of the behavior of his patients, Freud sometimes found much sense of guilt. Hence he had to postulate a Super Ego besides the Id and Ego.

Like the conscience this Super Ego tries to oppress Ego by several rules and taboos. It tries to direct Ego regarding what is has to do and what it has not to do. These directions are not based on practical needs. They are categorical imperatives.

There is another significant difference between the Super Ego and the Ego. The super ego develops only in the human beings while the Ego is found in some form in all the developed animals. This is because man has to pass through a very long period of infancy and his sexual power takes much time to arrive at its object in the adult sexual life. According to Freud, the Ego develops in the life of the individual whereas the sources of the Super Ego can be traced from the primitive man. Thus man gets the Super ego not only in his own life, but through traditions as well. Yet most of the part of the Super Ego develops anew in every child. Freud has traced its origin to the frustrated sexual desires in the child. According to Freud in the child there is a real sex-impulse which searches for a person of different sex. According to this view the boy loves the mother and the girls love the father. Not only this but the boy finds rival in the father while the girl finds a rival in the mother. Thus the mind of the child is a field of terrible conflict which creates so many mental complexes. If is through these conflicts that the Super Ego develops.

The above views regarding the nature and interrelations of Id, Ego and Super Ego are held as such according to Freud. Adler and Jung differ from Freud in certain aspects. For example, whereas for Freud the Ego follows the reality principle, according to Adler it

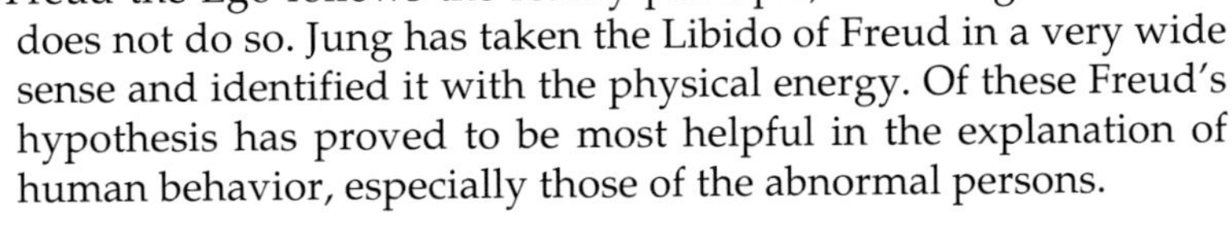
does not do so. Jung has taken the Libido of Freud in a very wide sense and identified it with the physical energy. Of these Freud's hypothesis has proved to be most helpful in the explanation of human behavior, especially those of the abnormal persons.

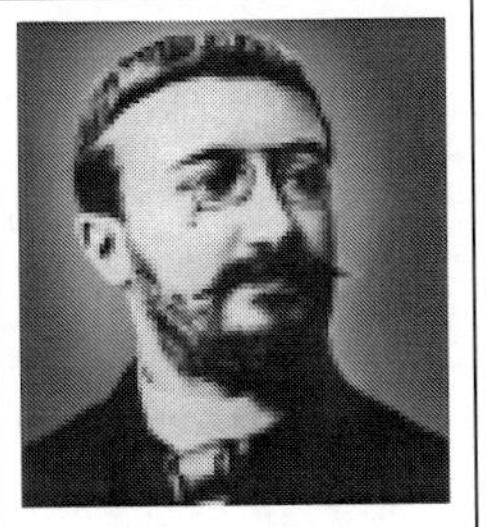
Alfred Binet

ALFRED BINET (BORN 1857)

A French Psychologist. He has the singular distinction of being the Father of the Intelligence Testing movement. He constructed the first Intelligence Tests as a Psychologist. He has also made contribution to our understanding of the Thought process.

CE SPEARMAN (BORN 1863)

A British Psychologist and was associated with the Department of Psychology of the University of London. He devoted himself mainly to the application of Statistics to the analysis of intelligence test results. Through his work he came to propose his theory of two factors in explaining 'intelligence.'

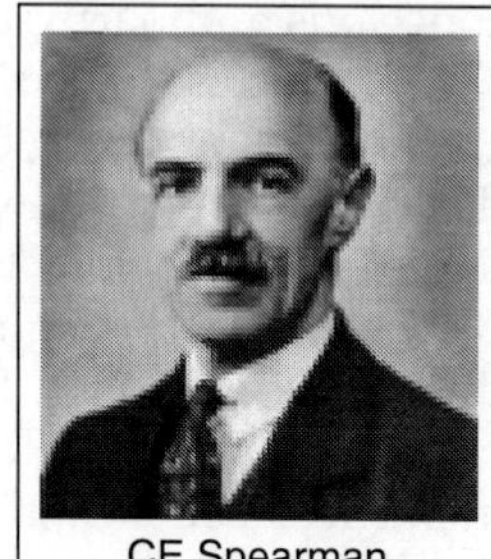

CE Spearman

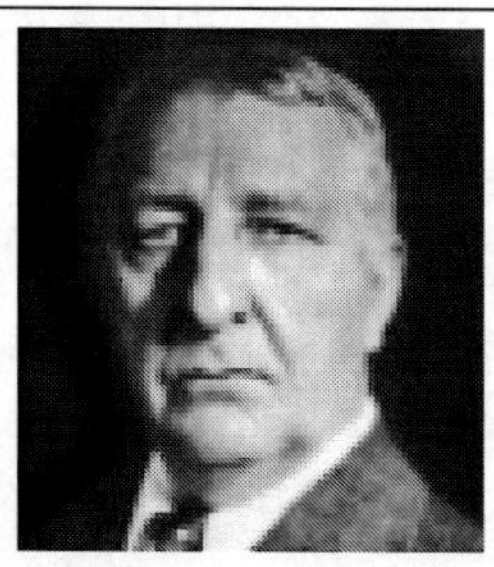

William McDougall

WILLIAM MCDOUGALL (1871-1938)

An Englishman by birth, but worked during the latter part of his life in America and made his name there as a great psychologist. He was the founder of the school of psychology called "Hormic School." This school in also called "Purposevism." McDougall was an opponent of the views expressed by Watson and his followers as contained in behaviourism. He has contributed a good deal to our knowledge of instincts and emotions. He was also the first psychologist to apply the science of psychology to social behavior and relationships.

2 CHAPTER

Nature and Scope of Psychology

Meaning

The word "Psychology" used by Rudolf Goekle in 1590. This word is derived from the combination of the Greek words "Psyche" and "logos". 'Psyche' means "soul or spirits", 'logos' means "discursive knowledgc or study", 'logy' means 'denoting a subject of study or interest'. Thus literally Psychology means the 'study of soul'. The term psychology itself comes on the scene because of the original belief that the special activities and powers of the human being were expression of an entity called "soul" working in through man. The soul or Atma is 'psyche' and the 'logos' means 'science. So psychology is a science of soul. It was believed that "life of human being has no meaning without soul", but people could not successfully explain the relation of the soul with the body. The problem persisted presenting itself on the main problem of the relation between body and soul. So later, the spiritual aspect was altogether left out of account and in view of its mystical characteristic, causing obstacle in the comprehension of the concrete facts of life, the word 'soul' substituted by a more comprehensive word "mind" because the term 'mind' has certain philosophical implications referring to the nature of matter and mind. William James (1890) used the term "mind" in place of soul. Some ancient Greek philosophers called psychology as the 'science of mind' because it was held as a branch of mental philosophy.

Modern psychology does not concede existence of mind, so mind has been substituted by mental processes or modes. Even those who use the word mind are not unanimous about its nature. Later, scholars felt that main work of psychology was to study the human conscious experience. Generally people are aware of most of what they do, be it motor activity or mental activity. Taking clue form this, they called psychology as "science of consciousness". This concept was objected by many experts, that study of the unconscious part of the mind within the jurisdiction of psychology. Later psychologists, during the time psychology was becoming a science, wanted to discard as far as possible philosophical concepts and ideas stating that psychology does not believe in consciousness. Consciousness has been substituted by "conscious process, the word consciousness does not include animal or human behavior; and psychology also studies unconsciousness and subconscious processes. As psychology claims berth in science, some of the experts in the field called psychology as a science of behavior.

It was JB Watson, the founder of the school of behaviorism popularized psychology as 'science of behavior'. Even before the Watson, Pillsbury said Psychology may be most satisfactorily defined as the science of human behavior. This concept of psychology takes behavior in a very narrow sense. Behavior as Watson saw it, was merely stimulus—responses. Behavior on the modern psychology takes it, includes the external behavior as well as the inner experiences of the human beings, and of the animals of higher species. In psychology the term behavior to include only behavior such as running and eating, but also activities such as perceiving, remembering or learning. In fact, all these processes are activities of the human organism. It is in the light of this concept that they are studied in modern psychology. The term behavior is used in a very wide meaning. It includes the behavior of men, women as well as of animals, of normal as well as abnormal and of children as well as of adults. Behavior does not imply merely the physical activity but it also includes internal processes. Modern psychology includes all types of experiences in internal behavior. Thus behavior is not only motor, but also cognitive and conative. The term behavior would also include motives that determine and direct our overt behavior. Thus using the term behavior in a very broad sense to cover our overt behavior and innate experience and the more definitely psychological activities such as thinking, reasoning, etc. Now, psychology is the scientific study of behavior and mental processes. Behavior includes all of our outward or overt actions and reactions such as talking, facial expression, and movement. Mental processes refer to all the internal, covert activity of our minds such as thinking, feeling and remembering, etc.

Nature of Psychology

Psychology is a positive science because it studies facts. The psychological judgments are factual. Science is a systematic study of limited field of experience. This study can be called a science only when it has limited field to study and systematic method to use. Psychology a science because it uses only the scientific method. Modern psychology admits only those methods which are strictly scientific and which gives is the knowledge that can be verified anywhere. Psychology as a science should be strictly confided to the scientific methods of study. It is however not the subject matter of a study that it makes a science, but its methods. It is the method of science which distinguishes it from art and philosophy. This to understand science, it is relevant to analyse the necessary steps in scientific method.

Psychology possesses a well-organized theory, which is supported by the relevant psychological laws and principles. It deals with the mind and its working and the knowledge of psychology helps in studying other persons mind. Since it is a science deals systematically with human behavior, with motives, feelings, emotions, thoughts and actions of men and women.

Psychology helps us to understand the behavior of people around us, to find out how and why they behave differently and what forces have worked to make them so different from us, and to study human nature and the manifold ways in which it expresses itself in the life of different individuals. Psychology has been defined in many different ways. It has been called the science of mental life, the science of mental processes, states, activities or functions, the study of behavior in its mental and bodily aspects, a systematic inquiry into man's relations with his environment and the like. In short there are as many definitions of psychology as there are textbooks and a beginner is often confused as to the nature and scope of this science. But in spite of these differences psychologists are agreed that the chief purpose of the study of psychology is to know more about human nature and human activity.

Definitions of Psychology

- Psychology is the study of human nature (Edwin G Boring)
- Psychology is the scientific study of activities of individuals in relations to his environment (RS Woodworth)
- Psychology today concern itself with the scientific investigation of behavior, including from the standpoint of behavior, much of which earlier psychologists dealt with experience (NL> Munn)
- Psychology is a positive science of behavior
- Psychology is the science of behavior and experience (Skinner)
- Psychology is the study of human behavior and relationships (Crow and Crow)
- Psychology undertake to make a scientific study of the individual considered as a unit as he really is in his dealings with other individuals and with the world (Woodworth).

Thus psychology may be defined as the science of behavior, a systematic study of all that man does in response to a world of things and persons. In this definition there are two terms which need explanation, *science and behavior.*

- **Science:**The term *science* describes any systematically arranged body of verified knowledge. It deals with a particular type of subject, or with certain kinds of facts or events. For example, physics deals with energy, with facts about heat, light, sound, electricity; chemistry deals with matter, with how material things are composed and decomposed; biology deals with living things, plants and animals, with how they grow and develop; and psychology deals with human behavior, with the thoughts, feelings and actions of men and women. Thus each science deals with a group of related facts and principles. Secondly, the subject-matter or the body of facts dealt with by each science is obtained by means of carefully controlled observations made by specially trained observers, (scientists). Thirdly, each science tries to formulate general principles governing facts included in its field of study. These general principles are very necessary for without them it is not possible to understand new facts, to explain them by relating them to already known facts, to foresee their occurrence and to control their recurrence. These laws are not axioms like those laid down in geometry, they are verified statements regarding the relations which exist among observed events. Fourthly, all knowledge called scientific must be definite, accurate, reliable and verifiable. Psychology as a science concerns itself with facts of behavior. Its specific subject-matter consists of facts about an individual organism activities in relation to environment. These facts it obtains, like other sciences, through carefully planned observations. Among these facts it tries to discover relations so that some general statement about their occurrence and recurrence can safely be made. These are the laws of psychology which tell us in broad outline the nature and course of human activity, and they help us not only to understand human behavior but also to predict and control it.

Human activity may be studied in two ways. Commonly people study it in terms of goodness and badness and describe it as right or wrong. This is an appreciative approach in which they try to judge behavior in the light of some standard of worth or value and the sciences which follow this method of study are called *normative* sciences. For example, ethics is a normative science of behavior; logic is a normative science of thought. Another method of studying human activity is what may be called descriptive and all that people do is to describe human activity as it is observed in different stages, aspects or phases without any regard to its moral worth. Right or commendable behavior is an interesting and important as true thinking. Sciences which follow this method of study are called positive sciences. Psychology is a positive science. It is concerned not with how people ought to behave but with how people actually do, not with facts as they ought to be but with facts as they are. It does not seek to influence or improve behavior but only to describe it as it is observed in the life of an adult, a child, a lunatic or a genius. Behavior in all its aspects is interesting to the psychologist and questions of worth do not enter into his methods of observation and study.

- **Behavior** The word behavior is used in a very broad sense. It includes not only motor activities like walking, playing, digging or building but also such activities as give us knowledge, for example, perceiving, imagining, remembering, thinking or reasoning, and emotional activities like feeling happy, sad, angry or frightened. They are all activities of the individual, his life depends on them and it is difficult to think what the individual would be without them. They all are included in the term behavior. 'Any manifestation of life is activity' says Woodworth and behavior is a collective name for all such manifestations. Whatever an individual does from the most passive state of sitting still and looking at the wall to the most active striving after a goal like chasing a thief or writing an article, is included in behavior. Movements of limbs and acts of hearing, seeing and smelling are as much behavior as thoughts, emotions and memories. Behavior expresses the entire life of an individual. The individual is both a body and a mind. It is a psychophysical organism whose life is an integral unity of mental and bodily activity. Though for purposes of study and description we distinguish between mental processes and bodily changes, between thoughts, memories and emotions on the one hand and movements and actions on the other, in actual experience there is no mental activity separate and isolated from physical activity. Life is one single continuous flow of activity and its mental and bodily aspects though distinguishable are not really separable. They are two ways of looking at the same object. Behavior is both mental and bodily.

Now the individual cannot be studied apart from the environment in which he lives, moves and has his being. He does not exist in isolation and his activity does not take place in vacuum. Science behavior is the activity of the individual organism in relation to its environment and that psychology helps in understanding and predicting behavior, it mean that an individual's activities are to be studied as responses to definite situations or environment. Walking on the road a child sees a big dog rushing towards him is frightened and thinks of running away and hiding himself. His behavior cannot be understood apart from the situation in which it has been aroused. Now the influence which the environment exercises on the organism and rouses it to activity called stimulus and the activity that is so aroused is called the *response.* A pin-prick makes us jump. The pin-prick is the stimulus and jumping is the response. A noise makes us turn our heads. The noise is the stimulus and the act of turning our heads is the response. All forms of behavior are responses or reactions to stimuli. The environment in which behavior takes place need not necessarily be material or physical. It may consist of other organisms and their behavior. The stimulus may not be a pin-prick or a noise but a question, a frown or a sneer will be the response. Man not only walks, puts on clothes, takes tea or shaves his beard in response to physical stimuli but he does them in a manner approved and commended by other individuals who are members of his group or society. Many of our activities are responses to physical environment, such as breathing, keeping our balance against a strong wind, eating food to sustain ourselves or closing our eyes to avoid dust, and they fulfill individual needs. But there are other activities which are essentially social, though on that account the individual does not need them the less. They take place in a group. We love some people and hate others. Our likes and dislikes are influenced by those of our group. The stimuli of such responses are social and are derived from our interactions with other members of our group. Fashions, etiquette and customs are forces which we cannot ignore in our conduct and they form a part of our social environment. Thus each act of behavior is a response to a stimulus which is a force or action affecting the organism.

Individual does not come into his behavior all at once. It has been a matter of slow growth and development from the early years of infancy to maturity and old age. What a grown-up man is able to do think and feel today is the result of a number of changes that have come about in his physical and mental life. His limbs have grown, his sense organs have matured and his abilities have become more definite and perfect. In fact, life is growth, maturity and decline, and its span is marked by certain stages such as infancy, childhood, adolescence, youth, maturity, and old age, at each of which behavior is marked by certain characteristic features. Psychology studies this growth and its several stages. It compares child and adult, youth and old age so as to obtain a full view of behavior in all its stages of growth and development.

Essentials of Psychology as a Science

As stated earlier the science of psychology tries to explain how behavior of one individual differs from that of another. But while it is interested in differences between one individual and another, it seeks to formulate, as far as possible, the general laws of behavior holding good even of very different individuals. To that end it compares not only child and adult or youth and age but also man and animal. The behavior of man under different diseases and defects like insanity and hysteria is also studied to obtain a complete picture of the subject-matter. Thus whether definitions of psychology as the science of mental life, the study of interactions of the individual with his environment or the science of the activities of an individual, we are not for from the common objective of understanding, explaining, predicting and controlling behavior in a systematic and scientific way.

Modern psychology studies man from prenatal stage up to old age, from the cradle to the grave. Thus, in the ultimate analysis, psychology is the positive science of behavior taking behavior in the widest possible sense. Since Psychology is a positive science. Before discussing the claims of psychology to be called an exact science it is necessary to find out the meaning of the term 'science' itself. Thus a study can be called a science only when it has a limited field to study and a systematic method to use. It is however not the subject matter of a study that makes it a science, but its method. It is the method of science which distinguishes it from art and philosophy. Thus to understand science, it is relevant to analyse the necessary steps in the scientific method. Scientific method requires much creative imagination, objectivity, patience and hard labor. It requires a scientific attitude or spirit in study. The following are the main steps in a scientific method:

1. *Observation:* The first step in a scientific method is to observe the object of study closely and carefully. This observation requires various types of apparatuses and instruments. These apparatuses and instruments must be correct and exact.
2. *Recording:* Another step in the scientific method is the recording of whatever is observed. This requires detached objectivity.
3. *Classification:* After the data are gathered, the scientist classifies it according to facts. As Karl Pearson writes, "The classification of facts, the recognition of their sequence and

relative significance is the function of science". The classification is done in such a way that a certain relation and pattern may be observed in the scattered data. Thus by classification the data are organized on a particular pattern.

4. *Generalization:* The fourth step in the scientific method is generalization. By generalization, scientific laws are discovered in the classified data.
5. *Verification:* The fast and yet the most important step in the scientific method is the verification of the laws that have been discovered. Scientific facts are veridical. They can be verified by anyone under suitable conditions.

From the discussion of the steps in the scientific method as given above, it is clear that a science must have the following essentials:

1. *Scientific method:* It goes without saying that no study can be called a science without having a scientific method.
2. *Factuality:* Science is factual. The scientist studies the facts with an objective attitude.
3. *Universality:* Scientific principles are universal. They are found true in all times and in all climes.
4. *Veracity:* Scientific principles are veridical. They are subject to verification and are verified through scientific methods.
5. *Discovery of cause-effect relationship:* Science finds out cause-effect relationships in the subject-matter of its study and discovers universal principles.
6. *Predictability:* On the basis of these cause-effect relationships, the scientist predicts the future course in various phenomena and these predictions come true because they are based on universal factual principles.

After elaborately discussing the nature of science, the claim of psychology to be called a science can be easily examined. It will be found in sequence that psychology has all the above-mentioned essential characteristics of a science. The main points in his connection are as follows:

- *Psychology uses scientific method:* Almost all the methods of psychology are more or less scientific in their nature. Of these the experimental method is the most exact. It is no less scientific than any other method, used in other sciences. Modern psychology widely uses this method in all its branches. In the experimental method dependent and independent variables are distinguished, the dependent variables controlled and the effect of the independent variables observed. Thus, in the experiment, the psychologist observes a certain phenomenon in strictly controlled situations. He also uses various types of instruments, e.g. chronoscope, a highly sensitive clock, used to determine the interval of time down to the thousandth part of a second in reaction experiments. The psychological laboratories are continuously developing and new and more exact instruments are being constantly put to use. With these instruments the psychologist observes the phenomenon, notes it, compares and classifies it and discovers various principles through generalization. These general principles in psychology are much veridical as a science demands. It should be noted here that all others methods used in psychology are not as exact as the experimental method, but more and more efforts are being made to secure as much exactness as possible. Whatever difference of opinion may there be among the psychologists regarding the merits and demerits of a particular method, all agree that the methods utilized in psychology must be scientific.
- *Psychology is factual:* Psychology studies the facts of behavior. The psychologist is detached and objective in his observations and experiments. The proper field of psychology is not values but facts.

- *The laws of psychology are universal:* The laws of psychology have been found to be correct in every time and place, under the same conditions. The general principles of human psychology are universal, whatever differences there may be in the psychology of different individual, e.g. the psychological fact that human beings and animals are emotionally disturbed by any obstacle in the satisfaction of their impulses, is applicable everywhere.
- *The laws of Psychology are veridical:* Thus by verification and reverification psychological principles have been found to be true everywhere. They can be verified by any one. To illustrate, it is a psychological fact that wherever there is some mental abnormality, there are some frustrations behind it. This fact has been verified by the clinical psychologists. By discovering these frustrations and traumas, one can trace the causes of the particular abnormality.
- *Psychology discovers the cause-effect relationship in human behavior:* Psychology not only observes behavior, but also finds out cause-effect relationship in it, e.g. psychology has discovered why and in what circumstances a child becomes a delinquent or a degenerate. These findings have been put to use and found correct. Thus psychology discovers the 'how' of behavior together with its 'what'.
- *Psychology predicts human behavior:* By discovering the cause-effect relationship, psychology also predicts human behavior and these predictions are generally correct. Thus in the modern progressive countries, appointments to different government posts are made by relying on the predictions made on the basis of psychological tests. On the basis of these psychological tests, it is predicted that such and such person will be a good soldier and so a good administrator; and generally this proves true in actual experience.

From the analysis of the nature of psychology as given above, it is clear that its claims as a science are justified. Thus psychology is an exact science. This however, does not mean that its exactness is the same as that of physical sciences. As a matter of fact the demand of identical exactness from widely different sciences is unjustified. The exactness of a science very much depends on its subject-matter. It is clear that a science which studies mind or behavior cannot be as exact as the science studying the physical things, because behavior is a complex, changeable and dynamic subject of study. Hence while calling psychology an exact science, the limitations also are never fixed and perfectly determined. With the invention of new instruments and the discovery of new methods, psychology will become more and more exact, though it can be called as science but cannot be compared with natural sciences.

Scope of Psychology

Psychology in a science which aims to give us better understanding and control of the behavior of the organism as a whole. Since it is a science of human and animal behavior it includes the application of this to human problems.

The history of psychology has witnessed ever widening scope of its field. Psychology to-day does not only study the animal behavior, but it also studies the behavior of man in all the stages of his development. Not only does it study different types of behavior but it also compares it and finds out general principles useful in the understanding as well as the control of behavior. In brief, where there is behavior, one finds the scope of psychology. A survey of the different contemporary branches of psychology will give a rough picture of its present scope.

It is customary to give the scope of a subject apart from the definition. But this may not be quite necessary with regard to psychology. Instead of giving a short definition, we have actually given descriptions of the subject in our attempt to define it. Thus, a good part of the scope of the subject has already been referred to. It deals with the physiological mechanism, which is part and parcel of the human being. It deals with all our conscious, mental activities. It lays great emphasis on the various factors that work from within the unconscious regions of our mind. The reader would have already noticed that this science deals with almost all aspects of human life. It sometimes merely describes our activities. Sometimes it lays down correct principles for our thinking, feeling and imagination. It helps us in our attempt to learn, giving us the most efficient principles of learning. Thus psychology is a descriptive science which very closely affects the welfare of man. "Know thyself", is certainly one of the maxims. It is absolutely essential for a person to know how his mind works, how various motives interact within the depths of his mind, how easily susceptible he is to external influences, etc. before he can attain high levels of efficient living. A knowledge of this science helps him to regulate his conduct, to appreciate other people's behavior, to guard himself from prejudicial thinking and in short, to be a man. The vast scope of the subject implied in these possibilities of this branch of knowledge can be appreciated if we mention some of the many fields of applied psychology.

1. *Animal psychology:* Psychology studies animal behavior. This branch of psychology is known as animal psychology. Sometimes it is called comparative psychology, because it also compares human psychology and animal psychology. Animal psychology is useful for understanding the human behavior as well, because there is no absolute gulf between the two. Many experiments which cannot be performed on men may be easily performed on men may be easily performed upon animals, e.g. no one can study the effect of heredity as Weismann has studied in his experiments on mice. He cut down the tails of mice from generation to generation and concluded that this defect is not inherited even after several generations. Many psychologists who had equal interest in biology or zoology have been doing a good deal of work studying the behavior of animals. This has been done both for the sake of understanding the behavior of animals and also for understanding to some extent the behavior of man. It has been found that there are certain aspects common to both man and some of the animals. A good deal of our knowledge of the psychology of the learning process has been obtained from experiments with animals.
2. *Child psychology:* Psychology studies man from birth to death. Thus child psychology is an important branch of psychology. It studies the child from the prenatal state upto the adolescent stage. It studies the development of the child, its behavior, as well as various aspects of its personality. Thus, it is very useful for the educationists as well as for the parents. It discovers the secrets of the child world and so gives us an insight into the ways of controlling it as well as to mould it according to accepted social values. Within the scope of child psychology is the adolescent psychology. It studies the man from the age of 12 to 21 years. It studies the physical, mental and social growth of the adolescent individuals. This stage is known as full of stresses and strains. It is a stage through which man passes from childhood to adult stage. Hence the knowledge of its laws is very much helpful for the guidance clinics as well as for the parents, teachers and all others who have to deal with the adolescent. Many psychologists have devoted all their time to the study of the child. A study of the child has developed as a separate branch mostly because it calls for new and

particular types of methods suitable to children. Further, it is during this period of childhood that the developmental processes are at work with greater vigor. So the important part of child psychology is to deal with the various developmental processes such as motor, intellectual, emotional, social, etc. The ways in which factors of heredity and environment interact in the developmental processes of the child are also studied as an important problem in child psychology.

3. *Abnormal psychology:* Psychology not only studies the normal behavior but also the abnormal. It studies different types of psychoses, neuroses and other abnormalities, finds out their causes and general principles and utilizes them to cure these abnormalities. This branch of psychology is known as abnormal psychology. In recent years, abnormal psychology apart from clinical psychology as such, has developed into a major branch. Ever since Freud, Jung and Adler founded their schools, the working of the unconscious mind has attracted the attention of many psychologists. Thus a vast discipline dealing with the nature of the unconscious mind, its working, concepts of abnormality, types of abnormal behavior, theories of abnormal behavior, etc. has been developed. The literature available on this subject is really vast. When the teachings of abnormal psychology are applied to actual treatment of psycho-pathological cases, we call it either as medical psychology or as clinical psychology. An important branch of abnormal psychology which is well known to layman is *psychoanalysis.* The founder of this school, Sigmund Freud, has been very famous for his analysis of dreams, day dreams, various types of errors of pen, slips of tongue, forgetting, humor, art and religion, etc. Psychoanalysis provides the most interested literature in psychology, though it is not so much scientific and exact. One of the practical applications of psychoanalysis has been in the field of psychiatry.

4. *Physiological psychology:* Some other psychologists have been devoting their time mostly to a detailed analysis of the physiological structure of the human being in relation to the working of his mind. Though the physiological and the psychological systems should be really taken as one single unit, yet it sometimes pays to make a detailed analysis of the functions and structure of our nervous system, particularly the brain. As we mentioned earlier, people like Lashley and Sherrington have contributed greatly to our understanding of human behavior from the point of view of the structure of the brain. Thus the branch of physiological psychology has acquired a distinct status of its own. Psychology studies physiological processes from the psychological standpoint. This particular branch of psychology is known as physiological psychology. This includes the study of brain, spinal cord, the sense organs, muscles and nerves, etc. An important example of this field of study is the Weber Fechner law, which studies the least noticeable differences in different stimuli.
5. *Analytical psychology:* Psychology not only studies the various stages of the development of the individual, but it also analyses his different activities. This field is known as analytical psychology. In this branch of psychology the psychologist analyses the various complex processes into their components, finds out their genesis and the general laws regarding them. One of the branches of the analytical psychology is known as *genetic psychology,* which studies the species of men and animals from the psychological point of view.
6. *Psychology of individual differences:* Psychology studies the general principles which are universally applicable to the behavior of human beings, but it also studies the individual differences. This study is known as psychology of individual differences.

An important branch in this field is the *individual psychology* which is mainly concerned with the psychological types. An excellent example is the classification of men into introverts, extroverts and ambiverts attempted by Jung. The psychology of individual differences studies how different individuals differ in their personality, intelligence and other important traits. It studies the role of heredity and environment in creating individual differences.

7. *Dynamic psychology:* An important branch of abnormal psychology and psychoanalysis is known as dynamic psychology or psychology of normal motivation. It studies the conflicts, the frustrations and various types of complexes in infancy, childhood, adolescence and adult stage. It also finds out how these maladies may be removed so that one may become a normal and adjusted person in society.
8. *Experimental psychology:* The most important method of contemporary psychology is the experimental method and one finds it today particularly is the experimental method and one finds it today particularly used in a growing branch of psychology, known as experimental psychology. This is one of the most valuable branches of psychology since it uses strictly scientific methods in its study. Experimental psychology studies external behavior as well as the internal processes of the different stages of human development as also of animals. Only those phenomena fall outside its field which cannot be studied in controlled situations. But the scope of experimental psychology is gradually widening with the invention of new tools and instruments for experiments.
9. *Developmental psychology:* Psychology is dynamic. It studies man as a dynamic and developing being. Developmental psychology studies the various stages of the development of man, compares the developments of different individuals, finds out the causes of the differences and searches for general laws governing them. The study of the development processes helps to find out ways to control and reform them.
10. *General psychology:* The different branches of psychology hitherto described, are included in general psychology which does not go into the details of these processes but studies them from a general standpoint. Thus general psychology includes the study of sensations, perceptions, motives, memory, imaginations, thinking, personality and all other normal human activities and mental processes.
11. *Social psychology:* Psychology studies the behavior of man as individual as well as his behavior in social situations. The latter has been specialized by a branch of psychology, known as social psychology. Social psychology studies the behavior of men as members of crowd, group and audience, etc. Hence its knowledge is necessary for the leaders, the generals and the reformers. The social psychologist studies social problems, finds out their laws and employees them for the solution of those problems. The social psychology has been proved to be useful in almost every field of social life.
12. *Folk psychology:* A branch of psychology which studies superstitions, mythologies, culture, music, art and religion in their psychological aspect, is known as folk-psychology. This branch is gradually becoming important in more developed countries.
13. *Applied psychology:* Psychology is not only a theoretical study but also helps in the solution of various problems concerning different aspects of human behavior. This is known as applied psychology. Applied psychology today is, however, divided into different special branches, e.g. clinical psychology, educational psychology, legal

psychology and industrial psychology, etc. To have an idea of the scope of applied psychology, a brief survey of its important branches is useful. The following are some of the most important branches of applied psychology.

i. *Clinical psychology:* In recent years, particularly after the teaching of Freud, all mental disorders have been viewed from the psychological viewpoint. Most of the disorders have been found to be due to psychological or emotional conflicts. Here, the psychology of the unconscious mind is greatly emphasized. The formation and the workings of the unconscious mind are studied through an analysis of dreams, abnormal symptoms and other strange aspects of one's behavior. Psychotherapy has now won an important place among the methods for the treatment of all psychological disorders. The total psychological study of the abnormal person, all these form the scope of clinical psychology. Principles of mental hygiene also find a place within this field of applied psychology. Clinical psychology is concerned with the cure of various types of abnormalities, psychoses and neuroses, etc. One of the pioneers in this field was Sigmund Freud. Since his time clinical psychology has progressed so much that now every next modern hospital in the western countries has clinical psychologists attached to it. An American survey in 1951 showed that clinical psychology is being used in about 43 percent of the American hospitals.

ii. *Counseling and vocational guidance:* One of the most valuable applications of psychology is in the field of vocational guidance. Psychology helps young men and women to choose their career according to their capacities and talents. Thus the universities, the colleges, the industrial centers and the employment exchanges profit by the counseling of the psychologist. This helps them in finding the right man for the right job. Besides giving guidance to the youth in vocations, the psychologist also guides the parents in tackling with the problems of the child truancy, delinquency, etc.

iii. *Educational psychology:* It hardly needs to be pointed out that psychology would be greatly applied to the problems of education. Every teacher during his period of training has to study psychology and its application to educational problems. The psychology of learning, psychology of remembering and forgetting, assessment of pupils on the basis of tests, training the personality of the pupil, all the major problems of education can be effectively dealt with the help of psychology. So today educational psychology has developed as an advanced branch of applied psychology. Now psychology has almost revolutionized our approach to education. Not only the teacher but also the taught and parents have profited by psychology. As Clifford T Morgan puts it, "the study of the development of the child shows us what to teach, when to teach and how to teach". Educational psychology helps the teachers to bring about the utmost development of the faculties of the educand and to educate him according to his psychological capacities.

iv. *Selection for government services:* Modern Governments employ the services of the psychologist for the selection of suitable personnel for different public services, specially in the naval, land air forces. In the Second World War, army alpha tests and army beta tests were utilized for the recruitment of men in the army and the soldiers were given work according to the results of these tests. In the Second World War, engineering psychology, a new branch of psychology, was developed.

Engineering psychology helps to devise such machinery as may be operated with the least fatigue. Thus it has helped men in designing the autovehicles, engines, etc.

v. *Industrial psychology and commercial psychology:* The most useful application of psychology has been in the field of industry and commerce. By the study of the psychology of the consumer, the industrialists can know about the requisite qualities of the commodities as well as the methods of buying, selling and advertising. It is the field of advertisement that one notices most interesting application of psychology. Psychology has helped the industrialists in their relation with the laborers as well as in the recruitment of the laborers and in finding the suitable jobs for them. In the modern factories one finds wide use of different types of tests, e.g. tests of steadiness, tests of alertness, tests of special qualities, etc. In industry, there are several problems which could be mastered efficiently with the help of psychology. We have to select proper men who have the requisite aptitude for a particular job. Then only the job will be well done. This can be ensured by selecting men on the basis of vocational aptitude and vocational selection tests. In any industry, a finished product has to be sold and it must be advertised. A good advertisement is based directly on the psychology of attention. In any industry, the workers and various grades of officers will have to work as a team. Strikes and other such disturbances will affect the output in any industry. This means corporate life of the firm or factory should be properly ordered. Findings of modern social psychology make a great contribution towards this. These and so many other problems, major and minor, connected with industrial or business organizations can be effectively managed with the help of psychology. It is towards this that industrial psychology has gradually developed in recent years.

vi. *Military psychology:* During the last two World Wars a number of problems cropped up for which answers were sought from the psychologists. Quick selection of suitable men both for the ranks and at the officers level became a necessity during war time. Adequate personality qualities in an officer that would stand stress and strain in the battle-front had to be assessed in the shortest time possible during selection period. Psychologists came forward with suitable tests for such purposes. All war propaganda was carried on the basis of the psychology of suggestibility. Whether it be to maintain the morale of one's own side or to break the morale of the opponents, principles of psychology were used. What came to be called the "cold war" was mostly fought with the help of psychologists and psychology. Quick and efficient methods of treatment were necessary for cases for nervous breakdown at the battle-front. Thus even psychiatry and psychotherapy came to be developed along particular lines to meet the conditions of war.

vii. *Legal psychology:* Psychology has been used in the field of law and justice. It is useful for the judges, lawyers, witnesses and all others who are concerned with the law or justice. It has helped in the detection of crimes, false witnesses and other complex phenomena. Besides the above-mentioned applications of psychology, it is being very much used in almost every branch of the political field. In elections, administration, legislation, and all other fields, the knowledge of psychology is paying good dividends. As a matter of fact as psychology grows, its application in the different fields of human activities will also grow. The scope of psychology, theoretical as well as applied, includes every aspect of human behavior. Thus the scope of psychology includes the study of conscious, unconscious, subconscious; child, adolescent, adult; individuals, mobs and audiences; leaders and followers; laborers, students and men in all walks of life and also the different types of animal behavior. In short, where there is behavior, there is the field of psychology and this field is widening with the ever-increasing knowledge of the psychologists.

Aims of Psychology

Psychology is the positive science of behavior. It aims at the study of the facts of behavior, their collection, classification and comparison, and finds out general hypotheses based upon them. Thus the aim of psychology is the study of man's behavior. Behavior not only includes the overt activities, but also the inner processes. Thus psychology studies man's external as well as internal activities.

The aims of psychology are not only theoretical but also practical, though the theoretical and the practical fields have been specialized by different branches of psychology in different spheres. Whereas the theoretical studies aims at finding out general laws regarding behavior in their own field, the applied psychology aims at finding out the applications of these general laws. Thus psychology not only adds to our knowledge of human nature, but also makes life better. Not only does it aim at studying the personality of man, but it also aims at making it more balanced and adjusted.

Psychology's Goals

Psychology is the scientific study of behavior and mental processes. Behavior includes all of our outward or overt actions and reactions, such as talking, facial expression and movement. Mental processes refer to all the internal, covert activity of our minds, such as thinking, feeling, and remembering. Why "scientific"? To study behavior and mental processes in both animals and humans, researchers have to observe them. Whenever a human being is observing anyone or anything, there's always a possibility that the observer will see only what he or she expects to see. Psychologists don't want to let these possible biases cause them to make faulty observations. They want to be as precise and measure as carefully as they can, so they use the scientific method to study psychology.

Every science has goals. In physics, the goals concern learning how the physical world works. In astronomy, the goals are to chart the universe and understand both how it came to be and what it is becoming. In psychology, there are four goals that aim at uncovering the mysteries of human and animal behavior: description, explanation, prediction and control.

Description: The first step in understanding anything is to give it a name. Description involves observing a behavior and noting everything about it: what is happening, where it happens, to whom it happens, and under what circumstances it seems to happen. For example, a teacher might notice that a young girl in his second-grade classroom is behaving oddly. She's not turning in her homework, her grades are slipping badly, and she seems to have a very negative attitude toward school. That's *what* she is doing. The description of what she is doing gives a starting place for the next goal: *why* is she doing it?

Explanation: Explanation gives us why is it happening for example: To find out why the girl is doing all these things, the teacher would most likely ask the school counselor to administer some tests. Her parents might be asked to take her to a pediatrician to make sure that there is no physical illness, such as an allergy. They might also take her to a psychologist to be assessed. In other words, they are looking for an explanation for her behavior. Finding explanations for behavior is a very important step in the process of forming theories of behavior. A theory is a general explanation of a set of observations or facts. The goal of description provides the observations, and the goal of explanation helps to build the theory. For example, if all the tests seem to indicate that the young girl has a learning problem, such as dyslexia (an inability to read at expected levels for a particular age and degree of intelligence), the next step would be trying to predict what is likely to happen if the situation stays the same.

Prediction: Determining what will happen in the future is a prediction. In the example, the psychologist or counselor would predict (based on previous research into similar situations) that this little girl will probably continue to do poorly in her school work and may never be able to reach her full learning potential. Clearly, something needs to be done to change this prediction, and that is the point of the last of the four of psychology: changing or modifying behavior.

Control: Control, or the modification of some behavior, has been somewhat controversial in the past. Some people hear the word control and think brainwashing, but that is not the focus of this goal. The goal is to change a behavior from an undesirable one (such as failing in school) to a desirable one (such as academic success). Goal of control helps to how can it be changed.

In the example of the young girl, there are certain learning strategies that can be used to help a child (or an adult) who has dyslexia improve reading skills. The psychologist and educators would work together to find a training strategy that works best for this particular girl. Not all psychological investigations will try to meet all four of these goals. In some cases, the main focus might be on description and prediction, as it would be for a personality theorist who wants to know what people are like (description) and what they might do in certain situations (prediction). Some psychologists are interested in both description and explanation, as is the case with experimental psychologists who design research to find explanations for observed (described) behavior. Therapists, of course, would be more interested in control, although the other three goals would be important in getting to that goal. These goals have not really changed in the years since psychology's beginnings, but the methods of achieving them certainly have changed. In the next section, we'll take a look at the early pioneers in psychology.

Significance of Psychology in Nursing/Relevance to Nursing

There are many fields of knowledge which deal with human nature. History tells us of the changing thoughts and habits of nations and of the individual men and women who helped to bring about these changes. Economics tells us of the ways in which people work, earn, sell or buy. Politics rests upon our understanding of human nature. Biology tells us how the body is made, how it works and performs several acts of seeing, moving and holding things and how the body varies from one person to another. But the science of psychology is concerned with human nature as no other science is. It studies the several activities of man directly and for their own sake, not to understand the course of history or of social changes nor, like biology, to learn the functions of the several parts of the bodily organism but to obtain general laws about the activities and behavior of human beings. Men and women live in a world and respond to its influences. The world is composed of things and persons, and they interact with this world, accepting some influences and resisting others. This interaction between the individual and the world calls for scientific study, and psychology is the science which seeks to study all human activities with a view to obtaining general laws about them.

Everyone is interested in understanding themselves and other. They want to know the reasons for their actions like angriness, sadness, happiness, and different actions and reactions, likes and dislikes, interests and attitudes, etc. Psychology will enable us to know the reasons for all actions. Psychology not only helps to understand why other people do things they do, but it also helps better understand ourselves and our reactions to other people. Psychology can help us to understand how our brain and body are connected, how to improve our learning abilities and memory and how to deal with stresses in life both ordinary and extraordinary.

The nurses play an important role in health care delivery system, in which nurses are always working with their client, in hospitals, and other health care centers and institutions and they have to work with the medical team, health team and nursing team itself. So nurse needs to understand themselves and also wants to understand other people who come across the field of nursing including patients, and their relatives, friends and also the members of the collaborative team. Everyone of these people can be understood better if the nurse knows something of human behavior and how it is caused through the study of psychology. The nurses who takes the trouble to study, understand and use psychology in their work becomes a better team member. Nurses have to deal mostly with sick persons. The success of in their work depends upon their efficient understanding of psychology of patients. Nurses required to deal with patients in tender care. Besides dealing with patients nurses need to cooperate with medical team. So nurses must have very good knowledge of human psychology for proving better care to their clients and to become better nurses.

Psychology is the study of human behavior and the knowledge about the why's and wherefore's of human behavior is of immense value of the student nurse because in her job she comes across a wide variety of human behavior. The study of Psychology will help the student nurse in the following ways:

1. ***Psychology helps nurses to understand oneself:*** Self-knowledge is the key to success in all human endeavor. By understanding oneself we mean that the student nurse should know her motives, desires, emotions and ambitions. She must have a clear perception of the goal of other life. She should know what are her interests, what are their likes and dislikes and whether she is temperamental or cool-headed. For example if you are prone to be easily hurt it is better to avoid difficult situations and persons. Everyone must analyze her feelings, thinking and reasoning and how one goes about to solve the difficulties. This will give her an idea that she is highly complex but unique and individualistic. Therefore one must not try to follow the behavior patterns of others. Even the good features of others personalities must be subjected to critical appraisal in the light of one's own weak and strong points and not try to ape others. Psychology also reveals the basic needs which govern a person's life such as the value of food and sex in life. There are also social motives, cultural factors and religious compulsions. One does not live in a vacuum. One is subject to as many influences—the family, school, community and so on. A good grasp of various

influences controlling one's behavior will give the student nurse an insight into her own behavior and what are the factors controlling it. This understanding will cultivate in her a sense of self-discipline.

2. ***Psychology helps nurses to understanding others:*** Understanding others is as vital for happy life as understanding oneself. The student nurse has to work, study and live with her mates and teachers, doctors and helping staff. Besides she has to deal with most complicated personalities—the sick men and their guardians. Armed with a clear perception and insight into human nature she will be well-equipped to understand others better and thus be successful in interpersonal relationships, and this is key to one's success. If you know why others are different from you and that it is not necessary that all should adhere to a uniform set of values and that others can very well be fond of things which repel us, all this will help you to adjust easily even with difficult persons. Besides idiosyncracies, which all have in some measure, there are factors like cultural, religious and social background which make men different from each other. Such knowledge is of immense help in leading a contented and successful life. The study of Psychology is thus of great value in understanding ourselves as well as others.

3. ***Psychology help nurses to appreciate value of change:*** The study of Psychology tells us that man is a creature of habits and that his attitudes are generally rigid and inflexible. But unless there is flexibility and readiness to change one cannot be successful in one's life. The change in one's social milieu and physical environs is sometimes necessary for better adjustment and happiness. For example a nurse should not stand on prestige and false sense of pride in not using glasses or hearing aids if she is deficient in any of these. Artificial aids to make up natural deficiency must be used to achieve optimum performance and success in work. A girl who depends too much on her parents may benefit from living in hostel. An urban dweller may soothe her nerves by a sojourn in a village. Similarly, periodic relaxation by an outing or picnic is desirable.

4. ***Psychology help to know importance of interdependence of body, mind and spirit:*** A human being works as a close-knit unit in which the various parts of human personality, namely, body and mid affect each other. In modern medicine the psychosomatic concept is generally accepted. This means that the role of mind is disturbed or if he is emotionally depressed all kinds of physical ailments follow. It is common knowledge that due to anxiety people lose appetite or experience headache. Therefore while working with sick persons it will be a primary task of a nurse to soothe them, give them assurance that they will recover and are not badly ill. The success in nursing career depends very much on tactful handling of the patients. In this matter her knowledge of Psychology can be of immense value.

5. ***Psychology help for readjustment:*** Every profession and career requires readjustment. A nurse needs to make the following kinds of adjustments for success in the nursing career:-

1. Overcoming of home-sickness and self-reliance is needed if she has to live smoothly in hospital.
2. Adjusting to tolerate sick persons who may cry or be desperate or may even ventilate their anger by making the nurse a target of their abuses and curses.
3. Not to be taken in by show of affection, love and sympathy. Some patients may even make passes or indulge in indiscretion. She must keep her cool under these trying circumstances.
4. Trying to work and study together.

In these efforts knowledge of psychology can be helpful. An insight into the emotions will make clear lots of problem. After a discussion of the value of psychology for nurse, we will now discuss the definition, nature and scope of Psychology.

6. *Psychology helps to provide better nursing to clients:* The study of Psychology can help the nurse to gain an insight into her desires, motives, emotions and attitudes as well as the motives, attitudes and emotional complexities of patients and other persons she comes in contact with. It also explains to the interaction of mind and body and the impact of this upon human behavior. Psychology is a scientific study of human behavior and its dynamics, its physiological and other causes, the role and importance of sense perception, thinking and learning in it. A general knowledge of Psychology is very essential and useful in the art of effective nursing.

The act of effective nursing does not consist merely in mastering the knowledge and technique of nursing. Surely effective nursing is more than the knowledge of nursing techniques. It is also more than the possession and practice of certain skills and more than the mechanical performance of routine operations and duties in hospital. Undoubtedly a sound knowledge of physiology, anatomy and other discipline and mastery over techniques and procedures of nursing are essential for a competent nurse. But in as much as she has to deal with living human beings, she must have a sound knowledge of human nature if she is to perform well. There are certain elementary facts about human nature with which every nurse must be conversant and her practice should take account of these. These insights and understandings can be had by a careful study of Psychology. Nurses have to deal with a large cross section of human nature and it is, therefore, imperative to make an inquiry into factors and principles that make for effective nursing. Following are the principles which must be borne in mind by every nurse:

i. The whole patient and not the particular disease be attended to
ii. Individualized approach
iii. Sympathy and consideration
iv. Effective health teaching
v. Effective adjustments.

i. *The principle of whole patient:* An efficient and understand nurse does not treat the patient for a particular illness only. A sick man is not merely a diseased entity with a fractured limb, a nervous stomach, pyrexia and some other disease. Besides his diseases he is a human being with his likes and dislikes, prides and prejudices. The disease may not be so hurtful to him as a harsh word. A sweet remark may hasten his recovery whereas a taunt may thwart it. Every sick man has some permanent interests, desires, ambitions, capacities, family and religious affiliations, certain attitudes and aptitudes and a certain temperament. It is this background that a good nurse will weight and consider these intellectual and emotional factors as well as the physical implications of the particular disease. A nurse should bear in mind that every patient is an interaction of mind and body and that a scrupulous watch should be kept on the moods and emotions of the patient. According to Jessie Williams, "It is necessary to recognize that each individual patient is a unique personality who reacts to illness with his body, mind and emotions on his own individual way. It follows that one must remember always that one is not called up to nurse an appendix or a septic throat or whatever the physical illness may be, but a sick person". For example a patient who is to undergo an operation he must not only physically and clinically prepared but should also be mentally and emotionally prepared.

ii. *Individualized approach:* It is better to impress upon the patient that the attitude and approach of the nurse towards him is human and not professional and that he is being cared as an individual person. Indeed no two patients will be the same and it will be much advised if they are approached according to their unique personality. The right approach will aim at establishing a complete rapport with the patient and put him at ease in the strange environs of a hospital ward or room. In order to achieve this the nurse should remember the following things:
   - The patient should be treated warmly and courteously and receive him as a guest. He should be shown all possible care and affection.
   - The patient should be gently introduced to the peculiarities of a ward and well-oriented with the physical environs, facilities available and the people he is likely to come across. All this should be done with a touch of kindness.
   - The patient usually is tense when he comes to a hospital. He should be made to relax and all his fears and doubts gently allayed.
   - The over modest patients should be made to lose their self-consciousness and by gentleness their confidence should be won over.
   - Be a patient listener. Let the patient come out with his story in his own words. "When he finds that he is being listened embarrassment". Nursing should be an art of personal service to the sick. It should not degenerate into professionalism and become impersonal.

iii. *Sympathy and consideration:* By sympathy and consideration we can have a correct appraisal of the patient. A critical outlook is not helpful. Understanding the patient is the most important single factor in the art of effective nursing. After establishing a rapport with the patient an attempt should be made to understand him. The first and fore most thing to be done in order to understand a patient is to know his name. It is only if you are able to refer to the patient by his first name that you can inspire confidence in him. This cannot be done by calling the number of his bed or the name of his affliction. The sense of security of the patient is restored if he or she is addressed by his or her name. Calling persons by their first names and children by their nicknames inspires in them confidence an any feeling of estrangement is removed. If barriers of strangeness are broken the nurse can tend to the patients much better. The second factor which helps in understanding the patient is an ability to read faces. She should be able to guess from the appearance whether the patient is tense or relaxed. It is very helpful if by careful observation of the facial lineaments the nurse is able to guess if the patient is tense or relaxed, dejected or excited, bold or timid. A nurse with an acute sense of observation can obviously handle the patients efficiently. No two individuals are alike. A sober recognition of this fact is very helpful in successful dealings with others. Some patients are expansive, cordial and friendly while others are withdrawn and aloof and even antagonistic. Some patients are not quite cooperative; they are selfish and demanding, expecting to monopolize the attention of the nurse. Some patients tend to be anxious, tense and apprehensive while others are, on the whole, cheerful, calm and quiet. Some patients are quite sharp and intelligent and they grasp things quickly. They would follow the instructions easily and cheerfully. There are others who are slow and dull-witted. They do not understand the instructions carefully and are slow in following them. Their grasp is poor and they seem to be unable to think and reason even at a very elementary level. Indeed all individuals are different. Therefore it is impossible to come across two patients with identical nature. These differences may be due to heredity, cultural milieu, training and education and socio-economic status they enjoy. The patients react differently due to age, nature of illness and also due to the type of nurse's personality. Indeed it is the wide differences in humanity that makes the nursing profession both interesting and demanding.

On account of their different personality patterns, patients react in different ways to their illness and to their hospitalization. Accordingly patients can be classified into two main types—the tough and tender patients.

a. The tough patients know what they are suffering from; they have an idea of their illness. They are not easily posture at bed and bear well pain and discomfort. Their attitude to life is detached. The ebb and tide of their lives does not overwhelm them. They are rather lacking in imagination and are therefore calm and unworried. Their attitude toward life is that of resignation of unemotional acceptance of the vicissitudes of life. They are realists and face dangers squarely.
b. The tender patients fall into four subgroups: — (1) The anxiety-prone, (2) Obsessional, (3) The histrionic, self-dramatizing type and (4) The inadequate. Of these the anxiety prone patients are habitual worries. They are scrupulously conscious of their duties and usually display a great sense of responsibility. Being given to worry they generally remain tense, apprehensive and unable to relax. They feel easily and acutely even the slightest pain or discomfort. They are difficult to manage and are uncooperative.

- Obsessional patients also suffer from anxieties, worries and fears. But their worry is not general but confined to a particular subject and their worry has no basis whatsoever in reality. They may be constantly disturbed by the fear of catching some disease. They may not like to shake hands lest they contaminate themselves and fall ill.
- The histrionic or self-dramatizing type of patients have fertile imagination and dramatize the life events as these happen to them. They also exaggerate their suffering and consider themselves victims of some malignant agency. They weep easily and lament loudly their sufferings. They are childish and immature and their reactions to their illness and hospitalization are irrational. They behave like children and want to be coaxed and cajoled.
- The inadequate patient has a poor personality. He keeps aloof and is afraid to mix up with others in ward. He is a person who has been cared too much by his parents and relatives and, as a consequence, has lost all initiative. He does not face his illness objectively and has little desire to get well. He is pessimist and is apathetic towards his problems. He needs to be coaxed and cajoled to eat, to consume medicine and to exercise. These patients require special care and treatment. It is only an insightful, benevolent nurse who can make successful adjustments with all sorts of persons. These are the broad types, but is should not be expected that patients will neatly fit into these categories. As a matter of facts no patient will correspond one by one to the characteristics described above. Indeed the same patients may show the symptoms of anxiety and obsession. One may react toughly to one disease but may be tender in the face of another disease.

*7. **Psychology help nurse to provide age-wise care to clients:*** Age is an important factor in determining and explaining the individual variations and differences. The old patients will of course be different from the young patients. Each age has its own peculiar problems with which the nurse should be well-acquainted. A child of eight and a man of sixty-five may both be suffering from pneumonia, and the general principles underlying the nursing care in their disease may be the same, but there is a gulf of difference in mental and emotional needs of these two patients. A thorough knowledge will enable the nurse to gain an insight into the growth patterns and psychological needs of different age groups. The needs of the child, the adolescent and the adult and old will be different.

i. A nurse who is given the assignment of looking after the infants should be very careful about their growth requirements. The growth of an infant is all round—physical, mental, social and emotional. All phases of growth are interconnected. Growth is integral and is characterized by unification and wholeness. An infant needs security, love, and affection above all and these facts should be appreciated by the nurse. This must be provided by close personal attention on the part of the nurse. She should frequently pet and fondle the child. Of course there should no pampering as this encourages feeling of dependency among children. A child is ego-center and this fact should be always remembered while looking after the child. This ego-centrism is heightened during illness. But if this tendency towards ego-centrism is carefully kept in check the personality of the child is likely to permanently change or warp the developing personality. Many a times children do not like to become well and they malinger. It is sometimes the case that a child looks upon his illness as a welcome experience. This may happen because he is able to receive attention and get consideration during illness that he does not normally get. A good nurse can avoid this kind of situation.

   A nurse who is to take care of infants must realize that the primary task of an infant is to grow. The growth and development of an infant is all round—physical, mental, social and emotional. In nursing children following facts may well be remembered:

   - The surrounding of the child should be pleasant and cheerful.
   - If possible the members of the family of the child should visit him frequently.
   - A close rapport with the child should be established by understanding and appreciating his special needs.
   - If possible the child should be given suitable toys.
   - The use of force and violence should be scrupulously avoided in dealing with the child.
   - The child should be given love, affection and care.
   - The nurse should be patient in dealing with children.
   - The child should be encouraged to develop a spirit of independence.
   - An anxious child does not recover well. Therefore his emotional problems should be taken care of and he should be made to feel cheerful.
   - Personal involvement with the child should be avoided.

   The parents of sick children are likely to be anxious and worried. They may be very much upset if the child happens to be their only offspring. There is need to reassure parents and make them feel well and cheerful. An intelligent nurse will not allow herself to be upset by the irrational attitude of some parents. She should be tactful in handling difficult and delicate situations. If she can inspire confidence among parents and convince them, she is their well-wisher, everything will be well.

ii. The adolescent patient is helped best if his growth pattern and needs are fully understood. An adolescent is subject to mood variations. He may sometimes be over energetic and at other times be lethargic. Sometimes he is sociable and sometimes withdrawn and aloof.

The adolescent patient needs cheerful surroundings. He should have magazines and books to read. The over energetic display of adolescents needs to be appreciated and given room for manifestation. It is better if they are visited by friends besides their relatives. The adolescent wishes to be treated as a grown-up and does not like to be fondled and petted. An adolescent feels secure if he is treated as an equal, if difficulties are discussed with him, if he is given a chance to express his opinion and his opinion respected. It is advisable to provide for their hobbies and interests.

iii. The adult patient may be desperate and may be nursing some secret fears and anxieties. It is desirable if a nurse tries to probe into the causes of behavior in adults. The aged patients have their peculiar problems. Age brings about many physical, mental and emotional changes in the old person such as wrinkled skin, the loss of teeth, graying of hair, stooping shoulders, decrease in muscular strength, increase in tremors of hands and legs, the weakness of voice, decline in sensory and perceptual powers, particularly, in the acuteness of vision and hearing. Besides these in old age there is general infirmity. There is mental deterioration, memory is weak, the power of adjustment poor. A widower old age patient has additional drawbacks. He is generally depressed and lonely. Some old persons find life futile and a burden. The nurse should be well-versed with the knowledge of old age. She should be tender and sympathetic toward old patients.

As a rule illness and hospitalization are disturbing events and they upset the equilibrium of man. There are some who repeatedly fall ill and have gradually reconciled with their fate. But those who are suffering for the first time and are having their first experience of hospital life may be fearful, anxious and different. They may be unacquainted with the hospital routine. Of course the behavior of a patient in the hospital is governed by his temperament and educational and cultural background. Some patients are apparently very quiet and accept everything passively. They may seem to be ideal patients. But the appearances may be deceptive. They may be guilt-ridden. A wise nurse would not go by appearances alone but would find out the reasons for unusual passivity. She should try to discover and remove inward tensions and anxieties.

8. ***Psychology helps to adjust to the general effects of hospitalization:*** The general effects of hospitalization are as follows:

a. Illness is both painful and discomforting. It lowers ones activity and makes one despair of life. It interferes with the normal processes of rest and activity. The nurse must know that people differ in their capacities to bear pain and suffer. Some are highly upset by even small amount of suffering while others withstand gracefully even acute pain and suffering. The nurse should render help keeping in view these natural variations.
b. Illness restricts the life of all patients irrespective of their age, socioeconomic status or profession. Normal routine is disturbed, responsibilities have to be temporarily given up. This makes the patients anxious and disturbed. They must be given sufficient recreation to overcome their feeling of inadequacy.
c. Illness produces in patients decline in self-regard. Some patients feel the loss of self-regard too much and make attempts to restore it. They do this by finding faults with others. They become critical, complaining or openly hostile.
d. Illness makes the patients feel insecure and uncertain about their future. The nurse can lessen these feelings of insecurity by frank explanation of hospital conditions and procedures and reassure him by her sincere interest. The patient should be helped to

accept cheerfully the temporary break in his routine and reassured about his recovery. A hopeful patient recovers quickly.

e. In illness there is infantile regression. This tendency is shown is the behavior of adult patients who are highly demanding or excessively dependent. Adults who are reluctant to accept treatments are showing the symptoms of childish behavior.

f. Some patients are malingerers. They use the illness as a weapon to secure attention. Therefore they unnecessarily complain of pains and aches just to be able to secure the attention and sympathy of hospital staff. This malingering behavior serves a number of purposes. They reduce the demands made on the patients and, secondly, win for them a certain amount of extra sympathy and attention.

g. There are some patients who, on account of good food, personal care and attention, find hospitals a much better place to live in. They find in it a refuge from adverse family circumstances and the need to do hard work.

The patients for whom the hospital becomes an escape from hardships and responsibilities of home become acutely nervous when they are required to leave the hospital. The idea of going back to their work or to their home where they have to fulfill many obligations becomes disgusting to them in as much as it involves the loss of attention and care they receive from nurses and doctors, and that of freedom from responsibility which has characterized the period of sickness in the hospital. Such patients may find out excuses and false complaints in order that they may continue in the hospital. The nurse should try to explain politely the harsh facts to these patients. These patients need to be helped in a realistic manner.

9. ***Psychology helps to provide effective health teaching to clients:*** Streeter in her article *The Nurses Responsibility for Teaching Patients*, remarks that effective teaching (about health) will help the patient understand the hospital and its routine, the nature of diagnostic examination and treatment, principles of preservation of health and prevention of disorders, the nature of disease conditions, the after-care program and rehabilitation. An understanding of psychology can be of great help to a nurse to become a teacher. A nurse if she is to be an effective teacher, must understand that patients differ in their abilities to learn. Therefore her coaching should suit the individual need of the patient. In order to teach well an interest in the topic to be learned must be created. The patients if they understand the value and utility of what they are to learn will feel motivated. Without strong motivation there can be no learning. A nurse should know when the patient is ready to learn and to what extent he is prepared to learn. This can be known by nurse easily. With this knowledge she can easily impart knowledge which will be readily absorbed by the patient. As far as possible new ideas should be introduced in relation to what the patient knows already. As one author puts it: "While teaching, all new knowledge should be introduced slowly, simple things to precede more complex things". The golden rule is to suit your teaching to the needs and interests of the patient. Patient and other illustrated material is useful in teaching, whenever necessary it should be made us of. Above all it is better to gain the patients confidence and good will. The nurse should teach only when she has gained the confidence of the patient.

10. ***Psychology helps for successful personal and professional adjustment:*** A successful nurse is one who is well-adjusted and has interest in her job. The life of nurse needs to be characterized by a zest for living and an outgoing nature and cooperative attitude. Not everyone can make a good nurse. Only those who are sympathetic by nature, love, humanity and are not afraid of hard work can take to nursing profession. A nurse should have four following qualities:

a. Like people
b. Active mind and habits. Acute observation
c. Enjoy work
d. Emotionally mature.

The successful nurse must make good adjustment to her profession. In India nurses are not given their due respect by the society. Therefore only those who are innately dedicated to the service of humanity can become good nurses. The best nurses learn from their environment. Constant advances in medicine, sociology, psychology and public health must keep her alert. She needs to have an accurate and wise skill in self-evaluation and an intense interest in improvement. She must extend these abilities for the growth of her individual and professional life. The life of a nurse is very demanding. She has little time to spare for herself. Nonetheless it is necessary that she must carefully plan to meet her recreational needs. For success as a nurse it is essential to have a capacity for judicious relationship. The nurse must be well-adapted to teamwork. She has to work with all types of persons. Her conduct must be professionally correct. This is possible if she can be judicious in her dealings with other persons.

In addition to the above psychology also helps the nursing to in following aspects:

1. *Understanding behavioral factors:* Psychology is study of behavior, helps to identify behaviors and experiences that promote health, and influence the effectiveness of health care. It develops the way to reduce smoking and improve daily nutrition.
2. *Studying the relation of contextual factors with biology:* The contextual factors like economic, cultural, community, social and lifestyle factors that influence health people at high psychological workload at prone to cardiovascular diseases. For example, however, seductive advertising also contributes to psychological dependency on tobacco.
3. *Effects of disease:* It investigates how disease affects individual's psychological well-being. An individual who becomes seriously ill or injured problems meeting medical and other bills; problems obtaining proper care when a home away from the hospital; obstacles to caring for dependents; having one's sense of self-reliance compromised; gaining a new, unwanted identity as a sick person and so on.
4. *Preventing illness:* Health psychologist work towards promoting health through behavioral changes in an attempt to prevent illness. Say, stress-reduction interventions at the workplace can be effectively with patients in ways that overcome to understanding, remembering and implementing effective strategies for reducing exposures to risk factors and making health enhancing behavioral changes.
5. *Critical analysis of health policy:* It explores how health policy can influence inequities, inequalities , and social injustice. It expands the scope of health psychology beyond the level of individual health to an examination of the social and economic determinations of health both within and between regions and nations.
6. *Improving nurse/doctor-patient relationship:* It attempts to aid in the process of communication between health professionals and patients during consultations. It helps to overcome anxiety in hospital or related to disease, focusing on the patient's need, listening to the patient completely before making a decision and involving the patient in the process of choosing treatment and finding a diagnosis.

7. *Improving adherence to medical advice:* Getting people to follow medical advice and adhere to their treatment regimens is a difficult task. People often forget to take their pills or are inhibited by the side effects of their medicines. Failing to take prescribed medications is costly and wastes millions of usable medicines that could otherwise help other people. Therefore, the adherence can be improved by tailoring treatment programs to individual's daily lives. However, the adherence rates are difficult to measure.
8. *Managing pain:* It attempts to fine treatment to reduce and eliminate pains, as well as understand pain anomalies such as analgesia, administered analgesia, acupuncture (e.g. inosteoarthritis), biofeedback and cognitive behavior therapy.

3 CHAPTER Methods of Psychology

Method derived from a Greek word 'methodos' pursuit of knowledge. It means to particular procedure for accomplishing or approaching something. It is a systematic procedure involved in the investigation of facts and concepts. In any science, several different methods of study must sometimes be applied to a problem before all the pieces fit together properly. Each method contributes in its own way to the final solution. In planning a study, the scientist attempts to select the method or methods most appropriate to the particular problem under consideration.

Every science employs methods peculiar to its subject matter. As the subject matter changes so the methods. For example, physics studies physical things. These physical things are gross and can be handled with instruments. Hence physics uses experimental method. Psychology is the science of behavior. Behavior includes inner processes and experiences along with external and overt activities. Inner processes and experiences cannot be handled with instruments. Hence psychology uses introspection method also. Besides introspection, psychology uses observation and experimental methods which are widely used in other sciences.

Introspection Method

Introspection is one of the most important method of psychology. The psychoanalysis school has widely utilized this method, but the behaviorists are vehemently opposed to it. Watson, the founder of the school of behaviorism was absolutely opposed to this method. As he said, "Introspection forms no essential part of it's (of psychology) methods nor is the scientific value of its data dependent upon introspection in terms of consciousness". This criticism of introspection has however not been accepted by most of the modern psychologists. Woodworth and others have defended introspection method with elaborate arguments. But to assess the real value of this particular method and to find out its limitations, it is necessary to examine it.

To introspect means to look within. Thus interpretation is internal perception. In it the psychologist himself observes his internal activities and processes. This method is indispensable in the description of individual experiences, e.g. if a man goes to see a movie film and returns after seeing it, it is only through introspection that he can tell others how he feels about it. It is said that the advent of youth changes the behavior, mental conditions and the psychological processes of the individual. But how a young man feels is only a matter of introspection and can be explained only by him who has passed through this stage. Thus in the field of feelings, emotions, sentiments, prejudices and various types of internal experience, e.g. love, hate, pleasure, pain, fear, memory, thought and effort, etc. a man know them only by introspective analysis. No man can known another by the observation of his overt behavior. The pangs of separation from someone dear to us is not a matter of understanding or logic or observation, but purely of introspection. Thus introspection is indispensable for the study of internal behavior.

Psychology not only studies the overt behavior, but also the internal processes. It is the science of behavior. Behavior, as it is taken today, includes the internal experiences. Internal experience cannot be known by external observations. They can be known only through introspection by the subject himself. In introspection the individual himself systematically observer cannot take the help of the instruments or of the observations of another person. The observer can introspect his mental processes wherever and whenever he likes to do so. Thus the method of introspection has been proved to be very valuable in the field of psychology. Introspection is a unique method of psychology. Introspection is a physical or social. In spite of what the behaviorists say against it, psychology cannot dispense with introspection.

As started earlier introspection means to look within. It is internal perception or self-observation. The individual himself observes his internal activities and processes whenever and wherever he likes to do so. For example, a patient after surgery may be asked to report how he feels. The patient will try to look within and recall what happened and how he is feeling now.

Advantages

- It does not involve any expenditure as no need of any laboratory or apparatus
- Direct knowledge of mental experience of an individual is taken.

Disadvantages

But every method has its own limitations peculiar to itself. Hence introspection method also has its own limitations. Roughly its limitations are as follows:

1. It is truly said that the mental processes can be directly observed through introspection. But these data cannot be the basis of generalization since it is not necessary that experience of other persons should be identical with that of the observer.
2. By introspection one cannot known the experience of others and so cannot compare one's own experience with that of others, the experiences of other can only be known through observations or experiments. Hence, introspection alone is neither sufficient nor the most important method of psychology. Observation and experiments are definitely more valuable and important methods of psychology.
3. It cannot be used by children or mental defectives.
4. It is purely a private affair and cannot be verified by other observers. In many cases, the patients may not have the insight to know about their conditions or language to describe them accurately.
5. *It is difficult to attend the mental processes:* There is a difference between the perception of the object and the observation of the mental processes. The objects are material and concrete while the mental processes are psychic and abstract. Hence, it is not easy to attend the mental processes. One cannot observe them without much effort

in concentration, and concentration is a difficult feat. Thus to observe the mental processes through introspection, is a difficult effort.

But this difficulty in introspection is not unsurmountable. Introspection undoubtedly requires more concentration and the newcomer has only a few chances of success in it. But this difficulty can be removed by adequate practice and training. As a matter of fact introspection requires long training. Training and practice improve the capacity for abstraction and concentration. It makes introspection more valid.

6. *It is difficult to grasp mental processes:* Mental processes are changeable. The thoughts, feelings, desires, etc. are constantly changing. But observation requires a fixed objects. It is only then that one can easily observe the external object. But as soon as one attends to the mental processes, they disappear. Then how can they be observed? If a psychologist wants to know his mental state in fear, it is likely that fear may disappear as soon as he introspects.

   This difficulty in introspection is really valid to some extent, but it can be removed with the help of memory. In the example of fear it is a fact that it disappears as soon as one attends to it, but the feelings, in the state of fear, can be recalled with the help of memory and analysis. By practice and sufficient training, even the changing mental processes can be grasped. Besides, various observers can coordinate their observations and thus arrive at some general conclusions. A psychologist may introspect his own experience in the state of fear and other psychologists may also do the same. Now these statements may be gathered together and compared leaving out the uncommon elements and generalizations can be made on the basis of common findings. Thus memory, mental alertness and the comparison of the data given by the different observers may help one in grasping the changing mental processes during introspection.

7. *Many psychologists cannot study the same mental state:* Another difficulty which has been pointed out against introspection is that many psychologists can study similar but not the same mental processes, e.g. in the case of the study of fear, every individual psychologist will study only his own personal experience of fear. How can anyone arrive at some general principles by the comparative study of the data supplied by different individual psychologists? Such a description will not be the study of fear as a general state, but a collection of the experiences of fear in different individuals.

   But a careful observation of this difficulty will make it clear that it is more logical than practical. From the logical standpoint, it is right to say that many persons cannot observe the same mental state, but generalization in science depends on the common element found in different phenomena of the same species. Uniformity of human psychology is a postulate on which the entire edifice of psychology as a science has been built up. It is a fact that no two men are the same and yet there are laws universally applicable to all human beings. It is for this reason that the results of the experiments performed on the Germans are equally applicable to Americans. Thus it is clear that the foregoing difficulty is not genuine.

8. *In introspection, the mind is divided:* Another argument against introspection is that in it the same man is the observer as well as observed and so the mind is divided into two parts, since mind cannot look to itself without such division. It is on the basis of this argument that Comte has rejected introspection as impossible. But practically this objection seems to be baseless. In practice we do experience the inner states of fear, curiosity and lust, etc. A man says that he feels fear; another says that he feels

pain. In both these states, these men are observing their mental processes. As a matter of fact, self-consciousness is a characteristic of the human mind. We are self-conscious and we know that we are self-conscious. This fact may not be proved by logic, but is amply demonstrated by experience. Direct experience is self-evident and it requires no logical proof for its validity. Just as we can observe things outside us, similarly, though not exactly, we can observe our internal experiences as well. This observation can be made more exact with practice and training.

9. *It is impossible to observe the object and the mental processes at the same time:* In introspection sometimes one has to observe a mental state which is the result of some external stimulus. As Stout points out, "If a man observes the object of perception he will have to attend the object of perception as well as the activity of perceiving it". In this situation the difficulty is that if one attends to the object, one cannot attend to the mental state and *vice versa*. Hence, introspection is impossible in such situations.

   This argument against introspection method is valid to some extent because mind can attend to only one thing at a time, but even this difficulty can be removed by certain measures. One way is the rapid oscillation of attention between the object and the mental state and this process should be so quick that both may be observed continually, if not simultaneously. Another way is to attend to the object with the aid of memory and to remember the mental state in such attention.

10. *The knowledge of introspection is subjective and personal:* Another argument against introspection is that knowledge gained by it is subjective and personal. Hence the introspective data cannot be the basis of scientific principles. This difficulty, however, can be removed, on the one hand, by training and practice and, on the other, by collaboration of different psychologists in a particular study. These efforts will remove the subjective and personal elements from psychological data.

    Thus, a critical analysis of the different difficulties pointed out against introspection makes it amply clear that it is a useful method in psychology and can be made still more useful. But this should not make one forget the limitations of this method. In many situations introspection method is entirely useless, e.g. in the study of the psychology of the children, insane and abnormal, patients and animals, the method of introspection cannot be used. It is clear that here other methods, particularly those of observation and experiment, are useful. Introspection is an indispensable method in psychology, but modern psychology uses it only sparingly since its results are not as exact and verifiable as those gained by other methods. The method of introspection has thus its own limits and is less factual than other. Introspection method, however, cannot be eliminated from the field of psychology. Not only from the historical point of view but from the practical point of view also, its value stands unquestioned in its own field.

Observation Method

Observation means collection of data by means of observing behavior by somebody other than that person. For instance, a nurse gives an observational report on a patient with undiagnosed illness, she reports her observations such as patients temperature, pulse, color, facial expression, restlessness, etc. This method is very useful in studying the behavior of children and animals.

Observation is one of the oldest techniques that man has made use of. Even today, it is our common experiences to notice farmers feel the breeze, watch the sky, sun, moon and stars—all to determine what the whether is likely to be and what season is approaching.

Observation has been defined as "measurement without instruments". In education, observation is the most commonly employed of all measurement techniques. In the present as well as in the past, students have been labeled as good, fair or poor in achievement and lazy or diligent in study, etc. on the basis of observation. Similarly teachers have listened to speeches and ranked students 1, 2, 3 and so on.

The uses of observation includes:

- Being a record of the actual behavior of the child, it is more reliable and objective.
- It is a study of an individual in a natural situation and is therefore more useful than the restricted study in a test situation.
- The method can be used with children of all ages; of course, the younger the child, the easier it is to observe him. This method has been found very useful with shy children.
- It can be used with a little training and almost all teachers can use it. It does not require any special tool or equipment.
- It can be used in every situation; physical activities, workshop, classroom situations as well.
- It is adaptable both to individuals and groups.

There are some limitations which are:

- There is a great scope for personal prejudices and bias of the observer.
- Records may not be written within hundred percent accuracy as the observation is recorded after the actions of the observed. There is some time lag.
- The observer may get only a sample of student behavior. It is very difficult to observe everything that a student does or says. As far as possible, observations should be made from several events.
- It reveals the overt behavior only—behavior that is expressed and not that is within.

Principles to be Followed in Making Observations

1. The whole situation should be observed
2. One student should be selected to observe at a time
3. Students should be observed in their regular activities, such as in classroom, on the playground or in passing from class to class
4. Observations should be made over a period of days.

Requisites of Good Observation

i. Proper planning
ii. Proper execution
iii. Proper recording
iv. Proper interpretation.

Recording the observation: Generally two methods are employed for recording observation. Which of the two methods to be used depends upon the nature of the activities or behavior of the group to be observed. The skill of observer also plays an important role in deciding upon the method.

The first method is to record is to the observation simultaneously. It is useful in the sense that a time-gap may distort facts. However, at times, this may not be feasible when the action or activity performed is very swift. Moreover this is likely to distract the subjects.

Facts may be recorded soon after the observation is over. This is helpful as this does not distract the mind of the subjects. But the investigator may not be recall facts accurately after the interval of a few minutes.

The devices used in observation are:

i. Checklists
ii. Rating scale
iii. Score cards
iv. Blank form for tallying frequencies.

Results should be interpreted cautiously and judiciously after taking into account various limitations of the procedure.

Observation can be done by naturalistic way or using laboratory as follows:

Naturalistic observation: Sometimes all researchers need to know is what that happening to a group of animals or people. The best way to look at the behavior of animals or people is to watch them behave in their normal environment. That's why animal researchers like Jance Goodall went to the areas where chimpanzees lived and watched them eat, play, mate and sleep in their own natural surroundings. With people, research might want to observe them in their workplaces, homes, or on playgrounds. For example, if someone wanted to know how adolescents behave with members of the opposite sex in a social setting, that researcher might go to the mall on a weekend night.

The advantage of naturalistic observation includes it allows researchers to get a realistic picture of how behavior occurs because they are actually watching that behavior. In a more artificial setting, like a laboratory, they might get behavior that is contrived or artificial rather than genuine. Of course, there are precautions that must be taken. In many cases, animals or people who know they are being watched will not behave normally anyway, in a process called the *observer effect*, so often the observer needs to remain hidden from view. When researching humans, this is often a difficult thing to do. In the mall setting with the teenagers, a researcher might find that pretending to read a book is a good disguise, especially if one wears glasses to hide the movement the teens without them knowing that they were being watched. In other cases, researchers might use one-way mirrors, or they might actually become participants in a group, a technique called *participant observation*.

One of the disadvantages of naturalistic observation is the possibility of *observer bias*. The happens when the person doing the observing has a particular opinion about what he or she is going to see or expects to see. If that is the case, sometimes that person sees only those actions that support that expectation and ignores actions that don't fit. A way around is and, therefore, have no preconceived notions about what they "should" see. It's also a good idea to have more than one observer, so that the various observations can be compared. Another disadvantages is that each naturalistic setting is unique and unlike any other. Observations that are made at one time in one setting may not hold true for another time, even if the setting is similar, because the conditions are not going to be exactly the same time after time—researchers don't have that kind of control over the natural world. For who set traps for the animals of the poachers affected the normal behavior of the gorillas she was trying to observe.

Laboratory observation: Sometimes observing behavior in animals or people is just not practical in a natural setting. For example, a researcher might want to observe the reactions of animals to a mirror image of themselves and record the reactions with a camera mounted behind the one-way mirror. That kind of equipment might be difficult to set up in a natural setting. In a laboratory observation, the researcher would bring the animal to the equipment, controlling the type of animal, the number of animals, and everythingelse that goes in the laboratory.

As mentioned previously, laboratory settings have the disadvantage of being an artificial situation that might result in artificial behavior—animals and people often react differently in the laboratory than they would in the real world. The main advantage of this method is the degree of control that it gives to the observer.

Both naturalistic and laboratory observations can lead to the formation to hypotheses that can later be tested.

Every society has some taboos regarding the sex behavior. These taboos influence the development of males and females in the particular society. What shall be the influence on human development if all these taboos were removed? This cannot be known by actually abolishing all the taboos since that will lead to disorganization of society. This phenomena can be examined only by observation of the development of persons in the societies where there are very few or almost all taboos on sex activities. Similarly, facts regarding the insane and mentally abnormal persons cannot be determined either by introspection or through experiment. In such cases the method of observation alone is useful.

STEPS IN OBSERVATION METHOD

The above mentioned examples regarding observation method exhibit some of its particular traits. Roughly speaking, various steps in the method of observation are as follows:

1. *Observation of behavior:* Observation literally means the examination or perception of some behavior or processes. In observation everything or phenomenon is directly perceived, e.g. the psychologist perceives the behavior of the animals. If someone has to study the social behavior of monkeys, he should go where the monkeys are assembled and observe their behavior.
2. *Noting of behavior:* Observation in psychology is a scientific method. Hence it is not sufficient to perceive a certain behavior and to remember it. The observation, on the other hand, should be carefully noted down. In the examples of the study of the social behavior of the monkeys, the observer should carefully note down their various activities.
3. *Interpretation and analysis of behavior:* When the behavior has been noted down, it can be analyzed at leisure and the effect underlying it certified. The movements of hands and legs, the sound, the gestures and other external activities, express the internal conditions of the person. In the case of animals their mental conditions are inferred from their external activities. The basis of this inference is not the experience of the psychologist himself but the behavior of other animals and his insight into animal psychology. Thus the behavior is interpreted on the basis of analysis and inference.
4. *Generalization:* Scientific principles are based upon generalizations. Psychology is a science, hence its principles are also of the same nature. In observation, as a method of psychology, the purpose is to find out general principle. In the examples of the social behavior of monkeys, various psychologists will observe their behavior, note down their observations, analyse them, interpret them and finally find out general principles through generalization.

The observation method has also some defects. The main defects are as follows:

1. *Influence of personal interest:* In the observation method the psychologist himself observes, hence it is more likely that his personal interest should also influence his observation.

In the example of the observation of the social behavior among the monkeys, if a psychologist has an excessive interest in sex behavior, he will mainly attend to their sex activities and conceive them as more general than they actually are. Along with the observation, the personal interest also influences his interpretation. An excessively sexual person often interprets nonsexual behavior of others as sexual. A wicked man finds some wicked purpose even behind the sympathetic actions of others. A religious man would interpret even the sexual behavior of others as pure and religious. Thus the behavior is often interpreted wrongly due to the personal interests and attitudes of the observers. In the study of child, insane and mentally abnormal persons, this difficulty is very much observed, because there is much difference in the mental activities of these persons and those of the psychologist.

The above mentioned difficulty in the observation method is undoubtedly real, but can be removed through scientific detachment. The mental conditions of others can be understood through constructive imagination. It is true the few have scientific detachment and constructive imagination, but these can be developed through long practice and training.

2. *The possibility of bias:* Due to the personal views and tendencies of the psychologists, there is a possibility of bias and prejudice in the interpretation of behavior, e.g. in the countries where prejudices based on color are largely prevalent, the white psychologists seldom find good or higher traits in the behavior of black subjects.

But in spite of the above mentioned limitations and difficulties in the method of observation, it is indispensable in psychology. As has already been pointed out in many cases other methods are entirely useless and only the observation method works. In fact it requires training and practice to observe correctly and accurately. The observer should first analyze his own tendencies and remove preconceptions, prejudices, attachments and aversions and develop scientific detachment. Many of the things will be left without observation in the beginning or will be wrongly observed, but practice will make observation more accurate. It is experience, and practice which make observation scientific. An expert psychologist can train the new corners in observation. Personal bias, prejudice and errors may be removed by comparison of the notes of several psychologists and through mutual discussion.

INTROSPECTION AND OBJECTIVE OBSERVATION

Psychology is the positive science of behavior. Behavior includes external activities as well as internal experiences and feelings. Psychology studies both these external and internal aspects of behavior. Hence it requires the methods of introspection as well as that of external observation. Internal behavior or internal experiences and feelings are known through the method of introspection. External behavior or activities are known through external observation.

Thus neither introspection nor observation can replace each other. In some cases the introspection method is entirely useless, e.g. a religious man cannot understand through his introspection what a man can do under the impulse of sex or hate. His imagination, based on his own experience, cannot take him far, because he cannot even imagine all things which are actually possible. Hence here he must take recourse to external observation. Similarly most of the phenomena in child psychology, animal psychology and abnormal psychology are known only through external observation, since neither the child, animal or abnormal person can introspect, nor the psychologist can know their experiences through his own introspection.

Similarly, the method of external observation is useless in many cases, e.g. the differences between the feelings in fear, love, affection and jealousy, etc. cannot be known through external observation. It is only the introspective method which will work here. Thus it is clear that both the methods of external observation and that of introspection are equally necessary in psychology.

These statements makes it clear that "introspection and objective observation supplement each other". Where one method fails another method works and because every behavior has an internal and external aspect, its study requires both these methods, except in the cases in which either of these methods is entirely useless. Again both these methods mutually examine each other, e.g. if the experience of the majority of normal persons regarding a certain object is of a particular type, we can examine the validity of our own introspective experience by it. If it differs from the experience of almost of all persons, it should be classed as abnormal, if not wrong. Similarly, if someone is sure about his own introspective experience, he examines the experience of others on its basis and declares them as normal or abnormal, true or untrue. For example, a man who has experienced divide bliss or most intimate love, can judge the validity of attachment and concerned emotions in others. Thus, in brief, the methods of introspection and observation are mutually complementary.

Interview Method

An interview is a face-to-face relationship in which the interviewer and the child carry on some conversation with some purpose. During the interview (in school setting), the teacher or the school counselor tries to know the attitudes, interests and the motives of the child. The interview can be arranged or organized with an individual child or a group of children. The interview can supply information about the child which cannot be obtained from other approaches like experimentation and observation. Certain points may become more clear after interview. While conducting an interview—

Who is to interview: The interviewer or the teacher must be clear in his mind of his strengths and weaknesses.

Whom: He should understand the child thoroughly.

How: He should know the techniques of interviewing.

Why: He should be very clear in his mind of the purpose of interview.

Where: Suitable place should be selected for this purpose. It should be free from noise.

When: Proper motivation and the child should be developed.

What to ask: He should prepare his questions thoughtfully.

TECHNIQUES OF INTERVIEWING

- Rapport should be established. Rapport is a technical term used to denote the feelings of friendliness, security and mutual confidence between the investigator and the subject.
- The nurse should try to ease the patients fear by encouraging him that information will be kept confidential.

- The nurse attempts to ease tension in the mind of the patient with humorous remarks.
- All evidence of fatigue, pressure, irritation and anxiety should be avoided.
- On the whole, the interview should be confined to issues at hand. There might be a temporary shift in the discussion.
- The nurse may stop occasionally for giving patient time for recapitulation.
- Nothing should be done to undermine the self-respect of the patient.
- Moralizing should be avoided.
- The nurse should very carefully observe the physical reactions, bodily tensions, blushing, excitability and dejections, etc. of the client.
- The clients number of thought-provoking questions should be asked in a simple language and with a sweet tone and a pleasing voice.
- The interview should be terminated tactfully when it is felt that more time is needed for constructive help. The ending should be planned, not sudden; clear-cut and not indefinite.
- Salient points of the interview should be immediately recorded.

Limitations of the Interview includes the following

1. This method is subjective
2. The child may not unfold situation
3. The child is placed in an artificial situation
4. Sometimes it becomes difficult to interpret the results of an interview.

Experimental Method

The experimental method is generally regarded as the most sophisticated research method for testing hypotheses.

In the words of WS Manro and MD Engelhast, "Experimentation is the name given to the type of educational research in which the investigator controls the educative factors to which a group of children is subjected during the period of inquiry and observes the resulting achievement".

JW Best describes it as, "Experimental research is the description and analysis of what will be, or what occur, under carefully controlled conditions". Thus the keywords in an experimental research are:

1. What will be
2. What will occur
3. Carefully controlled conditions.

This method, made popular by Wundt, the psychologist studies the effects of a dependent variables on changes in independent variable (s). Many experiments are being conducted on people and animals dealing with learning, forgetting and many other mental activities. The tremendous progress of psychology during the 20th century is mainly due to this method.

Advantages of Experimentation

Among the main uses of experimentation in education are:

1. Determining and evaluating the adequacy and effectiveness of educational aims and objectives through the measurement of outcomes.

2. Serving as basis for the formulation, execution and modification of educational policies and programs.
3. Ascertaining the effect of any change in the normal educational programs and practices.

Experimentation in education is not a perfectly precise method. There are many variables in education which are extremely difficult or even impossible to control. The basic condition of other things being equal is difficult for fulfillment in educational research. There are many areas in which experimental studies in education can approximate strictly empirical research. For example, the teaching of spelling through different methods, difference between the effect of the authoritarian and the democratic set-up in education are problems which have been handled in a scientific way through the experimental approach.

For experimentation purposes, the teacher may divided the class into two groups. Students in each group should consist of more or less equal abilities and similar socio-economic background. One group will be the experimental group, while the other group will be called the control group. In order to find out the effect of the student learning on account of the new method to be used, the teacher has to determine the knowledge of the students prior to experimentation. This is called a 'pre-test'.

Psychology is the positive science of behavior. Science is distinguished from philosophy on the basis of methodological differences. Science is the study of any object by scientific method. Hence, if psychology is to be called a science, it should use scientific methods, e.g. introspection, case history and observation, etc. But experimental method is the most important in the study of psychology. It is the method which has the credit of bringing psychology to the level of an exact science. Hence modern psychology places the greatest emphasis on experimental method.

Experiment is a question asked systematically: Thus in experiment, the experimenter has a problem before him. He experiments to find out the answer to this problem. The clarity of the answer depends upon the clarity of the question. The question is based on hypothesis. This hypothesis is proved or disproved by the experiment, e.g. suppose that while studying or teaching someone thinks that motivation has its role in study. This is merely a hypothesis. To examine it, it is placed in the form of a question; 'Does motivation affect study?' To get an answer to this question, it requires psychological experiments. Suppose by experiments one arrives at the result that motivation is useful in study; this proves the hypothesis. Now another question might be raised as to how far motivation helps in study. This question will lead to further experiments in this line. In this way various types of enquires can be made through the method of experimentation, e.g. experiment regarding the effect of motivation on study. Similarly, the effect of intelligence and practice in learning, etc. may be put in the form of questions and experiments can be performed to get answers to them. In the experimental method, the observation is held in certain predetermined conditions. *The experiment is a controlled observation.* It is the observation of the behavior or activity in fixed circumstances. A characteristic of this observation is that it can be repeated in different places and times without difference in results.

Disadvantages of Experimentation

Like other methods, experimental method also has its own disadvantages. The following are the most important disadvantages of experimental method:

1. *Artificial situations of laboratory*—Artificial situation of laboratory is the characteristic of experimental method as well as its limitation. In the experimental method the experimenter leaves some variables independent, but controls other variables. But it is

very difficult to ascertain all the variables working in a particular situation, e.g. in the attainment of scholarship, the hours of work, the hours of extracurricular activity, anxiety for future, interest in social work, motivation for social work, hours of study, etc. were controlled and the time given for students' study was increased and decreased. The result achieved by the increase and decrease of the hours of study shows its effect on scholarship. As a matter of fact, it is very difficult to ascertain all the factors affecting the attainment of scholarship in a man and the result is that the effect of some of the factors might be ascribed to some others.

2. *Difficulty in the control of the attitude of the subject:* Another limitation in the experimental method is the difficulty in the control of the attitude of the subject. In experiments upon human beings it is often very necessary to control their attitudes, since if the subject is opposed to the experiment or careless towards it, he might give wrong answer to keep silent. But it is not always easy to control the attitudes of the subjects specially when they are children or students. This makes the result of the experiment unreliable.
3. *Difficulty of securing the cooperation of the subject:* Experimental method is impossible without the cooperation of the subject but the cooperation is not always easily forthcoming. It is possible that the subject may show himself fatigued or not-fatigued according to his attitude or give false replies. This difficulty makes the experimental method unreliable.
4. *Limited field:* The last but not the least important limitation of the experimental method is the limitation of its field. In several matters it cannot be applied at all, e.g. if one has to know the effect of bad environment on child's development, it is not possible to place some children in bad environment and wait for the results. Again in the case of the mental states, like love, etc. it is neither possible to control them nor to create them in the laboratory. These and many other phenomena can be studied only through observation or introspection, etc.

In spite of the above limitations of the experimental method, it is undoubtedly the most important and valuable method in psychology. It is by this method that the psychologist arrives at the most exact conclusions about behavior. On the other hand, some aspects of human behavior are so changeable and complex that one should be satisfied with their observation and arrive at some workable conclusions. The field of experimental method, however, is gradually being widened with the advent of new invention regarding tools and instruments. If observation and introspection methods have widened the field of psychology and made it come useful in daily life, it is the experimental method which has secured a respectable place for it among the sciences. In the word outside the limits of laboratory, man will always learn by experience and observation, but it is on the experimental method alone that the future of psychology as a science depends.

STEPS IN EXPERIMENT

The following are the steps in a typical experiment:

1. *Raising a problem*—The first step in an experiment is the raising of the problem, e.g. it is said that smoking is harmful to students. On the other hand, some say that it helps in concentration. Those who are neither for nor against smoking, may say that it is not smoking, but the personality of the student which is relevant to his achievements in examinations. This discussion creates a problem about the effect of smoking on physical or mental capacity. This problem may lead to further experiments.

2. *Formulation of a hypothesis:* In the example of smoking, the problem of its effect on physical and mental capacity can be put in the form of a hypothesis. This hypothesis will be like this "Smoking is harmful for physical and mental capacity". Now this hypothesis will be tested by experiments.
3. *To distinguish independent variables and dependent variables:* In the example of smoking, the physical and mental capacity will be the dependent variables, since these will be fixed in experiment. Smoking will be an independent variable since the aim of the experiment is to find out the effect of its presence and absence.
4. *Controlling the environment or situations:* There are several difficulties in the above mentioned experiment on smoking. It is just possible that the subject may try to prove that smoking has no effect on physical or mental capacities. But to neutralize these possibilities, the experimental situation is controlled. In the experiment on smoking, the eyes of the subject were bandaged. Two exactly similar holders were used. One of these holders had an electric wire through which the subject might inhale the warm air, while the other holder had a common cigarette. In all the sessions of the experiment, all types of sound produced by smoking were made, e.g. the rubbing of the match, etc. At the end of the experiment there were matchsticks and ashes lying around, so that the subject might think that he really smoked. The subject could not touch the cigarette at any time. The experimenter himself put and took away the holder from his mouth. In the sessions, when cigarette was not given to the subject, the experimenter himself smoked. To stop the signs received by the smoking and notsmoking were kept irregular. These special arrangements in the case of experiment on smoking are not necessary in all types of experiments. The arrangements of control differ according to the nature of experiment. In the case of man some special types of controls are necessary so that subject may not know the principles of the experiment, since it is feared that this might make difference in his mental attitude. But in the case of experiments on animals that difficulty is not there. There are different types of controls in the experiments on animals, e.g. Pavlov, in his experiment on conditioned reflex in the dog, made special arrangement for the flow of saliva and to gather it outside the dog's mouth.
5. *Analysis of the result:* Generally, the subjects of the experiment are divided into two groups one controlled and another experimental. In the experiment on smoking every subject was also his controlled subject. All smoked half the time and in the remaining half they inhaled warm air. The experimental group is often called independent variable, since the experimenter can stop it or modify it. In the experiment on smoking, cigarette is an independent variable and the result of its presence have been compared with the results of its absence. For the analysis of the results of the experiment, statistical technique is used.
6. *Verification of the hypothesis by the result of the experiment:* The result of the experiment exhibits whether the hypothesis was right or wrong. In the experiment on smoking, it was found by the comparison of the sessions of smoking and nonsmoking that there was very little difference in the results. Smoking increased heartbeat and the trembling of the hand. This effect was observed more in nonsmokers that the smokers subjects. No influence was observed on mental capacities known by mental tests. After 18 days of smoking it was concluded that it had very insignificant effect. This result disproved the hypothesis.

ROLE OF CONTROL IN EXPERIMENTAL METHOD

In an experiment, the subject is studied in controlled situations. The experimenter divides different factors in the experiment into dependent and independent variables and controls the former to watch the influence of the latter. Without such a control, the result of the experiment can never be dependable, e.g. in the experiment to determine the effect of smoking on study, the constancy of the stage of the subjects, their intelligence, work at school, etc. are necessary because all these factors influence the study. If these do not remain the same or constant, the difference by the influence of either of them may be misinterpreted at the difference due to smoking or nonsmoking. In ordinary life the importance of such a controlled observation is not so much emphasized. Hence most of the conclusions are far from being accurate. They are, at the most, merely workable inferences. By seeing some smokers in good health. Similarly, when a patient is cured, no effort is made to ascertain whether he has been cured by the medicine or owing to cold after the third day, but some people do not give the credit of are influenced in great measure by certain factors, e.g. the age, intelligence, motive, intention, education and the physical and the result of the experiments. Hence no definite conclusions can be drawn without controlling all these factors.

Thus every experiment has certain conditioning factors. In them, the general condition of the subject is very important. In the psychological experiment the attitude must be controlled. For example, if an experiment is being conducted with regard to learning, it is necessary that the subject should not be averse to learning since that will lead to the failure of the experiment. In such experiment the subjects are told that they should attend to such and such stimuli and leave such and such. Sometimes the subject is kept in illusion. He is told that a certain thing is being examined, while actually it is somethingelse which is under examination, e.g. in order to determine the influence of a certain medicine, sometimes the water and sometimes the medicine is injected. In experiments on animals, the attitude of the subject is injected. In experiments on animals, the attitude of the subject need not be controlled. But in experiments on human being, especially adults, it is necessary to control the attitudes of the subjects.

Side by side with the internal attitude, the external stimuli should also be controlled. Stimuli include all those internal and external factors which have some effect on the subject to be studied, e.g. light, sound, touch, temperature, smell, etc. are external stimuli and nervous excitements are the internal stimuli. Both these types of stimuli affect the subject. Hence they are controlled. The external stimuli are controlled with the help of various types of rooms and apparatuses. The internal stimuli are controlled by administering certain medicines or particular type of flood or by keeping the subject hungry, etc.

In certain experiments, the heredity should also be controlled, e.g. if the psychologist has to determine the effect of training and maturity on the development of the child, he should take two types of subjects, i.e. trained and untrained. Along with this both these subjects should also be the same. Similarity of heredity is found only in identical twins. Hence in such experiments the psychologist should take identical twins. Now one of these should be trained the other untrained. The comparison of the development of both these will exhibit the influence of training on development. Thus in the experiment upon human beings, many factors are to be controlled. In the experiment upon animals, sometimes some external or internal organ has to be removed through operation, e.g. in order to determine the influence of certain endocrine gland the behavior of the animal is noted, the endocrine gland is removed and the behavior is again noted. Now a comparison of the behavior with and without the particular endocrine gland will show the influence of that gland on behavior.

As has already been pointed out, the different factors in an experiment are divided into independent and dependent variables. Independent variables are stimuli or particular states of the subject which can be changed as desired. Often the independent variable is one because the experimenter has to see the effect of every factor separately. But if the effect is due to two factors, which are not separated from each other, it will be difficult to determine how much influence is exercised by each of them. In the statistical method, there can be more than one independent variable because statistical analysis separates the influence of each factor.

Dependent variable, as is clear from its name, depends on the independent variable. The experimenter keeps all the factors of experiment constant and changes some one factor. This change results in a certain effect in the subject. These factors are the dependent variables. These include the external behavior of the subject, e.g. speaking, hearing, laughing, weeping, etc. as well as internal processes. The internal processes are determined with the help of certain instruments.

The analysis of various factors of control in an experiment, as given above, clearly shows that the method of experiment very much depends on the control of the various factors in the particular experiment.

The analysis of various factors of control in an experiment, as given above, clearly shows that the method of experiment very much depends on the control of the various factors in the particular experiment.

Psychology is a study of behavior. Behavior has both external and internal aspects. Of these the external aspect can be observed, but the internal aspect can be explored only through the method of introspection. Some internal processes, e.g. blood pressure, heart-beat, etc. can be measured by certain instruments. But an instrument to measure the feeling has neither been invented nor can one hope of the invention. Hence experimental method cannot afford to ignore introspective data. To take an example, in the experiment of size-weight illusion, the subject raises different tins one by one. He begins with the tin which seems to be lighter than the standard tin. Thus he goes on raising the tins one by one till he declares a tin as having double the weight of the standard tin. This examination is carried on in the ascending and descending order. The experimenter depends upon the introspective data given by the subject. The subject does not actually weigh a tin to tell its weight, but tells it only on the basis of his own experience through introspection. Obviously, this introspective data cannot be ignored.

STATISTICAL CONTROL AND ANALYSIS

Sometimes it is not possible or even desirable to rule out the differential effects of all relevant variables by means of experimental control. In such instances psychologists are often able to simulate controlled conditions by mathematical methods. This is called *statistical control.*

Suppose, for example, that an experimenter is studying the effects of age on golfing ability. In designing his experiment, he would want to study players who were in different age groups but as nearly alike as possible in such other respects as golfing experience, the kind of coaching received, the type and difficulty of the courses played on, and desire to play golf. Obviously, with so many variables involved, it would be extremely difficult to obtain groups perfectly matched in all respects. The experimenter might, for example, obtain groups which were equated on all variables except amount of previous experience.

If this variable were left uncontrolled, the results of the experiments would be ambiguous. By using appropriate statistical formulas, however, the experimenter could determine the degree of relationship between playing experience and playing ability and then cancel out the effect of this uncontrolled variable on his results. In effect, a freely operating variable can thus be held "constant" mathematically.

Statistical analysis is used by psychologists in identifying the component abilities involved in complex tasks and skills. Consider, for instance, the separate abilities required to solve a simple story problem in arithmetic, such as "Mahesh has 4 apples and gives half of them to his sister. Gaanashrii is Mahesh's only sister. How many apples does Mary get?" Although this problem seems extremely simple to you, the statistical technique of factor analysis has shown that your ability to solve it involves such distinct factors as reasoning and numerical ability. Factor analysts identify these abilities by constructing and administering test and analyzing the relationships among the scores. Tests having no consistent relationship to one another are presumed to be measuring different abilities.

The Guidelines for Experiments in Human Subjects

Universities and colleges (where most psychological research is carried out) usually have ethics committees, groups of psychologists or other professionals who look over each proposed research study and judge it according to its safety and consideration for the participants in the study. These committees look at all aspects of the proposed research, from the written materials that explain the research to the potential subjects to the equipment that may be used in the study itself.

There are quite a few ethical concerns when dealing with human subjects in an experiment or other type of study. Here is a list of the most common ethical guidelines:

1. *Rights and well-being of participants must be weighed against the study's value to science.* In other words, people come first, research second.
2. *Participants must be allowed to make an informed decision about participation.* This means that researchers have to explain the study to the people they want to include before they do anything to them or with them—even children—and it has to be in terms that the participants can understand. If researchers are using infants, their parents have to be informed and give their consent. This is known as *informed consent.*
3. *Deception must be justified.* In some cases, it is necessary to deceive the participants. If that happens, it has to be because the study wouldn't work any other way, and the participants have to be told after the study exactly why the deception was important. This is called *debriefing. Debriefing* participants helps them understand why they were deceived and the importance of their responses to that deception.
4. *Participants may withdraw from the study at any time.* The participants must be allowed to drop out for any reason. Sometimes people get bored with the study, decide they don't have the time, or don't like what they have to do, for example. Children are particularly likely to decide not to play. Researchers have to let them go, even if it means getting more participants.
5. *Participants must be protected from risks or told explicitly of risks.* For example, if researchers are using any kind of electrical equipment, care must be taken to ensure that no participant will experience a physical shock from faulty electrical equipment.
6. *Investigator must debrief participants, telling the true nature of the study and expectation of results.* This is important in all types of studies but particularly in those involving a deception.

7. *Data must remain confidential.* Freud recognized the importance of confidentiality, referring to his patients in his books and articles with false names. This is also why psychologists and other researchers today tend to report only group results rather than results for a single individual, so that no one could possibly be recognized.

Survey Method

A survey is designed to obtain information from populations regarding prevalence, distribution and interrelations of variables within these populations. Survey is done by means of self-report, personal interviews and telephonic interviews by using questionnaire, checklists, rating scales, ranking and inventories. It assesses different aspects of behaviors, emotional experiences, aptitudes, knowledge, opinions, attitudes and values.

When it is not feasible or desirable to spend a long period of time in the field or to obtain data about all the individuals in a group, much valuable information may be obtained by conducting a *survey*. In this method the investigator, by using written questionnaires or oral interviews, obtains data from a selected group. It is important that he choose his group carefully so that it will constitute a *representative sample* of the larger group, or *universe,* in which he is interested. A representative sample is one drawn in such a way that every person in the universe from which it is drawn has an equal change of being selected. If the sample is not representative, the data collected will be of little value.

One of the best-known types of survey is the *opinion poll.* Political opinion polls are perhaps the most widely used kind, particularly in election years, but the opinion poll has many other uses. It is being used increasingly in industry as a means of determining consumer preferences and of improving employee management relations.

Advantages

- Flexibility
- Can be applied to many populations
- Broadness of scope
- Can focus on wide range of topics/can be used for many topics
- Better suited to extensive rather than intensive analysis.

Disadvantages

- Tends to be relatively superficial
- Rarely probe deeply into such complexities or contradictions of human behavior and feelings.

Test Method: Abilities, interest, attitudes and intelligence are measured by this method by making use of carefully devised and standardized tests. It can be administered to a large number of personnel at the same time saving a lot of time, energy and dislocation of routine work.

Case History Method

Case history/clinical method: It is a research method that involves a thorough, in-depth analysis of an individual, group, institution or other social units. It uses case histories, interviews, home visits and psychological tests. It aims at studying the causes and basis of people anxieties, fears and personal maladjustments. It is scientific biography consisting of collecting all the information about the individuals' past. This can be done by interviewing the individual himself and/or his family members, friends, classmates, teachers and others who knew him and who can provide information about his past. Documents like cumulative records, personal diaries and articles directly or indirectly can be used.

It is a mode of investigation into the casual relationship of complex educational phenomena. It is an intensive investigation of a unit—of a child, an individual, a community, a race, a nation, a family a club or a teenage gang.

The purpose of a case study is to understand the child/individual/unit/subject in-depth. Most case studies emerge out of a desire to assist to adjust. The datas are obtained with regard to the child's present status, his past experiences, his environment and the related factors so as to understand his behavior thoroughly.

Steps in case study includes the follows:

1. Determination of the status of the problem under investigation through direct observation or measurement.
2. Determination of he most probable antecedents of the case.
3. Formulation of a definite hypothesis or a set of hypotheses through a knowledge of similar cases.
4. Verification of the hypothesis.
5. Remedial steps for removing the causes for maladjustment.
6. Follow-up of the case.

Characteristics of a good case study include:

1. Data should be complete
2. Data should be valid
3. Recording should be kept confidential
4. Synthesis of data should be scientific.

In making a case study of a child, information has to be collected about his home background, attendance, participation in various activities, his assets and short-comings, his health and social relation, etc. Information should be collected from as many sources as possible. A large number of tools are used to collect information. These include school records, interviews with the child, his parents and others.

Psychology today is widely used for the cure of various types of abnormalities. The parents as well as the teachers seek guidance from the psychologist in their dealings with the children and students. They complain of the abnormality of the child and student, to the psychologist who with their help finds out the causes and tries to remove them. Thus today one finds a flourishing branch of psychology in the form of abnormal psychology. In the more developed Western countries, the frequency of nervous diseases is gradually growing as the rush of life is increasing with industrialization and urbanization. This has increased the importance of abnormal psychology. Abnormal psychology and psychiatry use a certain method known as case history in their study of abnormal cases. As is clear by the name of the method, in it the psychologist traces the whole history of the cases. This tracing of the history requires not only the statement of his story by the patient, but also whatever can be gathered from his relatives. The psychologist interviews all the new relatives of the patient and also his friends. By this interview much is known about the habits, routine, thinking, nature, etc. views also make the psychologist know the various types of relation asked to relate his life history. He is also asked to relate his dreams, etc.

and they are interpreted by the psychologist as they reveal the infantile life of the patient. All the data gathered through the patient as well as those related to him in some way, give an outline of the history of the case. By the analysis of this history the psychologist taken to whose behavior is not normal, or who are bad-tempered. He does not bother about punishment or dictates of the elders. The psychologist interviews the parents and other the child with him into a room and sympathetically tries to know various things about his life. He enquires about his conditions in school and about his friends. In short, he enquires about everything all the data gives him an idea of the causes of abnormality, truancy teachers are guided accordingly and the malady is removed.

Like other methods in psychology, case history method has also its own difficulties and limitations. One of the limitations is that it is very difficult to know the whole history of any patient and to observe it objectively. It is possible that while relatives are interviewed they may be prejudiced in their answers or try to hide some unpleasant thing. In the case of children it is difficult to know their history through them, because their memory is neither strong nor reliable and the psychologist has to depend upon the lose sight of something which is very important for the case. These and other limitations make it difficult for the clinical psychologist to arrive at a proper diagnosis. In the case of adults, abnormal, etc. however, the psychologist gets the data of their dream, analyses them and finds out some unconscious causes. He may also ask the patient to explain things about his childhood and tell the psychologist his story. The psychologist may question him from time to time and can get much out of his statements. Thus in the case of the child. This, however, does not mean absence of ultimate analysis the case history method has proved to be very valuable for the diagnosis of mental abnormalities. As a matter of fact it all depends upon the experiences and ability of the psychologist as to how far he is able to gather a history and analyse it to find the real causes. A psychologist like Sigmund Freud can very well make use of a case history to discover the causes of the most complex type of abnormality.

Developmental Method

Psychologist not only studies human behavior at a particular time, but also its development from birth to death. Thus it traces the mental and behavioral development of the individual from the cradle to the grave. In such a study the psychologist has to face many difficult problems which have much importance, e.g. the influence of heredity and environment in the development of the person, the conditions favorable and unfavorable to normal can be satisfactory decided only when the psychologist observes human development in perfectly controlled conditions. It the psychologist observes the development of child in controlled situations, he can be sure about the influence of different factors in it. This, however, is very difficult to put into practice, e.g. in order to know the influence of the unfavorable conditions on the development of the child the psychologist cannot put him unfavorable condition since that will be contrary to the ethical principles. Thus the psychologist will take the help of the observation of the development of the child in backward communities and of the child placed in unfavorable circumstances, e.g. orphans, etc. such an observation, obliviously, will not give them decisive knowledge as in the case of the experimental method and yet much valuable information will be collected.

Another difficulty in the developmental method is caused by the complexity and variety in development. As Prof. Woodworth aptly puts it, "the child behaves so much that an observer cannot record more than small samples." Again, mere observation of the child's development will not help the psychologist in arriving at any definite conclusions. To get at some definite questions and definite hypothesis in his mind. The more he is clear about his question, the he shall be clear in getting its answer.

Thus it is clear that the developmental method is less accurate that the experimental method and has more limitations and difficulties, but efforts are being made to make it more and more useful. The development of animals and valuable information has been gathered by comparing the development of the animals with that of the human beings. The chief value of this method is that it helps in keeping a firm eye on the dynamic aspect of behavior which is often missed in other methods. Human personality is a complex whole which goes on developing from birth through maturity till death. A dynamic approach to psychology requires that a particular human behavior should be studied separately as well as in the light of the entire process.

It studies the growth and changes in behavior in terms of its development from birth, death, influence of heredity and environment in the development of the person and conditions favorable and unfavorable for normal development and abnormality.

Life history methods of psychological research involve making intensive studies of individuals over a considerable period of time, usually in the attempt to trace the development of a particular form of behavior being investigated. In other words, the psychologist studies the conditions in peoples lives which have led to their becoming whatever they are, be they criminals, physicians, spinsters, or political agitators. By studying the antecedents of a specific form of behavior, he hopes to find its causes. The three basic life-history methods are the *daybook method*, the *clinical method*, and the *biographical method.*

- The *daybook method* is most often used in child study. The child's development is carefully observed and recorded day by day. A daybook record might contain descriptions of when a baby first sits, stands, walks and begins to talk. Accumulated records of this kind give us standards by which we are able to judge the normality of the development of individual children.
- The *clinical method* represents an elaboration and extension of the daybook method. Here the past life history and present life situation of a person are explored on the basis of any information available, usually in an effort to discover the cause of—and solution to—some emotional or social adjustment problem. The most effective clinical study usually requires at least three professional functions. A physician examines the individual for signs of physical illness; a social worker examines the home conditions which surround and have surrounded the patient; and a psychometrician administers and scores various tests of aptitude and personality. When a full record has been obtained of the important past and present influences in the patients' life, this information is put together and discussed at a staff meeting and recommendations are made. In some cases extensive therapy is undertaken, in other special training of some kind or a change in the home situation may be called for. A good psychological clinical provides for a follow-up to see whether its recommendations have been carried out and whether progress has been made.

  The clinical method has two important functions. First, it *compiles information* concerning the emotional and personality adjustments of human beings and is thus an additional means of observing and interpreting facts. Second, this method involves attempts to *modify behavior* in the interest of greater personal and social welfare.
- The *biographical method* is simply an attempt to obtain psychological understanding from an analysis of the records of men's lives as set down by themselves or others. An example

of the use of the literary biography for psychological research is found in a study by the famous psychologist and educator Edward L Thorndike, who made personality analyses of ninety-one famous men on the basis of information contained in their biographies (Thorndike, 1950). Using evidence drawn from the writings, speeches, and actions of these men, Thorndike undertook to rate each man in terms of forty-eight different personal characteristics, such as intelligence, sensitiveness, sociability, agreeableness, liking for beauty, liking for exercise, and so on.

The results of such biographical studies can be useful in giving insight into the characteristics which underlie the achievement of greatness in various professional fields. There are certain important limitations, however, to the scientific value of this method. In the first place, the biographer's motivation is always a matter of question. The writer may strive for a true record, but if his interest is great enough to motivate him to write, he is likely to be biased either for or against his subject. In the second place, biographical accounts are not always sufficiently complete or accurate, for most biographers are not psychologists and may over look seemingly insignificant incidents which actually were important in determining the course of the person's actions and achievements. Lewis M Terman, a psychologists who devoted much of his life to a study of mental development, complained of "the utter inability of a majority of otherwise competent biographical writers to appraise and interpret the facts which they themselves have recorded with reference to the early mental development of their subjects".

Field-Study Method

The field study method is the oldest research technique used in any science. It is not a substitute for the experimental method but is often applicable where experimentation is impossible. The field study method might be described as making direct observations of nature. The investigator simply goes into the field with a definite question (or set of questions) and makes observations, without trying to hold constant or even to know all the conditions under which his subjects are operating. Often the observer does not even need the direct cooperation of his subjects—in fact, some field studies are most successful when the subjects are not aware of being observed. In other instance the investigator finds it helpful to join in the day to day life of his subjects of their ways of living.

CHAPTER 4

Body-Mind Relationship

Mind is the faculty of consciousness and thought. It is the person's ability think and reasons the intellect and memory. Individual identified with their intellectual faculties. So mind is the faculty by which one is aware of surroundings and by which one is able to experience emotions, remember, reasons and make decisions. Mind is an abstract component which arises out of the CNS and develops along with other developments in the human body. It has two components namely physiological and psychological. So it involves organs, faculties and qualities of various sorts. The brain is the organ, intelligence is the faculty and consciousness is the quality. Behavior is the way in which someone behaves (act or conduct oneself in a specified way). Behavior means all the convert and overt activities of human beings that can be observed. It may be cognitive (knowing), affective (feelings), and psychomotor (doing). There is an interaction of mind and body in behavior which effects of the body on mind, i.e. physically identifiable events on psychological functioning on behavior for example taking stimulants (caffeine, nicotine) increases CNS activity particularly by enhancing dopamine activity, and increases alertness, suppress appetite, etc. similarly effects of mind on body can influence physical functioning and behavior. For example effects of stress, the body may respond to stress by producing excessive stress hormones (catechol amines and corticosteroids) leads to increased heart rate, increased blood pressure, increased oxygen intake, increased mental activity, increased skeletal blood flow, decreasing splanchnic blood flow, etc. and increasing cortisol-increasing gluconeogenesis, increases proteins and fat metabolism, increased aldosterone—sodium and water reabsorption, decreased urine output, and increased thyrodine—increasing metabolic rate.

Every individuals development into a unique personality is determined by a very complex process of interaction between his heredity and his environment through time, each level of development depending partially on the levels previously reached. The process by which heredity continues to function after birth is called maturation. Environment influences development by supplying stimuli which elicit patterns of response already prepared by maturation and by presenting situations that require the learning of new responses or the changing of old ones. An instinctive behavior pattern which is inborn, appears full-blown upon the first occasion that an adequate stimulus is presented, without previous opportunity for learning. Although such behavior is sometimes found in the lower animals, it is very rare in man. His behavior patterns fall on a continuum between pure instinct and pure learning, depending upon the degree to which learning has interacted with maturation in their development.

At the time of conception, the characteristics of both parents, and of many preceding generations, are passed on to the new individual through the union of the father's sperm cell and the mother's ovum. The zygote, or fertilized egg, from which the child develops receives exactly the same number of chromosomes (twenty-three) from each parent. The many thousands of genes within the chromosomes are the real determiners of heredity, being responsible, alone or in combination, for every hereditary characteristic. The way in which the genes function is becoming better understood as the complex DNA molecules of which they are a part are being studied. When unlike genes are paired, the dominant one determines what characteristics will appear in the offspring, recessive genes take effect only when both in a pair are identical. Sex is determined by whether a female—producing X chromosome or a male producing Y chromosome from the father is joined with the X chromosome provided by the mother. No two individuals except monozygotic (identical) twins have the same heredity. Fraternal, or dizygotic, twins are no more closely related than ordinary siblings.

Under the guidance of heredity, the organism living in a normal environment undergoes a process of growth involving the nervous system, the muscles, and the endocrine glands. The child improves in ability to make adequate adjustments through two important changes in his nervous system: (1) an increase in the size of his brain and (2) an increase in the complexity of the neural patterns connecting receptors and effectors. Structural connections established by maturation may become functional through learning.

Although the infant has his total number of muscle cells at birth, they grow in size and strength through both maturation and exercise. The period of most rapid muscular growth is during adolescence.

The endocrine glands most closely involved in development are the pituitary, the thyroids, the adrenals, and the glands. Improper functioning of the pituitary, which is the most important glands in influencing development, may lead to dwarfism, gigantism, or acromegaly, the latter being an overgrowth of portions of the skeleton caused by over secretion of the pituitary growth hormone in adult life. Thyroid deficiency results in cretinism, a peculiar type of dwarfism usually accompanied by subnormal intelligence. The adrenal glands produce adrenal androgens which regulate the development of adult sexual characteristics, particularly those associated with masculinity. Over activity of the adrenal cortex produces virilism, excessive masculinity. The gonads also produces secondary sex characteristics even before beginning to produce sperms or eggs at puberty. The gonads of the male produce testicular androgens; those of the female produce estrogens, which promote growth of the reproductive organs, and progesterone, which prepares the uterine tissues for supporting fetal life. Menarche, the stage when menstruation first appears, occurs between the ages of twelve and fourteen.

Although the rate and pattern of maturation differ significantly from child to child, the maturation process always follows an orderly sequence, proceeding along the physiological gradient from head to limbs. According to the principle of motor primacy, the neuromuscular structures must reach a certain stage of maturation before they can respond to stimulation. Maturation is characterized by a pattern—of development from whole to part, from general to specific.

The forty-week prenatal period includes a two-week germinal period followed by a six-week embryonic period, the remainder of the time being called the fetal period. During this time the organism receives nourishment through the umbilical cord from the mother's placenta. The fetus makes spontaneous movements and can also respond to external stimuli.

There is some evidence that it can learn. It may develop abnormally as a result of such conditions as emotional disturbances in the mother, improper medication, excessive smoking by the mother, or radiation.

The newborn infant or neonate is differently proportioned from an adult. His senses of taste, smell, and touch, including sensitivity to temperature, are well-developed as compared to those of hearing and vision. He makes general responses involving large portions of the body as well as specific, automatic responses known as reflexes. From birth he is a social creature, and his relationship with his mother has a great deal to do with his later personality.

Restricted environment in infancy, such as that experienced in institutions, often causes serious handicaps in later social adjustment and may also affect intelligence. Sensory restriction in a normal environment, such as a temporary hearing defect at a crucial stage in development, may also have permanent bad effects. Lower animals reared in restricted environments suffer a loss in ability to learn and even to perceive painful stimulation normally. Studies have also shown that early social contact may be essential for the development of normal adult sexual patterns. Enriched environment, on the other hand, improves intelligence and heightness social adjustment.

At each period of life, developmental tasks are imposed on the individual by his society and by his own needs. Successful performance of these tasks, which vary from culture to culture, is made possible by past learning and by maturation.

Studies have shown that there is no one prime of life for all abilities. Two methods may be used to study the growth and decline of human abilities. In using the cross-sectional method, investigations need only one set of tests to study subjects of different ages, but it is difficult for them to obtain representative samples of subjects, to find tests that will be fair to all age groups, and to equate the factor of motivation for all groups. The longitudinal method, while making it possible to determine the initial abilities of all subjects, has the practical difficulty of requiring an elaborate research organization. Also, numerous forms of each test are needed in order to avoid the effects of practice. Studies made using both methods indicate that performance on tests containing visual and motor factors declines most rapidly with age, whereas performance on verbal and informational tasks may actually improve throughout the individuals productive years.

Psychology is the science of human behavior which expresses and depicts mental processes and experience or the mind. Mind is the some total of various mental processes such as observing, knowing, thinking, imagining, remembering, judging and others. Psychology studies the relationship between mind and body. In any act mind and body affect each other. The mind operates at the levels of thinking, emotions and action. Mind and body cannot act independently, cannot be separated from each other.

Psychology studies human behavior which involves both body and mind. They interact each other. As stated earlier mental functions and physical states affect each other. In many occasions bodily emotions affecting mental functioning in a normal healthy individuals. For which quoting few examples are given below:

- It is observed that increase in blood pressure leads to mental over activity.
- Fatigue of the body leads to difficulty in concentrates and reduces a sense of proportion.
- Constipation can cause irritability and depression.
- Increased secretions of thyroid gland leads to mental restlessness and over activity.
- Decreased or under secretion of thyroid gland leads to dull lethargy of mind and body.

In the same way, mind also affect bodily functions which includes for example:

- Mind motivates all physical and motor activities.
- Unpleasant emotions such as fear, anger, worry causes headache, insomnia, indigestion, etc.
- Emotional conflicts are responsible for various mental illnesses such as, hysteria, neurasthenia, and GI problems such as peptic ulcer, ulcerative colitis, or flatulence.
- Deep thinking and concentration can cause physical fatigue.

We have just noticed the tripartite functioning of our mind. It operates at the levels of thinking, emotion and action. The mind operates in conjunction with the body. Psychology studies the relations of mind and body. There is an interaction between mind and body. Mind and body affect each other. The interactionism, according to which mind and body affect each other, is the current accepted view. The old idea of parallelism between mind and body has been rejected.

The nervous system and glands have potent effect upon our thinking and feeling. The over action of certain hormones in our body give us excitement. Let us illustrate the effects of body upon mind and mind upon body.

i. *Action of Body Upon Mind*
   a. Rise in blood pressure leads to mental excitement.
   b. Fatigue interferes with intellectual activity.
   c. Sudden emotion causes mental imbalance.
   d. Constipation can make us irritable.
   e. Dyspepsia can make us gloomy.
   f. Over action of thyroid gland leads to excitement and its under action to lethargy.
   g. Bad throat and septic tonsils can weaken concentration.

ii. *Action of Mind Upon Body*
   a. All physical and motor activity begins by the motivation of mind.
   b. The negative emotions like fear, anger, jealousy produce illness. They make us depressed. Emotional conflicts lie at the root of much gastrointestinal ills and neuroses.
   c. Deep thinking and concentration can cause physical fatigue.

According to an eminent writer, "A man's body and mind in all reverence, I say it—are, like a jerkin and its lining, rumple the one you rumple the other".

The practice nature of mind is not yet fully understood but it is safe to assume that mind is intimately connected with the brain. Therefore, a review of bodily functions with brain or cortical functions will help us to appreciate better the relation between mind and body.

i. Compared to all other creatures the brain of man is most developed. In gross weight the brain of elephant weights more than that of man. But in proportion to body weight man's brain weights most comparatively.
ii. An injury to brain interferes with the mental processes.
iii. Our nerves carry the impulses of the physical changes to the brain and only then does the mental process start. When a person pricked by a thorn. His nerves convey the message to the brain and the mental experience of pain is felt.

The above discussion is very much useful to the nurses in understanding the etiology of diseases.

Biopsychology or the study of the biological bases of behavior and mental processes, is not really as new a perspective as one might think. In the biological perspective, human and animal behavior is seen as a direct result of events in the body. Hormones, brain chemical, tumors and diseases are some of the biological cause of the behavior and mental events. For example, evidence is mounting for a biological cause (perhaps even genetic) for schizophrenia, a mental disease involving delusions (false beliefs) hallucinations (false sensory perceptions) and extremely distorted thinking.

Analysis of Mental Phenomena

The conscious experience reveals itself in three separate and distinct mental processes. These are cognition, affection, and conation, that is, the knowing process, the feeling process and the process of action. For example, you are witnessing an operation. Here you know certain facts, feel certain emotions and lastly may force yourself it by another example. A child cries. The mother listens to the cries and knows that the child is hungry. She feels compassion for the baby and immediately proceeds to feed him.

These three mental processes are also called modes of consciousness or the modes of becoming conscious. In every conscious process we know something; it either induces the feeling of pleasantness in us and we strive towards something.

It must be recognized that knowledge, emotion and action do not always follow a set serial order. It is not the case that we first know and then feel and thereafter act. We may first feel and then act and know in the last. For example something is irritating our skin. Immediately our hand hits the spot and we catch a mosquito or an ant. Here knowledge came in the last. Therefore, it is well to remember that in the conscious phenomena the order of occurrence of knowing, feeling and willing is not always the same.

It must also be remembered that all conscious experience is admixture of all the three modes of our consciousness. There is no conscious phenomenon which is not at once cognitive, affective and conative. We are only able to analyze our conscious experience into these elements. These do not exist independently and distinctly.

When we know something we are not devoid of the elements of feeling or striving. We call a mental process cognitive not because it consists purely of knowing and is bereft of the other elements. We call it so because the knowing element predominates and the other two are in the background.

Similarly a feeling process is not devoid of cognitive and conative elements. These are there but these are in the background while the feeling element is in the fore. Therefore, we may sum up by affective depending upon the conscious element of cognition, conation or affection dominating. This may be explained with the help of few examples. Reading of these liens is a cognitive process because here the primary interest is understanding. Enjoying a symphony or a song is an affective process because knowing or doing are not vital here. Similarly, arranging a bed or dressing up for date is a conative process though the element of feeling may be quite dominant. Getting annoyed with a person is an affective experience because the element of feeling is predominant though the elements of knowing and willing are also there. A swimmer running a race in the pool knows that he is running for a prize and there is an element of hope and despair in his heart. But nonetheless this is a conative experience, because the element of action overshadows both elements of cognition and affection.

Mind as Conscious-Unconscious Dynamic Whole

In psychology the human mind was sometimes considered as a mere collection of many faculties. Thus according to faculty psychology, human mind has many powers and there are different centers of these powers in the mind. But gradually, researchers in the field of mental activities discovered that the mind works as a whole. Researchers concerning the localization of brain functions showed that if a certain part of the mind receives injury, the other parts being to do the function.

Mind is not a collection but a dynamic whole. It is changing. The mental powers and processes constantly develop owing to interaction with the environment. In the interpretation of mental behavior Freud has given the hypothesis of three elements—Id, Ego and Superego. Of these there the Id is inborn, but both Ego and Superego develop within the environment.

Previously it was thought that the entire mind is conscious. Activities and processes which are now considered due to unconscious were thought to be influenced by divine or supernatural powers. From the psychological researchers gradually the existence of unconscious was proved and according to modern psychologists most of the mental processes in man are directed by his unconscious mind.

There are however, no water tight compartments between conscious and unconscious levels of the mind. Both these are continuous and constantly interact upon each other. For example according to Freud ego is partly conscious and partly unconscious and thus mediates between these two levels of mental consciousness.

Thus in modern psychology the mind is a conscious, unconscious dynamic whole. This is a basic concept whose outlines are gradually becoming more and more clear. The psychologists have achieved much in this field, but as more and more researchers will be conducted regarding the mental behavior, the outlines of this dynamic form of the mind will be more and more clear.

The Consciousness

Mental life is a continuous process, but in it certain concentric fields can be observed. For example, everyone knows that mental life of the dream or sleep is different from the life of the waking stage. Even in the waking state itself, man's mental life is not always of the same type. He distinctly sees some object, but other objects he knows only indistinctly. Something he forgets, some he remembers and some other things are recalled after being forgotten for sometime. Analyzing all these different forms of mental life the psychologists have admitted two fields of consciousness—

1. Focus of consciousness
2. Margin of consciousness.

In the focus of consciousness, everything can be seen clear and distinct from other objects. This is also called the field of attention. In it the span of mental activity is represented. In it the focul consciousness is very clear. For example while seeing the moon, the moon is seen as distinct from the stars and planets.

Round about the focus of consciousness there is the margin of consciousness. In it the attention is not fixed. Hence it is also called failed of inattention. Its consciousness is known as marginal consciousness. In it things are seen as hazy and indistinct. For example, while seeing the moon there is an indistinct consciousness of the presence of stars as well. Stout has called this area as the subconscious.

Both the above mentioned levels of consciousness are included in the threshold of consciousness. Below the threshold of conscious there is the subconscious. The existence of the subconscious is proved by may indirect testimonies. Hoffding and Freud called it unconscious. It is the reservoir of past experience and impressions. Its consciousness is not direct.

These levels of consciousness are entirely separate from each other. The different parts of our conscious life are not separated from each other by anything whose nature is different from consciousness. Hence this division of mental life is only a hypothesis for the interpretation of mental behavior which helps in understanding the various mental processes.

Conscious and unconscious are two levels of consciousness. On the conscious level the object remains in the field of our attention. We know it directly and it is clear. On the other hand the unconscious impulses are below the threshold of consciousness and so do not fall within the field of our attention. Their existence is known indirectly through hypnosis and posthypnotic suggestions, etc. The objects of unconscious are not known directly. As compared to the conscious level it is more complex, dynamic and instinctive. According to Freud, the conscious and the unconscious levels are opposed to each other. On the conscious level the desires are manifested. The unconscious is the level of repressed desires. It is irrational. According to Freud the unconscious is more important in mental life, than the conscious level.

The Unconscious

Freud emphasized the role of unconscious mind in human behavior. According to Freud almost the entire mental life is directed from the unconscious forces. The conscious level is a very small part of the unconscious mind. The unconscious is the reservoir of the unfulfilled motives. It stores repressed desires do not disappear but go to the unconscious of the man, and there await suitable chances for manifestation. Of these almost all the desires are sexual. It is these sexual desires which are the cause of much of the behavior of human beings. Freud calls the universal form of these sexual desires with the name libido. Libido is the motivating force in human life.

Most of us know by our everyday experience, that our conscious mind is not the only field of the mental activities. There are many things which we forget and cannot remember even after trying, though after sometime we again recall those things without making any effort. Sometimes one is sure that he has definitely seen a particular person somewhere-else, but even after trying his best he fails to recall the past acquaintance though after sometimes he suddenly recognizes him. The perception of certain things arouses some of our emotions. In the dreams, the past experiences are often recalled. There are many difficult questions which one fails to solve even after trying for hours and hours and at last leaves off the effort to solve it but after sometime he suddenly arrives at their solution. Sometimes, when we determine before sleep that we have to get up at 2 o'clock at night, we suddenly get up at the appropriate time, though our conscious mind was not working to that effect. These and many other experiences of our everyday life as well which performs many important functions in our life. This mind is not conscious, because we do not know it directly. It does many thing which the conscious mind fails to do. This is the unconscious in man.

Existence of unconscious: The following are the main proofs advanced by psychologists for the existence of unconscious—

i. *Hypnotism:* In the hypnotic state the consciousness of the hypnotized person appears to be entirely different from his waking consciousness. As seen from outside he appears to be sleeping, but he is particularly conscious of the instructions of the hypnotizer. After he gets up from this sleep, he does not remember anything about the hypnotic state of mind. All this proves that in the hypnotic state the man was on a level of consciousness which is other than the waking consciousness and outside its reach. This is the unconscious in man.

ii. *Posthypnotic suggestion:* A more convincing proof for the existence of unconscious is in that of posthypnotic suggestions. In the hypnotic state the hypnotizer directs the hypnotized person to perform a particular action at a particular time. As the man wakes up from his hypnotic state, he forgets everything regarding this direction, but as the appointed hour arrives he infallibly follows the directions. Bernheim has described an experiment in which he instructed a person to do an action a definite time and the man involuntarily did the same. In American, in the inquiry of a famous murder case, it was found that the real murderer was not the person who shot, but a doctor who directed the person in the hypnotic state to shoot the particular man at an appointed hour. The man exactly followed the instruments, but he did not know anything about the murder either before or after the incident. He did it only as an instrument in the hands of the doctor. Thus, it is clear that he was controlled not by his conscious mind, but by the consciousness which was controlled by the directions of the doctor in the hypnotic state. This is the conscious.

iii. *Proofs from mental abnormalities:* Freud and other psychoanalysts and clinical psychologist have proved the existence of unconscious by the analysis of mental abnormalities. In his New Introductory Lectures on Psychoanalysis, Freud describes a lady who developed a strange behavior. She used to overturn an inkpot of red ink at a white table cover, ring the bell to call the servant and stood at a corner of the table in such a way so that the red spots of the ink might be visible to others. This abnormal action was almost daily repeated in a state of fit. After a detailed analysis of this abnormal behavior, Freud disclosed that it was related with the first night of the lady's marital life. It happened that the husband failed to perform the usual sexual act and at last threw red ink on the bed sheet as a sign of bleeding so that his failure might not be disclosed to others. The lady kept this frustration in her unconscious mind and used to satisfy it through this abnormal behavior. The whole act was a repetition of the incident and the unconscious effort was to show that everything was normally done. As this unconscious cause was revealed to the lady, i.e. as it was made conscious, her abnormal behavior disappeared. The main technique which Freud adopted in curing mental patients was to analyse the unconscious causes and to bring them into consciousness.

iv. *Psychopathologies of everyday life:* In his famous book Psychopathologies of Everyday Life, Freud has described the different types of slips, i.e. slips of pen, slips of tongue, etc. and other errors committed in daily life. Freud has tried to show by analysis that all these slips and errors have their cause rooted in the unconscious. To give an example, a doctor wrote to a medicine manufacturing firm that he had applied their medicine to human beings and found them workable. This was a slip of pen because testing poison on human beings mean murder and no murderer would like to reveal his crime by writing it to someoneelse. As a matter of fact the doctor wanted to write guinea pigs in place of human beings, but failed owing to slip of pen. Freud has shown that this slip was not uncaused, but had its cause in the unconscious. When Police enquired into the matter, it was found that the doctor had actually administered poisons to human being. It should be remembered here that it is not necessary that there should be some unconscious cause behind every slip or error, but abnormal slips or errors as the one committed by the doctor, generally do have some powerful unconscious cause behind them.

v. *Free association:* Take a list of words and ask different persons to give words by free association. You will find that everyone responds differently, e.g. if the given word is diamond, one will respond by saying ruby, other 'money' while some other may say 'knife'. The association of the word knife with diamond appears rather abnormal and strange. Generally such abnormal associations have some unconscious causes by analyzing which even thefts have been discovered by means by free association.

vi. *Dream analysis:* Though psychologists do not agree that all the dreams have unconscious causes, yet no one denies that unconscious causes have an important role in the formation of dreams. Thus dreams point out to that unconscious world in which the repressed desires and tendencies of man remain lying for the suitable occasion to manifest themselves.

vii. *Other proofs:* Besides the above mentioned proofs, many other proofs of the existence of unconscious can be found in our daily life, e.g. sudden forgetting of anything or sudden recall, unknown inspirations in art, etc. solution of such difficult problems during sleep which could not be solved even while waking and finally sudden change in the behavior of individuals, etc.

Views on Unconscious

Before 18th century, the unconscious was not seriously discussed or explored. Many did not accept even its existence. Most of the phenomena which are now assigned to unconscious were formerly thought to be due to supernatural beings. This history of the exploration of the nature of unconscious in the West can be of the exploration of the nature of unconscious in the West can be divided into the two periods, viz. from Leibnitz to Morton Prince and from Morton Prince to the Psychoanalysts, like Freud, etc. and the modern psychologists. Of these the second period is the more important. In the first period besides Leibnitz, Hartmann, Schopenhauer and Herbart, discussed about unconscious, Dr. Morton Prince removed many false conceptions regarding the nature of unconscious. But it was Sigmund Freud, the father of psychoanalysis who has given the most comprehensive and scientific revelations regarding the unconscious and its functions.

Freud's views: Just as only 1/10th part of an iceberg remains above the water, while the 9/10th is concealed below the water, similarly the conscious level of the man's mind is a very small part of the unconscious. Thus according to Freud most of the human activities are motivated from the unconscious and it is the unconscious which should be explored to find out their causes. Freud devised many methods to explore the unconscious. It was this technique which came to be known as psychoanalysis.

According to Freud our unconscious mind includes those experiences which were repressed, because of their being painful or contrary to social norms. Along with these of the unconscious consist of instinctive desires which were not allowed to be expressed on the conscious level. These desires are mostly sexual while few are concerned with the ego as well. According to Adler most of the unconscious tendencies are concerned with the mastery motive.

Jung's views: According to Jung, Freud's concept of unconscious is too much limited. The unconscious is so vast that it can never be fully described. What Freud has described as unconscious, is only a small part of it which is formed in the life time of the individual. According to Jung we are born with a racial unconscious. Jung defines unconscious as 'the totality of psychic phenomena that lacks the quality of consciousnesses. Thus according to Jung there are two types of unconscious: Personal and Collective. The person unconscious of Jung includes all that which Freud described in Foreconscious and Unconscious. It includes all those experiences which have been forgotten or repressed.

The concept of collective unconscious is Jung's contribution to psychology. It is inborn. It includes the archetypes of thousands of years of experience of human race. It includes all those reactions and tendencies which are characteristic of human race. In it there are all the instincts peculiar to man. There are no thoughts in it. It has rather the natural and primitive methods of thinking.

Importance of Unconscious in Human Life

Researchers in the field of unconscious have revealed that it is very important to human life. Most of our behavior in everyday life has its causes in the unconscious. Dreams are controlled by the unconscious. In the day dreams, unconscious plays a vital role. Mental abnormalities have their roots in the unconscious. The causes of forgetting are in the unconscious. Unconscious takes an important part in our imagination. Many of man's slips and errors, e.g. as that of writing, speaking, other of physical and mental activities, etc. are due to unconscious causes. Thus all our desires which are not satisfied, remain in the unconscious and manifest on the conscious level through dreams, day dreams, errors and abnormal behavior. These can be understood by the analysis of the unconscious and many mental abnormalities can be removed through this understanding. Many of the things learnt by us which appear to be forgotten remain in the conscious. Insight is a result of this depth of experience and it very much helps in further learning. It is due to this that some men have so much insight in art, literature or science, etc. It is these unconscious urges which motivate man in fine arts because through them the repressed desires are satisfied.

The powers of unconscious can be used for much good in human behavior. Generally there is conflict between the conscious and the unconscious tendencies which lead to much abnormal behavior in man. But if unconscious is controlled or its cooperation is achieved, much improvement can be made in our capacities and activities. By future researchers in this field, more light will be thrown on the importance of unconscious in human life and behavior.

The dreams: Dream is an everyday experience of human life and the man has always been curious to know its meaning. In modern times, the psychoanalysts have done much work in the direction of the analysis of dream and many hypotheses have been formulated to explain it. According to Freud dreams are wish-fulfillment. Most of our desires, i.e. the antisocial desires or such desires the fulfillment of which is beyond our capacity cannot be satisfied in the waking stage. For example, if a promise desires to get out of prison, he cannot do so. In such state his desires are not satisfied, but repressed. These repressed desires do not disappear but manifest themselves in the form of dreams.

Thus, dreams are the means of the expression of our repressed desires. These repression desires manifest themselves in the form of dreams, because at that time the waking reason of the man does not hinder them. But still to avoid the social conscience in man in the form of censorship, the repressed desires express themselves in the form of dreams only in a changed form. According to Freud most of the desires expressed in the form of drams are sexual by nature. The society does not allow their expression. For example if a boy wants to meet a girl, to talk with her and to have romances, he cannot do so for fear of the society and represses this desire. But this desire does not leave his mind, it only goes to the unconscious. From the unconscious it cannot manifest itself as it is, because even while sleeping, the censorship does not allow him to do so. Just as a cinema film, before it is exhibited, is examined by the censor of the Government and shown only after undergoing it, similarly the dream can manifest itself only after passing censorship of the Superego.

According to Jung it is the unconscious attitudes of the person towards the present difficulties and problems of life which manifest themselves in the form of dream. According to Woodworth it is not the unconscious desire which manifests in the dream but the un-satisfied desire. According to Adler the desires expressing themselves in the dream are those of unsuccessful self assertion and related with the power motive. All these views agree that dreams are the manifestation of repressed desires though they differ about the nature of these desires.

But as has been pointed out by Woodworth and others, all dreams are not wish-fulfillment. Some dreams are meaningless and some are due to physical cause, while some other express our reactions to particular things in life. Even in the wish fulfillment dreams all desires cannot be labeled as sexual or concerned with power motive or with the difficulties of life. Human psychology is a complex phenomenon and so is the dream. Some dreams might be entirely self-contradictory. Hence the view that all dreams are wish fulfillment is one-sided though not wrong.

Dreams have an important place in mental life. Repressed or restrained and frustrated desires remain in our unconscious. This is the state of latent dreams. When these desires manifest themselves in the form of dreams it is known as manifest dream. The mechanism of converting a latent dream into manifest dream is known as dream work. In it the desires are expressed in various ways. By the expression of repressed and frustrated desires, the person achieves mental peace.

i. *Dreams are helpful in sleep:* Common man says that he cannot sleep because of dreams. But Freud pointed out that we sleep because of dreams. Thus dreams help in the continuation of sleep. For example, sometimes while sleeping, we feel very thirsty. In such condition had there been no dream we could not have slept. What happens is that we dream of drinking water and go on sleeping at least for sometime with the help of the dream water. But when it fails to quench the thirst, we wake up and have to drink the real water. It is an example of the physical need. Mental desires and tendencies are also satisfied through dreams and the sleep continues. For example, a student engrossed in the fear and worries of the examination dreams about it and continues to sleep. If these dreams were not there, the student could not sleep. If these dreams were not there the same desires would express themselves in some abnormal behavior and there may be many difficulties in the individuals adjustment. Dream is the most harmless way of the expression of desires. In it neither the time is wasted, as it is in the case of day dreams nor there is any harm, as in the case of error not any difficulty in adjustment, as in the case of abnormal behavior.

ii. *Abnormalities detected through dreams:* In psychoanalysis many of the abnormalities are discovered through the analysis of dream. In this analysis the method of free association is widely used. In it the individual, without using his reason associates ideas with his experiences of dream. This association shows the unconscious cause, by which mental abnormalities are detected.

Generally speaking there are following differences between night dreams and day dreams–

1. Night dreams are seen while sleeping and day dreams are seen while waking.
2. Hence day dreams are more conscious than the night dreams. They have more play of imagination.
3. Day dreams are generally about the future. Night dreams may be connected with any time past, present or future.

Theories of Dreams

Though man has always been inquisitive about the meaning of dreams, it was Aristotle who for the first time took dreams as a psychological problem. Before Aristotle, persons generally traced dreams to supernatural power. Aristotle for the first time emphasized that dream is a mental process. Since then psychologists have continually searched for the causes of dreams and tried to interpret them. The first systematic interpretation of dreams was presented by Sigmund Freud, a physician-psychologist of Vienna. Various theories about interpretation of dreams can be classified as follows—

1. Physiological theories of dreams.
2. Psychoneurological theories of dreams
3. Psychoanalytical theories of dreams.

Of these the last is the most important one. In it the main theory has been presented by Freud, though the theories of Adler and Jung are also worth mentioning. Now all these various theories regarding the interpretation of dreams will be systematically dealt with.

1. *The physiological theory of dreams:* The physiological theory of dreams, as is clear from its name, admits internal and external physical stimuli as the causes of dreams. Man cannot see dreams in the absence of these stimuli. But because man is never free from these stimuli, dreams are often seen. Thus dream is a mere response to the physical stimuli created in sleep. Besides this, it has neither any meaning nor use. In the words of Binze, "All the facts as we see them, urge us to characterize the dream as a physical process, in all cases useless and in many cases definitely morbid". Besides Binze the most important advocates of the physiological theory include Mourie, Robert and Delege. According to Delege, dreams are caused by the sensory impression collected in the brain due to the suppression in day time. Thus man's suppressed sensory impressions manifest themselves in dreams. According to Robert it is the unfulfilled thoughts of waking life and the sensory influences which create dream. About the utility of dreams the views of Robert are different from those of Binze. According to Robert the dreams make man's life more balanced. In the waking state a whole load of sensory influences is gathered on the brain. This load is lightened in the dream state. Thus dreams save brain from the load of the sensory influences is gathered on the brain. This load is lightened in the dream state. Thus dreams save brain from the load of the sensory impression.

No one can deny the influence of physiological sensations in the process of dream, but physiological interpretation alone is not sufficient. The dream has a mental and psychological aspect as well. It is hence that something which happens in the childhood is seen in dreams even after twenty years. It is true that the physical sensations bear some influence on dream, but due to psychological difference the same physical sensations can create different expressions in the dreams of different persons. For example, if a knife or some hard thing is placed on the neck of some sleeping person, a farmer may dream of the stroke of his sickle while a student of French History may dream of guillotine. The theory of Robert regarding the utility of dreams is more real than that of Binze, etc. The dreams however, not only remove the load of the sensory impressions, but also manifest mental frustrations.

2. *Psychoneurological interpretation:* The psychoneurological theory of dreams has been presented by Harton. According to this theory, dream is an apperception of trial and error, i.e. the dreamer tries to understand and perceive the sensation, sometimes he succeeds in it sometimes does not succeed and sometimes partly succeeds. For example, if some water is poured on the feet of a sleeping man or if the feet of a sleeping man are uncovered in some winter night, the person can dream of walking on snow. Similarly, a man sleeping in the running train may dream of hurricanes, owing to the physical sensations of the noise of the train. Thus according to Harton's theory, the man sees a dream in accordance with external stimuli working on his body. Sometimes when the man wakes up after hearing some terrible sound in his dream he really finds some object falling outside. According to Harton it is the sound of this falling object which makes the dreamer. Harton has explained his theory on the basis of psychoneurology.

The psychoneurological interpretation of dream is also one-sided because it fails to interpret many dreams. For example how can any one interpret the dreams related to the childhood memories on the basis of this theory? It also does not explain why some dreams are meaningless. In spite of these failings of this theory, no one can deny that there is an element of trial and error in dreams.

3. *Psychoanalytic interpretation:* As has already been pointed out, the best interpretation of dreams is the psychoanalytic theory. The psychoanalytic of dream was first presented by Sigmund Freud. Later on Adler and Jung presented interpretations different from those of Freud. Hence here it shall be relevant to discuss Freud's theory as the best specimen of psychoanalytic interpretation.

Freud's Theory of Dreams

People say that we cannot sleep because we dream, Freud tried to prove that we sleep because we dream. Thus according to Freud dreams are not impediments in sleep, but rather a help to it. All dreams, according to him, are wish-fulfillment. This theory of dreams has been elaborately discussed by Freud in his famous book, 'The Interpretation of Dreams'. The general outline of Freud's theory of dream is as follows:

1. *Dreams are wish-fulfillment:* Freud emphasized that man's desires which are not satisfied in the external world or which are repressed due to some causes, do not get extinguished, but go to the unconscious and from there try to manifest themselves on suitable occasions. The manifestation of dreams is one of the suitable means of the expression of these unconscious desires.

It can be questioned here that if dreams are wish-fulfillment, why does one see painful and traumatic dreams? Freud has explained this difficulty by pointing out that these dreams are the distorted forms of the latent content of the dreamer. For example, if a young man dreams that a lady severely gets hurt and the lady resembles his mother, Freud will interpret the dream by pointing out that the young man actually desired that his mother should get hurt. Every young man would revolt against this interpretation. But according to Freud, in man's mind there are mutually conflicting desires. Where there is love there is hate, where there is an urge for life, there is a desire for death as well. But some time in the state of traumatic neurosis the dreams often stop in the state of worry and appear to be unsuccessful in the fulfillment of desire. Hence later on Freud modified his theory and called the dream. 'Attempted wish-fulfillment' and not wish-fulfillment itself. Thus later on Freud divided dreams into three classes. (a) Wish dreams, (B) Anxiety dreams and (C) Punishment dreams.

2. *The importance of sexual desires in dreams:* According to Freud the most common, most dominant and most frustrated desires of man are sexual desires. On the one hand the man wants to satisfy his sexual impulses, while on the other hand he also wants to preserve the social and moral norms. Thus there are two conflicting tendencies in man's mind—Id and Ego. Id is the reservoir of frustrated desires. It seeks the satisfaction of sexual desires. The superego is the representative of social morality and tries to control sexual impulses. This is the dream censor to escape which the latent dream manifests itself in different forms.
3. *Dream work:* The latent content of the dream is the frustrated desire. Due to censorship this desire cannot manifest itself in the dream in its real form. The censorship resists the dream wish due to which it assumes distorted forms. Thus dream work is the process by which the latent content becomes manifest content of the dream. As has already been pointed out the latent dream cannot manifest in a distorted form. This work is done with the help of the following five mechanisms:
    i. *Condensation:* In the condensation much of the part of the latent dreams disappears before manifesting. May accident assume the form of symbols and many images merge together and become one. For example, a man may dream of a person who has characteristics of many of his acquaintances all in one.
    ii. *Displacement:* In this mechanism the primary things in the latent dream become secondary in manifest dream and the secondary become primary. Hence the censorship fails to recognize the real desires.
    iii. *Dramatization:* In this mechanism the abstract desires of the latent content manifest themselves in concrete form in the dream. This dramatization is not in the real form, but in changed form. Thus in dreams the feelings and emotions, etc. manifest in concrete form.
    iv. *Symbolization:* In this book on dreams, Freud has given a detailed description of different symbols of various sexual organs and tendencies. For example, a tree in a dream may symbolize a male organ. In this form the censorship has no objection in it. Hence frustrated desires manifest themselves in the form of symbols.
    v. *Secondary elaboration:* Man wants to see a continuity and meaningfulness in everything. Hence while awaking after dream he elaborates the dream and there and tries to make it more logical and meaningful. This mechanism is known as secondary elaboration. This conceals the real form of the dream.

Criticism of Freud's Theory

As has already been pointed out Freud's theory is the most important among the psycho-analytic theories regarding the interpretation of dream. Hence while criticizing psychoanalytic theory most of the criticisms have been leveled against Freud's theory. Of these, the most important objections are as follows:

1. *Excessive emphasis on unconscious:* It has been pointed out by Woodworth that Freud has laid too much emphasis on the role of unconscious in the dream. Most of the desires which are ignored and rejected still remain conscious. It is not true that all the frustrated desires are unconscious. The desires expressed in dreams are not so much conscious, as frustrated and the frustrated desires can be even absolutely conscious.
2. *Too much emphasis on sex impulse:* It has been pointed out by many Freud has laid too much emphasis on the role of sexual impulse in the dream. On this point the views of Adler and Jung are as much true as that of Freud. Again, some dreams are meaningless. Only a small number of dreams can be labeled as sexual.
3. *The interpretation of normal through abnormal:* Mcdougall has pointed out against Freud's interpretation of dreams that in it the normal has been explained by abnormal. Freud's formula regarding the interpretation of dreams may be helpful in the understanding of some dreams specially those of neurotics. But there is no sufficient ground to apply this formula on every dream. In fact Freud's interpretation of dream was mostly build up on the data supplied by his patients. Freud tried to interpret every normal dream by this theory. It is more scientific of interpret abnormal by the normal than the *vice versa.*

In spite of all the objections against Freudian hypothesis, it should be remembered that Freud's interpretation proves to be most successful and useful in the interpretation of many dreams. For example, proofs have been found regarding the manifestations of the repressed desires in dreams, wish fulfillment in dreams, symbols in dreams and the dreams mechanism, etc. In fact Freud's interpretation is not so much wrong as limited and one-sided. It cannot explain all the dreams. Similarly, the views of Adler and Jung are equally one-sided. It should be remembered in this connection that of all the theories of these three psychologists, Freud's interpretation of dreams was definitely most successful.

In fact all the theories regarding the dream interpretation are one-sided. There, one should admit that a dynamic and integral standpoint is necessary. No common theory can be built up for the interpretation of all the dreams. Dream is a complex process which may be connected with any of the time, past, present future; in which sex, hatred, self-assertion, any of the conscious or unconscious impulse may work. Hence, Woodworth has rightly said "No interpretation really conveys the dream. Speaking for myself, I have grave doubts of the validity of any dream interpretation. What underlies a given dream is certainly much more than what finds place in any interpretation".

5 CHAPTER

Genetics and Behavior

The term 'genetics' has been derived from Greek word 'gene' which means 'grow into' or 'to become'. Gene is a unit of heredity which is transferred from parent to offspring and is held to determine some characteristics of offspring in particular, a distinct DNA forming part of chromosome. Genetics is the scientific study of heredity in which it deals with how specific traits or predispositional one transmitted from parents to offspring.

Heredity involves all those physiological and psychological peculiarities which inherit parents. These peculiarities are transmitted to us through the gene. In this way the children of white parents are fair while those of dark parents are generally dark. In one of parents is fair while other is dark the child may be either fair dark complexioned. It is the heredity which determines the structure, color of the skin, the hair structure, height, facial features, nasal index, eyetie index, etc. Heredity is passing the traits to the offspring. This is the process by which an offspring cell or organism acquires the characteristics of its parent cell or organism. Through heredity, variations among individuals prevail and cause the species to exist. It is seen that particular genes influence the development of human traits like intelligence, personality.

Since, there was any scientific investigation, in earlier days it was believed that the effect of heredity arises from the mixing of the bloods of parents. But in later part of 18th century, a priest Mendal proved the fallacy of this theory by his experiments on the seeds of pea. Mendals experiments and the investigation of other scientists proved that the effect of heredity is transferred from one generation to the next through the gene. By the intercourse between male and female, the sperm cell of the male meets the egg cell of the female, and the child is conceived. These cells are made of protoplasm and they have chromosomes in their nucleus. There are genes inside the chromosomes. The heredity of the child is formed through these genes, determining his physiological and some psychological peculiarities. In human being every physiological trait has a definite gene corresponding to it. This gene is never found single because both the parents contribute one gene each. Thus the person gets is pair of gene from his parents of every physiological trait. This is heredity. If these two genes are similar the child inherits that quality but if the two are dissimilar it is the dominant of the two genes which gives it qualities to the child.

In actual sense life begins with the conception, approximately nine months, before birth. The mechanism of conception is as mentioned in brief as follows:

The male and female reproductive organs produce germ cells. In the male their teste produce the male germ cells, the spermatozoa, while in the females, their ovaries produce the female germ cells, the ova. Life is the result of the union of these male and female cells. As a result of coitus at the time of mating the male germ cells, numerous in number try to come in contact with female germ cells. The male germ cells are deposited at the mouth of the uterus and try to make contact with the single ovum (normally only one ovum is produce in each menstrual cycle). Out of so many spermatozoa only one sperm establishes contact with the ovum and makes it fertilized. The fertilized ovum is technically known as Zygote. Actually fertilization of the ovum is the beginning of the life which starts the process of the child development in the mother's womb. The fertilized ovum consists of a semifluid mass called cytoplasm and within the cytoplasm there is the nucleus which contain the chromosomes. The chromosomes exist in pairs. In the fertilized ovum (Zygote) there are 23 pairs of chromosomes, 23 of which one contributed by the father and 23 by the mother. Each chromosome consists of number of minute particles called "gene". These genes are the physical substances passed on from parent to offspring and thus are the real carriers and determiners of heredity traits. What we get out of the heredity is the net result of the traits and characteristics of the parents and forefathers transmitted to the zygote through the respective genes.

Therefore the inherited characteristics are always transmitted through respective genes at the time of the fertilization of the ovum by the sperm and consequently heredity refers to a biological mechanism as a result of which the child gets something from his ancestral stock through his parents. It points out the native capital and endowment of an individual, the some total of the traits potentiality present in the fertilized ovum at the time of conception.

Need of Studying Genetics

All nurses need to be able to understand language of genetics, be able to communicate with others using it appropriately, interview clients and take an accurate history over three generations, recognize the possibility of a genetic disorder in an individual or family.

History taking of patient: All nurse need to understand the language of genetics and its disorders, be able to take an accurate history over three generations, recognize the possibility of a genetic disorder in an individual or family. She takes comprehensive relevant family histories by interviewing the clients and their families.

Dealing with patients with genetic disorder: Nurses come in contact with children and adults with childhood genetic disorders and will have to deal with how these disorders will influence and be influenced by the common health problems of adults as their age. Nurses, also will see the usual health problems of adults superimposed on the genetic background of a childhood genetic disorder such as cystic fibrosis. And other genetic disorders. For which nurses has to performs following activities mentioned below:

- Nurse plans, implements, administers or evaluates screening or testing programs
- Nurse monitors and evaluates clients with genetic disorders
- Nurse works with families under stress produced by problems related to a genetic disorder
- Nurse coordinates care and services
- Nurse assess needs and interactions in clients and families
- Nurse assesses the client and family's cultural/ethnic health beliefs and practices as they relate to the genetic problem

- Nurse assesses the client and family's strengths and weaknesses and family functioning
- Nurse relates the heredity and environment for the client's health status.

Communication and counseling: Nurses take part in communicating and counseling with regard to the following.

- Nurses explain and interpret correctly the purpose, implications and results of genetic tests
- Nurse serves as an advocate for a client and family affected by a genetic disorder
- Nurse educates the public about genetics
- Nurse reinforces and interprets genetic counseling and testing information
- Parents and other family members can be explained about the importance and link of heredity and environment on the growth and development of the child.

Genetic Influences on Health

With the beginning of the new millennium we have witnessed the completion of the international Human Genome Project (HGP) to map and sequence the human genome. The information from this project about the 3 billion base pairs of the human genome will open the possibility of changes in every aspect of biology and medicine and have a major impact on health care in the future (International Human Sequencing Consortium, 2001).

Much effort is being focused on identifying gene variations. Although as a human species we are 99.9 percent alike, it may be the 0.1 percent variation that will help us understand the genetic risk for illnesses. It is hoped that treatment strategies can be devised that are specific to an individuals diseases mutation. Another new field of study created by the HGP is the study of how inheritance affects the body's responses to drugs, called Pharmacogenetics. The hope is that better, safer, and in some cases more powerful drugs can be developed. The information from the HGP may influence more areas than we can currently imagine. Because of this, part of the total budget for the project was allotted to the Ethical, Legal and Social Implications (ELSI) program to deal with the new genetic discrimination, privacy and education. It will continue to look at new issues generated by information about our human genome.

Nurses will increasingly be faced with interpreting genetic information in client histories and diagnostic testing, and with assuming responsibility for protecting client privacy (Scanlon and Fibison, 1995). To better counsel families and to anticipate likely problems, the nurse needs a fundamental understanding of the principles of genetics and the importance of heredity and the prenatal environment as etiologic factors in diseases and disorders of childhood.

Genetic diversity: It is the amount of variation seen in a particular population. The differences occur in different communities, races or ethnic groups that lead to individual differences among populations. The genes have an impact on the characteristics of human beings. Like the Japanese and Chinese have significant appearance than Whites and Indians. The study of individual differences helps to study variations among people at a particular time and situation. Studies show that various diseases are influenced by genetic factors and family history. For example, diabetes mellitus is inherited as a heterogenous, multigenic trait. It carries a risk of 25-50 percent in identical twins, whereas siblings have a 6 percent risk and offspring a 5 percent risk. An association exists between diabetes and several antigens (HLA).

Genetic Variability: It is a measure of the tendency of individual genotypes in a population to vary from one another. The genetic variability describes the susceptibility of organisms to diseases and sensitivity to toxins or drugs. Various sources of variability in a population are:

- *Genetic recombination is one source of variability:* During meiosis, two homologous chromosomes from male and female crossover one another and exchange gene sequences. The chromosomes then split apart and are ready to form an offspring. The crossover is random and is governed by its own set of genes that code from where crossovers can occur. Being controlled by genes means that recombination is also variable in frequency and location. Thus, it can be selected for fitness by nature because the more recombination, the more variability and the easier it is for the population to handle changes.
- *Immigration, emigration and translocation:* Each of these is the movement of an individual into or out of a population. When an individual comes from a previously genetically isolated population into a new one, it will increase the genetic variability of the next generation if it reproduces.
- *Polyploidy:* Having more than two homologous chromosomes allows for even more recombination during meiosis, and allowing for even more genetic variability in one's offspring.
- *Diffuse centromeres:* Being diffuse causes the chromatid to split apart in many different ways allowing for chromosome fragmentation and polyploid hence creating more variability.
- *Genetic mutations:* Contributed to the genetic variability within a population and can have positive, negative or neutral effects on the individuals fitness.
- *Correlated traits:* Although some genes have only an effect on a single trait, many genes have an effect on various traits. So, a change in a single gene will have an effect on all those traits.
- *Resemblance between relatives:* When individual differences are studied by estimating the variations among various components is called the *principle of relatedness.* A child has a father and mother. Thus, the child and father share 50 percent of their alleles, as do the child and the mother. However, the mother and father normally do not share genes as a result of shared ancestors. Similarly two full siblings share on average 50 percent of alleles with each other while half sibs only 25 percent.

Heredity in Health Problems

Contained within the nucleus of every somatic cells in the human body are approximately 35,000-70,000 *genes*, the genetic material responsible for programming the body's physiologic process and characteristics (International Human Genome Sequencing Consortium, 2001). These genes are composed of segments of DNA (deoxyribonucleic acid) and are organized into structures called *chromosomes*, which are visible only during certain stages of cell division. Alterations of a whole chromosome, a part of a chromosome, or even a single gene can manifest as a genetic disorder. Important to this concept is that this alteration or mutation may have been passed from one or both parents and previous generations, or it may be a new alteration in that individual. It is misleading to regard all genetic disorders as having been "passed through the family".

Environment: Though there are many evidences for genetic influence on the human variability, but still it is not very clear. So, many believes that the environment of the person effects the human's body. It can be natural, built, social, internal/external environments. The pollutants in the environment have been linked to chronic diseases such as cancer, asthma, and cardiovascular health problems. For instance, the relationships exist between global warming and malaria, ozone depletion and skin cancer, habitat fragmentation and Lyme disease, and the health impact of persistent organic pollutants such as DDT.

Now *'Nature versus nurture'* ignores the only separate effects of genes and environment on individual difference. It studies the contribution of interactions between genetics and environment. In reality, gene expression is environment dependent and one could not exist without the other. The 'quantitative genetics' studies the continuous traits (such as height, weight) and its underlying mechanisms. For example, the phenotypic value (P) of an individual is the combined effect on the genotypic value (G) and the environmental deviation (E).

$$P=G+E$$

The genotypic value is the combined effect of all the genetic effects, including nuclear genes, mitochondrial genes and interactions between the genes. It is often subdivided in an additive (A) and a dominance component (D). The additive effect describes the cumulative effect of the individual genes, while the dominance effect is the result of interactions between those genes. The environmental deviation can be subdivided in a pure environmental component (E) and an interaction factor (I) describing the interaction between genes and the environment. This can be described as:

$$P= A+D+E+1$$

Examples:

- Phenylketonuria (PKU) is a human genetic condition caused by mutations to a gene coding for a particular liver enzyme, disturbs brain development and other problems.
- Low monoamine oxidase (MAOA) activity due to functional polymorphism in MAOA gene promoter is a significant risk factor for aggressive and antisocial behavior in adults who report victimization as children.

Genes and Chromosomes

Genes are the basic units of heredity. The term 'gene' was used previously to mean the hereditary factor (s) that determined a characteristic or trait.

Today, a gene can be more precisely defined as a segment of deoxyribonucleic acid (DNA) that encodes or determines the structure of an amino acid chain or polypeptide. A polypeptide is a chain of amino acids connected to one another by polypeptide bonds. The vast majority of genes are located in the cell nucleus but genes are also present in the mitochondria of the cells. Genes direct the process of protein synthesis; thus they are responsible for the determination of such products as structural proteins, transport proteins, cell membrane receptors, gap junction proteins, ion channels, hormones and enzymes. Genes not only determine the structure of proteins and enzymes, but are also concerned with their rate of synthesis and regulatory control. Ultimately, genes guide development of the embryo. One consequence of altered enzyme or protein structure can be altered function. The capacity of genes to function in these ways means that they are significant determinants of structural integrity, cell function, and the regulation of biochemical, developmental and immunological processes.

The normal human chromosome number in most somatic (body) cells and in the zygote is 46. This is known as the diploid (2N) number. Chromosomes occur in pairs, normally one of each pair is derived from the individuals mother and one of each pair is derived from the father.

There are 22 pairs of autosomes (chromosomes common to both sexes) and one pair of sex chromosomes. The sex chromosomes present in the normal female are two X chromosomes (XX). The sex chromosomes present in the normal male are one X chromosome and one Y chromosome (XY). Gametes (ova and sperm) each contain one member of a chromosome pair for a total of 23 chromosomes (22 autosomes and one sex chromosome). This is known as the haploid (N) number or one chromosome set. The fusion of male and female gametes during fertilization restores the diploid number of chromosomes (46) to the zygote normally contributing one maternally derived chromosome and one paternally derived chromosome.

The Twin Mechanism

Life is the result of fusion of two cells. In a normal case, when a single ovum is fertilized by sperm cell of the male, it results in the birth of a single offspring. However, in some cases, this normal function is disturbed and there are cases of multiple births, i.e. the birth of two or more offsprings at a time. There are two types of twins, are as follows:

1. **Monozygotic twins:** Have been called the most common human structural defect. They are derived from the cleavage of a single fertilized ovum. In the process of fertilization of the ovum by sperm, the ovum is made to split into two parts. In a normal process, these parts are again united. Sometimes, however, it so happens that these two split parts fail to unite together. The result is that each part is developed into a complete individual in the form of a pair of identical twins.

   Nurses should carefully assess the twins of any monozygotic twin with a malformation for overlooked or subtle defects. The nurse should send the placenta and membranes of any apparent singleton born with malformations for analysis for any evidence of a deceased co-twin or an incomplete twin.
2. **Dizygotic twins** (fraternal, binovular) result from fertilization of two ova, most likely ruptured from two distinct graafian follicles usually of the same or one from each ovary, by two sperms during a single ovarian cycle. Their subsequent implantation and development differ little from those of a single fertilized ovum. The dizygotic twins, may result from both autosomal recessive and autosomal dominant inheritance. Once a woman has had a pair of dizygotic twins, her chances of having another pair is increased fourfold without correction for age.

Genetics and Behavior

The brain is the most complex organ, and thousands of genes are involved in some way with brain function. Cell-to-cell communication occurs through a large number of neurons, nerve cell connections and various known neurotransmitters. About 30 percent of the known genetic diseases involve nervous system defects. The genetics of cognitive abilities, mental functioning, social attitudes, psychological interests, psychiatric disorders, learning disorders, behavior, addiction, mood and personality traits have been complicated by the complexity of brain function as well as the social, ethical, legal and political factors. The genetic factors in the major types of mental illnesses such as schizophrenia, mood or affective disorders has resulted in behavioral, learning and emotional conditions.

Various genes affect the behavior of a person through genetic influence on structure and pattern of anatomical configuration such as regulation of neurotransmitters. Many studies show that behavior of a person largely depend upon the interaction of heredity and environment. Some studies are described below:

- In one large family, a defect in the gene for monoamine oxidase. A (MAOA) leading to deficiency resulted in an X-linked recessive mild mental retardation and a pattern of aggressive, impulsive and violent behavior.
- Persons with certain genotypes might create high stress environments, thus increasing the probability of mental illness.
- The gene make-up of an individual responsibility for personality, social attitudes, psychological interests and religiousness.
- Families have been studied for generations past from the point of the unique presence, or absence of some personality attributes. It has been found that family members and their descendants show a remarkable resemblance. For example, a family known to be rich and of repute may consistently display healthy signs and wealth and intelligence while a family of ill-repute may exhibit a record of the characterless, poor and defamed persons.

Similarly such studies and many of the abnormalities and diseases have been found to be there from generation to generation and consequently, heredity plus environment has been made responsible for subsequent development and behavior of an individual.

There is probably a genetic component in all disease processes. In some disorders the genetic defect is known; in others the precise nature of the genetic component is more obscure. In some the disorder is apparent at birth; in others the manifestation do not appear for weeks, months, or years. Some diseases and disorders are determined by the genetic constitution of the individual, such as muscular dystrophy, Marfan syndrome, and Down syndrome. Other diseases, although genetically determined, do not become clinically apparent until environmental factors precipitate the onset of symptoms. For instance, phenylketonuria is a disorder in which the enzyme to metabolize the protein phenylalanine is lacking. Deleterious effects in the infant are exhibited subsequent to sufficient ingestion of phenylalanine-containing substances, such as milk. Also, the acute symptoms of sickle cells disease are precipitated by certain conditions such as lowered oxygen tension, infection, or dehydration.

Another area in which this interplay of genetic and environmental factors is being investigated is cancer genetics. All cancer is genetic in the sense that cancer cells result from a "sporadic" gene malfunction (acquired mutation). However, only 5 to 10 percent of all cancers are inherited, which means the gene mutation that predisposes to cancer was present in the germline. Therefore the individual is prone to cancerous development much earlier in life.

Other disorders result primarily from environmental factors. These include most infectious diseases and trauma. Development of the disease depends on environmental contact with the etiologic agent, but there is strong evidence to indicate a decided genetic element in the susceptibility to most diseases (e.g. tuberculosis, poliomyelitis, and measles in some populations).

Table 5-1: Characteristic age of onset for manifestations of some genetic diseases	
Age of Onset	*Condition*
Lethal during parental life birth	Some chromosome aberrations Some gross malformations Congenital malformations Chromosome aberrations (e.g. Down syndrome) Some forms of adrenogenital syndrome Some forms of deafness
Soon after birth	Phenylketonuria Galatosemia Cystic fibrosis (sometimes) Maple syrup urine disease
Infancy	Sickle cell anemia (sometimes later) Tay-Sachs disease Werdnig-Hoffmann disease
Early childhood	Cystic fibrosis Duchenne muscular dystrophy Fragile X syndrome
Near puberty	Limb-girdle muscular dystrophy Some forms of adrenogenital syndrome Turner syndrome
Young adulthood	Acute intermittent porphyria Hereditary juvenile glaucoma
Variable-onset age	Diabetes mellitus (0 to 80 years) Huntington chorea (15 to 65 years) Myotonic dystrophy (birth to old age)

Genetic diseases can usually be classified into one of the following broad categories according to the hereditary factors that produce the observed effect: cytogenetic, mitochondrial, monogenetic, or multifactorial. Prenatal environmental influences, such as alcohol exposure and placental abnormalities, are also regarded as being within the realm of genetics because these effects can produce congenital structural, functional, or growth defects. In such cases the chromosomes would be normal although anomalies produced might be indistinguishable phenotypically from a genetically determined anomaly. The important difference is that the defects would not be inheritable because they would not have been caused by a genetic mutation.

Congenital Malformations

The development of an organism, especially during embryogenesis, is an intricate process in which all parts must be properly integrated to ensure a coordinated whole. The rate must be such that one part is ready when needed by another part; otherwise, either part may cease to grow or may deviate from its normal path. Congenital anomalies, or birth defects, occur in 2 to 4 percent of all liveborn children and can arise at any stage of development. There is wide variability in etiologic factors, as well as in type, extent, and frequency of defects. Some defects result when a state present in one phase of development as a normal condition persists into another phase as abnormal. For example, a cleft lip is normal is young embryo, and a patent ductus arteriosus is essential during fetal life. Any agent that interferes with these complex processes will produce a defect in development ranging in severity from an insignificant local anomaly to complete degeneration.

A few congenital defects are clearly caused by a single gene mutation, some are associated with chromosome abnormalities, and others are produced by known intrauterine environment factors. However, many of the more common and severe defects (e.g. pyloric stenosis, central nervous system malformations, cataracts, and congenital heart disease) appear to be consistent with multifactorial inheritance.

The types of malformations that can result from genetic and/or prenatal environmental causes can be major structural abnormalities with serious medical, surgical, or quality-of-life consequences, or they can be minor anomalies or normal variants with no serious consequences, such as sacral dimple, an extra nipple, or an umbilical hernia. Malformations can occur in isolation, such as congenital heart defect, or multiple anomalies may be present. A recognized pattern of malformations due to a single specific cause is called a syndrome, such as Down syndrome or fetal alcohol syndrome. A nonrandom pattern of malformations for which an etiology has not been determined is called an association, such as VATER (vertebral defects, imperforate anus, tracheoesophageal fistula, and radial/renal defects) association. Neural tube defects, cleft lip and /or cleft palate, deafness, congenital heart defects, and mental retardation are examples of anomalies that can occur in isolation or as a part of a syndrome or association and can have different etiologies, such as single-gene or chromosome abnormalities, prenatal exposures, or multifactorial causes.

Chromosome (Cytogenetic) Disorders

Chromosome or cytogenetic disorders deviations in either structure or number of a chromosome; the consequences in either situation can be readily observed in the affected individual and are often severe or even lethal. The reason for this is that a numerical or structural chromosome abnormality involves a duplication or loss of at least a few genes, or up to thousands of genes. Although the types of cytogenic disorders are not as varied as those caused by a single-gene, the incidence for many of the specific abnormalities is significantly higher than that for any of the single-gene (monogenic) disorders.

A structural abnormality involves loss, addition, rearrangement, or exchange of some of the genes of a chromosome. If there is sufficient remaining genetic material to render the organism viable, structural alterations can produce an endless variety of clinical manifestations. These deviations are usually a result of an error in cell division in the sperm or ovum that resulted in that individual, but the parents are chromosomally normal.

Sometimes, however, the chromosomes abnormality can be inherited from a parent who is a balanced translocation carrier. Also, fragile or weak, sites have been identified on both autosomes and on the X chromosome. An X chromosome fragile site has been associated with physical and mental abnormalities termed fragile X syndrome.

Another relatively rare structural abnormality that can occur is a ring chromosome. If a break occurs in the terminal end of both arms of a chromosome, the ends may fuse together, forming a circle. Like any structural alteration of a chromosome, the clinical manifestations depend on which genes are lost.

The normal number of chromosomes in a somatic cell is 23 pairs, or 46 total. Deviations in chromosome number involve the gain or loss of a chromosome and are designated with the suffix–somy. A cell that contains one fewer that the total number of chromosomes is called a monosomy because of the loss of one member of a chromosome pair; a cell that contains one more than the total number of chromosomes resulting from the addition of an extra member to a normal pair is called a trisomy. A number of deviations compatible with life occur in humans, especially those involving the sex chromosomes; the more serious outcomes are related to abnormalities of the autosomes. Trisomies are the chromosomes aberrations encountered most commonly by health care workers. Monosomies may occur as often in conceptuses but are usually nonviable. A relatively rare but clinically recognized variation is triploidy, in which there are three chromosomes in every pair, so that the total chromosome number is 69. This condition is lethal in early infancy.

The clinical consequences that attend variations in chromosome number frequently consist of discrete, identifiable syndromes, particularly in regard to the trisomies. The chromosome structural anomalies form a more diverse group of reported physical deviations with few recognized syndromes. Some of the chromosomes disorders, such as Down syndrome, can be identified on the basis of physical characteristics but require chromosome analysis to rule out the less common situation of translocation Down syndrome.

Causes of Chromosome Defects

There is considerable speculation regarding the precise cause of chromosome errors. Ionizing radiation—especially large doses or from occupational exposure—has been found to be a cause of chromosome breaks, rearrangements, and nondisjunction. Autoimmune diseases appear to have a role in the pathogenesis of nondisjunction during cell division. Viruses have also been implicated, especially in relation to chromosome breakage. However, only germ cell chromosome errors or breaks have the potential to cause chromosome abnormalities in offspring. Somatic errors do not have reproductive consequences.

Most of the information regarding factors that cause chromosome errors is related to parental age. The incidence of trisomic births corresponds strongly with increasing maternal age, regardless of the number of pregnancies. For example, the risk of trisomy 21, or Down syndrome, increases dramatically for mothers more than 35 years of age. There is no positive explanation for this observation. However, throughout a lifetime the germ cells are vulnerable to a variety of exogenous influences and to the normal effects of the aging process. Increasing paternal age is not associated with most chromosome abnormalities, but it is associated with an increased risk for new mutation cases of autosomal dominant disorders, such as skeletal dysplasias.

A. AUTOSOMAL ANOMALIES

The first known case of a chromosomal anomaly associated with a clinical disorder was described by Lejeune, Gautier and Turpin in 1959 in Down's syndrome or mongolism. Characterized by mental retardation and a few other clinical symptoms, the condition is due to trisomy (presence of an extra chromosome so that a certain pair is represented by three homologous instead of two) of an autosomal chromosome. So far three clinical syndromes have been found to be associated with trisomy of autosomal chromosomes. A few genetic disorders are related to some other aberrations of the autosomes and are described below.

1. Down's syndrome: This is frequently due to trisomy of the G group chromosome 21 arising from nondisjunction during meiosis in one of the parents. The karyotype thus shows 47 chromosomes. G trisomy is the most common of all autosomal trisomies.

Sometimes a translocation between a D group chromosome and 21, or between two G group chromosomes is associated with the syndrome. Some patients of Down's syndrome show mosaicism. Metaphase spreads of such patients show two cell lines in peripheral blood, one cell line with normal chromosomes, another with 21 trisomy.

About one in 700 births of both sexes could show Down's syndrome. The disorder is characterized by a typical mongoloid facial appearance, webbed neck, a flat nasal bridge, epicanthal fold (small folds of skin over inner corners of eye typical of the mongoloid race), brushfield spots around the iris, short fingers, and a gap between the first and second toe. Their striking feature is mental retardation with IQ ranging between 25 and 50 (normal average humans have an IQ of 80). Congenital heart disease and leukemia occur in many cases. Many have poor muscle tone during infancy. There is a higher incidence of Down's syndrome among children of older mothers. The patients live for a variable number of years. A Down's male is usually sterile, females are fertile and rarely have produced offspring. The dermatoglyphic pattern (arrangement of lines on palm and fingers) shows in many cases a line called simian crease and distal axial triradius. Frequently all the ten fingers show ulnar loops.

As in most genetic diseases there is no cure for a Down's patient. Affected individuals are usually institutionalized. However, after the birth of a Mongol child it is necessary for the parents to have proper genetic counseling to prevent the birth of another child with Mongolism. An accurate diagnosis through karyotype analysis of the affected child and both parents could provide an estimate of the recurrence risk. When mongolism is due to a translocation, the abnormality can be passed on to future generations through the gametes. A child that inherits the translocation is affected and could in turn produce victims of Down's syndrome. In contrast, Down's syndrome due to nondisjunction, which is a rare event during gametogenesis, is not familial and the condition is not inherited.

2. Edward's syndrome: Edward and his colleagues in 1960 described a syndrome due to trisomy of an E group chromosome (16-18) and occurring more often in females than in males. The individual may also be a mosaic having a normal cell line and an 18 trisomic line. The incidence is about 1 in 3,500 live births.

   The physical and mental growth is much retarded and death usually occurs in early childhood. Patients have hypertonicity of skeletal muscles resulting in a peculiar characteristics by which the affected person keeps the fingers tightly clenched against the palm of the hand. The typical features also include micrognathia (small jaws), deformed ears, small sternum and pelvis, a characteristic dermatoglyphic pattern and severe retardation.
3. Patau's syndrome: In 1960 Patau and his associates described a clinical disorder originating from trisomy D group chromosome (13-15). Most of the affected persons have a small head and abnormalities of the face, eyes and forebrain, cleft lip and palate, low set deformed ears, small chin, and the hands are often clenched in the manner described for Edward's syndrome. In general the individual appears more severely malformed than in the previous two syndromes and the mean life span is only about 4 months.
4. Cri du chat (cat cry) syndrome: An interesting abnormality in which the affected newborn cries in a manner resembling the mewing of a cat, was first described by Lejeune in 1963 in France, hence the same cri du chat (cat cry). A small head, widely spaced eyes,

receding chin and congenital heart disease are some other typical features. The condition is due to a deletion in the short arm of the B group chromosome 5, and is very rare.

5. Wolf syndrome: Another very rare syndrome is caused by a deletion in the short arm of a B group chromosome (No. 4). It is distinct from the cat cry syndrome.
6. The Philadelphia (Phl) chromosome: This is one the best known cases of a specific association between a chromosomal anomaly and a human disorder. The bone marrow cells of most of the patients with chronic granulocytic leukemia show a deletion of the long arm of a G group chromosome (No. 22) called Philadelphia or Phl chromosome. The banding technique has further revealed that a portion of the long arm of chromosome 22 is actually translocated to a longer chromosome.
7. Chromosome 13 and retinoblastoma: A deletion in the long arm of chromosome 13 is specifically associated with retinoblastoma, an autosomal dominant trait.

Both numeric and structural abnormalities of autosomes account for a variety of syndromes usually characterized by mental deficiencies. A few are associated with a group of characteristics that clearly indicate the precise chromosome anomaly. The first and the most common disorder in which an associated chromosome abnormality was demonstrated is Down syndrome. The most viable trisomies are trisomy 21 (Down syndrome), trisomy 18 (Edward syndrome), and trisomy 13 (Patau). Nurses often note dysmorphic facial features, behavioral characteristics such as an unusual cry and poor feeding behavior, and other neurologic manifestation such as hypotonia or abnormal reflex responses, which may alert them to these and other chromosome abnormalities.

Partial chromosome abnormalities involve a missing (deletion) or extra (duplication) segment of a chromosome. The features of classic deletion and contiguous gene (microdeletion and microduplication) syndromes are usually less recognizable at birth. Phenotypic effects of these syndromes may include a cluster of known single-gene disorders. The ***classic deletion syndromes*** can be detected on a routine chromosome analysis and include cri du chat (Table 5.2), Wolf-Hirschhorn, and chromosome 18 deletions. ***Contiguous gene syndromes*** are disorders characterized by a microdeletion or microduplication of smaller chromosome segments, which may require special analysis techniques or molecular testing to detect. Microdeletion syndromes are more common and may have more clinically obvious phenotypic effects than microduplication syndromes. Examples of these syndromes include Prader-Willi, Angelman, DiGeorge, and Beckwith-Wiedemann.

B. SEX CHROMOSOME ABNORMALITIES

The possible mechanisms by which sex chromosome abnormalities may occur are the same as those previously described (i.e. prefertilization nondisjunction during one the meiotic divisions of gametogenesis in either parent or in the early postfertilization divisions of the zygote). An alteration in the number of sex chromosomes usually does not produce the profound effects that are associated with the autosomal trisomies. Intelligence may be normal or low-normal, or the child may have some learning disabilities, but moderate or severe mental retardation is less common.

1. ***Turner syndrome*** (45, X) is essentially the only viable monosomy. It is still extremely lethal prenatally, with 99 percent of these fetuses being spontaneously aborted. Most girls have one + X chromosome missing from all cells (45, X). Some have mosaic cell lines with some cells 45, X and others 46, XX. The syndrome should be suspected in the

Table 5-2: Common autosomal aberrations			
Syndrome	*Chromosome abnormality and nomenclature*	*Average incidence (Live birth)*	*Major clinical manifestations*
Cri du chat	Deletion of short arm of No.5 chromosome—56, XY, 5p –	1:50,000	Distinctive weak, high-pitched, mewlike cry resembling the cry of a cat; small head; hypertelorism, failure to thrive; severe mental retardation—profound with age
Trisomy 13 (Patau)	Trisomy of No. 13 chromosome—47, XY, +13	1:4000-15,000	Cleft lip and palate (frequently bilateral); ear malformations; microphthalmia; polydactyly; eye defects; cardiac defects; mental retardation; early death
Trisomy 18 (Edward)	Trisomy of No. 18 chromosome—47, XY, +18	1:3500-8000	Deformed and low-set ears; micrognathia; rocker-bottom feet; overlapping (index over third) fingers; prominent occiput; hyper-telorism; cardiac defects; mental retardation; failure to thrive; early death
Trisomy 21 (Down)	Trisomy of No. 21 chromosome—47, XY, +21 (trisomy); 46, XY, + (14:21) (translocation); 46, XY/47, XY, +21 (mosaic.	1:700+	Brachycephaly with flat occiput; inner epicanthal folds; small ears, nose and mouth with protruding tongue; muscular hypotonia; broad, short hands with stubby fingers and transverse palmar crease; broad, stubby feet with wide space between big and second toes; cardiac defects; mental retardation; variable life expectancy

newborn period by the presence of lymphedema of the hands and feet and a low posterior hairline, in childhood by a webbed neck and short stature, and at puberty by delayed development and primary amenorrhea (Tables 5.2 and 5.3). The reason for the growth retardation is unknown. The child's growth is usually normal until 3 years of age and then slows, gradually drifting away from the normal growth curve. There is no prepubertal growth spurt, and girls with Turner syndrome are generally infertile. These girls may have difficulty with peer relationship and with understanding social cues. They may exhibit behavioral problems, especially in relation to immature, socially isolated behavior. Most, however, lead productive lives and function as independent adults.

2. ***Klinefelter syndrome,*** the most common of all sex chromosome abnormalities, is caused by the presence of one or more additional X chromosomes. The majority of males with this syndrome have a chromosome complement of 47, XXY, but there are numerous variants in the number of extra sex chromosomes. There are no distinctive physical characteristics that are helpful in detecting Klinefelter syndrome before the advent of puberty. Mental impairment of varying degrees is a frequent finding and appears to have a direct relationship to the number of X chromosomes in the cells. The severity of retardation increases with the number of X chromosomes. Characteristic features of the Klinefelter syndrome are listed in Table 5.3.

   The milder physical and mental deficiencies of children with sex chromosomes abnormalities compared with children with autosomal abnormalities are due in part to a phenomenon called *X inactivation or Lyon hypothesis.* In all body cells one X

Table 5-3: Common sex chromosome abnormalities				
Syndrome	*Chromosome nomenclature*	*Phenotype*	*Occurrence*	*Clinical manifestations*
Turner	45, X	Female	1:2500 female births	Short stature; webbed neck' low posterior hairline; shield-shaped chest with widely spaced nipples; usually infertile
Triple X	47, XXX (can also be 48,XXXX or49,XXXXX.	Female	1:850-1250 female births	Normal female characteristic; usually tall; variable mental capacity and behavior, at risk for impaired language, neuromotor problems, learning skills and psychosocial adaptation; fertile
Klinefelter	47, XXY (48,XXYY 48,XXXY, 49,XXXXY and so on, mosaics)	Male	1:850 male births	Tall with long legs; hypogenitalism; sterile; male secondary sex characteristics may be deficient; gynecomastia (30%); poor psychosocial adjustment
XYZ male	47, XXY (can also be 48,XYYY or mosaic)	Male	1:900 male births	Usually normal sex development; tendency to be tall with long head; poor coordination; may demonstrate poor impulse control; at risk for learning disabilities

chromosomes is biologically active; if more than one X chromosome is present, most (but not all, as previously thought) of the other (s) are in some way "switched off", or inactivated, during the very early divisions of the zygote and remain so throughout life. Because of the milder effects of sex chromosomes abnormalities, many individuals are phenotypically normal and may remain undiagnosed. Sex chromosomes mosaicism occurs, which also accounts for some variation in phenotype. The aberrant social behavior described as typical of multiple-Y chromosome abnormalities is thought to have been exaggerated and is more limited to poor impulse control, hyperactivity, and learning disability.

Multiples of the X and Y chromosomes exist, in trisomic or greater numbers (see Table 5.3). Regardless of the number of X chromosomes, the presence of a Y chromosome appears to be a male determining factor. Therapy of sex chromosome disorders consists primarily of hormone treatment to initiate appropriate pubertal sexual development. Growth hormone therapy may be used in girls with Turner syndrome to increase growth velocity and, hopefully, final height.

In 1942 Klinefelter described this condition in phenotypic males which turned out to be due to an extra X chromosome (47, XXY). The affected individuals appear normal in childhood, the abnormalities becoming visible only in adult males. The syndrome is characterized by absence of spermatogenesis, gynecomastia, and excessive secretion of gonadotropins in the urine. Since smears of Klinefelter's males show Barr bodies, they are referred to as chromatin-positive males. Most of the patients are mentally retarded and develop a variety of psychiatric problems. Although many have the karyotype 47, XXY, some may have 48, XXXY, 49, XXXXY, or 48, XXYY, or they may be cytogenetic mosaics.

3. ***The XYY male:*** In 1965 Jacobs et al found that many of the men kept in institutions for the retarded due to aggressive and antisocial behavior have 47 chromosomes with XYY sex chromosomes. They are usually tall but not always mentally retarded, frequently show hypogonadism and are sterile. The presence of two Y chromosomes can be recognized as two brightly fluorescent bodies by proper staining. The discovery of this syndrome received publicity because of the possible association of a chromosome anomaly with human behavior.

4. ***The triple-X syndrome:*** These are individuals with 3X chromosome designated superfemales. They are mentally retarded, sexually normal and fertile. Although most triple-X females have 47, XXX karyotype, some may have 48, XXXX, 49, XXXX, and still others may be mosaics. They show 2, 3 or 4 Barr bodies in their buccal smears (always one Barr body less than the total number of X's).

5. ***Intersex:*** Individuals with both male and female gonadal tissues are called hermaphrodites (from Greek Hermaphrodites, the son of Hermes and Aphrodite). Their karyotype analysis shows that they are mosaics having both X and Y chromosomes in their cell lines. Their buccal smears may or may not show a Barr body. Their external genitalia are often ambiguous, and they are almost sterile.

The condition of pseudohermaphroditism is also included among intersexes. Such individuals are cytogenetically normal with 46, XY (male pseudohermaphrodites) or 46, XX (female pseudohermaphrodites) chromosomes and normal buccal smears for one sex only. But phenol-typically they show both male and female characters. There are two classes. Male pseudohermaphrodites that have testes and either ambiguous or female-like external genitalia. The female pseudohermaphrodites have ovaries and either ambiguous or male like external genitalia. The pseudohermaphrodites have some defect in the biosynthesis of testosterone in the testes or in the adrenal glands or in both.

C. CHROMOSOMES AND SPONTANEOUS ABORTIONS

About 15 percent of all human pregnancies terminate before the 22nd week by spontaneous abortion. A study of aborted fetuses by D.H. Carr (1967, 1971) has shown that 5-6 percent of abortions are due to chromosomal aberrations. Triploidy is frequently observed in aborted fetuses. In fact the first cases of triploidy in humans were discovered from two aborted fetuses by Penrose and Delhanty in 1961. A characteristic clinical feature of triploid abortions is the hydatidiform mole of the placenta. Trisomy is also very common in abortuses. Trisomy for all the 22 autosomal pairs has been observed in abortuses. The most frequent however is trisomy 16. The XO constitution is common in abortuses, and unbalanced translocations are also observed.

D. CHROMOSOMES IN DISORDERS WITH DNA REPAIR DEFECTS

There are four inherited disorders with DNA repair defects which show chromosomal anomalies. The affected persons are also predisposed to cancer. The most well-studied is Xeroderma pigmentosum (XP described elsewhere). This is characterized by defects in repair of DNA lesions caused by UV rays and other mutagens. The patients often develop skin cancers. In Bloom's syndrome (BS) there is slow rate of DNA chain maturation during replication. Patients are sensitive to sun's rays and retarded in growth. Their cultured cells show an increased frequency of sister chromatid exchanges. In ataxia telangiectasia (AT) the cells are not able to repair damage caused to bases in DNA by gamma rays. Fanconi's anemia (FA) affects bone marrow cells. There is faulty repair of cross links in DNA. In all the 4 disorders the cultured cells show one or the chromosomal abnormality.

Single-Gene (Monogenic) Disorders

Disorders that are the result of a defect or mutation of a single rather than a partial or whole chromosome abnormality, are called single-gene disorders. These disorders, which generally follow a simple, definite inheritance pattern, are rare individually, but collectively they constitute a significant portion of health problems seen in infants and children. They can involve any system in the body. They can be of such minor importance that they have little effect on the child or be so severe as to cause serious disability or to be incompatible with life.

The defective or mutated gene cannot be diagnosed by chromosome analysis, because it is at a more basic level of the chromosome, that of the DNA structure. These disease producing mutant genes are usually distributed or transmitted in families according to basic Mendelian principles of dominant or recessive behavior on the autosomes or sex chromosomes (usually the X chromosomes). Some generalizations can be applied to dominant and recessive inheritance patterns of the autosomes or sex chromosomes and the resultant diseases and malformations.

A number of variables are observed in many disorders that modify the basic inheritance patterns. In addition, there are genetic phenomena that are not explained by traditional Mendelian inheritance. These variations and concepts are discussed following presentations of traditional autosomal dominant, recessive, and sex chromosome X-linked patterns.

Autosomal Inheritance Patterns

Autosomal dominant inheritance: Children with an autosomal dominant disorder have usually inherited it from an affected parent, although the parent's care may have been mild and undetected (Fig. 5.1). When a first case in a family appears, it is usually as a result of a new mutation. It is being recognized, however, that in rare cases, especially when a second affected child is born, one parent could have germline mosaicism (i.e. the gene mutation for a disorder is only present in the egg or sperm cells). Depending on the degree of disability the condition imposes on the individual and the age of onset, the gene will either die out or continue to be passed on through several generations. For example,

		Affected parent	
	Gametes		a
Normal parent	a	a Affected	a a Normal
	a	a Affected	a a Normal

Fig. 5.1: Possible offspring of mating between normal parents and one heterozygous for an autosomal dominant trait

Huntington disease, a progressive incapacitating and fatal neuromuscular disease, is usually not manifested until age 40 or later, after the affected person may have passed on the defective gene to offspring. Incomplete penetrance of autosomal dominant disorders is common, and there is wide variability in expression. Regardless of penetrance or variable expression in the parent, there is a 50 percent risk of passing on the defective gene to offspring, where it may be fully expressed. Other examples of autosomal dominant disorders include achondroplasia, neurofibromatosis, and Marfan syndrome.

Characteristics of Autosomal Dominant Inheritance includes in following:

1. Males and females are affected with equal frequency
2. Affected individuals will have an affected parent, although expression may be variable (unless the condition is caused by a new mutation or germline mosaicism)
3. Children of a heterozygous affected parent have a 50 percent probability of possessing the defective gene, although it may be nonpenetrant.
4. Children of affected parents who did not receive the affected gene will have unaffected children.
5. Traits can be traced vertically through previous generations—a positive family history—unless it is new mutation, germline mosaicism, or nonpenetrant.
6. Autosomal dominant disorders are more common than recessive disorders and are usually less severe.

Autosomal recessive inheritance: Children who display an autosomal recessive disorder will always be homozygous for that trait. The heterozygous person, with only one gene for a rare recessive disorder, remains undetected in the population (Fig. 5.2). It is estimated that each person carries from three to eight genes for a severe genetic disease. For example 1 in 20 persons in the US and Northern European populations carry the recessive gene for cystic fibrosis. In the African-American population, 1 in 10 persons is a carrier for the sickle cell gene. For Phenylketonuria the general population carrier rate is 1 in 50. However, the probability of the mating of two persons who carry the same gene is highly unlikely. The chances are increased if the mating occurs in persons who select a mate because of geographic, ethnic, or religious restrictions or blood relationship. For example, 1 in 30 Ashkenazi Jews is a carrier of the Tay-Sachs disease gene. The age of onset for autosomal recessive disorders is early, and, because they are usually biochemical defects, heterozygote detection and prenatal diagnosis are often possible. Other examples of autosomal recessive disorders include the thalassemias, congenital adrenal hyperplasia, glactosemia, and cystic fibrosis.

		Heterozygous parent A/a	
	Gametes	A	
Heterozygous parent A/a	A	AA Normal	A Carrier
		A Carrier	Affected

Fig. 5.2: Possible offspring of mating between two parents with a recessive gene on an autosomes

Characteristics of autosomal recessive inheritance as shown below:

1. Males and females are affected with equal frequency.
2. Affected individuals will have unaffected parents who are heterozygous for the trait.
3. There is a 1 in 4 (25%) chance that any child of two unaffected heterozygous parents will be affected.
4. Unaffected siblings of an affected person have a 2/3 risk of being a carrier.
5. Affected individuals mated to normal individual will have normal children, all of whom will be carriers.
6. There is usually no evidence of the trait in previous generations—a negative family history—unless consanguinity.

X-linked Inheritance Patterns

Genes on the X chromosome differ from those on the Y chromosome; therefore the transmission of traits caused by these genes will vary according to the sex of the individual who carries the gene. The two X chromosomes in the female are alike in gene constitution, with two genes for each trait. Genes on the X chromosome have no counterpart on the Y chromosome; therefore a characteristic determined by a gene on the X chromosome is always expressed in the male. One of the most significant aspects of X-linked inheritance is the absence of father-to-son transmission. Although it is essential for development of the male phenotype, the Y chromosome carries no known medically significant characteristics.

X-linked Dominant Inheritance: Superficially this pattern resembles an autosomal dominant inheritance pattern (Fig. 5.3). This type of inheritance is relatively uncommon. An example of an X-linked dominant disorder is hypophosphatemic vitamin-D resistant rickets. The inheritance pattern of fragile X syndrome and may not follow the standard X-linked pattern.

Characteristics of x-linked dominant inheritance as given below:

1. Affected individuals will have an affected parent.
2. All the daughters but none of the sons of an affected male have the probability of being affected (although usually more mildly).
3. Half the sons and the half the daughters of an affected female will be affected.
4. Normal children of an affected parent will have normal offspring.
5. There are no carriers (although expression may vary).
6. The inheritance pattern shows a positive family history.

		Normal mother	
	Gametes	X	X
Affected father	Y	YX Affected daughter	YX Affected daughter
	Y	XY Normal son	XY Normal son

		Normal mother	
	Gametes	X	X
Normal father	Y	YX Affected daughter	XX Normal daughter
	Y	YY Affected son	XY Normal son

Fig 5.3: Sex difference in offspring ratios in X-linked dominant inheritance. Solid circle. Dominant allele on X chromosome

	Gametes	Normal mother X	Normal mother X
Affected father	Y	XY Carrier daughter	XY Carrier daughter
Affected father	Y	XY Normal son	XY Normal son

	Gametes	Carrier mother X	Carrier mother Y
Normal father	X	XX Normal daughter	YX Carrier daughter
Normal father	Y	XY Normal son	YY Affected son

Fig. 5.4: Sex difference in offspring ratios in X-linked recessive inheritance. Open circle. Recessive allele on X chromosome

X-linked Recessive Inheritance: The abnormal gene behaves as any recessive gene would; that is, its effect is hidden by a normal dominant gene. Therefore, two recessive genes are usually present if manifestations in the female are seen (Fig. 5.4). This rare situation would be a carrier. However, unequal X inactivation can also produce manifestations in a carrier female. New mutations are not uncommon. Examples of X-linked recessive disorders include hemophilia types A and B and Duchenne muscular dystrophy.

Characteristics of X-linked recessive inheritance

1. Affected individuals are principally males.
2. Affected individuals will have unaffected parents (except in the rare possibility that the father is affected and the mother is a carrier).
3. Half the female siblings of an affected male have the probability of being carriers of the trait.
4. Unaffected male siblings of an affected male cannot transmit the disorder.
5. Sons of an affected male are unaffected.
6. Daughters of an affected male are carriers.
7. The unaffected male children of a carrier female do not transmit the disorder.

Gene Variation and Nontraditional Inheritance

A number of variables have been observed that explain or modify basic inheritance patterns and the effects of chromosome abnormalities. Some of these variations have been recognized for some time; others are newly discovered phenomena that explain some apparent contradictions in the established patterns of inheritance. Some of the variations involve individual genes, and others involve whole-chromosome behavior but will still affect manifestations of single-gene disorders. Also, some disorders have been reported to follow more than one inheritance pattern in different families (e.g. a classifically recessive disorder may occasionally be reported as following a dominant or X-linked pattern in other families).

The most notable of these gene variations is mutation. A mutation is any heritable change in the DNA sequence of a gene. Mutation can be a deletion, duplication, or alteration in the base pair sequence. A mutation may cause the protein made by that gene to be produced in an altered, less functional form; to be produced in a decreased amount; or to be entirely absent. A gene mutation may have occurred generations ago and be passed down unchanged until it dies out because an individual does not reproduce, or a new gene mutation, such as the mutation that causes fragile X syndrome, and new mutations are seldom if ever identified. Other diseases are known to have a high new mutation rate, such as the 30 to 50 percent rate for neurofibromatosis and Duchenne muscular dystrophy. This type of definitive determination of a gene mutation is possible only for those single-gene disorders in which the gene site has been located and characterized. Some disorders previously described as exhibiting sporadic occurrence (e.g. Williams syndrome) not attributable to a traditional inheritance pattern may be new mutations with effects such that the individual does not reproduce and the mutation is not passed on to offspring.

Variable expression is an important concept that describes differences in the extent and severity of manifestations of genetic diseases. There is a continuum of expression for any affected person from undetectable (mild) to severe clinical manifestation. Therefore a phenotypically normal person may still possess the mutant gene. This situation most often applies to autosomal dominant disorders; for example, a parent of a child with neurofibromatosis may exhibit only a couple of café-au-lait spots. Genomic imprinting and X-inactivation, discussed later in this section, may account for some variation in expression and penetrance; a term used less often as these new discoveries explain in phenotypic manifestations.

The discovery of a new type of mutation in some genetic disorders has helped explain their variation in inheritance patterns and clinical expression. Within genes are sequences of DNA nucleotide repeats. A normal gene has a certain number of these repeats; for example, in the fragile X syndrome gene there are about 30 to 50 repeats. Some persons, however, have additional repeats of from 50 to 200, which have been termed permutations. These permutations in females are unstable and during meiosis can undergo amplifications, expanding to hundreds more repeats, thereby becoming a full mutation and causing the offspring to be affected. Because fragile X is an X-linked disorder, females are less likely to be affected because of the tempering effect of the second X chromosome. These expanding repeats have also been found to occur in myotonic dystrophy, Huntington disease, and spinocerebellar ataxia, which are autosomally transmitted disorders. This expanding gene discovery exhibits the old concept of genetic anticipation, in which certain dominantly inherited disorders tend to worsen or have an earlier age of onset with succeeding generations. It is believed that additional disorders may be discovered to exhibit this type of mutation. In fact, the first recessively inherited disorder to exhibit an expansion mutation is Friedreich ataxia. This disorder usually demonstrates an onset in puberty or early adulthood, depending on the repeat size of the smaller of the two expansion alleles. Recent evidence suggests genetic anticipation may be a factor for the presence of father-son testicular tumors.

Genomic imprinting and uniparental disomy are two genetic phenomena that consider the parental origin of genetic information (i.e. maternally or paternally derived). The concept of genomic imprinting refers to modification, in some instances, of genetic material, resulting in phenotypic differences based on whether the genes/chromosomes were from the mother or the father. Genomic imprinting is exhibited during pregnancy, when paternally derived chromosomes seem to positively influence placental development and maternally derived chromosomes seem to positively influence fetal development. It has also been shown to be a factor in some genetic disorders, most classifically Prader-Willi and Angelman syndromes. In both of these disorders, about two-thirds of affected individuals have a deletion of the same segment of chromosome 15. However, the clinical manifestation of Prader-Willi and Angelman syndromes are markedly different. If the deletion occurs on the paternally derived chromosome 15, the child exhibits Prader-Willi syndrome; if the deletion occurs on the maternally derived chromosome 15, Angelman syndrome is manifested.

Prader-Willi syndrome is characterized by central hypotonia, cognitive dysfunction, dysmorphic appearance, behavioral disturbances, hypothalamic hypogonadism, short stature and obesity, as well as abnormal low body temperature, and increased tolerance to pain, and diminished salivation. In contrast, Angelman syndrome (also called happy puppet syndrome) includes severe mental retardation, characteristic facies, abnormal (puppet like) gait, and paroxysms of inappropriate laughter. Children with Angelman syndrome are usually nonverbal, although they may vocalize.

In some cases both copies of a chromosome pair are determined to have come from one parent, either the mother or the father, instead of one from each, a phenomenon called *uniparental disomy*. Another example of uniparental disomy has been reported with cystic fibrosis, in which both chromosomes, each with a mutant recessive gene, came from the carrier mother; the father was not a carrier. In cases that appear to be nonpaternity, uniparental disomy may be a factor. One of the several theories about uniparental disomy is that the chromosome pair was originally a trisomy and the father's chromosome was randomly expelled, leaving two copies of the mother's chromosome. Because the chromosomes appear as a normal "pair", diagnosis of this situation is only possible with molecular (DNA) techniques. Uniparental disomy has also been reported with Beckwith-Wiedemann syndrome, which is characterized by overgrowth and hypoglycemia at birth.

Mitochondrial Disorders

Mitochondrial DNA mutations also account for nontraditional inheritance patterns. Mitochondria are components of the cell cytoplasm involved in energy production.

They perform many different functions in different tissues of the body. They are the only cellular organelles to have their own DNA distinct from nDNA and inheritance is exclusively maternal. A defect in the mtDNA can lead to altered functions of the proteins in some or all of the cells. Because the mitochondria perform so many different functions in the body, when a mutation has occurred, the spectrum of symptoms is enormous. Individuals with the same mtDNA mutation may be symptom-free or severely affected with seizures, pancreatitis, and metabolic disease. Even within the same family, different manifestations of the mitochondrial condition are seen. Mutations may be inherited or occur spontaneously. It is now believed that mitochondria are responsible not only for diseases occurring in childhood, such as Leigh disease (with symptoms of hypotonia, seizures, and failure to thrive), but they can be responsible for many common diseases associated with aging such as diabetes, parkinsonism, and dementia. Because there is such variability of expression with mitochondrial disorders, it can be very confusing to determine the diagnosis. However, when a child has an unexplained constellation of symptoms, a mitochondrial disorder should be considered.

Diagnosis of a mitochondrial disorder can be very difficult and therefore genetic counseling may be possible only in a small number of cases. Nuclear DNA mutations can also cause disorders of the mitochondria, and, with the advances in the detection of nDNA mutations, accurate diagnosis and therefore accurate information about recurrence risk and prenatal diagnosis is possible. Currently, treatment for these disorders is symptomatic and some patients show benefits from vitamin and cofactor supplementation. Referral to mitochondrial support groups can be very helpful to parents.

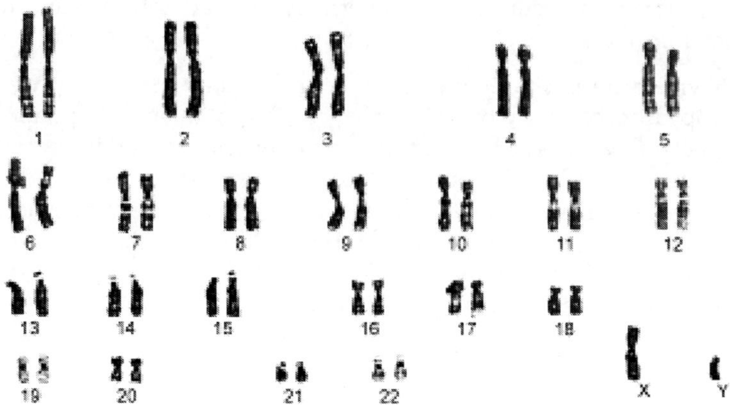

Fig. 5.5: Normal male karyotype

Cytogenetic and Molecular Genetic Diagnosis

Cytogenetic Diagnostic Techniques

Chromosome analysis by karyotyping, a pictorial representation of the chromosomes matched by size and banding patterns into pairs from 1 to 22 (the twenty-third pair are the sex chromosomes) is the basis of genetic diagnosis (Fig. 5.5). Numeric and structural abnormalities such as Trisomies and translocations are easily seen on chromosome analysis. The most common human cells used to analyze the chromosomes are skin tissue (including fetal skin cells), bone marrow and, most frequently, blood leukocytes obtained by venipuncture. The chromosomes are cultured and examined during mitosis, when they are most visible. Deletions, duplications, and translocations of larger segments of genetic material are visible on routine chromosome analysis. However, microdeletions, microduplication, and fragile sites usually require newer, enhanced resolution techniques that essentially "stretch out" the chromosome, thereby allowing detection of more subtle defects. Another new technique that has enhanced diagnosis of these subtle defects is ***fluorescence in situ hybridization (FISH),*** which uses radioactive or fluorescent probes in a variety of ways to identify chromosome and DNA abnormalities such as Williams and Prader-Willi syndromes.

Molecular Diagnostic Techniques

Diagnosis of genetic disorders at the gene level has experienced remarkable advances in technique. Identification of single-gene mutations responsible for some genetic disorders is now possible as more and more genes are being mapped (located on a specific chromosomes or segment of a chromosome) through efforts as part of the Human Genome Project. In some conditions, such as cystic fibrosis (CF), sickle cell disease, Huntington disease, and fragile X syndrome, the specific gene/DNA mutations are known and can be detected directly. For other disorders, while the exact gene location is not known, the particular chromosome and specific segment are known. By using "linkage" studies and mapping techniques, the likelihood that an individual has inherited the same chromosome segment as a known affected member of the family can be determined. Use of these techniques allows not only diagnosis of an affected individual but also determination of carrier status and prenatal diagnosis (i.e. whether a fetus is normal, a carrier, or affected). There are over 200 diseases that can be diagnosed by direct or indirect (linkage) DNA testing. DNA testing "enabling" technologies include Southern blotting and polymerase chain reaction (PCR) as the most common methods. Each method has advantages and disadvantages and is chosen depending on the characteristics of the mutation being tested.

Disorders Detected by DNA Based Testing

Achondroplasia
Apert syndrome
Becker muscular dystrophy
Congenital adrenal hyperplasia
Crouzon syndrome
Cystic fibrosis
Duchenne muscular dystrophy
Fragile X syndrome
Friedreich ataxia
Gaucher disease
Hemophilia A (factor VIII deficiency)
Hemophilia B (factor IX deficiency)
Huntington disease
Lesch-Nyhan syndrome
Maple syrup urine disease
Marfan syndrome
Myotonic dystrophy
Neurofibromatosis type I
Osteogenesis imperfecta
Phenylketonuria (PKU)
Sickle cell disease
Spinal muscular atrophy
Spinocerebellar ataxia
Tay-Sachs disease
Thalassemias (alpha and beta)
Tuberous sclerosis

Multifactorial Disorders

A number of diseases and defects that are encountered frequently in the population show an increased incidence in some families but have no clear cut affected unaffected classification. Although the incidence is higher than would be expected by chance, no specific mode of inheritance can be identified. In some, environmental appear to play an important role. These conditions are classified as multifactorial disorders, in which a genetic susceptibility and appropriate environmental agents interact to produce a disease state. Diseases considered to be multifactorial at least in isolation) include neural tube defects, cleft lip and cleft palate, many congenital heart defects, congenital hip dislocation, and pyloric stenosis. Determining risks of recurrence is more difficult than for single-gene disorders, but the risk is usually low, less than 10 percent. For example, anencephaly and/or spina bifida occur in 0.2 to 5 births per 1000 in the general population. The recurrence risk after the first affected child is 3 to 6 percent. Advances in genetics are enhancing knowledge of multifactorial inheritance to better understand familial risks.

Disorders of the Intrauterine Environment

The prenatal intrauterine environment can have a profound and permanent effect on a developing fetus, even when chromosome or single-gene abnormalities are not present. Sometimes, however, intrauterine effects occur in tandem with genetic factors. Intrauterine growth retardation (IUGR), for example, can occur with many genetic syndromes, such as Down, Russell-Silver, Prader-Willi, and Turner syndromes, or can occur from nongenetic causes such as maternal alcohol ingestion. Placental abnormalities are increasingly being found to be the etiologic factor in neurodevelopmental disorders (such as cerebral palsy and mental retardation) that were previously attributed to asphyxia during delivery.

Teratogens, agents that cause birth defects when present in the prenatal environment, account for the majority of adverse intrauterine effects not attributable to genetic factors. Types of teratogens include drugs (phenytoin [Dilantin], warfarin [Coumadin], tretinoin [Accutane]); chemicals (ethyl alcohol, cocaine, lead); infectious agents (rubella, cytomegalovirus); physical agents (maternal hyperthermia); and metabolic agents (maternal phenylketonuria). Many of these teratogen exposures and the resulting effects are completely preventable, such as ingestion of alcohol resulting in fetal alcohol syndrome/ fetal alcohol effects (FAS/FAE), which causes severe birth defects including mental retardation. The incidence of FAS is estimated at 5.2 per 10,000 live births.

Management of Genetic Disease

There is no cure for genetic disease at present, although preventive and corrective therapy is helping to reduce the harmful effects in an increasing number of conditions. Genetic research is making progress in the art of altering the genetic material directly. Meanwhile, the major goal of therapy is modification of the internal or external environment to correct or minimize the effects of the genetic defect.

Therapeutic Modalities

The therapeutic modalities available for genetic disorders are few when compared with the infinite variety of conditions affecting the population, but with increased understanding of the basic defects and the technical advances being made, an increasing number of genetic disorders are becoming amenable to treatment.

Surgical repair. Surgical repair of structural defects has made it possible to prolong life in a number of multifactorial disorders, such as congenital heart disease and pyloric stenosis. Numerous facial and limb deformities can be altered by plastic and reconstructive techniques. In cases of familial polyposis coli, surgical removal of the colon eliminates the countless polyps that invariably become cancerous. Splenectomy prevents the trapping of abnormal blood cells in that organ in several hereditary disorders of red blood cells. Early diagnosis and enucleation in retinoblastoma have reduced the mortality from this malignant eye tumor.

Diet modification. For disorders in which an enzyme deficiency causes a toxic accumulation of a substance or its by-products, restricting the intake of foods containing the offending substance often prevents irreversible damage from the improper metabolism of these compounds, this dietary control is a life-long recommendation. Examples include the low-phenylalanine diet prescribed for children with Phenylketonuria (PKU), elimination of dairy products containing lactose for infants and children with hereditary lactase deficiency, avoidance of foods containing or producing galactose for children with galactosemia, and a diet low in branched-chain amino acids for infants and children with maple syrup urine disease. Women with PKU who have not maintained dietary control must reinstitute a strict low-phenylalanine diet before conception and maintain it throughout pregnancy to prevent a high risk of adverse fetal effects. Folic acid supplementation preconceptionally has been shown to reduce the incidence or recurrence of neural tube defects (NTDs).

Folic acid. Folic acid supplementation before conception can have a major impact in the prevention of NTDs. Therefore in 1992 the US Public Health Service made the recommendation that all women capable of becoming pregnant should consume 0.4 mg of folic acid per day. The food and drug administration mandated that as of 1998 folic acid would be added to enriched grain produces. This would add 0.1 mg folic acid to the daily diet of the average person. Since that time there has been a 19 percent reduction in the incidence of NTDs.

Women who have previously had a pregnancy affected with an NTD are advised to take 4.0 mg of folic acid per day beginning 1 month before conception and continuing throughout the first trimester of pregnancy. The risk of recurrence in another pregnancy affected by an NTD is reduced by 72 percent in women following this regimen.

Product replacement: In some deficiency diseases, supplying the missing product that cannot be synthesized prevents undesirable effects. For example, thyroid extract is prescribed to prevent the damaging effects of hypothyroidism and providing the missing blood factors prevents life-threatening and debilitating hemorrhage in persons with hemophilia. Other examples are insulin for diabetes mellitus, growth hormone for growth hormone deficiency, and corticosteroids for adrenogenital syndrome.

Avoidance of drugs or other substances: In drug induced disease, such as glucose-6-phosphate dehydrogenase deficiency and the porphyrias, avoidance of the drugs that precipitate a reaction provides a simple preventive measure.

Removal of toxic substances: Removal of toxic substances that accumulate in vital tissues as a result of a hereditary disease can prevent disabling complications. Some of the deleterious effects of hemochromatosis, a hereditary disorder characterized by an excess accumulation of iron in the liver, heart, and pancreas, can be reduced with the removal of iron by administration of chelating agents or periodic phlebotomies.

Immunologic prevention: The administration of immunoglobulin to Rh-negative mothers following the birth of an Rh-positive infant is effective in preventing Rh-antibody formation that causes hemolytic disease of the newborn in subsequent births.

Transplantation: Replacement of nonfunctioning organs with normal organs is increasing the survival of children with defective organs because the problems of tissue incompatibility are better controlled. Examples of organ transplants include the kidneys in hereditary polycystic kidneys, the heart in severe cardiac myopathy, the liver in hepatic atresia, and bone marrow.

Cofactor administration: Diet supplements can be given when the body is unable to synthesize or effectively use some substances needed as cofactors in metabolism, such as vitamin B, in pernicious anemia, in which absorption of this vitamin is absent. Vitamin and cofactor supplementation may be used in the treatment of mitochondrial disease.

Recombinant DNA: The transfer of modified genetic material from one organism (a virus) to another cause the viral DNA to become integrated into the cellular DNA of a recipient cell, often a bacteria cell. This recombinant DNA multiplies, producing the missing substance in the host cell. This technology has been applied in growth hormone therapy and factor VIII synthesis.

Gene transfer: Fragments of DNA from a normal gene can be introduced directly into a recipient cell lacking such a gene. This approach has been attempted in humans with the transfer of normal gene copies of β-hemoglobin into bone marrow cells in a effort to treat a form of β-thalassemia and has been used in sickle cell disease. Gene transfer has also been successfully used in adenosine deaminase deficiency. Gene therapy research has suffered a number of setbacks in clinical research, and the search for safer, more effective ways to transfer genes into human cells continues.

Other therapies: Other methods such as enzyme repression and competitive inhibition are providing effective treatment in some metabolic disorders. Growth hormone therapy is used in Turner and Noonan syndromes. Future therapies include the possibility of replacement or stabilization by injection or oral administration of a substance that the patient lacks.

Environmental Manipulation

Inherited disease or defects for which there is no therapeutic modality can be modified to enhance the quality of life for the affected individual. Some examples of environmental manipulation include hearing aids for deaf children, glasses or vision enhancers such as enlarged print and books in Braille for the visually impaired, mobilizing devices such as braces and wheelchairs for persons with muscle and bone impairment, prosthetic devices for limb deficiencies, and infant stimulation programs to maximize the potential of children who are mentally retarded.

Impact of Hereditary Disorders on the Family

Genetic Screening

Tests to detect the presence of a defective gene are rapidly assuming greater importance in management of genetic disorders as more defects are identified and techniques are developed for easy application. It is probable that with improved technology, mass screening for numerous defects may eventually be a routine procedure. However, to be truly effective, screening programs depend on thorough education of both health professionals and the public regarding these programs and the limitations and implications of testing. The religious, moral, ethical, and legal issues revolving around screening and prenatal diagnosis are extensive and change over time.

Purposes of Screening

Genetic screening is presumptive identification of an unrecognized genotype in individuals or populations. There are several purposes for this screening: (1) to detect the presence of apparent or nonapparent disease, (2) to provide reproductive information, and (3) to gain information concerning the incidence of a disorder in the population.

Newborn screening. Newborn screening began in the 1960s when Dr. Guthrie devised the blood spot test to screen for PKU. Newborn screening for PKU was begun in all states, and currently each state offers screening for a number of additional disorders such as sickle cell anemia, galactosemia, hypothyroidism, congenital adrenal hypoplasia, and others. The disorders selected for newborn screening have been chosen because they meet the following criteria:

- The disease occurs with a significant frequency
- An inexpensive and reliable method of testing exists
- There is effective treatment and intervention
- If untreated, the baby will die or be severely mentally retarded
- An affected baby may appear normal at birth.

Because many of the conditions tested for are metabolic disorders, it is important that the first newborn screening blood sample be obtained at least 24 hours after the first protein feeding or within the first 72 hours of life. Infants found to be at high risk for a metabolic condition such as PKU or galactosemia are immediately referred to a medical center for testing to confirm the diagnosis and initiate treatment. Mass screening programs have indicated that many disorders are more prevalent than formerly believed. Other that are included in some screening programs are congenital adrenal hyperplasia, maple syrup urine disease, sickle cell disease and other hemoglobinopathies, tyrosinemia, adenosine deaminase deficiency, and various other aminoacidurias and urea cycle disorders.

Newborn screening for CF has been controversial and is offered in only a few states. The Wisconsin Cystic Fibrosis Newborn Screening Project found that identification of affected newborns prevented severe malnutrition and improved long-term growth.

A number of technologies are available for detecting disease—biochemical assays, protein iontophoresis, chromosome analysis, and testing with DNA molecular probes. It is sometimes recommended that the DNA of an affected family members at a later date, such as in a subsequent pregnancy.

Screening for reproductive information: Screening for heterozygotes (carriers) can detect unaffected persons with certain genes who, when they mate with an individual who carriers a similar gene, are at high risk of producing an affected offspring. These individuals are thus provided with the knowledge they need for use in decisions about family planning. Carriers of a number of diseases can be detected by laboratory tests, but, because of the rarity of these diseases, mass screening is not feasible except in persons or populations known to be at risk. Persons at risk include close relatives of those with an inborn error of metabolism or other detectable disorder, as well as certain ethnic populations known to have a high incidence of a specific disease, such as sickle cell anemia in African-Americans, Tay-Sachs disease in Ashkenazi Jews, and thalassemia in people of Mediterranean ancestry.

This type of screening is sometimes controversial. Screening for carrier status for CF is one such situation that has the potential to create ethical dilemmas. CF is caused by a gene mutation, but there are numerous variations that cause the same phenotypic effect. Only 90 percent of these mutations are known, meaning that an individual with a CF-causing gene mutation would not be identified as a carrier 10 percent of the time. Therefore, following screening, a couple may feel safe to proceed with pregnancy yet still have a child with CF. Other possible dilemmas with carrier status screening include marriage partner selection bias based on carrier status and misunderstanding of the implications of carrier status (i.e. that individuals are not affected themselves and that there is only potential risk to offspring if the partner is also a carrier). Carrier or presymptomatic testing of children is generally not recommended or performed except in conditions such as familial adenomatous polyposis because the humerous intestinal polyps can become malignant during adolescence.

Careful counseling is necessary with carrier screening to ensure that individuals understand the limitations of testing and the implications of results. Even with careful counseling, there may be significant misunderstanding or misuse of information.

Presymptomatic testing for individuals at risk of an adult-onset disorder, such as Huntington disease, presents different, but equally weighty, dilemmas. Huntington disease is an autosomal dominant inherited disorder characterized by progressive neuromuscular deterioration and dementia, with eventual complete incapacitation and death. The age of onset is approximately 40 (±12 years) years of age—ironically, after childbearing occurs. Individuals with an affected parent have a theoretic 50 percent risk of eventually becoming symptomatic. The emotional threat for these individuals as they face an unknown future can be devastating. Now, through DNA testing, it can be determined with 98 percent accuracy whether they inherited the Huntington gene mutation. For some individuals, the chance that they would find out that they will develop this distressing condition is unbearable, like a delayed death sentence. They would rather not know. Others do want testing in the hope that the news will relieve them of the dread of the unknown and provide direction for their life whether the news if good or bad. Because testing is often of family groups, even those who receive good news may experience survivor guilt if another family member receives bad news. An equally devastating situation has occurred with the discovery of a gene defect that causes inherited breast cancer. Women in these cancer-prone families face an 85 percent risk of developing breast or ovarian cancer. The dread in some women who have had family members die can be so great that they will undergo a prophylactic mastectomy.

The economic consequences of carrier status screening and presymptomatic testing are also foreboding. Technologic advances have outstripped policy making; therefore discrimination in the workplace and in insurance coverage has occurred on the basis of screening and testing results. Many states are enacting legislation to prevent such discrimination, but the complexity has hampered effective statutes, and many issues remain unresolved. Maintaining confidentiality of tests results while knowing the possible consequences is an additional sobering burden.

Screening for epidemiologic information: Public health officials may use screening as a method for monitoring the incidence of diseases or malformations in a population in order to detect environmental or other causes that might significantly influence the incidence of the disorders. For example, geographic and socioeconomic variations in the incidence of NTDs eventually led to research that determined that folic acid supplementation of 0.4 mg per day in women of childbearing age reduces NTD occurrence by as much as 50 percent.

Significance of Screening to Families

Mass screening programs have received mixed acceptance from health professionals and the general public. The reasons for controversy include lack of knowledge on the part of health professionals about the testing purposes and implications of results, the public cost of testing (if government funded), and the psychologic implications of learning about carrier status. However, with the success of several well-organized or legislated programs and their significance in the prevention of disease or of the damaging effects of disease, an increasing number of programs are gaining acceptance and support.

Much of family concern regarding screening centers around the issues of informed consent and the use of screening information. Some states require written consent; some specify the tests to be performed; and some describe the risks, benefits, and the right to be informed of uncertain results, including the implications of an abnormal finding. Institutions may provide classes for families to explain the screening program, provide verbal explanation, or distribute written materials. In some areas exemptions from mandated screening are allowed in certain situations, such as objections on religious grounds if there is a conflict with religious practices and beliefs of an established church.

The nature and purposes of the procedure should be clearly explained to clients in language that they can understand. The issue of divulging unexpected findings is subject to debate. If a genetic trait is detected in a child but not in a parent (such as the sickle cell trait), the question of paternity may be raised. It is also important to help families understand the meaning of **false-positive** test results (indicates a problem exists when it does not) and **false-negative** test results (indicates a problem does not exist when it does).

Release of information to persons other than the family is also subject to debate. At present the reporting of genetic findings is not mandatory as it is for certain contagious diseases and it is questionable whether this would be desirable. A family may not wish for other family members or even the family practitioner to receive the results of screening. Knowledge of screening results by third parties may lead to insurance or employment discrimination. All of these possibilities should be made clear to families in order to provide them with some selective control.

The social stigma of being the carrier of a defective gene may be a side effect of screening. In some families such knowledge is a source of embarrassment and is damaging to the self-esteem of tis members. Teenagers are especially vulnerable to the effects of knowing they carry a specific defective gene at a time when identify formation and peer approval are extremely important. Cultural views regarding this knowledge can have profound effects on the members of some ethnic groups. In some cases, social status within the cultural group can be impaired.

Probably the most important area for nursing practice is teaching. Families need an understanding of why the screening is proposed, what the results mean, and how the family can interpret false-positive and false-negative results. Anxiety is greater when families have not received sufficient information about the screening or testing process and its significance for their health. The need for further testing, no matter what the reason, can be extremely stressful to families, and they also have a right to know who assumes the cost of additional testing or retesting—the family or the state. The nurse is a valuable resource in ensuring that families are aware of alternatives and in helping them make the best decision.

Prenatal Diagnosis

Advances in technology have greatly increased the spectrum and accuracy of prenatal detection of genetic diseases and defects. Prenatal testing provides the means to detect defects that are best corrected soon after delivery, conditions that may require preterm delivery for early correction, conditions that may require cesarean delivery, conditions that may require medical or surgical treatment before birth, and conditions on which a decision may be based to terminate a pregnancy. In addition, a very important benefit is that normal results provide peace of mind for the expectant family. However, even with normal prenatal test results, the birth of a healthy baby cannot be guaranteed.

A variety of techniques are available for diagnosing a number of diseases and defects in the fetus. Some procedures are considered screening tests, meaning that the tests only indicates a higher risk than expected in the general population or an age-dependent risk. Other methods are diagnostic tests, meaning that they determine with a high degree of accuracy the presence or absence of a birth defect or genetic disorder (Table 5.4). Risks of prenatal testing vary, depending on the procedure.

There is approximately a 2 to 3 percent risk of a major birth defect or genetic disorder with each pregnancy in the general population regardless of other risk factors such as age

Purpose	Advantages	Disadvantages	Risks
Triple Marker Screen (Also called trisomy profile screen)			
Screening test for NTDs, ventral wall defects, and trisomy pregnancies (e.g. Down syndrome	Identifies women at higher risk who otherwise would not receive diagnostic testing	Is not diagnostic; only indicates need for further testing.False-positive and false-negative results occur	Venipuncture Minimal risk
Ultrasonography			
Assess gestational age, fetal growth, placental sufficiency. Detects multiple gestation and structural anomalies Screening and diagnostic test	Detects structural anomalies and effects of intrauterine environment that may not be detected by chromosome analysis	Accuracy depends on skill of ultrasonographer, quality of equipment, and size of defect. Does not detect biochemical abnormalities	Noninvasive
Amniocentesis			
Chromosome analysis of fetal cells DNA analysis Alpha-fetoprotein (AFP) analysis, other biochemical analyses	Diagnostic for chromosome abnormalities. Provides DNA for direct and indirect testing for single-gene disorders. High accuracy for detection of NTDs using biochemical analysis	Does not detect structural anomalies not caused by chromosome abnormalities except for neural tube or ventral wall defects (VWDs). Usually not performed until second trimester (14-16 weeks). Results are usually available in 1-3 weeks. Relatively expensive	Invasive ½% risk of spontaneous abortion. Nongrowth of fetal cells requires repeat procedure
Chorionic Villus Sampling (CVS)			
Chromosome analysis of chorionic (fetal) cells DNA analysis	Diagnostic for chromosome abnormalities. Provides DNA for direct and indirect testing for single-gene disorders. Test is done earlier than amniocentesis (9-12 weeks); therefore results are available earlier	Diagnostic accuracy may be less because of greater risk of maternal cell contamination and false evidence of mosaicism, which may require subsequent amniocentesis Does not detect structural anomalies. Relatively expensive. Less available than amniocentesis	Invasive. Risk of spontaneous abortion 1-2%. Controversial evidence of limb-reduction defects

Table 5.4: Types of prenatal genetic testing

or family history. Prenatal diagnostic testing of the general pregnant population is not justified because of the risks, cost, and specificity of diagnostic procedures. Certain general and specific risk factors determine those for whom diagnostic testing, such as amniocentesis, is indicated. Relatively inexpensive and safe screening tests, such as routine ultrasound and maternal serum Trisomy Profile Screen for the remaining population will determine those for whom diagnostic testing is advisable.

Prenatal screening tests: The maternal triple marker ***Trisomy Profile Screen*** blood test is a prenatal screening test offered to all pregnant women under the age of 35 and is performed between 15 to 21 weeks of pregnancy. Three chemicals, alpha-fetoprotein (AFP), human chorionic gonadotropins (hCG), and unconjugated estriol (uE3), are synthesized in the fetal liver or yolk sac. By diffusion across the placenta and amnion, these proteins are present in the maternal circulation. The levels can be measured from a blood sample and compared with the norms for that point in gestation.

Neural tube defects (NTDs) such as anencephaly and spina bifida and ventral wall defects (VWDs) such as gastroschisis and omphalocele are associated with exposed fetal membrane and blood vessel surfaces that increase the maternal blood. Therefore an elevated AFP level may indicate an increased risk for an elevated neural tube defect (NTD).

The Trisomy Profile Screen can also detect an increased risk for Down syndrome, which may be present when the AFP and uE3 levels are lower and the hCG is elevated.

Certain factors other than NTDs or Down syndrome can cause an abnormal triple marker screening level, such as multiple gestation, incorrectly estimated gestational age, fetal hemorrhage, fetal death, placental abnormalities, or normal variation in the level of protein in the blood. Other factors affecting results that may require correction include maternal diabetes, race, and weight. Further diagnostic testing is indicated for abnormal results that cannot be attributed to any of these factors.

Ultrasonography can also be a screening or diagnostic technique, depending on the sophistication of the equipment, the skill of the ultrasonographer, and the type of abnormality seen. Ultrasound screening of all pregnant women can potentially detect major or minor findings that indicate a need for further diagnostic testing. Routine Ultrasonography is noninvasive, safe and a standard screening practice in many countries, yet controversy exists in the United States over its actual benefits *vs* cost.

High-resolution ***Ultrasonography*** is especially useful for detecting birth defects in which the chromosome analysis is most likely normal, such as with teratogen exposure; in multifactorial conditions, such as isolated congenital heart defect; and in anatomic defects, such as skeletal dysplasias and IUGR. Although equipment and ultrasonographer skill may vary, accuracy can be greater than 90 percent for detecting major neural tube, cardiac, kidney and bladder anomalies.

Prenatal diagnostic procedures: There are general, specific, and ethnic risk factors that may be present in my pregnancy that are indicators for diagnostic testing. The specific testing recommended depends on the identified risk. These may be preexisting risks, personal characteristics, or a newly identified risk for this pregnancy. General risk factors include age and abnormal triple marker screen results. It is a standard recommendation that women 35 years of age or older be offered amniocentesis, rather than screening, based on an increased risk for Down syndrome, other Trisomies, and sex chromosome abnormalities with advancing maternal age. Recent information suggests that amniocentesis should be offered at 31 years of age in twin pregnancies. Specific risk factors are usually identified in the family history, previous pregnancy outcomes, or the mother's medical history. Ethnic risk factors are based on a higher carrier rate frequency for certain genetic diseases in selected populations, indications for prenatal diagnosis when any of these risk factors are present is based on a greater than general population risk that a genetic defect or disorder will occur in the pregnancy. The specific risk is, of course, different for each situation.

Amniocentesis is currently the basis of diagnostic prenatal testing. It is usually performed at 14 to 16 weeks of gestation under ultrasound guidance. Estimated fetal loss following amniocentesis is 0.5 percent amniocentesis provides several types of diagnostic information. First, viable fetal skin cells that have sloughed off and are present in the amniotic fluid are obtained and cultured for chromosome analysis to detect chromosome abnormalities. Chromosome analysis results are obtained in about 7 to 14 days in most facilities and are 99 percent accurate. Second, DNA may be extracted from the chromosomes for direct DNA and indirect linkage analysis to detect single-gene disorders. Testing for each single-gene disorder is unique, therefore testing of this type is done only when a pregnancy is at high risk for a specific disorders, such as CF. The third type of diagnostic information available from amniocentesis is amniotic fluid AFP levels (AF-AFP). The AFP level in the amniotic fluid is a much more reliable indicator of an NTD or VWD because interfering factors, such as placental diffusion differences, are minimized. Also, an additional test for an enzyme specific to neural tissue acetylcholinesterase (AChE) may be done, which, if positive in the presence of an elevated AF-AFP level, is diagnostic of an open NTD.

Chorionic villus sampling (CVS) is a less commonly used procedure to obtain cells for chromosome analysis. An advantage of CVS is that it may be performed between 9 and 12 weeks of gestation, either transcervically or transabdominally. The procedure is somewhat controversial because of a slightly higher rate of fetal loss following the procedure. When performed at centers with a large experience the fetal loss rate is approximately the same as for amniocentesis. The accuracy of the chromosome analysis may be slightly less than with amniocentesis because of a greater risk for contamination by maternal cells, and if mosaicism is detected, a confirmatory amniocentesis at 14 to 16 weeks is recommended. A few additional diagnostic tests are sometimes used. ***Fetal blood sampling*** can be performed after 18 weeks of gestation. This procedure is usually done for prenatal evaluation of fetal hematologic abnormalities, inborn errors of metabolism, fetal infection, and rapid chromosome analysis. Fetal blood cells grow rapidly and hematologic and chromosome test results are usually possible in less than 1 week. ***Fetal biopsy (FB)*** is sometimes used to diagnose certain genetic skin disorders and metabolic disorders when DNA studies are unavailable or are uninformative. ***Fetal echocardiography*** may be performed for further diagnosis when a cardiac defect is noted on ultrasound. Research is underway to improve prenatal diagnostic testing.

A relatively new option for parents at risk of having a child with a genetic disorder is **preimplantation genetic diagnosis**. Through the technique of *in vitro* (test tube) fertilization, the embryo can be tested at the six—to eight–cell stage for the presence of the specific genetic disorder. If found to be normal or a carrier but not affected, the embryo(s) can then be implanted. This technique has been used for Tay-Sachs disease, CF, and some X-linked disorders (Harper, 1996). It was used by a couple who wished not only to avoid the birth of another child affected with Fanconi anemia but also to have a healthy sibling who could provide a human lymphocyte antigen (HLA) match for an affected sibling who needed stem cell transplantation.

Genetic Evaluation and Counseling

In recent years the significance of genetics as an etiologic agent in disease and disability has assumed a more prominent place in the nursing care of infants and children. The expanded recognition of genetic diseases and defects and an increasingly well-informed public creating a justified demand for genetic evaluation and diagnosis, as well as information regarding risks to present and future generations. Unfortunately, however, persons who need expert genetic counseling often make uninformed decisions on their own or are the victims of well-meaning but equally uninformed relatives, acquaintances, or paraprofessionals. Nurses involved in infant and child care continually encounter families in which there is a risk that a disorder may be transmitted to an offspring, as well as children who may have an undiagnosed genetic disorder that needs expert evaluation. It is a nurse's responsibility to be alert to situations in which families could benefit from genetic evaluation and counseling, become familiar with facilities in their areas where these services are available, and learn basic genetic principles. In this way, nurses will be able to direct individuals and families to needed services and to be active participants in the genetic evaluation and counseling process. Nurses should be knowledgeable regarding special services that are available to help in the management special support of affected children. Early identification of a genetic disorder allows anticipation of associated conditions therapy to avoid potential complications and to actualize or enhance the child's health potential. It may also prevent the unexpected birth of another affected child in the immediate or extended family.

Clients

The clients, or persons who seek genetic evaluation and counseling, must first be aware that there is a genetic or potential problem. They may be referred by a family practitioner, a specialist, a nurse, a friend, or a relative, or they may seek counseling as a result of information in the media. Clients who seek counseling expect information, explanation, reassurance, advice and help in making decisions.

Genetic evaluation for diagnostic purposes may occur at any point along the life span. In the newborn period, birth defects are an obvious reason for referral. Beyond the newborn period, indicators for referral include metabolic disorders, developmental delays, growth delays, behavioral problems, cognitive delays, abnormal or delayed sexual development, and medical problems known to be associated with genetic diseases. For example, a preschooler with hyperactivity and autistic-like behaviors may need evaluation for fragile X syndrome, and a 17-year-old girl with primary amenorrhea should be tested for Turner syndrome. In adulthood an asymptomatic individual with a family history of Huntington disease may desire testing to determine his or her risk of becoming symptomatic in the future.

With so many recent advances in genetic testing, it is not at all unusual for a child or adult with long-standing medical problems, including mental retardation, to be referred for reevaluation of his or her condition as a possible genetic disorder that might not have been diagnosable a few years earlier, such as microdeletion disorders or single-gene mutations. If a genetic diagnosis is made, the client will usually be referred back to the primary care physician with recommendations for routine management.

Clients may or may not be affected themselves but may request genetic counseling about the heritability of a trait. Clients might be a young couple contemplating childbearing who are concerned about a disorder in one of their families or who may seek advice because they are related. A couple who are both members of a population at risk for certain diseases may wish to determine whether they carry the harmful gene (e.g. African-Americans and sickle cell anemia, Ashkenazi Jews and Tay-Sachs disease, or persons of Mediterranean ancestry and thalassemia). A couple planning adoption might seek counseling regarding a prospective child.

More often, persons who inquire about the possibility of recurrence of a disease or disorder have a child, or had a child who died, with a genetic disease or disorder. They are concerned about their likelihood of having another, similarly affected child and may want to know what reproductive choices are available to them. This advice might be sought before the couple initiates another pregnancy or after the mother is already pregnant. If practical diagnostic testing is not done, the history of a condition in an order sibling, such as galactosemia, alerts health personnel to initiate specific and thorough testing for the condition in a newborn. In this way, early therapy can be initiated when indicated, thus minimizing or eliminating the effects of the disease or defect.

Parents need to know the risk in their particular situation and how it relates to the random risk for any prospective parents. When families understand the risks involved, they can make informed decisions regarding family planning and available prenatal testing. Additional counseling is necessary if abnormal results are obtained so that the couple can decide to continue or terminate the pregnancy. They will need considerable support for either decision. Parents may also have concerns about risks to unaffected siblings and about reproductive implications for their affected and unaffected offspring.

Counseling Services

The most efficient counseling service consists of a group of specialists, which may include physicians, geneticists, psychologists, biochemists, cytogists, nurses, social workers, and other auxiliary personnel. The services are most often under the leadership of a physician trained in medical aspects of the problem. The counseling service may serve only as a referral group, or it may conduct a regular clinic services. Most often it is associated with a large medical center, which may have extensive outreach programs with satellite clinics throughout adjacent rural areas. There are also numerous speciality clinics that deal with specific genetic disorders (such as CF, muscular dystrophy, hemophilia, or diabetes) and provide their own genetic counseling services. Unfortunately, these units are concentrated in and around large metropolitan areas. As a result, counseling is not always accessible to the large number of persons who would benefit from the service.

Unlike a medical prognosis, which predicts the outcome of a disease, a genetic prognosis directly involves other persons; the affected child, members of the immediate family, other relatives, and future offspring. For genetic evaluation or follow-up, the geneticist and the counselor usually work together to obtain the family history and pedigree and the medical history of the person being evaluated (including pregnancy, labor and delivery information), perform a physical examination for dysmorphic features, and order appropriate testing such as biochemical and cytogenetic procedures. A genetic diagnosis may or may not be made initially. Genetic evaluation and counseling is a time-consuming and labor-intensive process. The pediatric nurse can help the family understand sometimes lengthy process in arriving at a diagnosis as well as help the family prepare questions for the counseling session.

Genetic counseling is a communication process that deals with the human problems associated with the occurrence, or risk of occurrence, of a genetic disorder in a family. This process involves an attempt by one or more appropriately trained persons to help the individual or family.

- Comprehend the medical facts, including the diagnosis, the probable course of the disorder, and the available management.
- Appreciate the way heredity contributes to the disorder and the risk of recurrence in specified relatives.

- Understand the options for dealing with the risk of recurrence.
- Choose the course of action that seems appropriate to them in view of their risk and family goals and act in accordance with that decision.
- Make the best possible adjustment to the disorder in an affected family member and to the risk of that disorder.

Estimation of Risks

Effective genetic counseling based on a diagnosis or known risk factors requires a thorough evaluation of each situation. The counselor derives risks of occurrence or recurrence from information acquired through a thorough family history, including known genetic information. A careful, detailed family history not only provides a picture of the ***proband*** (the affected person, or index case) in relation to other family members but also may serve to identify others who are similarly affected or who might be presymptomatic or at risk of producing affected children. Analyzing the pattern of affected members of the family can assist in confirming a tentative diagnosis or in determining the level of risk in multifactorial inheritance.

An accurate diagnosis is essential in order to provide specific risk figures. There are over 6000 known inherited disorders, many of which have similar clinical manifestations but different modes of inheritance. For example, symptoms in the early stages of severe X-linked muscular dystrophy appear much like those of the milder autosomal recessive and autosomal dominant varieties, autosomal recessive neurogenic muscular atrophies, and nongenetic poliomyelitis. The significance of the risks related to each type of disorder is readily apparent. For disorders with an unknown or multifactorial cause, recurrence risks are termed empiric, meaning they are based on observations of recurrence in similar situations, rather than theoretic, meaning they are based on Mendelian inheritance patterns.

The mode of inheritance determines the degrees of risk in the major categories of genetic disorders. In general, the more definite and clear-cut the genetics, the greater the risks; as the causative factors become more obscure, the risk of recurrence is less likely.

Interpretation of Risks

When explaining risk estimates, the counselor does not attempt to make recommendations or decisions for clients. The counselor provides appropriate and accurate information about the nature of the disorder, the extent of the risk involved, the probable consequences, and alternative solutions but remains nondirective, leaving the final decision to the persons concerned. In some instances genetic information will increase the family's distress; in others their anxiety will be reduced, depending on their personalities and the meaning that the disorder has for that particular family.

Role of Nurses in Genetic Counseling and Referral

Genetic counseling is a professional speciality that requires master's level preparation and board certification because of the crucial nature of the information these professionals provide. However, the number of board-certified genetic counselors is limited; therefore nurses killed in counseling techniques are in a unique position to help meet the counseling needs of families in which there is a genetic disease or disorder. Public health nurses work with a family in a close, sustained relationship and earn the family's confidence and trust. Genetics specialists, with advanced preparation on counseling teams, and practitioners in the speciality areas of maternity and pediatric nursing are often involved with families in which there is a genetic defect. New advances in genetic diagnosis have greatly increased opportunities for, and responsibilities of nurses in all levels of practice in terms of assessment, referral, education, and counseling.

It is often a nurse who first identifies a need for counseling and referral by identifying the presence of an inherited disorder in a family history or by noting physical, mental, or behavioral abnormalities when performing a nursing assessment. Guidelines for determining if a genetic referral is indicated are given below:

Major or minor birth defects (anomalies) and dysmorphic features – Cardiac defect, ear or eye abnormalities, micrognathia, forehead prominence, hairline low-set on forehead or nape of neck, wide-set eyes, epicanthal folds, low-set or unusually shaped ears.

Growth abnormalities—Short stature, overgrowth, asymmetric growth, IUGR.

Skeletal abnormalities – Limb abnormalities, asymmetry, scoliosis, hyperextensible joints, hypotonic or hypertonic muscle tone, pectus excavatum, finger or joint abnormalities

Vision or hearing problems – Coloma, cat's eye, haring loss, vision loss, congenital or early cataracts

Metabolic disorder – Unusual odor of breath, urine, or stool

Sexual development abnormalities – Ambiguous genitalia, small penis, delayed onset of puberty, primary amenorrhea, precocious sexual development, large testicles

Skin disorders – Unusual pigmentation, café-au-lait spots, dry and scaly skin, skin tumors

Recurrent infection or immune deficiency – Ear infections, pneumonia

Developmental and speech delays or loss milestones

Cognitive delays – Learning disabilities, mild to severe mental retardation

Behavioral disorders – Hyperactivity, attention deficit disorder, autistic-like behavior, aggressive behavior.

A genetic nurse or counselor usually contacts the family before the primary counseling session or diagnostic workup to assess the needs of the family and to attempt to reduce their anxiety. In the interview the nurse takes a family history for pertinent information and explains the clinic procedures carefully. Many families are concerned about such things as whether they will be required to undress, if blood is to be drawn, if they can accompany the child during the visit, or if they will be told what to do about reproduction. Families who know what to expect are able to gain more from a counseling session.

The person taking a family history during a genetic consultation must allow a liberal amount of time. When possible, it is best to include both parents in the interview in order to elicit information about relatives on both sides of the family. Medical records, birth and death records, family Bibles, and photograph albums are helpful resources, and persons being interviewed should be instructed to bring such items if they are available. It may be necessary to consult other members of the family. The level of education and the degree of understanding vary widely among informants and influence the reliability of the information. There may be reticence on the part of informants, particularly if they view the disorder as something true something to be ashamed of or in some way threatening. Sometimes true relationships may be concealed, such as illegitimacy or nonpaternity.

Skillful interviewing is necessary in order to obtain essential, but often embarrassing or private, information. Since many parents may not be married, they should be addressed as couples or partners and asked about other unions that may have produced a pregnancy.

In eliciting a birth history from the mother and father, the nurse should specifically ask about abortions, miscarriages, and stillbirths as well as live births. To identify all members of the family tree, it is best to ask about pregnancies even of young teenagers. When inquiring about family diseases, it is often necessary to ask the question in different ways. For example, if a client denies any mental retardation in the family, asking other questions, such as about learning problems, being in special education classes, and failing or not completing school, may uncover a family history of cognitive impairment.

Referral regarding genetic counseling includes:

1. Individuals with a family history of hereditary diseases, birth defects, or developmental problems.
2. Known balanced translocations carriers or parents who have previously had a fetus or child with a chromosome abnormality.
3. Couples with a history of multiple miscarriages, stillbirths, or infertility.
4. Individuals at risk for ethnic-related disorders.
5. Pregnant women exposed to teratogenic agents.
6. Pregnant women of advanced maternal age (≥ 35 years).
7. Disorder sin which pregnancy could threaten maternal or fetal life or health.

The family history is recorded in the form of a pedigree chart or family tree (in some disciplines the pedigree chart is termed as genogram), using standard symbols to indicate persons, relationships, and significant details related to them. Construction of a pedigree begins with the affected child (proband, index case, original patient) and all the mother's pregnancies. Next, the maternal family history is explored in a similar manner; then information about relatives on the father's side, as well as any children or pregnancies that may have occurred through the father's previous unions, is gathered in the same manner. It is important at this point to determine whether the couple might be related in any way; although contrary to popular belief, this is usually a concern only for first cousins or closer relatives. The first-cousin risk for birth defects is about 5 percent vs the general population risk of 2 to 3 percent. The primary risk increase is for autosomal recessive disorders, in which the chance that two individuals carry the same rare, deleterious gene is increased if they are related.

Information to be solicited includes information not only about other affected family members but also; (1) births (live birth, stillbirths, and abortions [especially spontaneous abortions], including gestational age of pregnancy); (2) infertility problems; (3) matings (legally sanctioned, consanguineous, multiple, unwed, and other complex relationships); (4) health of family members, including any other genetic diseases or disorders or birth defects; and death and causes of death, including early infant deaths. Sometimes the place of birth and ethnic background are significant. For example, the incidence of Tay-Sachs disease is higher in Ashkenazi Jews from Eastern Europe than in Jews from other geographic origins. Also, when a pedigree chart is being evaluated, a sister's death in infancy from a congenital heart defect might be genetically significant, whereas a healthy sibling's death from drowning at age 1 year would not. Information concerning first-degree relatives is most important and should be complete.

Follow-up Care

The success of counseling is measured by the way in which the family uses the information presented to them. Maintaining contact with the family or referral to an agency that can provide a sustained relationship—usually the public health agency in their locally—is one of the most important aspects of the counseling process. Some families choose not to have follow-up visits, but in most instances these visits make the family feel that they have not been abandoned and facilitate the process of adjustment to the problem. A summary letter of the interview or counseling session is helpful to review information presented and reinforce recommendations.

Follow-up visits to the counseling service or in the home provide the family with the opportunity to ask questions that have arisen since previous visits. Often the family members have not really "heard" the information presented to them or have misinterpreted what they have heard, so that it may be necessary to repeat and reinforce counseling. In some disorders a diagnosis in one family member places relatives at risk and is an indication for further testing.

One very important aspect of follow-up care is support and assistance in management of the affected child. For example, a disorder such as PKU requires conscientious diet management; therefore it is important to make certain that the family understands and follows instructions. Genetic and speciality clinics devote a great deal of time and effort to helping families cope with the consequences of genetic disease.

Guidelines

Pedigree Construction

1. Begin diagram in the middle of a large sheet of paper.
2. Represent males by a square placed to the left and females by a circle placed to the right.
3. Represent the proband (index case, original patient) with an arrow (if the couselee or patient is different, place a C under that persons symbol).
4. Use a horizontal line between a square and a circle for a mating or marriage.
5. Suspend offspring vertically from the mating line and place in order of birth with oldest to the left (regardless of sex).
6. Symbolize generations by Roman numerals, with the earliest generation at the top.
7. Include three generations: grandparents, parents, offspring, siblings, aunts, uncles, and the first cousins of proband.
8. Include name of each person, their age, health problem and date and cause of death. Due to privacy concerns, include only first names of the person you are interviewing.
9. Date the pedigree and update at subsequent visits.

Nurses should be prepared to help families arrive at tentative decisions regarding the future, including family planning, education or institutionalization of a child with a disability, plans for adoption, and any other problems related to the specific situation. Initial and ongoing assessment of the family's coping abilities, resources, and support systems is vital in order to determine their need for additional assistance and support. As with any family who has a child with chronic health care needs, nurses must teach the family to become the child's advocate. Also nurses should be alert for evidence of risk factors that indicate poor adjustment (e.g. child abuse, divorce, or other maladaptive behaviors). Locating agencies and clinics specializing in a specific disorder or its consequences who can provide services (e.g. equipment, medication, and rehabilitation), educational programs, and parent support groups is part of the nurse's role. Nurses can be instrumental in helping parents start a support group when none is available.

In brief nurse's role in genetic evaluation and counseling of families includes the following:

1. Identify infants and children at risk of a genetic disorder.
2. Obtain family, prenatal and health history.
3. Assess the family's understanding of the genetic condition.
4. Refer for genetic evaluation and counseling when indicated.
5. Establish a plan of care with the family and coordinate care with other health professionals.
6. Understand the benefits and risks of genetic testing. Educate families about available testing.
7. Maintain privacy and confidentiality of family records and information.
8. Facilitate family access to early child stimulation programs genetic resources and support groups.
9. Provide follow-up care and support throughout the lifespan of the child.

Supportive Counseling

It requires time and understanding to deal with the emotional tension and anxiety generated in families who are faced with the prospect of a genetic disorder. Knowledge of and the ability to deal with the range of psychologic responses and all their ramifications (e.g. the grief reaction, guilt, anger, and coping mechanisms) are essential components of the nursing role in genetic counseling. Many of these factors determine the degree to which a counselor's message is understood and influence the family's attitudes and the use they make of counseling information.

Timing of the counseling requires careful evaluation. Some families may not be ready to listen immediately after a diagnosis is made or the first time information is presented to them. Families who seek genetic counseling, spontaneously or by referral, are apprehensive and know that decisions made on the basis of the information they receive may alter their lives significantly and may even alter their view of themselves. There may be numerous blocks to getting information across to families. Often they are so angry or frightened that they do not hear what is being said to them; they may feel guilty, embarrassed, or somehow inferior or inadequate. It may take a week or more for the family sufficient time or absorb the initial impact of the situation before they are ready to assimilate any new information.

It is important early in counseling to get a clear understanding of the family's initial concerns, their state of knowledge about the disease, and their attitudes and beliefs concerning the condition, and to determine the kind and amount of information they need or want. Some are not sure they should be at a counseling service. Whether the persons needing help are parents who have given birth to an affected child, relatives of an affected individual, persons who have been identified as carriers of a deleterious gene, or a couple with a higher-risk pregnancy, their feelings, attitudes, and fears must be addressed.

Careful interviewing and assessment will determine the extent and type of information needed and desired by the clients. Misunderstanding of the counseling information can have many causes. It can be due to cultural differences, the disparity of knowledge between the counselor and the family and the heightened emotion surrounding genetic counseling. Information often needs to be repeated several times before the family understands the content and its implications.

Guilt and self-blame are natural and universal reactions. Nurses must deal with parents feelings of guilt about carrying "bad genes" or having "made my child sick". Depending on the type of cytogenetic disorder, the counselor may be able to absolve the parents of guilt by explaining the random nature of segregation during both gamete formation and fertilization and that errors in cell division unique to the pregnancy in question are not likely to happen again and are not inherited. Families often try to "reason" that some unrelated event caused the abnormality (e.g. a fall, a urinary tract infection, or "one glass of wine") before the mother was aware that she was pregnant.

Nurses can provide an opportunity for parents to mourn the loss of the "perfect baby" dreamed of during the pregnancy. Parents may experience emotions of shock and disbelief, denial, guilt, shame, sadness, anger, and hostility at the birth of a baby with a genetic disorder or at the time of diagnosis of an older child's genetic disorder. These reactions are normal responses to information that may permanently change how they view their world.

Parental attachment and adjustment to the baby can be supported and facilitated by nursing interventions. Assessing the parent's understanding of the child's disorder and providing simple and truthful explanations can help them begin to understand their child's health issues. Guiding the parents in recognizing their child's cues, responses, and strengths can be helpful even for experienced parents. A caring attitude conveys the value of their child and, by extension, their value as parents. Help the parents identify their strengths as a family and identify support that is available to them.

If after the genetic evaluation parents do not have an accurate understanding of their child's disorder, follow-up is appropriate. Parents may need to hear the information several times before they begin to understand it. Referral to local and national support groups can be helpful. Contact with a local family that has a child with the same condition can be very helpful for a new parents. Privacy and confidentiality are imperative, and both families must gives permission before their contact information is given (ANA, 1998).

Sometimes there is comfort in knowing that everyone carries defective genes and that it is mere chance that both members of a couple happen to carry the same abnormal gene. Reactions may be different in situations where one member can pinpoint the "blame" (dominant or X-linked disorders), whereas in recessive disorders there is some reassurance for the couple to know that both of them carry the defective gene. Anxieties generated by superstitions and misconceptions can be dispelled.

Families have a tendency to be more ashamed of a hereditary disorder than of other illnesses. The threat of a hereditary "taint" often creates intrafamilial strife, hostility, and marital and couple disharmony, sometimes to the point of family disintegration. Crisis intervention may be necessary to prevent progressive discord.

A family member may decide not to have children after the diagnosis of a hereditary defect, or the decision to marry may be deferred on the basis of a disorder, even a remote chance of one, in a partner's family. Often these decision may not be based on accurate information because these individuals may not have been involved in the proband family's counseling.

Although people may understand the situation intellectually, this may not help them emotionally. A large and vital part of the nurse's role in genetic counseling is that of sympathetic and supportive listener. In addition, ensuring that families have accurate and complete information on which to make an informed decision is a primary goal.

Health information on the internet is increasingly obtained by families. Nurses can help families evaluate the accuracy of the information. It will be helpful to remind families that frequently information is given about the severely affected child and there may be little available pertaining to the mildly affected child.

The way in which members of a family respond to the probability of a genetic disorder will depend a great deal on the nature of the condition and the burden, actual or perceived, that it may placed on them. A burden is considered to be the total amount of distress, economic and emotional, that is placed on persons, their families, and society by the birth of an affected child—the anticipated burden as well as the threat of disability. Various factors that are associated with disorders produce a burden in different ways to determine the total impact on a family. These include severity, chronicity, age of onset, mortality, morbidity, presence or absence of chronic pain, mental retardation, and cosmetic disfigurement. A long-term grieving process, sometimes called chronic sorrow, can plague parents of a child with a disability. It has been described as a normal response to an abnormal situation. Parents may feel acute grief during milestones such as the first day of school or when other children are receiving their driver's licenses. Parents need support throughout the lifespan of the child.

In some disorders, such as Down syndrome, the burden of the disease rests primarily on the family rather than on the affected child. In diseases with severe crippling effects, such as muscular dystrophy, the impact of the disease affects both the child and the family. When a genetic disorder is inherited and extended family members are at risk, such as with fragile X syndrome, the parents face the burden of informing the other members. They may be met with disbelief, blame, or hostility, and they may need support in this difficult task.

All of these matters confront a family when they must make a decision about whether to risk a pregnancy that might result in a child with a disability, and nurses should be prepared to explore these probabilities and the availability of prenatal testing with them. If a pregnancy does result in a fetus or child with a genetic defect or disorder and the family chooses to continue the pregnancy, education about the condition and treatment options helps to provide the best possible outcome for the child.

Barriers to Effective Counseling

Differences in the ability to comprehend what is said probably interfere most with effective use of counseling information. Clients vary in experiences, education, language, and intellectual level, and even with careful explanation may have difficulty understanding the fundamentals of inheritance. They may be able to repeat information but fail to grasp its significance.

Cultural, religious, and ethnic values determine our responses as well as those of our patients and their families. These values and beliefs influence perceptions of health, disease, sexuality, reproduction, and disability. Whether or not a family finds interventions and genetic testing appropriate is influenced by these beliefs.

Sometimes nurses creates barriers with their own biases and personal feelings. Some diseases have a special impact on individual nurses, and in such cases it is difficult to be nonjudgemental. For some families, the attempt to be neutral may be viewed as unhelpful rather than noncoercive. By clarifying areas of confusion it is possible to help families make decisions. The basic tenet of genetic counseling is that families should be given all the facts and possible consequences and then be assisted, without coercion, in their problem solving. The decision concerning a course of action must be left to them.

6 CHAPTER

Biology of Behavior

Introduction

Psychology is the scientific study of behavior. The scientific study of all over activities of the organism as well as all the internal processes that are presumed to underline them, e.g. thinking, learning, memory, motivation, perception and emotion. The scientific study of the Biology of behvior is called as "Biopsychology". Behavior is aroused by some change in the conditions. Such changes are commonly called "stimuli" or "stimulus". A stimulus is then anything that makes an organism do something and what the organism does is known as a response. Human behavior then consists of responses to stimuli. Different stimuli evoke different responses. Many have tried to understand behaviors by analyzing them into stimulus response combinations. These stimulus response combinations can be very simple as very compiled. For example, when hand touch matchstick give we automatically withdraw own hand. Scene, he writes the story of the events or scene. Sometimes stimulus response combinations are innate also. This is the case with reflex actions most of these S-R combinations in the adults are the request of learning and experience.

A stimulus can be external or internal. External stimulus are a sound, a pinprick, mobile sound, the sight of a person, etc. Internal stimulus includes some chemical changes inside the body, physiological changes, etc. And sometimes sudden memories of the past much also act on stimuli. So stimulus is anything that makes an organism to act. Thus, a stimulus can in defined as any object, events or experiences that causes a response, the reaction of an organism. Responses can be external or overt and response can be internal or covert. Overt responses are directly observable while covert responses are not observable directly. Again responses can see immediate or responses can be delayed, i.e. the response are also innate or acquired. Normal life is possible only because of the fact that certain stimuli are associated with certain response due to innate nature or due to the process of learning.

Response Mechanism

Response mechanism is that system which helps the organism to adjust itself with the environment and controls its activities. Thus it is due to response mechanism that one finds selection, adjustments, synthesis, etc. in human behavior. The response mechanism in animals is divided into the following parts:

1. **Receptors:** Eye, nose, ear, tongue and skin, etc. are receptors. They receive the sensation. Human behavior begins through the receptors. It is only after the receptors have received the sensation that the response in the organism begins.

2. **Effectors:** Effectors include muscles and glands. They make the actual response possible.
3. **Nervous system:** Nervous system controls the response. It connects the receptors and motor organs.

Human organism is affected by the environment. The sun, heat, cold, etc. affect our body responds to external stimuli. This response changes the external environment. When something pinches, the pinched one feels a sensation. The sensation is received by the nervous system through which the receptors and motor organs are connected and the muscles of the hand react immediately so that the pinching object is removed. Thus the receptors receive stimuli from the environment and the motor organs change the environment by response. The human organism has innumerable receptors cells. Similarly, the receptors organs, e.g. muscles, etc. have innumerable muscles fibers. The nerves connect the receptors and the muscles and thus make response possible. These nerves carry the message from the receptors to the muscles. This communication has a speed of 75 yds., a second. Thus response takes a very small fraction of a second. In times of emergency, it becomes even more rapid.

The functioning of stimuli response combinations is made possible by the nervous system. It is this nervous system which controls the stimuli response mechanism. The knowledge of the nervous system and glands valuable to a nurse. The main points in this connection are as follows:

- It helps the nurses in the understanding of the diseases of nervous system and glands. Examples of the diseases of the nervous systems are chorea, stammering, stuttering, hysteria, epilepsy, deafness and blindness. These diseases are very much hinder the cure of the patients. Hence efforts must be made to diminish their influences and to curb them. Excess or deficiency in glandular secretions also influences personality.
- It helps the nurses in the understanding- of the physiological basis of the patient's diseases.
- It helps the nurses in the understanding of the individual differences among patients.
- It helps the nurses in understanding the process of attainment of knowledge and learning, by knowing which he can make desirable changes.
- It helps the nurses in having correct expectations from the patients and in understanding limits of their attainments.
- It helps the nurses in predicting the course of the future development of the patients.

Nervous System

The nervous system is the master controlling and communicating system of the body. It has been usually compared to an intricate telephone system with messages to and fro between the various parts of the body. The nervous system consists of two divisions: the central nervous system (CNS), including brain and spinal cord and the peripheral nervous system which includes cranial and spinal nerves. The peripheral nervous system further divided into the somatic or voluntary nervous system and the autonomic or involuntary nervous system. For convenience sake, this nervous system can be divided into various parts and each part should be studied in detail. Here, it must be remembered that it is the whole system that acts every time. In spite of multiplicity of the parts the whole system acts as one unit and also it can act in many different ways even to the same stimulus. Every thought, action and emotion reflect, its activity. Its signalling device or means of communicating with body cells, is electrical impulses, which are rapid and specific and cause almost immediate responses.

The function of the nervous system is control of all motor, sensory, autonomic, cognitive and behavioral activities. The nervous system has approximately 10 million sensory neurons that send information about the internal and external environment to the brain and 500,000 motor neurons that control the muscles and glands. The brain itself consists of more than 100 billion cells that link the motor and sensory pathways, monitor the body's processes, respond to the internal and external environment, maintain homeostasis and direct all the psychological, biologic and physical activity through complex chemical and electrical messages. The nervous system does not work alone to regulate and maintain body homeostasis; the endocrine system is a second important regulating system. While the nervous impulse, the endocrine system organs produce hormones that are released into the blood. Thus endocrine system typically brings *about it effects is a mass ensure way.*

The basic functional unit of the brain is the neuron. It is composed of a cell body, a dendrite, and an axon. The dendrite is a branch-type structure with synapses for receiving electrochemical messages. The axon is a long projection that carries impulses away from the cell body. Nerve cell bodies occurring in clusters are called ganglia or nuclei. A cluster of cell bodies with the same function is called a center (e.g. the respiratory center). Neuroglial cells, smaller types of nerve cells, support, protect, and nourish neurons.

Neurotransmitters

Neurotransmitters communicate messages from one neuron to another or from a neuron to a specific target tissue. Neurotransmitters are manufactured and stored in synaptic vesicles. They enable conduction of impulses across the synaptic cleft. Each neurotransmitter has an affinity for specific receptors in the postsynaptic bulb. When released, the neurotransmitter crosses the synaptic cleft and binds to receptors in the postsynaptic cell membrane. The action of a neurotransmitter is to potentiate, terminate, or modulate a specific action, and it can either excite or inhibit the activity of the target cell. Usually, multiple neurotransmitters are at work in the neural synapse. Various substances serve as neurotransmitters; major neurotransmitters are described in Table 6.1.

Table 6.1: Major neurotransmitters

Neurotransmitter	*Source*	*Action*
Acetylcholine (major transmitter of the parasympathetic nervous system	Many areas of the brain, autonomic nervous system	Usually excitatory, parasympathetic effects sometimes inhibitory (stimulation of heart by vagal nerve)
Serotonin	Brainstem, hypothalamus, dorsal horn of the spinal cord	Inhibitory, helps control mood and sleep, inhibits pain pathways
Dopamine	Substantia nigra and basal ganglia	Usually inhibits, affects behavior (attention, emotions) and fine movement
Norepinephrine (major transmitter of the sympathetic nervous system	Brainstem, hypothalamus, postganglionic neurons of the sympathetic nervous system	Usually excitatory; affects mood and overall activity
Gamma-aminobutyric acid (GABA)	Spinal cord, cerebellum, basal ganglia, some cortical areas	Excitatory
Enkephalin, endorphin	Nerve terminals in the spine, brainstem, thalamus and hypothalamus, pituitary gland	Excitatory; pleasurable sensation, inhibits pain transmission

Many neurologic disorders are due, at least in part, to an imbalance in neurotransmitters–that is, an increase in gamma-aminobutyric acid (GABA) in alcohol withdrawal seizures, a decrease in dopamine in Parkinson's disease, and a decrease in acetylcholine in myasthenia gravis. In fact, probably all brain functions are modulated through neurotransmitter receptor site activity, including memory and other cognitive processes.

There are two types of receptors: direct and indirect. Direct receptors are also known as inotropic because they are linked to ion channels and allow passage of ions when opened. They can be excitatory or inhibitory and are rapid acting (measured in milliseconds). Indirect receptors affect metabolic processes in the cell, which can take from seconds to hours to occur. Receptor sites are an expanding area of research because they are often the target for the action and development of new medications. These medications either block or stimulate neurotransmitters at receptor sites and thus provide relief from symptoms. Receptor sites are also sites for the action of addictive drugs.

Another important area of ongoing research is diagnostic testing that can detect abnormal levels of neurotransmitters in the brain. Positron emission tomography (PET), for example, can detect dopamine, serotonin, and acetylcholine. Single photon emission computed tomography (SPECT), similar to PET, can detect changes in some neurotransmitters such as dopamine in Parkinson's disease.

Physiology of the Neurons

Nerve is the most important part of response mechanism. It joins the receptors and the effectors. The nervous system is divided into two parts: (1) Central nervous system and (2) Autonomic nervous system. In the human organism there is a whole network of nervous system. The central nervous system, too has two parts: (1) Spinal cord, (2) Brain, which has three parts: (1) Cerebrum, (2) Medulla oblongata, (3) Cerebellum. The autonomic system has two parts: (1) Sympathetic, (2) Parasympathetic.

A nerve network spreads throughout the body, similar to the telephone cable network spread over the city. These nerves reach every receptor and muscle just like the cables which reach every business center, office, hospital, college, etc. all the nerves of the body are connected to the spinal cord and this central body resembles a telephone exchange where all the wires from the different telephones meet. Information is sent from any telephone in the system to the telephone exchange and the desired telephone connection is got. Thus, the exchange of information between two centers is always through the medium of the telephone exchange. A similar state of affairs exists in the nervous system. Sensory nerves bring information to the center from the receptors and the motor nerves carry directions to the muscles. But there is a big difference between the telephone system and bodily nervous system. The telephone exchange is merely a medium which has no say in anything which goes on. On the other hand the nervous center is not merely a medium because it decides upon the response to the stimuli and the part of the body to obey it. So, in reality it is this center which controls the whole response mechanism.

The nerves of the central nervous system reach every sense organ and muscle. These nerves are connected with the central ganglia of the spinal cord. All the nerves meet at this center. The nerves carrying the message from the receptors to the center are known as sensory nerves. The nerves carrying the message from the center to the muscles are known as motor nerves. The response mechanism works by systematic working of the sensory and the motor nerves. Besides these two types of nerves there are nerves connecting them.

Thus various responses of the human body function through nerve centers. These nerve centers are very complex. When seen with the help of a microscope, many subtle fibers are seen in other nerves. Some of these are even some yards in length. The complexity of the nerve center can be imagined from the fact that the optic nerve alone has about 4,000,000 fibers. A nerve is made up of a bundle of fibers. Fibers are connected outside the nerve center, but again meet in the nerve center. It is not necessary that one fiber should carry one message. Sometimes an outgoing fiber takes several messages. When the nerves are broken and the muscles are unconnected with the centers, these become useless.

The nervous system is made up of nerves. The nervous system and the nerve cells are connected through the blood vessels. These nerves also include their branches. These branches are of two types—Axons and Dendrites. Axon is one and alone while dendrites are many. Axons are several feet long. The dendrites extend like the small branches of a tree. The axon is covered by an insulating substance. The axons of the sensory nerves are sensory while axons of the motor nerves are motor. A motor axon extends from the brain or spinal cord to the muscle or gland. The sensory axon extends from the nerve cells to the brain. Thus these axons connect the receptors and the nerve centers.

The connection between the two cells is known as synapse. In this synapse an axon of a nerve finishes in fine branches and these fine branches get connected with the dendrites of some other nerves, and a sensation is carried from one to another. The axon carries the sensation and the dendrites receive it. Thus, the message is communicated from the axon of the nerve to the dendrite of another nerve. This message is in the form of nerve impulse which is like an electrochemical current found in the nerve. The force of the reaction of any muscle depends on the total number of these electrochemical currents per second, as it increases and decreases simultaneously.

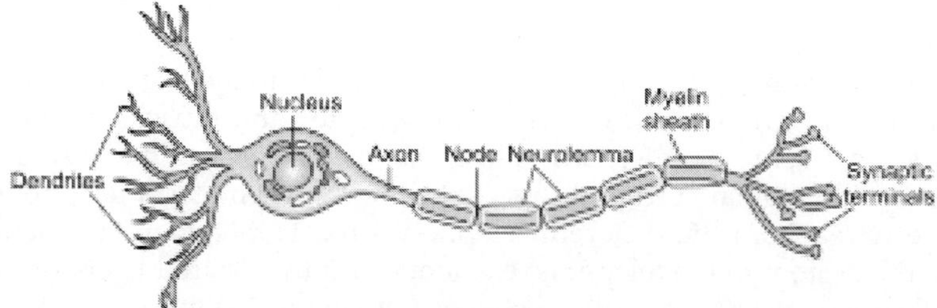

Fig. 6.1: Neuron

Nerve impulses: Neurons have two major functional properties (Fig. 6.1): Irritability, the ability to respond to a stimulus and convert it into a nerve impulse, and conductivity, the ability to transmit the impulse to other neurons, muscles, or glands.

The Central Nervous System

BRAIN

The brain is divided into three major areas: The cerebrum, the brainstem, and the cerebellum. The cerebrum is composed of two hemispheres, the thalamus, the hypothalamus, and the basal ganglia. In addition, connections for the olfactory (cranial

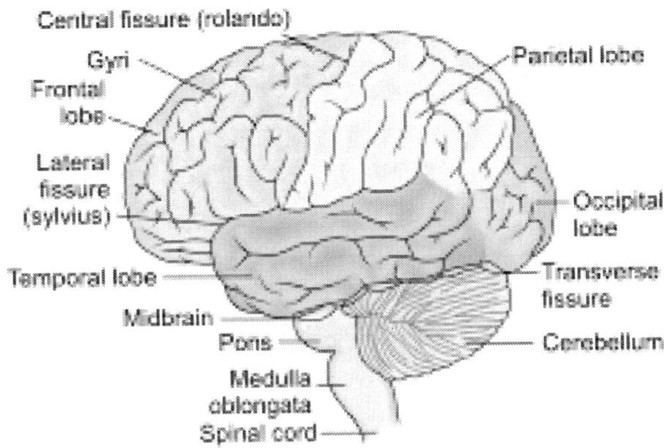

Fig. 6.2: External view of the brain showing lobes, cerebellum, and brainstem

nerve I) and optic (cranial nerve III) nerves are found in the cerebrum. The brainstem includes the midbrain, pons, medulla, and connections for cranial nerves II and IV through XII. The cerebellum is located under the cerebrum and behind the brainstem (Fig. 6.2). The brain accounts for approximately 2 percent of the total body weight; in an average young adult, the brain weighs approximately 1,400 g whereas in an average elderly person, the brain weighs approximately 1,200 g.

CEREBRUM

The cerebrum consists of two hemispheres that are incompletely separated by the great longitudinal fissure. This sulcus separates the cerebrum into the right and left hemispheres. The two hemispheres are joined at the lower portion of the fissure by the corpus callosum. The outside surface of the hemispheres has a wrinkled appearance that is the result of many folded layers or convolutions called gyri, which increase the surface area of the brain, accounting for the high level of activity carried out by such a small-appearing organ. The external or outer portion of the cerebrum (the cerebral cortex) is made up of gray matter approximately 2 to 5 mm in depth; it contains billions of neurons/cell bodies, giving it a gray appearance. White matter makes up the innermost layer and is composed of nerve fibers and neuroglia (support tissue) that form tracts or pathways connecting various parts of the brain with one another (transverse and association pathways) and the cortex to lower portions of the brain and spinal cord (projection fibers). The cerebral hemispheres are divided into pairs of frontal, parietal, temporal, and occipital lobes. The four lobes are as follows (Fig. 6.2):

- *Frontal:* The largest lobe, located in the front of the skull. The major functions of this lobe are concentration, abstract thought, information storage or memory, and motor function. It also contains Broca's area, critical for motor control of speech. The frontal lobe is also responsible in large part for a person's affect, judgment, personality, and inhibitions.
- *Parietal:* A predominantly sensory lobe located near the crown of the head. This lobe analyzes sensory information and relays the interpretation of this information to the thalamus and other cortical areas. It is also essential to a person's awareness of the body in space, as well as orientation in space and spatial relations.

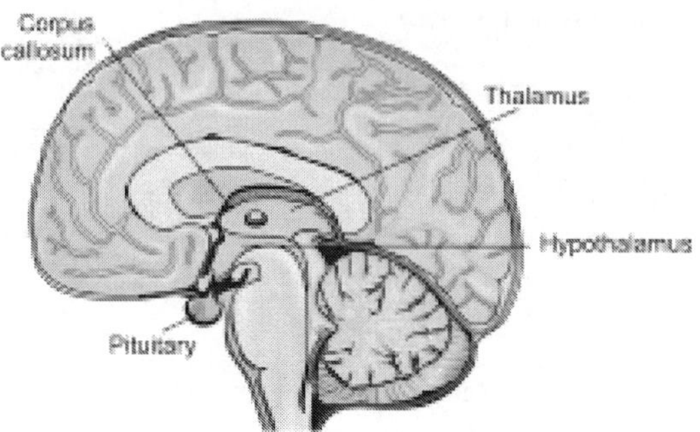

Fig. 6.3: Medial view of the brain

- *Temporal:* Contains the auditory receptive areas located around the temples. The temporal lobe contains a vital area called the interpretive area that provides integration of somatization, visual, and auditory areas and plays the most dominant role of any area of the cortex in thinking.
- *Occipital:* The posterior lobe of the cerebral hemisphere located at the lower back of the head, is responsible for visual interpretation.

The corpus callosum (Fig. 6.3) is a thick collection of nerve fibers that connects the two hemispheres of the brain and is responsible for the transmission of information from one side of the brain to the other. Information transferred includes sensation, memory, and learned discrimination. Right-handed people and some left-handed people have cerebral dominance on the left side of the brain for verbal, linguistic, arithmetical, calculating, and analytic functions.

The nondominant hemisphere is responsible for geometric, spatial, visual, pattern, and musical functions.

The basal ganglia are masses of nuclei located deep in the cerebral hemispheres that are responsible for control of fine motor movements, including those of the hands and lower extremities.

The thalamus (Fig. 6.3) lies on either side of the third ventricle and acts primarily as a relay station for all sensation except smell. All memory, sensation, and pain impulses also pass through this section of the brain.

The hypothalamus is located anterior and inferior to the thalamus. The hypothalamus lies immediately beneath and lateral to the lower portion of the wall of the third ventricle. It includes the optic chiasm (the point at which the two optic tracts cross) and the mammillary bodies (involved in olfactory reflexes and emotional response to odors). The infundibulum of the hypothalamus connects it to the posterior pituitary gland. The hypothalamus plays an important role in the endocrine system because it regulates the pituitary secretion of hormones that influence metabolism, reproduction, stress response, and urine production. It works with the pituitary to maintain fluid balance and maintains temperature regulation by promoting vasoconstriction or vasodilatation.

In addition, the hypothalamus is the site of the hunger center and is involved in appetite control. It contains centers that regulate the sleep-wake cycle, blood pressure, aggressive and sexual behavior, and emotional responses (i.e. blushing, rage, depression, panic, and fear). The hypothalamus also controls and regulates the autonomic nervous system.

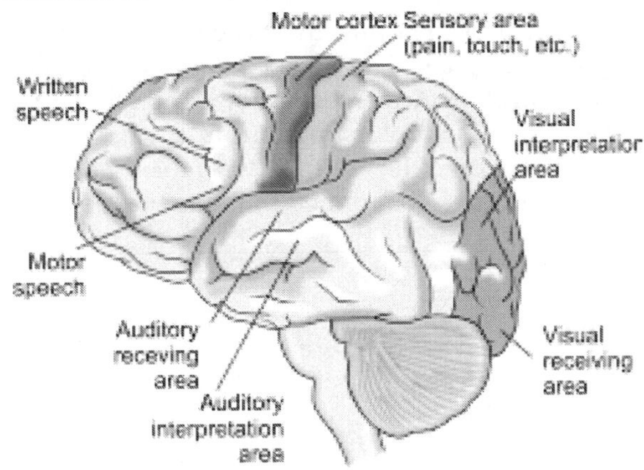

Fig. 6.4: Topography of the cortex as it relates to function

The pituitary gland is located in the sella turcica at the base of the brain and is connected to the hypothalamus. The pituitary is a common site of brain tumors in adults; frequently they are detected by physical signs and symptoms that can be traced to the pituitary, such as hormonal imbalance or visual disturbances secondary to pressure on the optic chiasm.

Nerve fibers from all portions of the cortex converge in each hemisphere and exit the form of a tight bundle of nerve fibers known as the internal capsule. After entering the pons and the medulla, each bundle crosses to the corresponding bundle from the opposite side. Some of these axons make connections with axons from the cerebellum basal ganglia, thalamus, and hypothalamus; some connect with the cranial nerve cells. Other fibers from the cortex and the subcortical centers are channeled through the pons and the medulla into the spinal cord. Although the various cells in the cerebral cortex are quite similar in appearance, their functions vary widely, depending on location.

The topography of the cortex in relation to certain of its functions is shown in Figure 6.4. The posterior portion of each hemisphere (i.e. the occipital lobe) is devoted to all aspects of visual perception. The lateral region, or temporal lobe, incorporates the auditory center. The midcentral zone, or parietal zone, posterior to the fissure of Rolando, is concerned with sensation; the anterior portion is concerned with voluntary muscle movements. The large area behind the forehead (i.e. the frontal lobes) contains the association pathways that determine emotions, attitudes, and responses and contributes to the formation of thought processes. Damage to the frontal lobes as a result of trauma or disease is by no means incapacitating from the standpoint of muscular control or coordination, but it can affect a person's personality, as reflected by basic attitudes, sense of humor and propriety, self-restraint, and motivations.

BRAINSTEM

The brainstem consists of the midbrain, pons, and medulla oblongata (Fig. 6.2). The midbrain connects the pons and the cerebellum with the cerebral hemispheres; it contains sensory and motor pathways and serves as the center for auditory and visual reflexes. Cranial nerves III and IV originate in the midbrain. The pons is situated in front of the cerebellum between the midbrain and the medulla and is a bridge between the two halves of the cerebellum, and between the medulla and the cerebrum. Cranial nerves V through VIII connect to the brain in the pons. The pons contains motor and sensory pathways. Portions of the pons also control the heart, respiration, and blood pressure.

The medulla oblongata contains motor fibers from the brain to the spinal cord and sensory fibers from the spinal cord to the brain. Most of these fibers cross, or decussate, at this level. Cranial nerves IX through XII conned to the in the medulla.

CEREBELLUM

The cerebellum is separated from the cerebral hemispheres by a fold of dura mater, the tentorium cerebelli. The cerebellum has both excitatory and inhibitory actions and is largely responsible for coordination of movement. It also controls fine movement, balance, position (postural) sense or proprioception (awareness of where each part of the body is), and integration of sensory input.

THE SPINAL CORD

The spinal cord and medulla form a continuous structure extending from the cerebral hemispheres and serving as the connection between the brain and the periphery. Approximately 45 cm (18 in) long and about the thickness of a finger, it extends from the foramen magnum at the base of the skull to the lower border of the first lumbar vertebra, where it tapers to a fibrous band called the conus medullaris. Continuing below the second lumbar space are the nerve roots that extend beyond the conus, which are called the cauda equine because they resemble a horse's tail. Similar to the brain, the spinal cord consists of gray and white matter. Gray matter in the brain is external and white matter is internal; in the spinal cord, gray matter is in the center and is surrounded on all sides by white matter.

The spinal cord is surrounded by the meninges, dura, arachnoid, and pia layers. Between the dura mater and the vertebral canal is the epidural space. The spinal cord is an H-shaped structure with nerve cell bodies (gray matter) surrounded by ascending and descending tracts (white matter). The lower portion of the H is broader than the upper portion and corresponds to the anterior horns. The anterior horns contain cells with fibers that form the anterior (motor) root end and are essential for the voluntary and reflex activity of the muscles they innervate. The thinner posterior (upper horns) portion contains cells with fibers that enter over the posterior (sensory) root end and thus serve as a relay station in the sensory/reflex pathway.

The thoracic region of the spinal cord has a projection from each side at the crossbar of the H-shaped structure of gray matter called the lateral horn. It contains the cells that give rise to the autonomic fibers of the sympathetic division. The fibers leave the spinal cord through the anterior roots in the thoracic and upper lumbar segments.

Sensory and Motor Pathways

The spinal tracts: The white matter of the cord is composed of myelinated and unmyelinated nerve fibers. The fast-conducting myelinated fibers form bundles that also contain glial cells. Fiber bundles with a common function are called tracts.

There are six ascending tracts. Two conduct sensation, principally the perception of touch, pressure, vibration, position, and passive motion from the same side of the body. Before reaching the cerebral cortex, these fibers cross to the opposite side in the medulla.

The two spinocerebellar tracts conduct sensory impulses from muscle spindles, providing necessary input for coordinated muscle contraction. They ascend essentially uncrossed and terminate in the cerebellum. The last two spinothalamic tracts are responsible for conduction of pain, temperature, proprioception, fine touch, and vibratory sense from the upper body to the brain. They are ascend, cross to the opposite side of the brain, and terminate in the thalamus.

There are eight descending tracts. The two corticospinal tracts conduct motor impulses to the anterior horn cells from the opposite side of the brain and control voluntary muscle activity. The three vestibulospinal tracts descend uncrossed and are involved in some autonomic functions (sweating, pupil dilation, and circulation) and involuntary muscle control. The corticobulbar tract conducts impulses responsible for voluntary head and facial muscle movement and crosses at the level of the brainstem. The rubrospinal and reticulospinal tracts conduct impulses involved with involuntary muscle movement.

Vertebral column: The bones of the vertebral column surround and protect the spinal cord and normally consist of 7 cervical, 12 thoracic, and 5 lumbar vertebrae, as well as the sacrum (a fused mass of 5 vertebrae), and terminate in the coccyx. Nerve roots exit from the vertebral column through the intervertebral foramina (openings). The vertebrae are separated by disks, except for the first and second cervical, the sacral, and the coccygeal vertebrae. Each vertebra has a ventral solid body and a dorsal segment or arch, which is posterior to the body. The arch is composed of two pedicles and two laminae supporting seven processes. The vertebral body, arch, pedicles, and laminae all encase and protect the spinal cord.

THE PERIPHERAL NERVOUS SYSTEM

The peripheral nervous system includes the cranial nerves, the spinal nerves, and the autonomic nervous system.

CRANIAL NERVES

Twelve pairs of cranial nerves emerge from the lower surface of the brain and pass through the foramina in the skull. There are entirely sensory (I, II, VIII), five are motor (Ill, IV, VI, IX, and XII), and four are mixed (V, VII, IX, and X), because they have both sensory and motor functions. The cranial nerves are numbered in the order in which they arise from the brain. For example, cranial nerves I and II attach in the cerebral hemispheres, whereas cranial nerves lX, X, Xl, and XII attach at the medulla (Fig. 6.5).

Most cranial nerves innervate the head, neck, and special sense structures. Table 6.2 lists the names and primary functions of the cranial nerves.

SPINAL NERVES

The spinal cord is composed of 31 pairs of spinal nerves: 8 cervical, 12 thoracic, 5 lumbar, 5 sacral, and 1 coccygeal. Each spinal nerve has a ventral root and a dorsal root (see Fig. 6.6). The dorsal roots are sensory and transmit sensory impulses from specific areas of the body known as dermatomes to the dorsal ganglia. The sensory fiber may be somatic, carrying information about pain, temperature, touch, and position sense (proprioception) from the tendons, joints, and body surfaces; or visceral, carrying information from the internal organs.

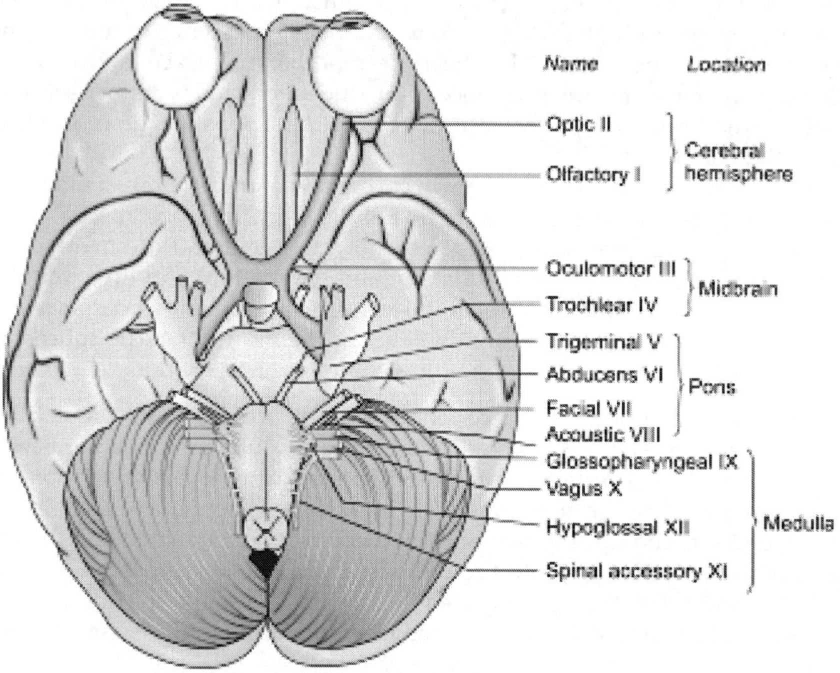

Fig. 6.5: Base of the brain showing entrance or exit of the cranial nerves

Table 6.2: Cranial nerves

Cranial Nerve	*Type*	*Function*
I (olfactory)	Sensory	Sense of smell
II (optic)	Sensory	Visual acuity and visual fields
III (oculomotor)	Motor	Muscles that move the eye and lid, papillary constriction, lens accommodation
IV (trochlear)	Motor	Muscles that move the eye
V (trigeminal)	Mixed	Facial sensation, corneal reflex, mastication
VI (abducens)	Motor	Muscles that move the eye
VII (facial)	Mixed	Facial expression and muscle movement, salivation and tearing, taste, sensation in the ear
VIII (acoustic)	Sensory	Hearing and equilibrium
IX (glossopharyngeal)	Mixed	Taste, sensation in pharynx and tongue, pharyngeal muscles, swallowing
X (vagus)	Mixed	Muscles of pharynx, larynx, and soft palate; sensation in external ear, pharynx, larynx, thoracic and abdominal viscera; parasympathetic innervation of thoracic and abdominal organs
XI (spinal accessory)	Motor	Sternocleidomastoid and trapezius muscles
XII (hypoglossal)	Motor	Movement of the tongue

The ventral roots are motor and transmit impulses from the spinal cord to the body, and these fibers are also either somatic or visceral. The visceral fibers include autonomic fibers that control the cardiac muscles and glandular secretions.

AUTONOMIC NERVOUS SYSTEM

The autonomic nervous system regulates the activities of internal organs such as the heart, lungs, blood vessels, digestive organs, and glands. Maintenance and restoration of internal homeostasis is largely the responsibility of the autonomic nervous system. There are two major divisions: the sympathetic nervous system, with predominantly excitatory responses, most notably the "fight or flight" response, and the parasympathetic nervous system, which controls mostly visceral functions.

The autonomic nervous system innervates most body organs. Although usually considered part of the peripheral nervous system, this system is regulated by centers in the spinal cord, brainstem, and hypothalamus. The autonomic nervous system has two neurons in a series extending between the centers in the CNS and the organs innervated. The first neuron, the preganglionic neuron, is located in the brain or spinal cord, and its axon extends to the autonomic ganglia. There, it synapses with the second neuron, the postganglionic neuron, located in the autonomic ganglia, and its axon synapses with the target tissue and innervates the effector organ. Its regulatory effects are exerted not on individual cells but on large expanses of tissue and on entire organs. The responses elicited do not occur instantaneously but after a lag period. These responses are sustained far longer than other neurogenic responses to ensure maximal functional efficiency on the part of receptor organs, such as blood vessels.

The autonomic nervous system transmits its impulses by way of nerve pathways, enhanced by chemical mediators, resembling the endocrine system in this respect. This accounts for the quality of these responses. Electrical impulses, conducted through nerve fibers, stimulate the formation of specific chemical agents at strategic locations within the muscle mass; the diffusion of these chemicals within the muscle is responsible for the contraction.

The hypothalamus is the major subcortical center for the regulation of visceral and somatic activities, serving an inhibitory-excitatory role in the autonomic nervous system. The hypothalamus has connections that link the autonomic system with the thalamus, the cortex, the olfactory apparatus, and the pituitary gland. Located here are the mechanisms for the control of visceral and somatic reactions that were originally important for defense or attack and are associated with emotional states (e.g. fear, anger, anxiety); for the control of metabolic processes, including fat, carbohydrate, and water metabolism; for the regulation of body temperature, arterial pressure, and all muscular and glandular activities of the gastrointestinal tract; for control of genital functions; and for the sleep cycle.

The autonomic nervous system is separated into the anatomically and functionally distinct sympathetic and parasympathetic divisions. Most of the tissues and the organs under autonomic control are innervated by both systems. Sympathetic stimuli are mediated by norepinephrine and parasympathetic impulses are mediated by acetylcholine. These chemicals produce opposing and mutually antagonistic effects. Both divisions produce stimulatory and inhibitory effects. For example, the parasympathetic division causes contraction (stimulation) of the urinary bladder muscles and a decrease (inhibition) in heart rate, whereas the sympathetic division produces relaxation (inhibition) of the urinary bladder and an increase (stimulation) in the rate and force of the heartbeat. Compares the sympathetic and the parasympathetic effects on the different systems of the body.

Sympathetic nervous system: The sympathetic division of the autonomic nervous system is best known for its role in the body's "fight-or-flight" response. Under stress from either physical or emotional causes, sympathetic impulses increase greatly. As a result, the bronchioles dilate for easier gas exchange; the heart's contractions are stronger and faster; the arteries to the heart and voluntary muscles dilate, carrying more blood to these organs; peripheral blood vessels constrict, making the skin feel cool but shunting blood to essential organs; the pupils dilate; the liver releases glucose for quick energy; peristalsis slows; hair stands on end; and perspiration increases. The main sympathetic neurotransmitter is norepinephrine (noradrenaline), and this increase sympathetic discharge is the same as if the body has been given an injection of adrenaline-hence the term adrenergic is often used to refer to this division.

Sympathetic neurons are located primarily in the thoracic and the lumbar segments of the spinal cord, and their axons, or the preganglionic fibers, emerge by way of anterior nerve roots from the eighth cervical or first thoracic segment to the second or third lumbar segment. A short distance from the cord, these fibers diverge to join a chain, composed of 22 linked ganglia, that extends the entire length of the spinal column, adjacent to the vertebral bodies on both sides. Some form multiple synapses with nerve cells within the chain. Others traverse the chain without making connections or losing continuity to join large "prevertebral" ganglia in the thorax, the abdomen, or the pelvis or one of the "terminal" ganglia in the vicinity of an organ, such as the bladder or the rectum (Fig. 6.6). Postganglionic nerve fibers originating in the sympathetic chain rejoin the spinal nerves that supply the extremities and are distributed to blood vessels, sweat glands, and smooth muscle tissue in the skin. Postganglionic fibers from the prevertebral plexuses (e.g. the cardiac, pulmonary, splanchnic, and pelvic plexuses) supply structures in the head and neck, thorax, abdomen, and pelvis, respectively, having been joined in these plexuses by fibers from the parasympathetic division.

The adrenal glands, kidneys, liver, spleen, stomach, and duodenum are under the control of the giant celiac plexus, commonly known as the solar plexus. This receives its sympathetic nerve components by way of the three splanchnic nerves, composed of preganglionic fibers from nine segments of the spinal cord (T4 to L1), and is joined by the vagus nerve, representing the parasympathetic division. From the celiac plexus, fibers of both divisions travel along the course of blood vessels to their target organs.

Sympathetic syndromes: Certain syndromes are distinctive to diseases of the sympathetic nerve trunks. Among these are dilation of the pupil of the eye on the same side as a penetrating wound of the neck (evidence of disturbance of the cervical sympathetic cord); temporary paralysis of the bowel (indicated by the absence of peristaltic waves and the distension of the intestine by gas) after fracture of any one of the lower dorsal or upper lumbar vertebrae with hemorrhage into the base of the mesentery; and the marked variations in pulse rate and rhythm that often follow compression fractures of the upper six thoracic vertebrae. Sympathetic storming, a syndrome that is associated with changes in level of consciousness, altered vital signs, diaphoresis, and agitation, may result from hypothalamic stimulation of the sympathetic nervous system following traumatic brain injury.

Parasympathetic nervous system: The parasympathetic nervous system functions as the dominant controller for most visceral effectors. During quiet, nonstressful conditions,

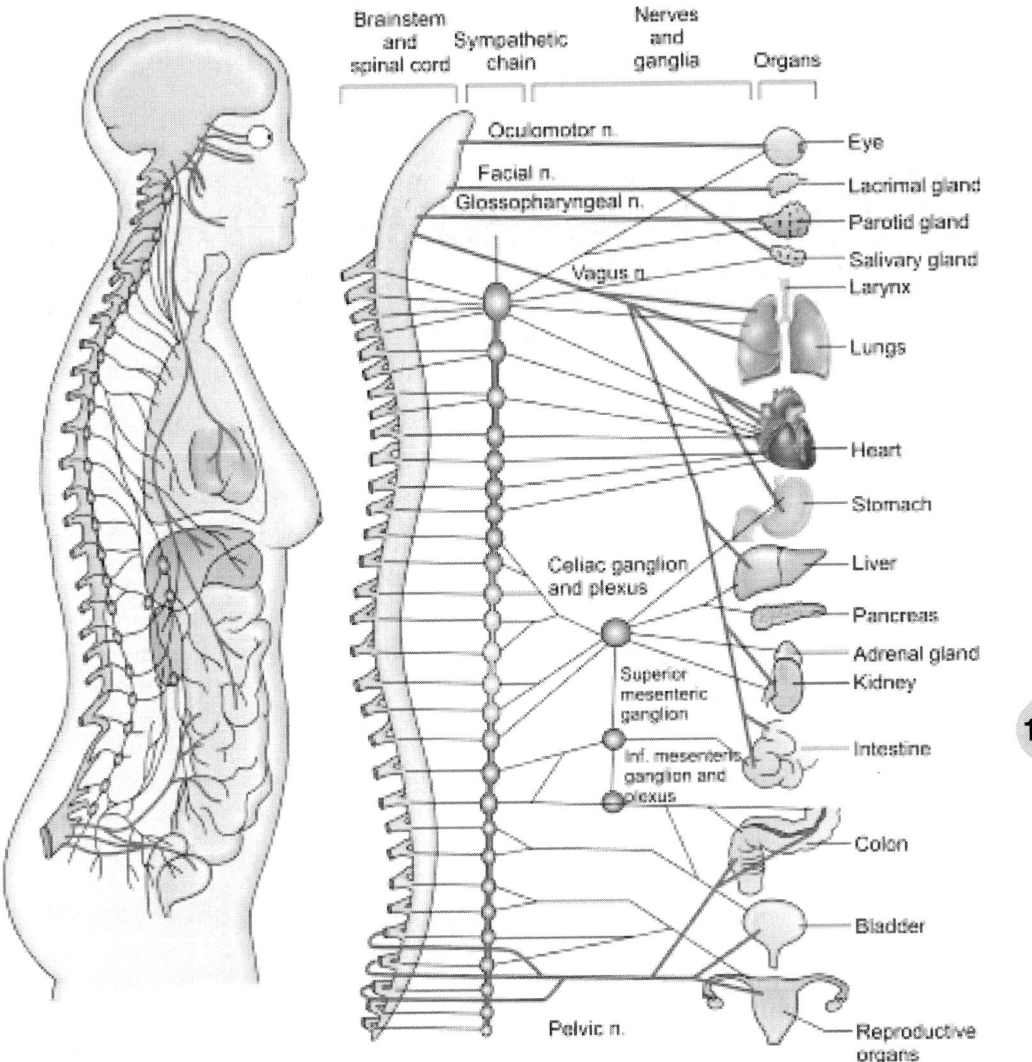

Fig. 6.6: Spinal nerves

impulses from parasympathetic fibers (cholinergic) predominate. The fibers of the parasympathetic system are located in two sections, one in the brainstem and the other from spinal segments below L2. Because of the location of these fibers, the parasympathetic system is referred to as the craniosacral division, as distinct from the thoracolumbar (sympathetic) division of the autonomic nervous system.

The parasympathetic nerves arise from the midbrain and the medulla oblongata. Fibers from cells in the midbrain travel with the third oculomotor nerve to the ciliary ganglia, where postganglionic fibers of this division are joined by those of the sympathetic system, creating controlled opposition, with a delicate balance maintained between the two at all times.

MOTOR AND SENSORY FUNCTIONS OF THE NERVOUS SYSTEM

Motor System Function

The motor cortex, a vertical band within each cerebral hemisphere, controls the voluntary movements of the body. The exact locations within the brain at which the voluntary movements of the muscles of the face, thumb, hand, arm, trunk, and leg originate are known. To initiate muscle movement, these particular cells must send the stimulus along their fibers. Stimulation of these cells with an electric current also results in muscle contraction. En route to the pons, the motor fibers converge into a tight bundle known as the internal capsule. A comparatively small injury to the capsule results in paralysis in more muscles than does a much larger injury to the cortex itself.

Within the medulla, the motor axons from the cortex form the motor pathways or tracts, notably the corticospinal or pyramidal tracts. Here, most of the fibers cross (or decussate) to the opposite side, continuing as a crossed pyramidal tract. The remaining fibers enter the spinal cord on the same side as the direct pyramidal tract. Each fiber in this tract finally crosses to the opposite side of the cord and terminates within the gray matter of the anterior horn on that side, in proximity to a motor nerve cell. Fibers of the crossed pyramidal tract terminate within the anterior horn and make connections with anterior horn cells on the same side. All of the motor fibers of the spinal nerves represent extensions of these anterior horn cells, with each of these fibers communicating with only one particular muscle fiber.

The motor system is complex, and motor function depends on the integrity of the corticospinal tracts, the extrapyramidal system, and cerebellar function. A motor impulse consists of a two-neuron pathway (described below). The motor nerve pathways are contained in the spinal cord. Some represent the pathways of the so-called extrapyramidal system, establishing connections between the anterior horn cells and the automatic control centers located in the basal ganglia and the cerebellum. Others are components of reflex arcs, forming synaptic connections between anterior horn cells and sensory fibers that have entered adjacent or neighboring segments of the spinal cord.

Upper and lower motor neurons: The voluntary motor system consists of two groups of neurons: upper motor neurons and lower motor neurons. Upper motor neurons originate: in the cerebral cortex, the cerebellum, and the brainstem. Their fibers make up the descending motor pathways, are located entirely within the CNS, and modulate the activity of the lower motor neurons. Lower motor neurons are located either in the anterior horn of the spinal cord gray matter or within cranial nerve nuclei in the brainstem. Axons of lower motor neurons in both sites extend through peripheral nerves and terminate in skeletal muscle. Lower motor neurons are located in both the CNS and the peripheral nervous system.

The motor pathways from the brain to the spinal cord, as well as from the cerebrum to the brainstem, are formed by upper motor neurons. They begin in the cortex of one side of the brain, descend through the internal capsule, cross to the opposite side in the brainstem, descend through the corticospinal tract, and synapse with the lower motor neurons. in the cord. The lower motor neurons receive the impulse in the posterior part of the cord and run to the myoneural junction located in the peripheral muscle.

Upper motor neuron lesions: Upper motor neuron lesions can involve the motor cortex, the internal capsule, the spinal cord, and other structures of the brain through which the corticospinal tract descends. If the upper motor neurons are damaged or destroyed, as frequently occurs with stroke or spinal cord injury, paralysis (loss of voluntary movement) results. However, because the inhibitory influences of intact upper motor neurons are now impaired, reflex (involuntary) movements are uninhibited, and hence hyperactive deep tendon reflexes, diminished or absent superficial reflexes, and pathologic reflexes such as a Babinski response occur. Severe leg spasms can occur as the result of an upper motor neuron lesion; the spasms result from the preserved reflex are, which lacks inhibition along the spinal cord below the level of injury. There is little or no muscle atrophy, and muscles remain permanently tense, exhibiting spastic paralysis or paresis (weakness).

Paralysis associated with upper motor neuron lesions can affect a whole extremity, both extremities, or an entire half of the body. Hemiplegia (paralysis of an arm and leg on the same side of the body) can be the result of an upper motor neuron lesion. If hemorrhage, an embolus, or a thrombus destroys the fibers from the motor area in the internal capsule, the arm and the leg of the opposite side become stiff, weak, or paralyzed, and the reflexes are hyperactive. If both legs are paralyzed, the condition is called paraplegia. If all four extremities are paralyzed, the condition is called quadriplegia or tetraplegia.

Lower motor neuron lesions: A patient is considered to have lower motor neuron damage if a motor nerve is damaged between the muscle and the spinal cord. The result of lower motor neuron damage is muscle paralysis. Reflexes are lost, and the muscle becomes flaccid (limp) and atrophied from disuse. If the patient has injured the spinal trunk and it can heal, use of the muscles connected to that section of the spinal cord may be regained. However, if the anterior horn motor cells are destroyed, the nerves cannot regenerate and the muscles are never useful again.

Flaccid paralysis and atrophy of the affected muscles are the principal signs of lower motor neuron disease. Lower motor neuron lesions can be the result of trauma, infection (poliomyelitis), toxins, vascular disorders, congenital malformations, degenerative processes, and neoplasms. Compression of nerve roots by herniated intervertebral disks is a common cause of lower motor neuron dysfunction.

Coordination of movement: The smoothness, accuracy, and strength that characterize the muscular movements of a normal person are attributable to the influence of the cerebellum and the basal ganglia.

The cerebellum (Fig. 6.2), described earlier, is located beneath the occipital lobe of the cerebrum; it is responsible for the coordination, balance, and timing of all muscular movements that originate in the motor centers of the cerebral cortex. Through the action of the cerebellum, the contractions of opposing muscle groups are adjusted in relation to each other to maximal mechanical advantage; muscle contractions can be sustained evenly at the desired tension and without significant fluctuation, and reciprocal movements can be reproduced at high and constant speed, in stereotyped fashion and with relatively little effort.

The basal ganglia, masses of gray matter in the midbrain beneath the cerebral hemispheres, border the lateral ventricles and lie in proximity to the internal capsule. The basal ganglia play an important role in planning and coordinating motor movements and posture. Complex neural connections link the basal ganglia with the cerebral cortex. The major effect of these structures is to inhibit unwanted muscular activity; disorders of the basal ganglia result in exaggerated, uncontrolled movements.

Impaired cerebellar function, which may occur as a result of an intracranial injury or some type of an expanding mass (e.g. a hemorrhage, abscess, or tumor), results in loss of muscle tone, weakness, and fatigue. Depending on the area of the brain affected, the patient has different motor symptoms or responses. The patient may demonstrate decorticate, decerebrate, or flaccid posturing, usually as a result of cerebral trauma. Decortication (decorticate posturing) is the result of lesions of the internal capsule or cerebral hemispheres; the patient has flexion and internal rotation of the arms and wrists and extension, internal rotation, and plantar flexion of the feet. Decerebration (decerebrate posturing), the result of lesions at the midbrain, is more ominous than decortication. The patient has extension and external rotation of the arms and wrists and extension, plantar flexion, and internal rotation of the feet. Flaccid posturing is usually the result of lower brainstem dysfunction; the patient has no motor function, is limp, and lacks motor tone.

Flaccidity preceded by decerebration in a patient with cerebral injury indicates severe neurologic impairment, which may herald brain death. However, before brain death is declared, spinal cord injury must be ruled out, the effects of all neuromuscular paralyzing agents must have worn off, and any other possible treatable causes of neurologic impairment must be investigated.

Tumors, infection, or abscess and increased intracranial pressure can all affect the cerebellum. Cerebellar signs, such as ataxia, incoordination, and seizures, as well as CSF obstruction and compression of the brainstem may be seen. Signs of increased intracranial pressure, including vomiting, headache, and changes in vital signs and level of consciousness, are especially common when CSF flow is obstructed.

Destruction or dysfunction of the basal ganglia leads not to paralysis but to muscle rigidity, with disturbances of posture and movement. The patient tends to have involuntary movements. These may take the form of coarse tremors, most often in the upper extremities, particularly in the distal portions; athetosis, movement of a slow, squirming, writhing, twisting type; or chorea, marked by spasmodic, purposeless, irregular, uncoordinated motions of the trunk and the extremities, and facial grimacing. Disorders due to lesions of the basal ganglia include Parkinson's disease, Huntington's disease, and spasmodic torticollis.

SENSORY SYSTEM FUNCTION

Integrating sensory impulses: The thalamus, a major receiving and transmitting center for the afferent sensory nerves, is a large structure connected to the midbrain. It lies next to the third ventricle and forms the floor of the lateral ventricle (Fig. 6.3). The thalamus integrates all sensory impulses except olfaction. It plays a role in the conscious awareness of pain and the recognition of variation in temperature and touch. The thalamus is responsible for the sense of movement and position and the ability to recognize the size, shape, and quality of objects.

Receiving sensory impulses: Afferent impulses travel from their points of origin to their destinations in the cerebral cortex via the ascending pathways directly, or they may cross at the level of the spinal cord or in the medulla, depending on the type of sensation that is registered. Sensory information may be integrated at the level of the spinal cord or may be relayed to the brain. Knowledge of these pathways is important for neurologic assessment and for understanding symptoms and their relationship to various lesions.

Sensory impulses convey sensations of heat, cold, and pain. The axons enter the spinal cord by way of the posterior root, specifically in the posterior gray column of the spinal cord, where they make connections with the cells of secondary neurons. Pain and temperature fibers cross immediately to the opposite side of the cord and course upward to the thalamus. Fibers carrying sensations of touch, light pressure, and localization do not connect immediately with the second neuron but ascend the cord for a variable distance before entering the gray matter and completing this connection. The axon of the secondary neuron crosses the cord and proceeds upward to the thalamus.

Position and vibratory sensations are produced by stimuli arising from muscles, joints, and bones. These stimuli are conveyed, uncrossed, all the way to the brainstem by the axon of the primary neuron. In the medulla, synaptic connections are made with cells of the secondary neurons, whose axons cross to the opposite side and then proceed to the thalamus.

Sensory losses: Destruction of a sensory nerve results in total loss of sensation in its area of distribution. Transection of the spinal cord yields complete anesthesia below the level of injury. Selective destruction or degeneration of the posterior columns of the spinal cord is responsible for a loss of position and vibratory sense in segments distal to lesion, without loss of touch, pain, or temperature perception. A lesion, such as a cyst, in the center of the spinal cord causes dissociation of sensation–loss of pain at the level of the lesion. This occurs because the fibers carrying and temperature cross within the cord immediately on entering; thus, any lesion that divides the cord longitudinally divides these fibers. Other sensory fibers ascend the cord for variable distances, some even to the medulla, before crossing, thereby bypassing the lesion and avoiding destruction.

Lesions affecting the posterior spinal nerve roots may cause impairment of tactile sensation, including intermittent severe pain that is referred to their areas of distribution. Tingling of the fingers and the toes can be a prominent symptom of spinal cord disease, presumably due to degenerative changes in the sensory fibers that extend to the thalamus (i.e. belonging to the spinothalamic tract).

CHAPTER 7

Psychology of Sensation

Introduction

The sensation is an extension of the physiological aspects of psychology, an understanding of the basic terms and concepts. The physiology of sensory systems provides an understanding of the basic terms and concepts. The physiology of sensory systems provides an understanding of thresholds and general psychophysiological concepts. This consists of knowledge of neural pathways and the ways in which sensory information is processed within them.

Sensation is the activation of receptors in the various sense organs. The nervous system enables us to get into contact with the environment and also to initiate and execute our responses. The world around us has complicated qualities. Many things are beautiful and enjoyable. Some may be unpleasant and annoying. A sweet scent delicious tastes of sweets, the jarring noise of traffic that disturbs us, the incessant barking of a dog next door irritating us, all these and myriads of other things form the external world around us. And our life mainly consists of reacting to this complex world in various ways. This contact with the outside worlds is obtained through what are known as the sense organs. Originally people believed that man has five sense organs, viz. smell, touch, hearing, sight and taste. But we now knew that there are some more senses and sense organs. The complete list may be given as visual, auditory, taste, smell, tactual, kinesthetic, static and organic. Of these, perhaps the first-two are most important deserving consideration in some detail.

Sensation is the process by which our sense gathers information and send it to the brain. A large amount of information is being sensed by any one time such as room temperature brightness of the lights, someone talking, a distant train, or the smell of perfume. With all this information coming into our senses, the majority of our world never gets recognized. People don't notice radiowaves, X-rays, or the microscopic parasites crawling on our skin, we don't sense all the odors around them. They only sense those things we don't have the sense of smell like bloodhound or the sense of sight like a hawk. Our thresholds are different from these animals and often even from each other.

Sense Organs

The various sense organs—eyes, ears, nose, skin and taste buds—are actually quite sensitive to stimulation. The famous British philosopher Locke has very appropriately described the sense organs as gateways of knowledge. Indeed without the vision, touch, hearing, smell and taste individual shall known nothing of external world. Indeed individuals will have no ideas, no concepts; person will not be able to communicate with each other nor recognize the faces. Individual cannot even imagine what the world would be like if he has no sense organs. By virtue of sense organs alone do people know the world around us. Sense organs are affected by the changes in the world around us and by our bodily conditions. These changes are called stimuli and sense organs are responsive to them. Sense organs consist of the receptors, specialized sensitive cells associated with the endings of sensory nerve fibers and various accessory apparatus tissues which contribute to the effectiveness with which the sense organs function. The sensory receptors are specialized forms of neurons, the cells that make up the nervous system. Instead of receiving neurotransmitters from other cells, these receptor cells are stimulated by different kinds of energy—for example, the receptors in the eyes are triggered by light, whereas vibrations trigger the receptors in the ears.

Each sense organ has a distinctive and specific function to perform. There is neither duplication nor overlapping of any function. The eye can only see but cannot hear or smell. The ear can hear but not smell or taste. It is impossible to have a sensation from an organ for which it is not specifically meant. For example people cannot smell with eyes. A blind person may know certain things by the sense of touch which people know through eyes; but he surely does not see. Though our sense organs are exclusive in their sensations yet they are not entirely independent in their functioning. They work in various combinations. Person will eat out food with the help of sight, smell, taste and temperature sensations. The kinesthetic and visual senses combine to given the body balance and coordination.

Sensation is the process of informing the brain about some experience occurring outside the central nervous system. These experience can be visual, auditory, somatosensory (touch, temperature, pain), olfactory, gustatory, kinesthetic (movement) and vestibular (orientation) senses.

The organs of sight, hearing, taste, smell, pressure, temperature and pain are sensitive to stimuli which are external. Some receptors, on the other hand, are found in the body cavity and in internal organs. These are sensitive to the internal stimuli. They give rise to taste, hunger, thirst, nausea, suffocation and other similar forms of sensitivity. Certain receptors are located between the internal and external surfaces, that is, muscles, tendons, joints and vestibules of the ears. They are responsible for our kinesthetic sensations. Some people believe that is a man loses one sense his other senses try to compensate this deficiency by becoming more acute and sharp. For example, a blind man usually has a heightened sense a touch. But this idea is mistaken. Infact what happens is that when one loses a particular sense, he tries to make more use of other sense organs. This exercise and training improves the functioning of the sense organs though the level of acuity or sharpness does not undergo change. Therefore, we can improve the capacity of a sense organ by use and exercise but we cannot in any way change its organic character.

Stimuli that are below the level of conscious awareness are called subliminal stimuli. (The word limin means "threshold", so sublimin means "below the threshold"). These stimuli are just strong enough to activate the sensory receptors but not strong enough for people to be consciously aware of them. Many people believe that these stimuli act upon the unconscious mind, influencing behavior in a process called *subliminal perception.*

1. THE SENSATION OF THE TASTE

Gustatory sense means the sense of taste and olfactory sense means the sense of smell. It is better to consider these two together because in actual life they often go together. Most of our taste sensations are really a combination of taste and smell. For example, coffee which we enjoy so much has the same bitter taste as quinine. If the flavor can be completely cut out, coffee will taste just as bad as quinine. Taste sensation occurs because of some small "taste buds" lying mostly below the surface of the tongue. Actually, it is these buds which form the taste receptors. In order that these buds are excited, the stimulus must be in form of a liquid. Before we can sense the taste of any object, it must be in the form of a solution so that it can come in contact with these buds. There are taste buds in certain parts of the mouth and the throat also. It is interesting to note that there are actually only four different kinds of primary tastes, sweet, sour, bitter and salty. All other tastes are combinations of these and of different smell sensations. The tongue has certain areas set apart for these four different tastes. The sides of the tongue are sensitive to sour, the back of the tongue to the bitter taste and the tip to sweet and salt. The total taste effect that we get when we actually eat something is a complex sensation arising from various other sense organs also, such as sense of touch and temperature in addition to smell.

The sense of taste, another evolved sense, manifests by means of certain nerves terminating in tiny cells of the tongue, known as 'taste buds. The taste buds are stimulated chemically by objects brought in contact with them, the impulse being conveyed to the nerves, and then transmitted to the brain. The sensations of taste are classified into five classes, i.e. sweet, sour, bitter, salty and hot (as in care of pepper, etc.)

The receptor cells for taste are located in the clusters of cells knows as the taste buds. Taste sensitivity is dependent upon a two-stage process that involves (i) the chemical stimulus penetrating the taste bud, and (ii) the chemical reaction that prompts the nerve impulse. Taste buds are served by branches of three cranial nerves (VII,IX, X), all of which terminate in the medulla or pons.

In 1916 a German psychologist named Hans Henning proposed that there are four primary tastes; sweet, sour, salty and bitter. In 1996, Lindeman proposed that there is a fifth kind of taste receptor that detects a pleasant "brothy" taste associated with foods like chicken soup, tuna, kelp, cheese and soy products, among others. Lindeman also proposed that this fifth taste be called umami, a Japanese word that describes the taste. The five taste sensations work together, along with the sense of smell and the texture, temperature and heat of foods, to produce thousands of taste sensations.

The sense of taste (taste in food, not taste in clothing or friends) and the sense of smell are very closely related. Have you ever noticed that when your nose is all stopped up, your sense of taste if affected, too? That's because the sense of taste is really a combination of taste and smell. Without the input from the nose, there are actually only four, and possibly five, kinds of taste sensors in the mouth.

Taste buds are the common name for the taste receptor cells, special kinds of neurons found in the mouth that are responsible for the sense of taste, or gestation. Most taste buds are located on the tongue, but there are a few on the roof of the mouth, the cheeks, and under the tongue as well. How sensitive people are to various tastes depends on how many taste buds they have; some people have only around 500, whereas other have 20 times that number. The latter are called "supertasters" and need far less seasoning in their food than those with fewer taste buds. Taste buds of little bumps those little bumps are called papillae, and the taste buds line the walls of these papillae. Each taste bud has about

20 receptors that are very similar to the receptor sites on receiving neurons at the synapse. In fact, the receptors on taste buds work exactly like receptor sites on neurons—they receive molecules of various substances that fit into the receptor like a key into a lock. Taste is often called a chemical sense because it works with the molecules of foods people eat in the same way the neural receptors work with neurotransmitters. When the molecules (dissolved in saliva) fit into the receptors, a signal is fired to the brain, which then interprets the taste sensation.

2. THE SENSATION OF SMELL

The sense of smell is a chemical sense. The ability to smell odors is called **olfaction, or the olfactory sense**. People do not actually smell with their noses. The outer part of the nose serves the same purpose for odors that the pinna and ear serve for sounds. Both are merely ways to get the sensory information to the part of the body that will translate merely ways to get the sensory information to the part of the body that will translate it into neural signals. So the external nose, like the outer ear, is just a collection device. The part of the olfactory system that turns odors into signals the brain can understand is located at the top of the nasal passages. This areas of olfactory receptor cells in only about an inch square in each cavity yet contains about 10 million olfactory receptors.

The sense of smell is manifested by means of delicate nerves termination in the mucous membrane of the nostrils. The mucous membrane contacts with minute objects entering the nostrils, and it registers the differences in the chemical composition of such particles. This message of the nerve ends is transmitted to the brain. The particles of the smelled objects must have actually entered the nostrils and have come in contact with these nerve ends in order to have been sensed. More nearness to the organ of smell is not sufficient, actual contact must be there, or we will smell nothing. We smell the rose only because minute particles of its substance are carried into our nostrils. We smell gas because some of its particles enter our nostrils.

The olfactory receptor cells each have about a half dozen to a dozen little "hairs" that project into the cavity. These "hairs" are called cilia. Like taste buds, there are receptor sites on these hair cells that send signals to the brain when stimulated by the molecules of substances that are in the air moving past them. When a person is sniffing something, the sniffing serves to move molecules of whatever the person is trying to smell into the nose and into the nasal cavities. That's okay when it's the smell of baking bread, apple pie, flowers, and the like, but when it's skunk, rotten eggs, dead animals—well, try not to think about it too much. Olfactory receptors are like taste buds in another way, too. Olfactory receptors also have to be replaced as they naturally die off, about every 5 to 8 weeks. Unlike the taste buds, there are more than five types of olfactory receptors. In fact, there are at least 1,000 of them. The sense of smell is different in some way from the other senses? Yes, the signals from the olfactory receptors in the nasal cavity do not follow the same path as the signals from all the other senses. Vision, hearing, taste, and touch all go through the medulla (where the signals from one side of the body crossover to the opposite side) and up through the brainstem, the thalamus, and finally to the area of the cortex that processes that particular sensory information. But the sense of smell has its own special place in the brain—the olfactory bulbs.

The olfactory bulbs are located right on top of the sinus cavity on each side of the brain directly beneath the frontal lobes. The olfactory receptors send their neural signals directly up to these bulbs, bypassing the entire lower brain and its selective attention filter, the reticular formation. If the olfactory signals bypass the part of the brain that lets us ignore constant and unchanging information, does that mean that we can not "ignore" smells? Fortunately, people can ignore a smell that is constant and unchanging, but it does not involve the reticular formation. The text stated that certain sensory receptors become less sensitive to a constant stimulus as time goes by, so that eventually a person no longer perceives the stimulus. This adaptation is why people don't continue to smell the odor of the kitchen garbage can after being home for a while.

Olfactory or the smell senses are received by what are called olfactory cells situated at the top inside of the nostrils. Here, the stimulus to be sensed must take the form of gaseous particles to be inhaled along with the air. These gas particles produce some chemical action in these cells which form the nerve current for the sensation. Attempts to classify smell sensation into different categories have not been on the whole successful. In fact our knowledge about the smell sensation is very much less than our knowledge of other senses.

3. THE SENSATION OF TOUCH

The sense of touch is really several sensations, originating in several different places in—and on—the body. Its really more accurate to refer to these as the body senses, or somesthetic senses. The first part of that word, soma, means "body", as mentioned in chapter two. The second part, esthetic, means "feeling", hence, the name. There are three somesthetic sense systems, the skin senses (having to do with touch, pressure, temperature and pain), the kinesthetic sense (having to do with the location of body parts in relation to the ground and to each other), and the vestibular senses (having to do with movement and body position). Skin is an organ. Its purposes include more than simply keeping bodily fluids in and germs out; skin also receives and transmits information from the outside worlds to the central nervous system. Information about light touch, deeper pressure, hot, cold and even pain is collected by special receptors in the skin's layers. There are about half a dozen different receptors in the layers of the skin. Some of them will respond to only one kind of sensation. For example, the pacinian corpuscles are just beneath the skin and respond to pressure only. There are nerve endings that wrap around the ends of the hair follicles, a fact people may be well aware of when they tweeze their eyebrows. These nerve endings are sensitive to both pain and touch. There are free nerve endings just beneath the uppermost layer of the skin that respond to changes in temperature and to pressure—and to pain.

The senses constitute the doors to the outside world. Which when opened permit the entrance of messages from that world. Human skin is not uniformly sensitive to different of stimuli. There are three skin/cutaneous senses.

- **Pressure (touch):** Pressure sensation is defined as tissue distortion, or the mechanical deformation of skin tissue. Pressure intensity is measured in grams per millimeter. As with other senses, the level of pressure sensitivity is different in different parts of the body. In general, the closure to the extremity, the more sensitivity there will be. The least sensitive is the back. Various receptors involved in pressure sensation are Merkel's disk, Meissner's corpuscle, free nerve ending, digital nerves and pacinian corpuscle.
- **Temperature**: This sensation explains about cold and heat sensitivity in different parts of the body. The body has receptors for cold and warmth. The receptors for small and more numerous that warmth receptors whereas warmth receptors are larger and less numerous.

- **Pain**: There are many questions relating to the nature of pain and how to stop it effectively. Initial thought that pain was a direct function of tissue damage was quickly proven to be incorrect (e.g. It was found that major tissue damage could go with minor pain sensation. Melzack and Wall explains "Gate theory" for pain that messages pass through a "gate" in the spinal cord and route to the brain. In effect, pain messages may or may not be sent depending upon other sensory experience and the moment's attention and activity. Pain can be reduced by endorphins counteracting the "pain messenger" neurotransmitter "substance P") and attention distraction (e.g. Lamaze method in childbirth).

There are pain nerve fibers in the internal organs as well as receptors for pressure. There are actually different types of pain. There are receptors (called proprioceptive receptors) that detect pain (and pressure) in the organs, a type of pain called visceral pain. But pain sensations in the skin, muscles, tendons, and joints are carried on large nerve fibers and are called somatic pain. Somatic pain is the body's warning system that something is being, or is about to be, damaged and tends to be sharp and fast. Another type of somatic pain is carried on small nerve fibers and is slower and more of a general ache. This somatic pain acts as a kind of reminder system, keeping people from further injury by reminding them that the body has already been damaged. For example, if you hit your thumb with a hammer, the immediate pain sensation is of the first kind—sharp, fast, and bright. But later the bruised tissue simply aches, letting you know to take it easy on that thumb. The best current explanation for how the sensation of pain works is called gate-control theory. In this theory, the pain signals must pass through a "gate" located in the spinal cord. The activity of the gate can be closed by nonpain signals coming into the spinal cord from the body and by signals a coming from the brain. The gate is not a physical structure but instead represents the relative balance in neural activity of cells in the spinal cord that receive information from the body and then send information to the brain.

Stimulation of the pain receptor cells releases a chemical called substances P (for pain, naturally). Substance P released into the spinal cord activates other neurons that send their messages through spinal gates (opened by the pain signal). From the spinal cord, the message goes to the brain, activating cells in the thalamus, somatonsensory cortex, areas of the frontal lobes, and the limbic system. The brain then interprets the pain information and sends signals that either open the spinal gates further, causing a greater experience of pain, or close them, dampening the pain. Of course, this decision by the brain is influenced by the psychological aspects of the pain causing stimulus. Anxiety, fear, and helplessness intensify pain, while laughter, distraction, and a sense of control can diminish it. (This is why people might bruise themselves and not know it if they were concentrating on something else). Pain can also be affected by competing signals from other skin senses, which is why rubbing a sore spot can reduce the feeling of pain.

Those same psychological aspects can also influence the release of the endorphin, the body's natural version of morphine. Endorphin can inhibit the transmission of pain signals in the brain, and in the spinal cord they can inhibit the release of substance P. The release of endorphins is perhaps one explanation for "runner's high" (the pleasurable feeing a runner may experience after running a long distance) and the effectiveness of acupuncture. Women are better able to tolerate higher levels of pain than men is a generalization that has no basis in fact. Some people also have heard that men are childish about pain and do not cope well with pain, but that is also a myth. The fact is that research has shown that women apparently feel pain more intensely than do men, and they also report pain more often men do. Men have been shown to cope better with many kinds of pain, possibly because men are often found to have a stronger belief than women that they can control their pain by their own efforts.

- **Tactual sensation:** These are referred to also by the terms cutaneous or simply, the skin senses. There are four kinds of cutaneous sensations, viz., touch, heat, cold and pain. The entire areas of our skin is not sensitive at all places to all these four sensations. These four sensations are actually different kinds of sensations, each having its own particular type of receptor. These four types of receptors are spread over different parts of the body. The receptors for all the cutaneous senses consist mainly of different types of small bulbs or corpuscles lying just below the surface of the skin. These corpuscles vary in their structure according to the regions of the body in which they are found. Some are sensitive to very light pressure and some are not. The pain receptors are sensitive only to pain. Similarly, the heat receptors are sensitive only to heat or warmth. Thus if we would still a warmth spot with a fine ice-cold point, we would still feel warm and not cold. But if we receive a blow or a large mass of body comes and dashes against our skin, simultaneously all these sensitive spots may be stimulated. With a fine pointed pencil or a proper apparatus called esthesiometer, we can map out different spots scattered an clustered over the different parts of the body. It has been found that the front parts of the body have more touch spots than the back. The lips and fingertips are also rich in touch spots.
- **Kinesthetic sense:** The kinesthetic sense is also known as the muscle sense. It is actually the sense of movement of our limbs. When our muscles and tendons move, the receptors connected with them communicate this movement to the brain. These receptors are called the kinesthetic sense organs. They are in the form of minute spindle-shaped organs located in the muscles and joints. These spindle-shaped receptors inform us of the position of our muscles and limbs and also the strain exerted on them.

  The proprioceptive receptors (proprioceptors) located in the skin, joints, muscles, and tendons, mentioned in the discussion of pain, are part of the body's sense of position in space—the location of the arms, legs and so forth in relation to one another and in relation to the ground. This sense is called kinesthesia, from the Greek words kinein (to move) and esthesis (sensation). When you close your eyes and raise your hand above your head, you know where your hand is because the proprioceptors tell you about the changes in pressure within the muscles.
- **Static sense:** This is also known as the sense of balance. We said in the previous chapter that the cerebellum is responsible for keeping our balance and posture. The first responsible which carry messages of disturbances in the balance, are the kinesthetic senses which we have mentioned. The semicircular canals of the inner ear also play an important part in this sensation. Details of the various parts of the ear will be mentioned later when we consider the auditory sensation. It may be mentioned here however, that these canals which are three in number are set in three planes, one in the horizontal position and the other two in the vertical position at right angles to each other. Any movement that shakes the head produces a disturbance in the fluid contained in these semicircular canals and each canal also contains a number of minute hair cells. When the fluid is disturbed, these hairs are affected and are swayed this way or that. It is this movement of the hairs that gives the static sense. So the real receptors for these sensations are these hair cells. Since the canals are set in three planes, movement in any plane can be reported accurately.

- **Organic sense**: Organic sensations are sometimes called body sensations. These refer mostly to sensations such as hunger, thirst, nausea, sex feelings, etc. We do not yet have the accurate knowledge of the location and nature of the various receptors pertaining to these senses. They are located inside the body in the various appropriate places.

4. VISUAL SENSATION

The ability to see the world clearly can easily be taken for granted. The eye is a sensitive, highly specialized sense organ subject to various disorders, many of which lead to impaired vision. Impaired vision may affect a person's independence in self-care, work and lifestyle choices, sense of self-esteem, safety, ability to interact with society and the environment and overall quality of life.

Since sight is very important, we must have some detailed knowledge about it. The organ which receives the light stimuli is itself very complicated and interesting. See the various objects. Through eyes, for example, we see a table, see a tree and so on. Actually the object as such is not seen by us. The only contact that we have with the object is through the light waves that come from the objects and strike a certain part of the eye. So, strictly speaking, people see only the light. The sense of sight is regarded as an evolution of the elementary sense of touch or feeling. It manifests through a most complex organism and nerve-arrangement. The eye, a sensory system, demonstrates the area and some of its basic concepts. When light energy reaches photoreceptors (rods and cones), neural signals are sent through the visual system, providing sensations. The travel route includes the neural layers through which the light must pass before being absorbed by the photoreceptors. A photochemical reaction is triggered in the photoreceptors, producing neural signals that are transmitted first to the bipolar cells and then to the ganglionic cells.

The human eye is well-planned camera and almost spherical. The eyeball is covered and made light-proof by three coats. The outer coat is called sclerotic. It is whitish in color. It is like the wooden or metal cover of the camera box. Attached to the sclerotic coat, almost like a lining, we have a layer called the choroid. The choroid is a black lining, and this black color ensures that the ball is absolutely light-proof. The third lining is the retinal which actually contains the receptors and plays the part of the sensitive film inside a camera. One difference is, unlike the case of the camera, this film (retina) is permanent and fixed and needs no change. The outer coating, sclerotic, gives place at the front of the eye to what is called cornea, a curved transparent lens-like substance. The choroid in its turn gives place to a circular muscle tissue called the iris. This iris leaves a hole in the center which we call the pupil of the eye. Just behind this hole is the actual lens. The ciliary muscles and the iris perform the function of the focusing mechanism. The eyeball is kept intact and spherical because of some liquid substance contained therein. The space between the cornea and the pupil is filled by a substance called aqueous humor and the space behind the lens and the entire outer cover of the eye is filled with a substance called vitreous humor. Both these humors are transparent and so, light easily passes through them. Now we can recapitulate as to what happens when we see an object. Light from the object reaches the eye at the point of the cornea and the cornea being transparent, the light is allowed to pass on inside to the lens through the pupil. The lends is adjusted to get a good focus of this light with the help of the ciliary muscles and the light is again passed on inside through the vitreous humor, to the retina. The retina is like a film which records light sensation.

Unlike most organs of the body, the eye is available of external examination, and its anatomy is more easily assessed than many other body parts. The eyeball, or globe sits in a protective bony structure known as the orbit. Lined with muscle and connective and adipose tissues, the orbit is about 4cm high, wide, and deep, and it is shaped roughly like a four-sided pyramid, surrounded on three sides by the sinuses: ethmoid (medially), frontal (superiorly), and maxillary (inferiorly). The optic nerve and the ophthalmic artery enter the orbit at its apex through the optic foramen. The eyeball is moved through all fields of gaze by the extraocular muscles. The four rectus muscles and two oblique muscles are innervated by cranial nerves (CN) III, IV, and VI. Normally, the movements of the two eyes are coordinated, and the brain perceives a single image.

The eyelids composed of thin elastic skin that cover striated and smooth muscles, protect the anterior portion of the eye. The triangular spaces formed by the junction of the eyelids are know as the inner or medial canthus and the outer or lateral canthus. With every blink of the eyes, the lids wash the cornea and conjunctiva with tears (Fig. 7.1).

Tears are vital to eye health. They are formed by the lacrimal gland and the accessory lacrimal glands. A healthy coid. If there is a defect in the composition of any of these layers, the integrity of the cornea may be compromised. Tears are secreted in response to reflex or emotional stimuli.

The conjunctiva, a mucous membrane, provides a barrier to the external environment and noursihes the eye. The goblet cells of the conjunctiva secrete lubricating mucus. The bulbar conjunctivae lines the inner surface of the upper and lower eyelids. The junction of the two portions is known as the fornix.

The sclera, commonly known as the white of the eye, is a dense, fibrous structure that makes up the posterior five-sixths of the eye. The sclera helps maintain the shape of the eyeball and protects the intraocular contents from trauma. The sclera may have a slightly bluish tinge in young children, a dull white color in adults, and a slightly yellowish color in the elderly. Externally, it is overlaid with conjunctiva, which is a thin, transparent, mucous membrane that contains fine blood vessels. The conjunctiva meets the cornea at the limbus on the outermost edge of the iris.

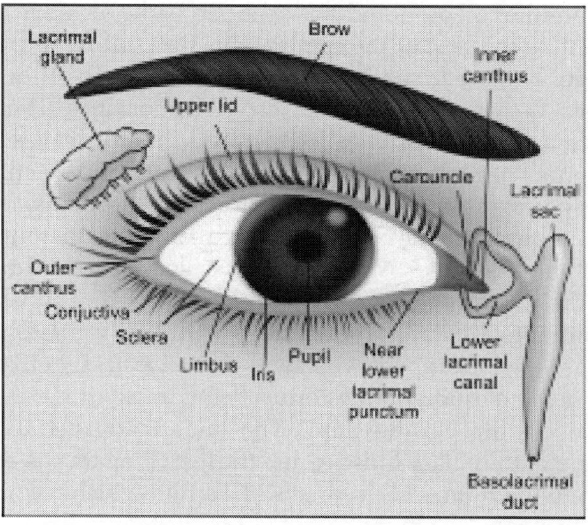

Fig. 7.1: External structures of eye

The cornea is a transparent, avascular, dome-like structure, forms the most anterior portion of the eyeball and is the main refracting surface of the eye. It is composed of five layers; epithelium, Bowman's membrane, stoma, Descemet's membrane, and endothelium. The epithelial cells are capable of rapid replication and are completely replaced every 7 days.

Behind the cornea lies the anterior chamber, filled with a continually replenished supply of clear aqueous humor, which nourshes the cornea. The aqueous humor is produced by the ciliary body, and its producation is realted to the intraocular pressure (IOP). Normal IOP is 10 to 21 mm Hg.

The uvea consists of the iris, the ciliary body, and the choroid. The iris, or colored part of the eye, is a highly vascularized, pigmented collection of fibers surrounding the pupil. The pupil is a space that dilates and constricts in response to light. Normal pupil are round and constrict symmetrically when a bright light shines on them. About 20 percent of the population have pupils that are slightly unequal in size but that respond equally to light. Dilation and constriction are controlled by the sphincter and dilator pupillae muscles. The dilator muscles are controlled by the sympathetic nervous system, eheras the sphincter muscles are controlled by the parasympathetic nervous system.

Directly behind the pupil and iris lies the lens, a colorless and almost completely transparent, biconvex structure held in position by zonular fibers. It is avascular and has no nerve or pain fibers. The lens enables focusing for near vision and refocusing for distance vision. The ability to focus and refocus is called accommodation. The lens is suspended behind the iris by the zonules and is connected to the ciliary body. The ciliary body controls accommodation through the zonular fibers and the ciliary muscles. The aqueous humor is anterior to the lens; posterior to the lens the vitreous humor. All cells formed thoughout life are retained by these, which makes the cell structure of the lens susceptible to the degenerative effects of aging. The lens continues to grow throughout life, laying down fibers in concetric rings. This gradual thikening becomes evident in the fifth decade of life and eventually results in an increasingly dense core or nucleus, which can limit accommodative powers.

The posterior chamber is a small space between the vitreous and the iris. Aqueous fluid is manufactured in the posterior chamber by the ciliary body. This aqueous fluid flows from the posterior chamber into the anterior chamber, from which it drains through the trabecular meshwork into the canal of Schlemm.

The choroid lies between the retina and the sclera. It is avascular tissue, supplying blood to the portion of the sensory retina closest to it.

The ocular fundus is the largest chamber of the eye and contains the vitreous humor, aclear, gelatinous substance, composed mostly of water and encapsulated by a hyaloid membrane. The vitreous humor occupies about two-thirds of the eys's volume and helps maintain the shape of the eye. As the body ages, the gel-like characteristics are gradually lost, and various cells and fibers cast shadows that the patient perceives as "floaters." The vitreous is in continuous contact with the retina and is attached to the retina by scattered collagenous filaments. The vitreous shrinks and shifts with age.

The innermost surface of the fundus is the retina. The retina is composed of 10 microscopic layers and has the consistency of wet tissue paper. It is neural tissue, an extension of the optic nerve. Viewed through the pupil, the landmarks of the retina are the optic disc, the retinal vessels, and the macula. The point of entrance of the optic nerve into the retina is the optic disc. The optic disc is pink; it is oval or circular and has sharp margins.

In the disk, a physiologic depression or cup is present centrally, with the retinal blood vessels emanating from it. The retinal tissues arise from the optic disc and line the inner surface of the through the opitc nerve, branching out through the retina and forming superior and inferior branches. The macula is the area to the retina responsible for central vision. In the center of the macula is the most sensitive are, the fovea, which is avascular and surrounded by the superior and inferior vascular arcades. Two important layers of the retina are the retinal pigment epithelium (RPE) and the sensory retina. A single layer of cells constitutes the RPE, and these cells have numerous funcitons, including the absorption of light. The sensory retina contains the photoreceptor cells: rods and cones. These are long, narrow cells shaped like rods or cones. The rods are mainly responsible for night vision or vision in lowlight, whereas the cones provide the best vision for bright light, color vision, and fine detail. Cones are distributed throughout the retina, with their greatest concentration in the fovea. Rods are absent in the fovea.

Visual acuity depends on a healthy functioning eyeball and an intact visual pathway. This pathway is made up of the retina, optic nerve, optic chiasm, optic tracks, lateral geniculate bodies, and optic radiations and the visual cortex area of the brain. The pathway is an extension of the central nervous system.

The optic nerve is also known as the second cranial nerve (CN II). Its purpose is to transmit impulses from the retina to the occipital lobe of the brain. The opitc nerve head, or optic disc, is the physiologic blind spot in each eye. The optic nerve leaves the eye and then meets the optic nerve from the other eye at the optic chiasm. The chiasm is the retina of each eye cross to the opposite side of the brain. The nerve fibers from the nasal retina of each eye cross to the opposite side of the brain. The nerve fibers from the temporal retina of each eye remain uncrossed. Fibers from the right half of each eye. Which would be the left visual field, carry impulses to the right occipital lobe. Fibers from the left half of each eye, or the right visual field, carry impulse to the left occipital lobe. Beyond the Chiasm, these fibers are known as the optic tract continues on to the lateral geniculate body. The lateral geniculate body leads to the optic radiations and then to the cortex of the occipital lobe of the brain.

The retina contains the actual sense cells or the receptors. There are two kinds of receptors in the retina called the rods and the cones. The retina contains a layer of pigment and these rods and cones are adjacent to the pigment. The light that comes in, produces some chemical and electrical changes in the pigment and this change in turn sets the rods and cones into activity. The rods and cones have different structures and different functions. The rods as the term indicates are long and comparatively thin. The cones are stumpy and stout. Physiologically the cones are more highly developed and complicated than the rods. It is important to remember how these rods and cones are distributed on the surface of the retina. Almost in the center of the retina, at the back of the eye, there is a point called fovea where only cones are present. This point happens to be the center of clearest vision. Outside this area of fovea rods and cones mingle and as we go further and further along the retina towards the front part of the eye, cones get less in number and rods increase until at lat in the very outer regions near the lens, there are practically only rods. We shall refer to this point later once again when we consider the problem of color vision.

It has been experimentally determined that the cones are responsible for color vision and the rods for vision of form and outline. The rods though less developed than the cones, have an important advantage. In twilight and in very dim light, we see outlines because of the presence of rods. We do not differentiate colors since the cones are not active. Yet we would see the form and shape. In darkness, the cones cannot respond at all. They need a fair amount of light to be active. But the rods can respond in dim light also. Rods and cones are connected by nerves called the optic nerves to the occipital lobes of the two cerebral hemispheres. Seeing the object instead of merely the light is because of the complex grouping and associating processes that go on in the cortex to which the light sensations are carried.

Right near the above, which is the center of clearest vision, there is a point at which the optic nerve pierces into the retina and sends out its branches all over. The nerve itself does not contain any receptors, viz. rods and cones. So this point almost at the center of the retina does not respond to any light stimulus. Hence it is called the blind spot.

Psychological Properties of Light

Light is a complicated phenomenon. Although scientists have long argued over the nature of light, they finally have agreed that light has the properties of both waves and particles. The following section gives a brief history of how scientists have tried to "shed light" on the mystery of light. Although Isaac Newton believed light to be a function of particles, in 1802 Thomas Young demonstrated that light behaves like waves. Research at the turn of the twentieth century provided evidence for both views—sometimes light behaves like particles and sometimes like waves. It was Albert Einstein who first demonstrated that light is actually both: He proposed tiny "packets" of waves called photons. These photons actually have wavelengths associated with them, hence, the wave-like properties.

When people experience light, they are not really aware of its dual nature. There are three psychological aspects to the experience of light: brightness, color and saturation. Brightness is determined by the amplitude of the wave—how high or how low the wave actually is. The higher the wave, the brighter the light will be. Low waves are dimmer. Color, or hue, is determined by the length of the wave. Long wavelengths are found at the red end of the visible spectrum (the portion of the whole spectrum of light that is visible to the human eye) whereas, shorter wavelengths are found at the blue end.

Saturation refers to the purity of the color people see: A highly saturated red, for example, would contain only red wavelengths, whereas a less saturated red might contain a mixture of wavelengths. For example, when a child is using the red paint from a set of poster paints, the paint on the paper will look like a pure red, but if the child mixes in some white paint, the paint will look pink. The hue is still red but it will be less of a saturated red because of the presence of white wavelengths. Mixing in black or gray would also lessen the saturation.

Light travels in the form of waves. The science of physics will give us many interesting details about this phenomenon. These waves can have different wavelengths which are responsible for different colors. Light also varies in its intensity. Sometimes different wavelengths can get mixed together to produce the various colors that are not the elementary colors of the spectrum. Color mixing is an interesting phenomenon as can be demonstrated by the fast rotation of a color wheel; when all the different colors are mixed together we get light gray. By mixing red and yellow, we get the various orange shades. By mixing blue and red, we get violet and the purple colors. When yellow and blue are mixed, the result is light gray or even white if properly done. So they neutralize each other when combined. Therefore the two colors, yellow and blue are called complementary colors. Similarly, red and green are also called complementary colors (actually when red and green are mixed we do not get white or gray as in the case of the other pair, but a kind of yellow). The problem of color vision has been studied by many physiologists to answer the question how exactly we see colors. Various theories have been offered to explain this phenomenon.

5. THE SENSE OF HEARING

The sense of hearing is manifested by means of delicate nerve terminating in the inner part of the ear. The eardrum, or "tympanum", vibrates in response to the air-vibrations or sound-waves reaching it from the outside. These vibrations are intensified, and the auditory nerve-ends take up the impression and pass it to the brain. Sound waves are sensed according to their characteristics of pitch, intensity, quality and harmony.

The name of this particular sense comes from a Latin word that means 'entrance or chamber'. The latter definition is probably the one that fits better here, as the structures for this sense are located in the innermost chamber of the ear. There are two kinds of vesticular organs, the otolith organs and the semicircular canals.

The otolith organs are tiny sacs found just above the cochlea. These sacs contain a gelatin-like fluid within which tiny crystals are suspended (much like pieces of fruit in a bowl of jello). The head moves and the crystals cause the fluid to vibrate, setting off some tiny hair-like receptors on the inner surface of the sac, telling the person that he or she is moving forward, back, sideways, or up and down. (It's pretty much the way the cochlea works with movement as the stimulus instead of sound vibrations).

The semicircular canals are three somewhat circular tubes that are also field with fluid and will stimulate hair-like receptors when rotated. There are three tubes so that there is one in each of the three planes of motion. Remember learning in geometry class about the x-, y- and z-axes? Those are the three planes through which the body can rotate, and when it does, it sets off the receptors in these canals. This disagreement between what the eyes say and what the body says is pretty much what causes motion sickness, the tendency to get nauseated when in a moving vehicle, especially one with an irregular movement. Normally, the vestibular sense coordinates with the other senses. But for some people, the information from the eyes may conflict a little too much with the vestibular organs, and dizziness, nausea and disorientation are the result. This explanation of motion sickness is known as sensory conflict theory. Actually, people can probably blame the dizziness for the nausea—in human evolutionary history, many poisons make a person dizzy, and the most adaptive thing to do is to expel the poison. So although there isn't any poison in a case of motion sickness, the person may "expel" something anyway.

One way some people overcome motion sickness is to focus on a distant point or object. That point won't seem to move like the objects closer to the car window, for example, and so this causes less conflict. This is also how ballerinas and ice skaters manage not to get sick when turning rapidly and repeatedly—they focus their eyes at least once on some fixed object every so many turns.

Psychological Properties of Sound

The properties of sound are indeed similar to those of light, as both senses rely on waves. But the similarity ends there, as the physical properties of sound are different from those of light.

Sound waves do not come in little packets the way light comes in photons. Sound waves are simply the vibrations of the molecules of air that surrounds us. Sound waves do have the same properties of light waves, though—wavelength, amplitude, and purity. Wavelengths are interpreted by the brain as the frequency or pitch (high, medium or low). Amplitude is interpreted as volume, how soft or loud a sound is. Finally, what would correspond to saturation or purity in light is called timbre in sound, a richness in the tone of the sound. And just as people rarely see pure colors in the world around us, they also seldom hear pure sounds. The everyday noises that surround people do not allow them to hear many pure tones.

Just as a person's vision is limited by the visible spectrum of light, a person is also limited in the range of frequencies he or she can hear. Frequency is measure in cycles (waves) per second, or hertz (Hz). Human limits are between 20 and 20,000 Hz, with the most accurate hearing occurring at around 1,000 Hz. (In comparison, dogs can hear between 50 and 60,000 Hz, whereas dolphins can hear up to 200,000 Hz). To hear the higher and lower frequencies of a piece of music on a CD, for example, a person would need to increase the amplitude—which explains why some people like to "crank it up".

The Structure of the Ear

The ear is a sensory organ with dual functions—hearing and balance. The sense of hearing is essential for normal development and maintenance of speech as well as the ability to communicate with others. Balance, or equilibrium, is essential for maintaining body movement, position, and coordination.

The ears are located on either side of the cranium at approximately eye level.

The external ear includes the auricle (pinna) and the external auditory canal. The external ear is separated from the middle ear by a disk-like structure called the tympanic membrane (eardrum) (Fig. 7.2A).

- The auricle, attached to the side of the head by skin, is composed mainly of cartilage, except for the fat and subcutaneous tissue in the earlobe. The auricle collects the sound waves and directs vibrations into the external auditory canal.
- The external auditory canal is approximately 2.5 cm long. The lateral third is an elastic cartilaginous and dense fibrous framework to which thin skin is attached. The medial

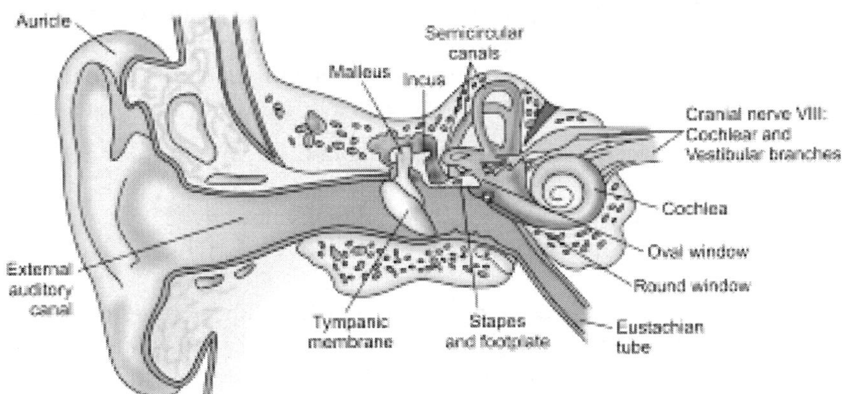

Fig. 7.2A: Anatomy of the ear

two-thirds is bone lined with thin skin. The external auditory canal ends at the tympanic membrane.

The skin of the canal contains hair, sebaceous glands, and ceruminous glands, which secrete a brown, wax-like substance called cerumen (ear wax). The ear's self-cleaning mechanism moves old skin cells and cerumen to the outer part of the ear.

Just anterior to the external auditory canal is the temporomandibular joint. The head of the mandible can be felt by placing a fingertip in the external auditory canal while the patient opens and closed the mouth.

The middle ear, an air-filled cavity, includes the tympanic membrane laterally and the otic capsule medially. The middle ear cleft lies between the two. The middle ear is connected by the eustachian tube to the nasopharynx and is continuous with air-filled cells in the adjacent mastoid portion of the temporal bone.

The eustachian tube, which is approximately 1 mm wide and 35 mm long, connects the middle ear to the nasopharynx. Normally, the eustachian tube is closed, but it opens by action of the tensor veli palatini muscle when the person performs a Valsalva maneuver, yawans, or swallows. It drains normal and abnormal secretions of the middle ear and equalizes pressure in the middle ear with that of the atmosphere.

- The tympanic membrane (eardrum), about 1 cm in diameter and very thin, is normally pearly gray and tranlucent. It consists of three layers of tissue; an outer layer, continuous with the skin of the ear canal; a fibrous middle layer; and an inner mucosal layer, continuous with lining of the middle ear cavity. Approximately 80 percent of the tympanic membrane is composed of all three layers and is called the parstensa. The remaining 20 percent lacks the middle layer and is called the pars flaccida. The absence of this fibrous middle layer makes the pars flaccida. The absecene of this fibrous middle layer makes the pars flaccida more vulnerable to pathologic disorders than the pars tensa. Distinguishing landmarks of the tympanic membrane include the annulus, the fibrous border that attaches the eardrum to the temporal bone; the short process of the malleus; the long process of the malleus, the umbo of the malleus,which attaches to the tympanic membrane in the center; the pars flaccida; and the pars tensa.
- The middle ear contains the three smallest bones (the ossicles) of the body; the malleus, the incus, and the stapes. The ossicles, which are held in place by joints, muscles, and ligaments, assist in the transmission of sound. Two small fenestrae (oval and round windows), located in the medial wall of the middle ear, separate the middle ear from the inner ear. The footplate of the stapes sits in the oval window, secured by a fibrous annulus (ring-shaped structure). The footplate transmits sound to the inner ear. The round window, covered by a thin membrane, provides an exit for sound vibrations.

The inner ear is housed deep within the temporal bone. The organs for hearing (cochlea) and balance (semicircular canals), as well as cranial nerves VII (facial nerve)and VII (vestibulocochlear nerve), are all part of this complex anatomy. The cochlea and bony labyrinth surrounds and protects the membranous labyrinth, which is bathed in a fluid called perilymph (Fig. 7.2B).

- The membranous labyrinth is composed of the utricle, the saccule, the cochlear duct, the semicircular canals, and the organ of Corti. The membranous labyrinth contains a fluid called endolymph. The three semicircular canals posterior, superior, and lateral, which lie at 90 degree angles to one another contain sensory receptor organs, arranged to detect rotational movement. These receptor end organs are stimulated by changes in

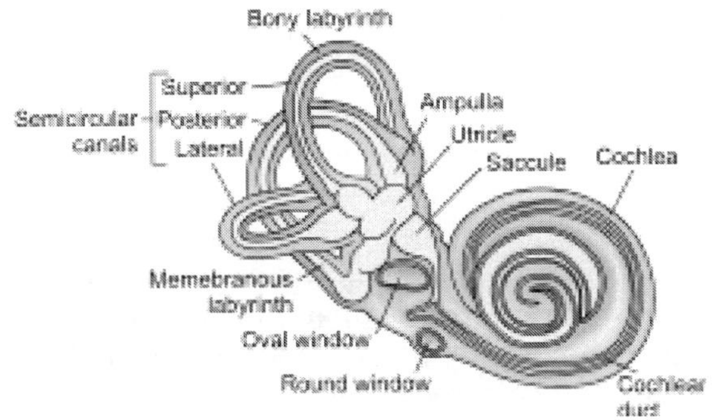

Fig. 7.2B: The inner ear

the rate or direction of a person's movement. The utricle and saccule are involved with linear movements.

- The organ of Corti is located in the cochlea, a snail-shaped, bony tube about 3.5 cm long with two and a half spiral turns. Membranes separate the cochlear duct (scala media) from the scala vestibuli, and the scala tympani from the basilar membrane. The organ of Corti is located on the basilar membrane stretching from the base to the apex of the cochlea. As sound vibrations enter the perilymph at the oval window and travel along the scala vestibuli, they pass through the scala tympani, enter the cochlear duct, and cause movement of the basilar membrane. The organ of Corti, also called the end organ for hearing, transforms mechanical energy into neural activity and separates sounds into different frequencies. This electrochemical impluse travels through the acoustic nerve to the temporal cortex of the brain to be interpreted as meaningful sound. In the internal auditory canal, the cochlear (acoustic) nerve, arising from the cochlea, joins the vestibular nerve, arising from the semicircular canals, utricle, and saccule, to become the vestibulocochlear nerve (cranial nerve VIII). This canal also house the facial nerve and the blood supply from the ear to the brain.

FUNCTION OF THE EARS

Hearing

Hearing is conducted over two pathways: air and bone. Sounds transmitted by air conduction travel over the air-filled external and middle ear through vibration of the tympanic membrane and ossicles. Sounds transmitted by bone conduction is the more efficient pathway. However, a defect in the tympanic membrane or interruption of the ossicular chain disrupts normal air conduction, which results in conductive hearing loss.

Sound Conduction and Transmission

Sound enters the ear through the external auditory canal and cause the tympanic membrane to vibrate. These vibration transmit sound through the level action of the ossicles to the oval window as mechanical energy. This mechanical energy is then transmitted through the inner ear fluids to the cochleam, stimulating the hair cells, and is subsequently converted to electrical energy. The electrical energy travels through the vestibulocochlear nerve to the central nervous system, where it is interpreted in its final form as sound.

Vibration transmitted by the tympanic membrane to the ossicles of the middle ear is transmitted to the cochlea, causing vibrations (waves) in fluids contained in the inner ear. These fluidwaves causes movement of the basilar membrane, stimulating the hair cells of the organ of Corti in the cochlea to move in a wave-like manner. The movements of the tympanic membrane set up electrical currents that stimulate the various areas of the cochlea. The hair cells set up neural impulses that are encoded and then transferred to the auditory cortex in the brain, where they are decoded into a sound message.

The footplate of the stapes receives impulses transmitted by the incus and the malleus from the tympanic membrane. The round window, which opens on the opposite side of the cochlear duct, is protected from sound waves by the intact tympanic membrane, permitting motin of the inner ear fluids by sound wave stimulation. For example, in the normally intact tympanic membrane, sound waves stimulate the oval window first, and a lag occurs before the terminal effect of the stimulus reaches the round window. However, this lag brane allows sound waves to impinge on the oval and round windows simultaneously. This effect cancels the lag and prevents the maximal effect of inner ear fluid motility and its subsequent effect in stimulating the hair cells in the organ of Corti. The result is a reduction in hearing ability.

Balance and Equilibrium

Body balance in maintained by the cooperation of the muscles and joints of the body (proprioceptive system), the eyes (visual system), and the labyrinth (vestibular system). These areas send their information about equilibrium, or balance, to the brain (cerebellar system) for coordination and perception in the cerebral cortex. The brain obtains its blood supply from the heart and arterial system. A problem in any of these areas, such as arteriosclerosis or impaired vision, can cause a disturbance of balance. The vestibular apparatus of the inner ear provides feedback regarding the movement and the position of the head and body in space.

Hearing Impairments

Hearing impairment is the term used to refer to difficulties in hearing. A person can be partially hearing impaired or totally hearing impaired, and the treatment for hearing loss will vary according to the reason for the impairment.

Conduction hearing impairment: Conduction hearing impairment can result from either a damaged eardrum (which would prevent sound waves from being carried into the middle ear properly) or damage to the bones of the middle ear. In the latter case, sounds cannot be conducted from the eardrum to the cochlea. Middle ear damage is often from ear infections that are not treated quickly enough or from chronic ear infections. In this case, hearing aids may be of some use in restoring hearing.

Nerve hearing impairment: In nerve hearing impairment, the problem lies either in the inner ear or in the auditory pathways and cortical areas of the brain. By the time most people are entering late adulthood, they have lost nearly half of their hair cells to the normal aging process. Exposure to loud noises during one's lifetime can cause the hair cells to break and speed up this loss, resulting in earlier hearing problems for many people in middle age.

Because the damage is to the nerves or the brain, nerve hearing impairment cannot be helped with ordinary hearing aids, which are basically sound amplifiers. A new technique for restoring hearing to those with nerve hearing impairment makes use of an electronic device called a cochlear implant. This device bypasses the outer and middle ears by sending signals from a microphone worn behind the ear to a sound processor worn on the belt or in a pocket, which then translates those signals into electrical stimuli that are sent to a series of electrodes implanted directly into the brain. The brain then processes the electrode information as sound.

With an implant, people can hear some speech and their own speech to a degree that allows more communication with others. See the psychology in the News section that follows for a report on this surgery as performed on former Miss America, Heather Whitestone.

Importance of Sensation in Nursing

Man acts with whole of his organism. There is an interaction of mind and body. Human behavior reveals the influence of both mental and physical factors. In order to understand human behavior fully we analyze its various aspects. When we analyze the bodily factors of human behavior, we find that the important elements involved in bodily functions are:

1. Receptors or the sense organs
2. Effectors or the muscles and endocrine glands
3. Integrating mechanism or nervous system.

Every sensory receptor has had the quality of being stimulated from outside the body and providing knowledge of events external to the body. *Sherrington* classified such senses as exteroceptors, interoceptors and proprioceptors. The exteroceptors receive direct stimulation from outside the body. The sensory field of the interoceptors is the gastrointestinal tract (making them the organic or visceral sensors). The sensory field of the proprioceptors is "in-betweens" (receptors in subcutaneous tissue, deeplying blood vessel, muscles, tendons and bone-coverings) having the common characteristics of being stimulated mainly by actions of the body itself.

Among the proprioceptors, Sherrington includes the labyrinthine balance function of the inner ear. This labyrinthine sense is unique in that no other sense can make good on a claim to yield no sensations of its own. If you feel dizzy, the sensations that you experience are kinesthetic, pressure, visceral-but not labyrinthine. The kinesthetic sense is also among the proprioceptors. An attributes of sensation are given below:

- **Quality:** Sensations differ in quality. For example, a sensation of sound differs from a sensation of color in quality. Also, sensation through same sense organ differ in quality.
- **Intensity:** The strength of sensation depends on objects strength of stimulus and the mental state of the individual.
- **Duration:** It depends on the continuity of the stimulus or its effect.
- **Extensity:** It means voluminousness or spreadoutness of sensation. As this increases, the sensation appears to be bigger. For example, the touch of a palm is more extensive than the touch of fingers.

Organic Sensations

Sensation is felt through the sense organs. We receive sensations through the eye, nose, tongue, skin and ear popularly known as five sense organs. There are many types of sensation but they can be divided in the following three categories.

1. Organic sensations
2. Special sensations
3. Motor/kinesthetic sensations.

The sensations which arise from the conditions of the internal organs are known as organic sensations. They do not need any external stimulation. Hunger creates organic sensation caused by the contraction of the walls of the stomach. These are divided into three on the basis of their location.

a. **Sensations whose location can be determined**: Some organic sensations can be easily located. The experience of cutting, burning, blistering, etc. is in the tissue. Its location is fixed.
b. **Sensations whose location is undermined**: The position of some sensations cannot be determined. The position of comfort and restlessness are spread over the entire body and no particular part of the body can be assigned to them.
c. **Sensations whose location is vague**: There are some more sensations about whose location, we have a vague notion. For example an hazy idea of the general location of some sensation like hunger, thirst, pain, though we do not know the exact location minutely.

The five sensations are those which are caused by the special sense organs like eyes, ears, nose, tongue and skin. As given below:

a. **Visual sensations:** Visual sensations, which are stimulated by light waves, are experienced through the medium of the eyes. They are of the two types- (i) Sensations of brightness, (ii) Sensations of color, of which the following four are primary red, yellow, green and blue. Color blind people do not feel these sensations.
b. **Auditory sensations:** These are received through the ears. They are the reactions of the ear to the vibrations in the air. Usually, the local symbol is absent in auditory sensations in which the power of discrimination is high. These sensations are important from the emotional viewpoint.
c. **Taste sensations:** It is the tongue which acquires these sensations. There are many papillae in the tongue. Mostly, there are taste pores in these papillae. There are bag-like structure called taste buds below taste pores, sensation of taste passes through the taste pores and reaches the taste bud, then the sensation is transferred to the brain resulting in taste experience. The central portion of the tongue cannot receive sensations of different tastes. The tip of tongue acquires the sweet taste, the rear the bitter taste, the edges the sour taste, while saline taste is spread uniformly all over the tongue.
d. **Olfactory sensations:** Receptor cells for the olfactory sensations are located in the nose at its apex. As only a part of the breath reaches them it is necessary to draw a deeper breath in order to smell the odor. The odor sensation is carried to strain and odor is perceived.
e. **Tactile sensation:** The skin contains the receivers of somesthetic sensations. There are two types of sensations.
   - *Cutaneous sensations* there are different areas for these sensations interspersed with insensitive areas of the body assigned to them.

- *Kinesthetic sensations* are felt in muscles, bones and various nervous joints and their covering membrane. Tensions, contraction, pulling, etc. are examples of motor sensations. They are caused by the muscles, tendons and joints. The nerves embedded in the joints move. The brain receives information of these sensations through the sensory nerves whose parts are in muscles, tendons and joints. The motor sensations put pressure upon the skin.

f. **Motor sensation:** Motor sensations are a means of the knowledge of the primary qualities of objects, e.g. their position, distance, direction, weight, etc. These sensations, take part automatically and generally pass by unnoticed.

The kinds of motor sensations are:

- *Sensations of position:* Such a sensation is generated when the arms are held motionless in a fully extended position.
- *Sensation of free movement:* If the arms are moved in all directions, then the arising sensations are those of free movement.
- *Sensations of impeded movement:* These can be experience by lifting some heavy weight.

Improper functioning of receptors result in sensory disorders or defects. As a consequence of this false or incomplete impressions of our environment. Happens, which includes:

1. *Visual disorders or defects:* The visual defects can be due to the defects in cornea or lens or due to deficiencies within the retina. Myopia, hyperopia, astigmatism and squint belong to the first type.

   The color blindness is due to retinal deficiency. The most commonly occurring type of color blindness is a failure to distinguish between red and green. The color blindness is not a disease. It cannot be cured by medicines. No amount of exercise and training can correct it. This visual deficiency is genetic. It is inherited.
2. *Disorders of the ear:* The sense of hearing is next only to vision in importance. It gives us the idea about the location of objects which cannot be seen. The defects of ear are: (i) varying degrees of deafness; (ii) deafness to certain specific tones and; (iii) ringing in the ear. The power of hearing can be impaired due to injury to the tympanic membranes, lesion of the auditory nerve, or a fixation or disengagement of the ossicles. The causes which lead to hearing defects are the running of ears, hardened wax and throat affections. The diseases like scarlet fever, measles, diphtheria, mumps, influenza, meningitis and injuries are produced by foreign objects. Naturally these conditions should be checked and corrected by prompt attention and treatment. Visual and auditory defects, if not corrected, interfere with learning process.
3. *Cutaneous or tactual disorders:* These defects include the absence of sensations of pressure, warmth, cold and pain.
4. *Olfactory disorders:* These disorders include the extreme sensitivity to certain odors and, on the other hand, insensitivity or failure to recognize certain odors. A man who smells rotten and foul odors everywhere is suffering from an olfactory disorder.
5. *Gustatory disorder:* The gustatory disorders refer to defects of taste. Certain persons suddenly lose all taste for food and, in particular, they lose sensitivity to salt. To some everything tastes bitter. These anomalies of taste are gustatory disorders.

In the light of the above knowledge regarding sensory processes, the following points should be borne in mind by the nurse while dealing with the patients:

1. Everyone reacts to colors; but the sick persons tend to over-react. Certain colors are stimulating and disturbing while others are soothing and balming to nerves. A nurse

will avoid those colors which are disturbing and stimulating and would use soft and subdued colors. The nurse may provide warm bright illumination and colors for those who need stimulation but will use only dim light and soft colors for patients who are highly strung.

2. The sick persons are usually hypersensitive to noise. The nurse should see to it that no loud noise is made in and around the sick rooms. No noise should be allowed when the patient is asleep.
3. In order that the patients eat well and relish their foods strong smells should be reduced as much as possible. Good and fresh food should be served with a smile. The patient should be encouraged to wash his mouth frequently.
4. The sick persons may be suffering from visual discomforts. Therefore the conditions which may aggravate eye stain should be scrupulously avoided.
5. According to Averill and Kempf the nurses should do something so as to control the foul and disagreeable smells or odors from the body, elimination and discharges from the foul be properly used and full ventilation allowed.
6. According to Averill and Kempf, "It makes a great difference to the patient whether the nurse's fingers are deft or clumsy in manipulating a dressing, whether her movements are jerky and incoordinated or whether they are smooth. Incoordinated and jerky movements of the nurse will result in discomfort to the patient".

In general a nurse should remember that sick persons undergo abnormal sensory experiences and as a result are irritable and disagreeable. They complain too much not because they wish to trouble others but because they are feeling uncomfortable. The emotional factors like fear, anxiety and worry make the patients distressful.

8 CHAPTER Glandular and Muscular Control of Behavior

Glandular Control of Behavior

The nervous system and the interconnected network of glands known as the endocrine system control body systems. Disorders of the endocrine system are common and have the potential to affect the function of every organ system in the body. Understanding the function of each of the endocrine glands and the consequences of hypofunction and hyper-function of each gland enables the nurse to anticipate physiologic changes and to plan interventions to address them. Nursing interventions that are essential in managing endocrine disorders are carried out in every setting, from the intensive care unit to the outpatient setting and the home.

Glands have a unique place and function in the body of the organism. They influence every aspect of the body. Beside influencing the body, human behavior and personality are also influenced by their activity. Life is active only because of the normal activity of glands. Infact bodily glands are structures formed by the special composition of cell molecules. Their function is also specific. The glands produce and secrete various chemical substances. Secretions of one class of glands are called hormones. Each gland of this group secrete a specific hormone. The hormone of various glands have very important influence on human behavior and his personality. For example, when insulin molecules, carried passively along in the blood, leave the blood and bind tightly to protein receptors of nearby cells, the response is dramatic: blood borne glucose molecules begin to disappear into the cells, and cellular activity accelerates. Such is the power of the second great controlling system of the body, the endocrine system. Along with the nervous system, it coordinates and directs the activity of the body's cells. However, the speed is very different. The nervous system is "built for speed". It uses nerve impulses to prod the muscles and glands into immediate action so that rapid adjustments can be made in response to changes occurring both inside and outside the body. On the other hand, the more slowly acting endocrine system uses chemical messengers called hormones, which are released into the blood to be transported leisurely throughout the body.

It is clear from the above discussion that the main function of glands is the discharge of secretion. There are some glands which do not pour their secretions into the blood but pour them out on the body surface through some tubes. Because of this characteristic, these glands are called duct glands or exocrine glands. The second type of glands have different characteristics. These second type of glands pour their chemical secretions directly into the bloodstream without the help of any duct (tube). Their secretions reach various organs of the body through blood and influence their activity. Because of this characteristic, these are called ductless or endocrine glands. These are two types of bodily glands:

1. Duct or exocrine glands
2. Ductless or endocrine glands.

ENDOCRINE GLANDS

Endocrine glands pour their secretions directly into the bloodstream without the help of any tube (duct). These glands have unique importance in animal and human body. These glands are located at different parts of the body. Chemical substances secreted by endocrine glands are known as hormones. These hormones influence various parts of the body and behavior. Hypo or hypersecretion from these glands have bad and good influences on body functions. Some of the hormones of these glands also take part in the metabolic processes in the body. Emotional behavior of human beings is also influenced by their action. A description of the general characteristics of endocrine glands will be given first before discussing their functions in detail.

The endocrine system has far-reaching effects in the human body because of its links with the nervous system and the immune system. The hormones secreted by the endocrine system are affected in large part by structures in the central nervous system, such as the hypothalamus. Other structures located in the brain, such as the pituitary gland, are endocrine glands that influence the function of a large number of other endocrine glands. Hormones secreted by the endocrine system affect the nervous system and are, in turn, mediated by the nervous system. The adrenal medulla, for example, secretes a number of substances (e.g. norepinephrine, epinephrine) that act as neurotransmitters. The immune system also interacts closely with the endocrine system. It responds to the introduction of foreign agents by means of chemicals (e.g. interleukins, interferons) and is regulated by hormones secreted by the adrenal cortex.

In addition to the hormones secreted by the major endocrine glands, other tissues produce hormones that are secreted into body fluids and act on nearby cells and tissues. The gastrointestinal mucosa produces hormones (e.g. gastrin, enterogastrone, secretin, cholecystokinin) that are important in the digestive process. The kidneys produce erythropoietin, a hormone that stimulates the bone marrow to produce red blood cells. The white blood cells produce cytokines that actively participate in inflammatory and immune responses.

Hormones are important in regulation of the internal environment of the body and affect every aspect of life. Some hormones target specific tissues; for example, adrenocorticotropic hormone (ACTH), or corticotrophin, is secreted by the anterior pituitary gland and targets the adrenal cortex to increase the secretion of the hormones of the adrenal cortex (i.e. glucocorticoids, mineralocorticoids, androgens). Other hormones affect a wide variety of cells and tissues of the body. Thyroid hormone is one example; it affects metabolic activity of cells throughout the body.

GLANDS OF THE ENDOCRINE SYSTEM

The endocrine glands include the pituitary, thyroid, parathyroids, adrenals, pancreatic islets, ovaries, and testes. Endocrine glands secrete their products directly into the bloodstream which differentiates them from exocrine glands, such as sweat glands, which secrete their products through ducts onto epithelial surfaces or into the gastrointestinal tract. The hypothalamus is the link between the nervous system and the endocrine system. The chemical substances secreted by the endocrine glands are called hormones. Hormones help regulate organ function in concert with the nervous system. This dual regulatory system, in which rapid action by the nervous system is balanced by slower hormonal action, permits precise control of organ functions in response to varied changes within and outside the body.

The endocrine glands are composed of secretory cells arranged in minute clusters known as acini. No ducts are present, but the glands have a rich blood supply, so the hormones they produce enter the bloodstream rapidly. In the healthy physiologic state, hormone concentration in the bloodstream is maintained at a relatively constant level. When the hormone concentration increases, further production of that hormone is inhibited. When the hormone concentration decreases, the rate of production of that hormone increases. This mechanism for regulating hormone concentration in the bloodstream is called negative feedback, and it is important in the regulation of many biologic processes.

Hormones are classified as steroid hormones (e.g. hydrocortisone), peptide or protein hormones (e.g. insulin), amine hormones (e.g. epinephrine), and fatty acid derivatives (e.g. retinoids). These different classes of hormones act on the target tissues by different mechanisms. Hormones can alter the function of the target tissue by interacting with chemical receptors located either on the cell membrane or in the interior of the cell.

Peptide and protein hormones interact with receptor sites on the cell surface, which results in stimulation of the intracellular enzyme adenyl cyclase. This causes increased production of cyclic 3', 5'–adenosine monophosphate (cyclic AMP). The cyclic AMP inside the cell alters enzyme activity. Thus, cyclic AMP is the "second messenger" that links the peptide hormone at the cell surface to a change in the intracellular environment. Some of the protein and peptide hormones also act by changing membrane permeability. These hormones act within seconds or minutes. The mechanism of action for amine hormones is similar to that for peptide hormones.

Steroid hormones, because of their smaller size and higher lipid solubility, penetrate the cell membranes and interact with intracellular receptors. The steroid-receptor complex modifies cell metabolism and the formation of messenger ribonucleic acid (mRNA) from deoxyribonucleic acid (DNA). The mRNA then stimulates protein synthesis within the cell. Steroid hormones require several hours to exert their effects, because they exert their action by the modification of protein synthesis.

Each endocrine gland has its own unique characteristics and functions. But there are some characteristics which are common in all the endocrine glands. Some of these common characteristics are given below:

- All endocrine glands pour their secretion directly into the blood without the help of any tube. These secretions reach the whole body through the blood vessels.
- Secretions of endocrine glands are called hormones. Hormones of each endocrine gland have its unique properties and functions.
- Whereas different glands have specific functions in the body, they also affect the activity of each. Infact different glands work as a system.
- Normal secretion of endocrine glands is beneficial for the body and behavior. But, on the other hand, their abnormal activity results into various symptoms in the body. Abnormal activity may be of two types. First, if secretion from the gland is more than normal, it is called hyperfunction. Secondly, if the secretion is less than normal, activity of the gland is low and it is known as hypofunction.

- Secretion of endocrine glands influence human body functions and behavior. Their hypo- or hyperfunctioning have different influences. These influences work on all cells, tissues and organs of the body.

Other hormone producing tissues and organs includes the following:

- The placenta is a temporary organ formed in the uterus of pregnant women. Its primary endocrine role is to produce estrogen and progesterone, which maintain pregnancy and ready breasts for lactation.
- Several organs that are generally nonendocrine in overall function such as stomach, small intestine, kidneys, and heart have cells that are secrete hormones.
- Certain cancer cells secrete hormones.
- Excluding pathology, efficiency of the endocrine system remains high until old age.
- Decreasing function of female ovaries at menopause leads to such symptoms as osteoporosis, increased chance of heart disease, and possible mood changes.
- Efficiency of all endocrine glands gradually decreases with aging, which leads to a generalized increase in incidence of diabetes mellitus, immune system depression, and lower metabolic rate.

Although hormones have widespread and varied effects, the major processes controlled by hormones are reproduction; growth and development; mobilizing body defenses against stressors; maintaining electrolyte, water, and nutrient balance of the blood; and regulating cellular metabolism and energy balance. As you can see, the endocrine system regulates processes that go on for relatively long periods and, in some cases, continuously.

Compared to other organs of the body, the organs of the endocrine system are small and unimpressive. Indeed, to collect 1 kg (about 2.2 pounds) of hormone-producing tissue, you would need to collect all the endocrine tissue from eight or nine adults! The endocrine organs also lack the structural or anatomical continuity typical of most organ systems. Instead, bits and pieces of endocrine tissue are tucked away in widely separated regions of the body. However, functionally the endocrine organs are very impressive, and when their role in maintaining body homeostasis is considered, they are true giants.

Major Endocrine Glands

There are various endocrine glands in the human body. Their location in the body and functions are different. Following are the major endocrine glands in the human body.

1. Pituitary gland
2. Thyroid gland
3. Parathyroid gland
4. Adrenal gland
5. Pancreas gland
6. Gonads
7. Pineal gland
8. Thymus gland

Location of these glands in human body has been shown in Figure 8.1. It is now believed that thymus and pineal glands have no importance in human behavior. A detailed discussion of the functions of other endocrine glands is given below.

The endocrine system is a major controlling system of the body. Through hormones, it stimulates such long-term processes as growth and development, metabolism, reproduction and body defense.

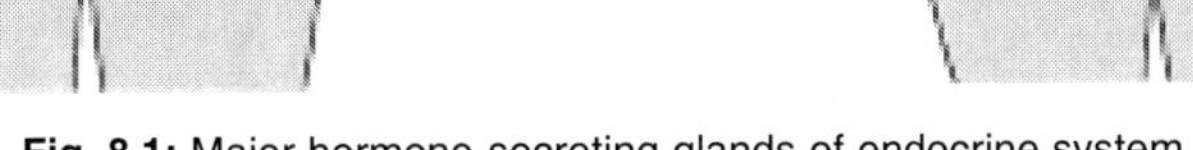

Fig. 8.1: Major hormone-secreting glands of endocrine system

Endocrine organs are small and widely separated in the body. Some are part of mixed glands (both endocrine and exocrine in function). Others are purely hormone producing. All hormones are amino acid-based or steroids.

Endocrine organs are activated to release their hormones into the blood by hormonal, humoral, or neural stimuli. Negative feedback is important in regulating hormone levels in the blood.

Blood borne hormones alter the metabolic activities of their target organs. The ability of a target organ to respond to a hormone depends on the presence of receptors in or on its cells to which the hormone binds or attaches.

Amino acid-based hormones act through second messengers. Steroid hormones directly influence the target cells DNA.

The embryonic development of the endocrine glands varies. The pituitary gland is derived from epithelium of the oral cavity and a neural tissue projection of the hypothalamus. The pineal body is entirely neural tissue. Most strictly epithelial glands develop as little sac-like outpocketings of the mucosa of the digestive tract. These would the thyroid, thymus and pancreas. Formation of the gonads and the adrenal and parathyroid glands is much more complex and is not considered here.

Barring outright malfunctions of the endocrine glands, most endocrine organs seem to operate smoothly until old age. In late middle age, the efficiency of the ovaries begins to decline, causing menopause (commonly called "the change of life"). During this period, a

woman's reproductive organs begin to atrophy and the ability to bear children ends. Problems associated with estrogen deficiency begin to occur, such as arteriosclerosis, osteoporosis, decreased skin elasticity, and changes in the operation of the sympathetic nervous system that result in "hot flashes". In addition, fatigue, nervousness, and mood changes such as depression are common. No such dramatic changes seem to happen in men. In fact, many men remain fertile throughout their lifespan, indicating that testosterone is still being produced in adequate amounts.

The efficiency of the endocrine system as a whole gradually declines in old age. Striking changes occur in aging women due to decreasing levels of female hormones, and there is no question that growth hormone output by the anterior pituitary declines, which partially explains muscle atrophy in old age. Elderly persons are less able to resist stress and infection. This may result from over-reproduction or underproduction of the defense equilibrium and alter general body metabolism. Older people are often mildly hypothyroid, and all other people have some decline in insulin production, and type II diabetes is most common in the elderly.

1. Pituitary Gland

Pituitary gland controls the functions of many other endocrine glands. It is located on the ventral side of the brain. It is connected to the posterior part of the hypothalamus. It has three main secreting parts:

1. Anterior pituitary gland
2. Posterior pituitary gland
3. Intermediate pituitary gland.

- Anterior pituitary is more important form the point of view of behavior. It is this part of the pituitary which regulates the activity of other glands. A number of hormones are secreted from anterior pituitary. These hormones are very complex and they have many influences on human behavior.
  - The pituitary gland hangs from the base of the brain by a stalk and is enclosed by bone. It consists of a glandular (anterior) portion and a neural (posterior) portion.
  - Except for growth hormone and prolactin, hormones of the anterior pituitary are all tropic hormones.
    - i. *Growth hormone (GH):* An anabolic and protein-conserving hormone that promotes total body growth. Its most important effect is on skeletal muscles and bones. Untreated hyposecretion during childhood results in pituitary dwarfism; hypersecretion produces gigantism (in childhood) and acromegaly (in adulthood).
    - ii. *Prolactin (PRL):* Stimulates production of breast milk.
    - iii. *Adrenocorticotropic hormone (ACTH):* Stimulates the adrenal cortex to release its hormones.
    - iv. *Thyroid stimulating hormone (TSH):* Stimulates the thyroid gland to release thyroid hormone.
    - v. Gonadotropic hormones
      - a. *Follicle stimulating hormone (FSH):* Beginning at puberty, stimulates follicle development and estrogen production by the female ovaries; promotes sperm production in the male.
      - b. *Luteinizing hormone (LH):* Beginning at puberty, stimulates ovulation, converts the ruptured ovarian follicle to a corpus luteum, and causes the corpus luteum to produce progesterone; stimulates the male's testes to produce testosterone.

- Releasing and inhibiting hormones made by the hypothalamus regulate release of hormones made by the anterior pituitary. The hypothalamus also makes two hormones that are transported to the posterior pituitary for storage and later release.
- Posterior pituitary gland secretion is called pituitrin. It has three hormones whose functions are different. First hormone is called oxytocin. It stimulates the contraction of smooth muscles of intestines and uterus. The second is called antidiuretic hormone. It helps the excretion of various substances from the body. This hormone regulates the level of water in the body. The third hormone is called vasopressin which affects the autonomic nervous system and controls the blood pressure.

The posterior pituitary stores and releases hypothalamic hormones on command, i.e. (i) Oxytocin: Stimulates powerful uterine contractions and causes milk ejection in the nursing woman. (ii) Antidiuretic hormone (ADH): Causes kidney tubule cells to reabsorb and conserve body water and increases blood pressure by constricting blood vessels. Hyposecretion leads to diabetes insipidus.

The activity of this part of the intermediate pituitary gland is concerned with the excretion of urine from the body. Its hormone controls the activity of urine excretion.

2. THYROID GLAND

The thyroid gland is located in the tissue of the neck around the wind pipe. Hormone secreted from this gland is called thyroxine. Activity of the thyroid gland influences various bodily activities. Its hormone thyroxine controls the rate of various metabolic processes. Various processes of oxidation going on in the body are regulated by this hormone. Thyroid gland gives enough cooperation in the activities of various tissues of the body and in the stimulation of the process of general growth in the body. Activities of various muscles of the body are influenced by the action of its hormone. Regulation of body temperature, control of blood pressure and rate of heart beating are influenced by the action of the hormone thyroxine. In some cases secretion of hormones from thyroxine gland is low. In this state of hyposecretion, metabolic process in the body are slowed down and energy production in the body is reduced. This state occurs in human beings when there is acute deficiency of iodine in their diet. Different diseases occur in children and adults as a result of hypofunction of the thyroid gland. Deficiency of thyroxine in children gives rise to an abnormality called cretinism. In cretinism body growth is arrested and there is weakness in it. Body is lethargic and change comes in many of its organs. Brain does not function normally and mental processes are slowed. Normal growth of sex organs is arrested. Resistance to various diseases is reduced in the body. In adults low secretion of this hormone gives rise to a disease called myxedema. In this disease skin of the body becomes fat and dry. Hair become brittle and begin to fall. Face becomes ugly and tongue becomes fat because of which the voice becomes hoarse. The person is usually very sluggish and sleepy. He lacks drive and is unemotional. His thinking power is reduced. For the treatment of this disease, medicines containing iodine are given.

Hypersecretion of this gland also gives rise to abnormal conditions. Metabolic processes in the body are speeded up because of increased thyroxine in the blood. Rates of heart beating and respiration are increased. The person becomes more active and seems to have more energy. The person suffering from this disease becomes irritable and restless. This disease is called exophthalmic goiter. There is slight temperature in the body and the skin remains wet. These symptoms can be eliminated by giving a thyroid-inhibiting drug.

i. The thyroid gland is located in the anterior throat.

ii. Thyroid hormone (thyroxine [T_4] and triiodothyronine [T_3]) is released from the thyroid follicles when blood levels of TSH rise. Thyroid hormone is the body's metabolic hormone. It increases the rate at which cells oxidize glucose and is necessary for normal growth and development. Lack of iodine leads to goiter. Hyposecretion of thyroxine results in cretinism in children and myxedema in adults. Hypersecretion results from Graves disease or other forms of hyperthyroidism.
iii. Calcitonin is released by C cells surrounding the thyroid follicles in response to high blood levels of calcium. It causes calcium to be deposited in bones.

3. PARATHYROID GLANDS

Parathyroid glands are situated in the neck near the wind pipe. They are four in number and two glands are attached to each thyroid. Secretion from the parathyroid is called parathormone. A major function of this gland is to regulate the level of calcium and phosphorus in the body. The growth of the body, bones and their strength depends upon this gland. Growth of teeth and their proper function is also influenced by the secretion of this gland. It is essential for the normal activity of muscles.

i. The parathyroid gland are four small glands located on the posterior aspect of the thyroid gland.
ii. Low blood levels of calcium stimulate the parathyroid glands to release parathyroid hormone (PTH). It causes bone calcium to be liberated into the blood. Hypersecretion of PTH results in tetany; hyposecretion leads to extreme bone wasting and fractures.

The normal amount of the hormone from parathyroid is essential of the growth and strength of bones and teeth. Hyposecretion of this gland in the human body gives rise to a disease called tetany. There is generally high temperature in the body. Muscles become weak and muscle twitches occur. Sometimes respiratory muscles fail, breathing and heart beating stop and the person dies. This abnormality is because of the loss of calcium from the blood as a result of the absence of PTH. For treating this abnormal condition, the person should be given calcium salts. Use of vitamin D is also helpful.

Hypersecretion of PTH results in excess of calcium in the blood. But excess of calcium is associated with a lowered supply of phosphorus in the blood and the result is the disturbance in the balance of calcium and phosphorus in the blood. Excess of calcium slows down the muscular activity. In this condition sensitivity of the body becomes low and there is nervous weakness. In this state of abnormality the person is sluggish and his appearance becomes ugly. Generally surgery is used for treatment very serious condition of abnormality because of the hypersecretion of parathyroids.

Hormone of this gland has an important influence of human behavior and personality. Its normal secretion leads to normal emotional behavior. Its adequate quantity is essential for body balance and normal neuromuscular processes. In the state of hypersecretion, the person becomes lethargic and sluggish and his sensitivity is decreased.

4. ADRENAL GLANDS

Adrenal glands are situated on the top surface of kidneys in the body. These are two in number and one gland is situated on each side in the body. Though these glands are near the kidneys but their function is not related with them in any way. Each adrenal has two parts. Both parts secrete different hormones and their activity has different influence on the body and behavior. The two parts of the adrenal glands are:

a. Adrenal cortex
b. Adrenal medulla.

a. Adrenal cortex: A number of hormones are secreted from adrenal cortex. These are called cortical steroids or corticoids. These hormones influence the metabolism of carbohydrates, water, sodium and other salts. The balance between sodium and potassium in the body is maintained by the function of steroids. Sodium-Potassium balance is essential in the body for normal physiological functions. In the absence of this balance, resting potential in the membrane is changed and neural processes are affected. Carbohydrate metabolism is increased by the function of these hormones. This is essential for many processes in the body. Blood sugar is deposited glycogen in the liver and the basal metabolic rate is increased.

In the case of hypofunction of adrenal cortex when the secretion of cortical steroids is low, many metabolic processes in the body, especially concerned with carbohydrates and sodium are slowed up. Excessive water and sodium are excreted through urine. The level of water and sodium is reduced in the body. On the other hand concentration of potassium in the body is increased. This results into a disturbance of this balance slows neural and muscular activities. Blood pressure is also affected. Level of glucose in the blood is reduced. Body weight begins to decrease gradually. Temperature of the body falls below normal. These are the symptoms of a serious disease called Addison's disease. The person may die due to this disease. Hypersecretion of cortical steroids interfere with the normal sexual development of the person. In females, excessive hair growth of the face and other masculine signs appear. Their general softness begins to disappear. Similarly over action in young boys gives rise to sexual characteristics of adult males.

Physiological effects of the hormones of adrenal cortex are clear from the above discussion. It is natural that personality and behavior of the person is affected by these physiological changes. Hyposecretion of this gland results in the low metabolism of carbohydrates and salts and the person becomes weak lethargic and easily fatigued. The person generally suffers from feelings of inferiority if this condition continues. On the other hand hypersecretion of this gland results into disturbance into the sexual development of the person and its creates changes the personality and behavior of the person.

i. The adrenal glands are paired glands perched on the kidneys. Each gland has two functional endocrine portions, the cortex and the medulla.

ii. Adrenal cortex hormones include:
   a. Mineralocorticoids, primarily aldosterone, regulate sodium ion (Na^+) and potassium ion (K^+) reabsorption by the kidneys. Their release is stimulated primarily by low Na^+ and/or high K^+ levels in blood.
   b. Glucocorticoids enable the body to resist long-term stress by increasing blood glucose levels and depressing the inflammatory response.
   c. Sex hormones (mainly androgens) are produced in small amounts throughout life.

iii. Generalized hypoactivity of the adrenal cortex results in Addison's disease. Hypersecretion can result in hyperaldosteronism, Cushing's disease, and/or masculinization.

b. Adrenal medulla: Adrenal medulla is the inner part of the adrenal gland. It is made up of neural tissues and has strong effects on the visceral functions controlled by the autonomic nervous system.

The adrenal medulla produces catecholamines (epinephrine and norepinephrine) in response to sympathetic nervous system stimulation. Its catecholamines enhance and prolong the effect of the "fight or flight" (sympathetic nervous system) response to short-term stress. Hypersecretion leads to symptoms typical of sympathetic nervous system overactivity.

In normal state adrenal medulla has no particular function. It has a special contribution in emergency situations. In emergency situations, adrenal medulla is stimulated by the activity of sympathetic nervous system and secretes hormones. Its two major hormones are (1) Adrenaline or epinephrine and (2) Noradrenaline or norepinephrine. Adrenaline has widespread physiological effects and thereby enables the organism to meet the emergency. It increases the heart rate and blood pressure. Pupils of the eyes are dilated and erection of the hairs on the body occur.

In the state of emergency the body needs more energy. The hormone adrenaline helps in this by raising the blood sugar level by stimulating the liver to convert glycogen into glucose level and release it into the blood. Neuromuscular activity is also increased by this change. Effect of this hormone increases the intake of oxygen in the body as a result of which the rate of metabolism is increased. In emotions like anger and fear, the secretion of adrenaline is especially increased.

Influence of adrenal medulla on behavior and personality: As has been discussed above, the activity of this gland has a direct relationship with a person's emotions and emergency situations. So it is natural that its hormones effect his personality and behavior. Normal activity of this gland helps in maintaining the emotional balance of the person. In the state of fear, anger and external emergency the hormone adrenaline is secreted from this gland. Activity of the liver, breathing and circulation of blood are increased. All these result in extra energy and drive in the body. Thus this gland has a special contribution in producing energy in the body in emergency situations. On the other hand, in some states the secretion of adrenaline from the gland is low. In the state of decrease of hormone the person becomes weak and apathetic. He loses appetite and normal sexual urge. The overall picture is that of a depressed personality.

5. PANCREAS

Pancreas is located near the small intestine. It acts both as a duct gland and ductless gland. Its outer portion is duct gland. Its center portion is composed of group of cells, called beta cells which have only endocrine functions. Their hormone is called insulin. The hormone insulin has a unique role in body functions. Carbohydrates present in the body are burned and converted sugar is utilized by the cells of the body through the influence of insulin. If the level of sugar in the blood becomes high because of various reasons, then insulin converts this extra sugar into glycogen which gets deposited in the liver and muscles. Various body organs like brain are able to get a constant supply of sugar because of the influence of glycogen. Thus the activity of the beta cells of pancreas regulates the sugar level in the human body as given below:

i. Located in the abdomen close to the stomach, the pancreas is both an exocrine and endocrine gland. The endocrine portion (islets) releases insulin and glucagon to blood.
ii. Insulin is released when blood levels of glucose are high. It increases the rate of glucose uptake and metabolism by body cells. Hyposecretion of insulin results in diabetes mellitus, which severely disturbs body metabolism. Cardinal signs are polyuria, polydipsia and polyphagia.
iii. Glucagon, released when blood levels of glucose are low, stimulates the liver to release glucose to blood, thus increasing blood glucose levels.

Abnormal activity of pancreas has disastrous effects on body functions. Hyposecretion of its hormone insulin increases the blood sugar level. In this state the amount of sugar in the urine of the person becomes high. This disease is known as diabetes. The person gradually becomes weak in this disease. He may die if the disease becomes serious. For the treatment of this disease it is essential to lower the blood sugar level. For this purpose insulin injections are given to the person and the intake of carbohydrates in the diet is reduced.In the state of hyperfunction, the amount of insulin secretion becomes high which results in the lowering of blood sugar level. The body does not remain normal. There are tremors and convulsions in the body. The person becomes relates restless from time-to-time. Glucose is given for the treatment of this disease.

6. SEX GLANDS OR GONADS

The female and male gonads produce sex hormones that are identical to those produced by adrenal cortex cells. The major difference are relative amounts produces.

The female gonads, or ovaries, are paired, almond-sized organs located in the pelvic cavity. Beside producing female sex cells (ova or eggs), ovaries produce two groups of steroid hormones, estrogens and progesterone. The ovaries do not really begin to function until puberty, when the anterior pituitary gonadotropic hormones stimulate them into activity. This results in the rhythmic ovarian cycles in which ova develop a-rid blood levels of ovarian hormones rise and fall.

Sex glands are also called gonads. These are known by different names in males and females. Female gonads are called ovaries and in male these are called testes. Sperms are produced in the testes and ova in the ovaries. Beside these cells various hormones are secreted directly into the blood from these sex glands. These hormones are responsible for the sex characteristics typical of men and women. Main hormones from the male sex glands are androsterone and testosterone. These hormones have three major functions in the body of males. First function is the normal development of male sex organs. Second function is the inhibition of mammary glands and other female characteristics in males. Third function is the development of other sex characteristics in males. In the case of female gonads, main hormones are esterone and progestin. Sex organs of females develop under the influence of esterone. Menstrual cycle of females is also regulated by it. Growth of mammary glands and other sex characteristics are under its influence. Hormone progestin has many functions in connection with the development of fertilized ovum in the female uterus.

a. The ovaries of the female release:
- **Estrogens:** Release of estrogens by ovarian follicles begins at puberty under the influence of FSH. Estrogens stimulate maturation of the female reproductive organs and female secondary sex characteristics. With progesterone, they cause the menstrual cycle.
- **Progesterone:** Progesterone is released from the corpus luteum of the ovary in response to high blood levels of LH. It works with estrogens in establishing the menstrual cycle.

b. The testes of the male begin to produce testosterone at puberty in response to LH stimulation. Testosterone promotes maturation of the male reproductive organs, male secondary sex characteristics, and production of sperm by the testes.

c. Hyposecretion of gonadal hormones results in sterility in both females and males.

Hormones of sex glands have special importance in human life. Sex characteristics of males and females develop under their influences. In the course of time a girl becomes a woman and a boy becomes a man because of the influence of sex glands. Attraction activity of these glands not only interferes with the normal sex functions but also sometimes results into the development of bodily characteristics of opposite sex. The voice of a woman becomes hoarse, increase of hair growth takes place on her body and softness of body organs of mammary glands may appear in males because of the disturbance in the activity of sex gland. Thus the secretions of gonads have important influences on the behavior and personality of human beings.

7. PINEAL GLAND

It is located in the third ventricle of the brain, releases melatonin, which affects biological rhythms and reproductive behavior. The pineal body, also called the pineal gland, is a small, cone-shaped, cone-shaped gland found in the roof of the third ventricle of the brain. The endocrine function of this tiny gland is still somewhat of a mystery. Although many chemical substances have been identified in the pineal gland, only the hormone melatonin appears to be secreted in substantial amounts. The levels of melatonin rise and fall during the course of the day and night. Peak levels occur during daylight around noon. Melatonin is believed to be a "sleep trigger" that plays an important role in establishing the body's day-night cycle. In some animals, melatonin also helps regulate mating behavior and rhythms. In humans, it is believed to coordinate the hormones of fertility and to inhibit the reproductive system (especially the ovaries of females) so that sexual maturation is prevented from occurring before adult body size has been reached.

8. THYMUS GLAND

It is located in the upper thorax, functions during youth but atrophies in old age. Its hormone, thymosin, promotes maturation of T lymphocytes, important in body defense. The thymus gland is located in the upper thorax, posterior to the sternum. Large in infants and children, it decreases in size throughout adulthood. By old age, it is composed mostly of fibrous connective tissue and fat. The thymus produces a hormone called thymosin and during childhood thymus acts as an incubator for the maturation of a special group of white blood cells (T lymphocytes, or T cells) that are important in the immune response. The role of the thymus (and hormones) in immunity.

Muscular Control of Behavior

The musculoskeletal system includes the bones, joints, muscles, tendons, ligaments, and bursae of the body. The functions of these components are highly integrated; therefore, disease in or injury to one component adversely affects the others. For instance, an infection in a joint (septic arthritis) causes degeneration of the articular surfaces of the bones within the joint and local muscle atrophy.

Diseases and injuries that involve the musculoskeletal system are commonly implicated in disability and death. The leading cause of disability is arthritis. Falls account for more hospitalizations yearly among the elderly. Musculoskeletal diseases and injuries can significantly affect overall productivity, independence, and quality of life in people of all ages. Nurses in all practice areas encounter patients with disruption in musculoskeletal function. The health and proper functioning of the musculoskeletal system is interdependent with that of the other body systems. The musculoskeletal system has important functions. It provides protection for vital organs, including the brain, heart, and lungs, and provides a sturdy framework to support body structures. It also makes mobility possible. Joints hold the bones together and allow the body to move. The muscles attached to the skeleton contract, moving the bones and producing heat that helps maintain body temperature. Movement facilitates the return of deoxygenated blood to the right side of the heart by massaging the venous vasculature. In addition, the musculoskeletal system serves as a reservoir for immature blood cells and essential minerals, including calcium, phosphorus, magnesium, and fluoride. More than 98 percent of total body calcium is present in bone. In addition, the red bone marrow located within bone cavities produces red blood cells, white blood cells, and platelets through a process referred to as hematopoiesis.

Muscles are attached by tendons (cords of fibrous connective tissue) or aponeuroses (broad, flat sheets of connective tissue) to bones, connective tissue, other muscles, soft tissue, or skin. The muscles of the body are composed of parallel groups of muscle cells (fasciculi) encased in fibrous tissue called fascia or epimysium. The more fasciculi contained in a muscle, the more precise the movements. Muscles vary in shape and size according to the activities for which they are responsible. Skeletal (striated) muscles are involved in body movement, posture, and heat-production functions. Muscles contract to bring the two points of attachment closer together, resulting in movement.

Our behavior involves action of different parts of our body. We move our limbs when we take bath, eat, dress, walk or run. Besides outward movements of our limbs there are movements of our internal organs. In digestion, breathing and blood circulation there are movements of internal organs and tissues. Our muscles are responsible for the bodily movements, internal and external. Because flexing muscles look like mice scurrying beneath the skin, some scientist long ago dubbed them muscles, from the Latin word mus meaning "little mouse". Indeed, the rippling muscles of professional boxers or weight lifters is often the first thing that comes to mind when one hears the word muscle. But muscle is also the dominant tissue in the heart and in the walls of other hollow organs of the body. In all its forms, it makes up nearly half the body's mass.

The essential function of muscle is contraction, or shortening—a unique characteristic that sets it apart from any other body tissue. As a result of this ability, muscles are responsible for essentially all body movement and can be viewed as the "machines" of the body.

Muscle Types

There are three types of muscle tissue—skeletal, cardiac, and smooth. These differ in their cell structure, body location, and how they are stimulated to contract. But, before we explore their differences, let's look at some of the ways they are the same.

Skeletal and smooth muscle cells are elongated. For this reason, these types of muscle cells (but not cardiac muscle cells) are called muscle fibers. Second, the ability of muscle to shorten or contract, depends on two types of myofilaments, the muscle cell equivalents of the microfilament of the cytoskeleton. Whenever you see the prefixes myo- and mys- ("muscle") sacro- ("flesh"), you will know that muscle cells the cytoplasm is called sarcoplasm.

1. Skeletal muscles: The muscles of the head, trunk and limbs are known as voluntary muscles, because they contract and produce movements in response to voluntary efforts. They are also called striped muscles, because under microscope their long thin fibers are seen to fine dark and light cross markings. The skeletal muscles enable the individuals to make movements by contracting and relaxing. These movements may be outwardly visible or not as in walking, running, gesticulating, eating, etc. Speed, strength and precision of movements involved in these activities depend on the coordination and control of the muscles. The muscle control is lost when the nerve centers or fibers are injured or diseased.

Skeletal muscle fibers are packaged into the organs called skeletal muscles that attach to the body's skeleton. As the skeletal muscles cover our bony "underpinnings", they help form the much smoother contours of the body. Skeletal muscle fibers are cigar-shaped, multinucleate cells, and the largest of the muscle fiber types—some ranging up to 30 cm (nearly 1 foot) in length. Indeed, the fibers of large, hardworking muscles, such as the antigravity muscles of the hip, are so big and coarse that they can be seen with the naked eye.

Skeletal muscle is also known as striated muscle (because its fibers appear to be striped) and as voluntary muscle (because it is the only muscle type subject to conscious control). However, it is important to recognize that skeletal muscles are often activated by reflexes (without our "willed command") as well. When you think of skeletal muscle tissue, the key words to keep in mind are skeletal, striated and voluntary. Skeletal muscle tissue can contract rapidly and with great force, but it tires easily and must rest after short periods of activity.

Skeletal muscle fibers, like most living cells, are soft and surprisingly fragile. Yet skeletal muscles can exert tremendous power—indeed, the force they generate is often much greater than that required to lift the weight. The reason they are not ripped apart as they exert force is that thousands of their fibers are bundled together by connective tissue, which as a whole. Each muscle fiber is enclosed in a delicate connective tissue sheath called an endomysium. Several, sheathed muscle fibers are then wrapped by a coarser fibrous membrane called a perimysium to form a bundle of fibers called a fascicle. Many fascicles are bound together by an even tougher "overcoat" of connective tissue called an epimysium, which covers the entire muscle. The epimysia blend into the strong, cord-like tendons, or into sheet-like aponeuroses, which attach muscles indirectly to bones, cartilages, or connective tissue coverings of each other.

Besides simply acting to anchor muscles, tendons perform several functions. The most important are providing durability and conserving space. Tendons are mostly tough collagenic fibers, so they can cross rough bony projections, which would tear the more delicate muscle tissues. Because of their relatively small size, more tendons than fleshy muscles can pass over a joint.

Many people think of muscles as always having an enlarged "belly" that tapers down to a tendon at each end. However, muscles vary considerably in the way their fibers are arranged. Many are spindle-shaped as just described, but in others, the fibers are arranged in a fan or a circle. In consequence of exercise the muscles become fatigued. In fatigue the muscles lose contractibility and by rest their strength and capacity are restored.

2. Smooth muscles: The muscles of intestines (as well as certain other structures, notably blood vessels and the uterus) called smooth muscle because under the microscope, unlike the skeletal muscles, it has no fine cross markings. In contrast to skeletal muscle it contracts automatically and cannot respond to an effort of will. It differs further in its relative slowness of action and in its nerve control. The smooth muscles are responsible for such vital processes as alimentation excretion and circulation. They function involuntarily and are not responsive to any effort of the will. They are solver to contract and slower to return to normal state. Smooth muscle has no striations and is involuntary, which means that we cannot consciously control it. Found mainly in the walls of hollow visceral organs such as the stomach, urinary bladder, substances along a definite tract, or pathway, within the body. We can best describe smooth muscle using the terms visceral, nonstriated and involuntary. Smooth muscle cells are spindle-shaped and have a single nucleus. They are arranged in sheets or layers. Most often there are two such layers, one running circularly and the other longitudinally. As the two layers alternately contract and relax, they change the size and the shape of the organ. Movement of food through the digestive tract and emptying the bowels and bladder are examples of "housekeeping" activities normally handled by smooth muscles. Smooth muscle contraction is slow and sustained. If skeletal muscle is like a speedy wind-up car that quickly runs down, then smooth muscle is like a steady, heavy-duty engine that lumbers along tirelessly.

3. Cardiac muscle: It is found in only one place in the body—the heart. The heart serves as a pump, propelling blood into the blood vessels and to all tissues of the body. Cardiac muscle is like skeletal muscle in that is striated and like smooth muscle in that it is voluntary and cannot be consciously controlled by most of us. Important key words to jog your memory (or this muscle type are cardiac, striated, and involuntary).

The cardiac fibers are cushioned by small amounts of soft connective tissue and arranged in spiral or figure 8-shaped bundles. When the heart contracts, its internal chambers become smaller, forcing the blood into the large arteries leaving the heart. Recall that cardiac muscle fibers are branching cells joined by special junctions called intercalated discs. These two structural features and the spiral arrangement of the muscle bundles in the heart allow heart activity to be closely coordinated. Cardiac muscle usually contracts at a fairly steady rate set by the heart's "in-house" pacemaker, but the heart can also be stimulated by the nervous system to shift into "high gear" for short periods, as when you race to catch a bus.

Functions of Muscles

Muscle plays four important roles in the body: it produces movement, maintains posture, stabilizes joints and generates heat.

- **Producing movement:** Just about all movements of the human body are a result of muscle contraction. Mobility of the body as a whole reflects the activity of skeletal muscles, which are responsible for all locomotion (walking, swimming, and cross-country skiing, for example) and manipulation. They enable us to respond quickly to changes in the external environment. For example their speed and power enable us to jump out of the way of a runaway car and then follow its flight with our eves. They also allow us to express our emotions with the silent language of smiles and frowns.

  These are distinct from the smooth muscle of blood vessel walls and cardiac muscle of the heart, which work together to circulate blood and maintain blood pressure, and the smooth muscle of other hollow organs, which forces fluids (urine, bile) and other substances (food, a baby) through internal body channels.
- **Maintaining posture:** People are rarely aware of the workings of the skeletal muscles that maintain body posture. Yet, they function almost continuously, making one tiny adjustment after another so that we can maintain an erect or seated posture despite the never-ending downward pull of gravity.
- **Stabilizing joints:** As the skeletal muscles pull on bones to cause movements, they also stabilize the joints of the skeleton. Indeed, muscle tendons are extremely important in reinforcing and stabilizing joints that have poorly fitting articulating surfaces (the shoulder joint, for example).

- **Generating heat:** The fourth function of muscle, generation of body heat, is a byproduct of muscle activity. As ATP is used to power muscle contraction, nearly three quarters of its energy escapes as heat. This heat is vital in maintaining normal body temperature. Since skeletal muscle accounts for at least 40 percent of body mass, it is the muscle type most responsible for heat generation.

Each of the three muscle types has a structure and function well suited for its job in the body. But since the term muscular system applies specifically to skeletal muscle. To sum up the activities of the muscles in relation to human behavior as follow:

- Skeletal muscle forms the muscles attached to the skeleton, which move the limbs and other body parts. Its cells are long, striated, and multinucleate. Skeletal muscle fibers are subject to voluntary control. Connective tissue coverings (endomysium, perimysium, and epimysium) enclose and protect the muscle fibers and increase the strength of skeletal muscles. Skeletal muscles make up the muscular system.
- Smooth muscle cells are uninucleate, spindle-shaped, and arranged in opposing layers in the walls of hollow organs. When they contract, substances (food, urine, a baby) are moved along internal pathways. Smooth muscle control is involuntary.
- Cardiac muscle cells are striated, branching cells that fit closely together and are arranged in spiral bundles in the heart. Their contraction pumps blood through the blood vessels. Control is involuntary.
- The sole function of muscle tissue is to contract or shorten. As it contracts, it causes movement, maintains posture, stabilizes joints and generates heat.
- The multinucleate cylindrical skeletal muscle fibers are packed with unique organelles called myofibrils. The banding pattern (striations) of the myofibrils and the cell as a whole reflects the regular arrangement of thin (actin-containing) and thick (myosin) filaments within the sarcomeres, the contractile units composing the myofibrils.
- Each myofibril is loosely enclosed by a specialized ER, called the sarcoplasmic reticulum (SR), which play an important role in storing and releasing calcium ions. Calcium ions are the final trigger for muscle fiber contraction.

Skeletal Muscle Contraction

Each muscle cell (also referred to as a muscle fiber) contains myofibrils, which in turn are composed of a series of sarcomeres, the actual contractile units of skeletal muscle. Sarcomeres contain thick myosin and thin actin filaments.

Muscle cells contract in response to electrical stimulation delivered by an effector nerve cell at the motor end plate. When stimulated, the muscle cell depolarizes and generates an action potential in a manner similar to that described for nerve cells. These action potentials propagate along the muscle cell membrane and lead to the release of calcium ions that are stored in specialized organelles called sarcoplasmic reticula. When there is a local increase in calcium ion concentration, the myosin and actin filaments slide across one another. Shortly after the muscle cell membrane is depolarized, it recovers its resting membrane voltage. Calcium is rapidly removed from the sarcomeres by active reaccumulation in the sarcoplasmic reticulum. When the calcium concentration in the sarcomere decreases, the myosin and actin filaments cease to interact, and the sarcomere returns to its original resting length (relaxation). Actin and myosin do not interact in the absence of calcium.

Energy is consumed during muscle contraction and relaxation. The primary source of energy for the muscle cells is adenosine triphosphate (ATP), which is generated through cellular oxidative metabolism. At low levels of activity (i.e. sedentary activity), the skeletal muscle synthesizes ATP from the oxidation of glucose to water and carbon dioxide. During periods of strenuous activity, when sufficient oxygen may not be available; glucose is metabolized primarily to lactic acid, an inefficient process compared with that of oxidative pathways. Stored muscle glycogen is used to supply glucose during periods of activity. Muscle fatigue is thought to be caused by depletion of glycogen and accumulation of lactic acid. As a result, the cycle of muscle contraction and relaxation cannot continue.

During muscle contraction, the energy released from ATP is not completely used. The excess energy is dissipated in the form of heat. During isometric contraction, almost all of the energy is released in the form of heat; during isotonic contraction, some of the energy is expended in mechanical work. In some situations, such as shivering because of cold, the need to generate heat is the primary stimulus for muscle contraction.

The contraction of muscle fibers can result in either isotonic or isometric contraction of the muscle. In isometric contraction, the length of the muscles remains constant but the force generated by the muscles is increased; an example of this is pushing against an immovable wall. Isotonic contraction, on the other hand, is characterized by shortening of the muscle with no increase in tension within the muscle; an example of this is flexing the forearm. In normal activities, many muscle movements are a combination of isometric and isotonic contraction. For example, during walking, isotonic contraction results in shortening of the leg, and isometric contraction causes the stiff leg to push against the floor.

The speed of the muscle contraction is variable. Myoglobulin is a hemoglobin-like protein pigment present in striated muscle cells that transports oxygen. Muscles containing large quantities of myoglobulin (red muscles) have been observed to contract slowly and powerfully (e.g. respiratory and postural muscles). Muscles containing little myoglobulin (white muscles) contract quickly (e.g. extraocular eye muscles). Most muscles contain both red and white muscle fibers.

Muscle Tone

Relaxed muscles demonstrate a state of readiness to respond to contraction stimuli. This state of readiness, known as muscle tone (tonus), is produced by the maintenance of some of the muscle fibers in a contracted state. Muscle spindles, which are sense organs in the muscles, monitor muscle tone. Muscle tone is minimal during sleep and is increased when the person is anxious. A muscle that is limp and without tone is described as flaccid; a muscle with greater than normal tone is described as spastic. In conditions characterized by lower motor neuron destruction (e.g. polio), denervated muscle becomes atonic (soft and flabby) and atrophies.

Muscle Actions

Muscles accomplish movement by contraction. Through the coordination of muscle groups, the body is able to perform a wide variety of movements. The prime mover is the muscle that causes a particular motion. The muscles assisting the prime mover are known as synergists. The muscles causing movement opposite to that of the prime mover are known as antagonists. An antagonist must relax to allow the prime mover to contract, producing motion. For example, when contraction of the biceps causes flexion of the elbow joint, the biceps are the prime movers, and the triceps are the antagonists. A person with muscle paralysis (a loss of movement, possibly from nerve damage) may be able to retrain functioning muscles within the synergistic group to produce the needed movement. Muscles of the synergistic group then become the prime movers.

Exercise, Disuse and Repair

Muscles need to be exercised to maintain function and strength. When a muscle repeatedly develops maximum or close to maximum tension over a long time, as in regular exercise with weights, the cross-sectional area of the muscle increases. This enlargement, known as hypertrophy, results from an increase in the size of individual muscle fibers without an increase in their number. Hypertrophy persists only if the exercise is continued. The opposite phenomenon occurs with disuse of muscle over a long period of time. Age and disuse cause loss of muscular function as fibrotic tissue replaces the contractile muscle tissue. The decrease in the size of a muscle is called atrophy. Bed rest and immobility cause loss of muscle mass and strength. When immobility is the result of a treatment modality (e.g. casting, traction), the patient can decrease the effects of immobility by isometric exercise of the muscles of the immobilized part. Quadriceps setting exercises (tightening the muscles of the thigh) and gluteal setting exercises (tightening of the muscles of the buttocks) help maintain the larger muscle groups that are important in ambulation. Active and weight-resistance exercises of uninjured parts of the body maintain muscle strength. When muscles are injured, they need rest and immobilization until tissue repair occurs. The healed muscle then needs progressive exercise to resume its preinjury strength and functional ability.

Activity of the skeletal muscles includes the following:

- All skeletal muscle cells are stimulated by motor neurons: When the neuron releases a neurotransmitter (acetylcholine), the permeability of the sarcolemma changes, allowing sodium ions to enter the muscle cell. This produces an electrical current (action potential), which flows across the entire sarcolemma, resulting in release of calcium ions from the SR.
- Calcium binds to regulatory proteins on the thin filaments and exposes myosin binding sites, allowing the myosin heads on the thick filaments to attach. The attached heads pivot, sliding the thin filaments toward the center of the sarcomeres, and contraction occurs. ATP provides the energy for the sliding process, which continues as long as ionic calcium is present.
- Although individual muscle cells contract completely when adequately stimulated, a muscle (an organ) responds to stimuli to different degrees, that is, it exhibits graded responses.
- Most skeletal muscle contractions are titanic (smooth and sustained) because rapid nerve impulses are reaching the muscle, and the muscle cannot relax completely between contractions. The strength of muscle contraction reflects the relative number of muscle cells contracting (more = stronger).
- ATP, the immediate source of energy for muscle contraction, is stored in muscle fibers in small amounts that are quickly used up. ATP is regenerated via three routes. From the fastest to the slowest, these are via a coupled reaction of creatine phosphate with ADP, via anaerobic glycolysis and lactic acid formation, and via anaerobic respiration. Only aerobic respiration requires oxygen.
- If muscle activity is strenuous and prolonged, muscle fatigue occurs due to an accumulation of lactic acid in the muscle and a decrease in its energy (ATP) supply. After exercise, the oxygen debt is repaid by rapid deep breathing.

- Muscle contractions are isotonic (the muscle shortens and movement occurs) or isometric (the muscle does not shorten, but its tension increases).
- Muscle tone keeps muscles healthy and ready to react. It is a result of a staggered series of nerve impulses delivered to different cells within the muscle. If the nerve supply is destroyed, the muscle loses tone, becomes paralyzed, and atrophies.
- Inactive muscles atrophy. Muscles challenged by resistance exercise to respond (almost) beyond their ability increase in size and strength. Muscles subjected to regular aerobic exercise become more efficient and stronger and can work longer without tiring. Aerobic exercise also benefits other body organ systems.
- All muscles are attached to bones at two points. The origin is the immovable attachment; the insertion is the movable bony attachment. When contraction occurs, the insertion moves toward the origin.
- Body movements include flexion, extension, abduction, adduction, circumduction, rotation, pronation, supination, inversion, eversion, dorsiflexion, plantar flexion and opposition.
- On the basis of their general functions in the body, muscles are classified as prime movers, antagonists, synergists and fixators.
- Muscles are named according to several criteria, including muscle size, shape, number and location of origins, associated bones, and action of the muscle.
- Muscles have several fascicle arrangements that influence their force and degree of shortening.
- Muscles of the head fall into two groups. The muscles of facial expression include the frontalis, orbicularis oris and oculi, and zygomaticus. The chewing muscles are the masseter, temporalis and buccinators (which is also a muscle of facial expression).
- Muscles of the trunk and neck move the head, shoulder girdle, and trunk and from the abdominal girdle. Anterior neck and trunk muscles include the sternocleidomastoid, pectoralis major, intercostals, rectus abdominis, external and internal obliques, and transverse abdominis. Posterior trunk and neck muscles include the trapezius, latissimus dorsi, and deltoid. Deep muscles of the back are the erector spinae muscles.
- Muscles of the upper limb include muscles that cause movement at the shoulder joint, elbow, and hand. Muscles causing movement at the elbow include the brachialis, biceps brachii, brachioradialis, and triceps brachii.
- Muscles of the lower extremity cause movement at the hip, knee, and foot. They include the iliopsoas, gluteus maximus and medius, adductors, quadriceps and hamstring groups, gastrocnemius, tibialis anterior, fibularis muscles, soleus, and extensor digitorum longus.
- Increasing muscular control reflects the maturation of the nervous system. Muscle control is achieved in a cephalic/caudal and proximal/distal direction.
- To remain healthy, muscles must be regularly exercised. Without exercise, they atrophy; with extremely vigorous exercise, they hypertrophy.
- As we age, muscle mass decreases, and the muscles become more sinewy. Exercise helps to retain muscle mass and strength.

Importance of Muscles in Nursing the Clients

Muscle tone means the readiness of the muscles to contract. It ensures smooth and ready responses. The tonus of muscle is responsible for the quickness and swiftness with which we perform our actions. It is the tonus of muscles of legs, trunk and neck which enables us to perform such activities as solving a problem, listening to a lecture or aiming at a target. However general muscular tension causes irritability and excitability. This is illustrated by the tense state of the statement who is unable to rest or relax or sleep. According to Crow and Crow, a patient convalescing from diseased muscle tone may find it difficult to overcome his inertia.

The diseased and sick persons are likely to have defective muscle tone which may cause in them difficulties in digesting food, in proper elimination and in resting and relaxing. The difficulties of the patient due to defective muscles tones should be appreciated and well known to the nurse.

Certain diseases result in hypotonic musculature. They affect adversely the muscular tone of the body. If the patient is to regain his muscle tone he must be made to rest, relax and sleep, eat wholesome and nutritious food, have plenty of sunshine and fresh air. A nurse should keep such things in mind. She should help the patient to remain physically quiet and serene in mental outlook. The patient must avoid negative emotions.

In order to regain the proper tonus of the muscles the convalescent patient need exercise of the muscles. He should be encouraged to move his limbs freely as far as possible, sit up and take a little walk. Above all the nurse should take good care of her own muscles and keep them in fit condition, because unless she is smart and radiates alacrity the patient is likely to feel discouraged.

Illness and fatigue are due to microbes and death of leukocytes. Rest, relaxation and cheerful outlook are necessary to combat this condition.

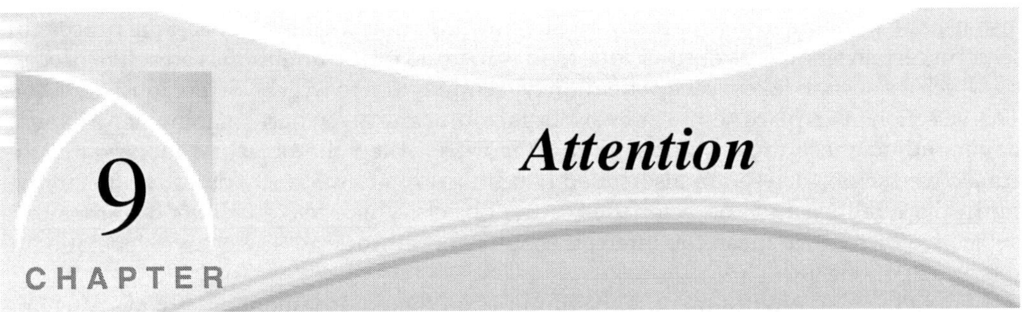

9 CHAPTER Attention

Introduction

Attention is the cognitive process of selectively concentrating on one aspect of the environment while ignoring other things. The physiological sensitivity of the organism sets a basic limit to know of our surroundings, our observation of the world is also dependent upon the closely related processes of attention and perception. Attention, a process of psychological selectivity, involves an adjustment of the body and its sense organs, clear and vivid consciousness, and a set towards action. The postural aspect of attention corresponds to the orienting or attitudinal reflex discovered in lower animals by Pavlov. Experiments have shown that the central nervous system selects some stimuli and suppresses reaction to others. This is made possible by the centrifugal or 'wrong-way' nerve pathways, which go from the brain down to the relay stations of the sensory pathways and also from the motor pathway (corticospinal or pyramidal tract) to the hindbrain. The centrifugal auditory pathway, a bundle of nerve fibers from the brain to the ear, is called the bundle of Oort. These and the other 'wrong-way' fibers act like electronic gates to block response to certain stimuli and allow the organism to pay attention to more important ones. Certain characteristics of the stimulus object—such as change, size, prepotency, and repetitiveness—help determine which stimuli win out over competing ones in attracting our attention. Equally important are such subjective factors as the organic condition of the individual, his interests, and his susceptibility to social suggestions. Attention shifts constantly from one aspect of a situation to another. It also fluctuates involuntarily, even when the sense organs are adjusted to a particular stimulus. Distractions interfere with attention, although the amount of interference depends greatly upon subjective factors.

People have been dealing so far with the various ways by which they have contact with the outside world. At every moment numerous stimuli from the outside environment come and call for our attention. But in fact, they cannot attend to all these. They always select. This selection is based on some conditions which will be mentioned presently. At any moment a certain area of the environment is thus selected. This area of which they are aware is called the field of consciousness. It can be quite rich and complicated. Even when reading book, we may be aware of the temperature, some noise that is heard outside, the contents in the room such as furniture, books, etc. and so many other things. All these form the field of our consciousness at the moment. But we are not aware of all of them with the same degree of intensity. We are most aware of what we read (provided you are really reading). This particular part of the field is called the "focus of consciousness". We also use the term the focus of attention. Thus by attention we simply mean the process by which a certain small area of conscious field is focused on. So attention is an active process by which a selection takes place. Attention determines that to which you are most attentive. This selection takes place because of various factors at any given particular moment. Experts have studied these factors under two categories, called the objective factors and the subjective factors. These are also called conditions of attention. By objective factors we mean the qualities and characteristics of the objects which make us attend to them. By subjective factors we mean the interests, habits and attitudes that we have developed in the course of our life.

Man lives in an environment. The stimuli from the environment are always affecting him. But these stimuli do not affect him equally. It is a common place observation that some stimuli affect us more than others. This shows that man selects out of environmental stimuli. This tendency of selection shows that there is a motivational process in him which is known as attention. This attention is affected by interest, attitudes and mental set. It is a selective process which includes motivation, mental set and selection. To take an example from human beings, if a student is not motivated, he will not attend to the class lecture. While a professor is delivering a lecture in the class, there are several other sounds being made in other rooms and the surroundings. The student who hears the lecture selects professor's voice out of the noise in the surroundings. While a student is attentively hearing the lecture, one can very well note his physical set which also indicates his mental set. Receptor adjustment, bodily adjustment, postural adjustment, muscular tension and central nervous adjustments are typical of bodily sets in attention. Thus, in brief, attention can be defined as a process which compels the individual to select some particular stimulus according to his interest and attitude out of the multiplicity of stimuli present in the environment.

Definitions of Attention

Attention appears to be a power or faculty which people can turn on or off at will or something which people can lend to this or that situation. In real sense, when individual try to examine the nature of attention on scientific line individual find attention is purely an act, a process or a function. It should never be considered as a force that makes us aware of one thing to the exclusion of others. Let us try to understand the nature of this process through the readings of distinguished writers. Definitions of attention are as follows:

Dumville states that "Attention is the concentration of consciousness upon one object rather than upon another".

Ross defines "Attention is process of getting in an object of thought clearly before the mind".

Morgan and Gilliland opines that "Attention is being keenly alive to some specific factor in our environment. It is a preparatory adjustment for response".

RN Sharma defined "Attention as a process which compels the individual to select some particular stimulus according to his interest and attitude out of the multiplicity of stimuli present in the environment".

So attention is the cognitive process of selectively concentrating on one as aspect of the environment while ignoring the things.

Nature of Attention

Definitions mention above point out the following important facts about the meaning and nature of the term 'attention':

1. Attention is focusing of consciousness on a particular object: Number of things of the environment at a particular time and are aware or conscious of many of them. Therefore, focusing of consciousness on a particular object, idea or activity makes us able to understand it and we become fully conscious or aware of it. Attention is the name given to this process of the focusing of consciousness or awareness that makes us become alive to one thing to the exclusion of others. Hence it is proper to define attention as the process of the concentration of consciousness upon one object rather than another.
2. Attention is constantly shifting: When we are attending to an object at a particular moment, person clearly aware or conscious of it as his consciousness is focused on it. What happens to other objects and activities which are not at the focus of our consciousness at that moment? Are we aware of them or not? Of course we are aware of many of them but not clearly as in the case of focused object. Why is it so? The reason lies in the division of the field or perception or consciousness at a particular moment. Consciousness at a particular moment may be divided into two parts, central and marginal. At the time when our attention is on the blackboard and consciousness is focused on it, the other objects and activities in the classroom remain within the reach of marginal consciousness. This helps us in becoming partly conscious or aware of them. Both these fields of perception or consciousness are interchangeable. The object which is at a moment within the focus of consciousness or even beyond that. Therefore, it is proper to realize attention as a flexible and dynamic process. The subject of attention generally goes on changing and the object of attention remains the same on which the consciousness is centered.
3. Attention is selective: At any moment, there are various stimuli in the environment of an individual which try to affect him. For example there may be music coming from the radio, some one talking and noises coming from the street. Instead or these stimuli affecting the same sense organ, there may be stimuli affecting us from other sense organs. Our reaction is selective. Only those stimuli which suit our interests and attitudes, are able to attract attention, others are ignored. The stimulus which is more important and useful than the other is attended at once whereas the less important and significant ones are attended later on. In this way represents a narrow field and is always selective.
4. Attention is a state of preparedness or alertness: Attention is considered as a process involving a preparatory adjustment for response. During this process, the organism tries to prepare himself or adjust himself to the stimulus situation. In other words he goes into a process of physical, mental and emotional alertness or preparedness. His sense organs adjust themselves to receive the stimulus more effectively. Individual may mark him turning his head, or fixing his eyes towards the object of attention. Besides this, the muscles of the body are also specially prepared to the object of attention or to engage in the activity that is in the focus as attention. At this stage of preparedness one may easily notice the state of tension in the muscles. Attention does not only involve motor preparedness but also brings mental alertness or preparedness. One becomes mentally alert and tries to exercise one's mental powers as affectively as possible at the time of paying attention to a task. In this way attention brings an all-round alertness and preparedness in the organism for accomplishing the task successfully.

Types of Attention

The classification given by Ross seems to be more agreeable as given below:

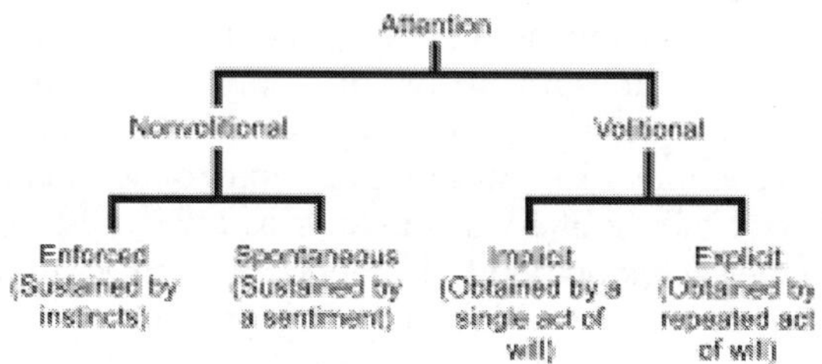

1. Nonvolitional or Involuntary Attention. This type of attention is aroused without the play of will. Here we attend to an object or an idea without making any conscious efforts on our part. Mother's attention towards her crying child, attention towards the members of opposite sex, sudden loud noise, bright colors, etc. are the example of nonvolitional attentions.

Nonvolitional attention can be aroused by our instincts as also by our sentiments. The attention which is aroused by the instincts is called enforced nonvolitional attention. For example. A youngman, when we make an appeal to his sex instinct or curiosity becomes quite attentive in his task. The type of attention which he plays at this time can be named as enforced nonvolitional attention.

The other subtype of nonvolitional attention, aroused by the sentiments is called 'Spontaneous nonvolitional' attention. It is the result of properly developed sentiments. It give somewhat automatic or spontaneous attention towards that object, idea, person round which our sentiments are formed.

As has been explained above, nonvolitional attention is not only direct by the individual desire or motivation, it may even be against it. It generally hinders the process of goal seeking. If, for example, your attention is attracted by a song while you are studying, your studies will suffer. Social adjustment is similarly obstructed by involuntary attention. The proper adjustment of a student can be the outcome, only of an undisturbed attention to his studies. On account of the fact that one can pay attention to only one thing at a time, the student will not be able to attend to his studies if his attention continually wanders in other directions. Obviously, a person forgets his goal owing to involuntary attention and cannot effect his adjustment.

2. Volitional or Voluntary Attention. Attention is volitional or voluntary when it calls forth the exercise of will. It demands the conscious efforts on our part. It is least automatic and spontaneous and not given whole heartedly like volitional attention. Usually in such type of attention, we have a clear-cut goal before us and for its accomplishment we, with all our efforts, make ourselves attentive. For example. Attention paid at the time of solving an assigned problem of statistics answering questions in examination hall, consulting the railway time table at the time of starting for a railway journey.

Voluntary attention (its name is indicative of it nature) is that which is willingly directed to an object. If, for example a student attends to his studies of his own accord and not as a result of any external pressure, his attention will be called voluntary. An analysis reveals elements of desire and interests, aim and social adjustment in voluntary attention. In the forgetting example the student directs his attention because of some particular aim like the passing of an examination, acquiring knowledge or one of a number of other goals. He takes interest in studying. By passing examination or acquiring knowledge he may be able to support a family or gain social standing. Like other activities, attention is just another form of adjustment. The difference between voluntary and involuntary attention is that while the former is secured by the motivational elements in the individual, the motivating elements exist outside in the latter case.

Volitional attention is further subdivided into two categories—Implicit volitional attention and Explicit volitional attention. Whereas in the former, a single act of volition sufficient to bring about attention, in the latter we need repeated acts of will to sustain it. When a child is assigned some mathematical sums in the classroom, and he does not attend to them, he is warned by the teacher that he will be punished if he does not do his assigned practice work. This can make him exercise his will power, attend to the assigned task and finish it properly. Here a single act of will is responsible for the arousing of attention. Hence we can take it as an example of implicit volitional attention.

In explicit volitional attention, attention is obtained by repeated acts of will. One has to struggle hard for keeping oneself attentive. It requires a strong will power keen attention and strong motives for the accomplishment of the task. The attention paid at the time of examination day for the required preparation against the heavy odds and distraction, is a glaring example of such attention.

Attention may be overt or covert. Overt attention is the act of directing sense organs towards a stimulus sources. Covert attention is the act of mentally focusing on one of several possible sensory stimuli.

3. Habitual attention: Besides the two types mentioned above, there is a third type, the habitual or nonvoluntary attention. The difference between nonvoluntary and in-voluntary attention is that the former type is the result of some habit or practice and the motivation is in the individual but the reason for the attention in the latter type is in the object. Habitual attention is different from voluntary attention because habitual attention has no need for a will as the latter does. But continued application of voluntary attention converts it into habitual attention. For example, a student pays voluntary attention to study in the beginning but it is gradually transformed into habitual attention is in between voluntary and involuntary types of attention.

Actually the above distinctions in attention are not very clear. The difference between voluntary and involuntary attention is often only just discernible. No attention can be said to belong to any one of the three types exclusively. A scholar has to exercise his will in spite of his involuntary attention is reading. There is an unconscious desires to pay attention to an object which involuntarily draws your attention. In this way the difference in the types of attention is small though it is of great importance from the psychological view-point.

The nature of attention permits of its concentration in only one direction at one time. Direction of attention to two or more objects means either their acceptance as one or such an oscillation of attention between all of them as gives the impression of simultaneous attention. But experiments have proved, beyond doubt, that a person can pay attention to only one object at a time.

Factors Associated with Attention

I. OBJECTIVE FACTORS

They may be brought under seven headings:
1. Intensity
2. Size
3. Repetition
4. Movement
5. Change
6. Systematic form
7. Novelty.

These are explained under external determinants of attention in this chapter.

II. SUBJECTIVE FACTORS

One who is interested in gardening may be attracted by the new kind of flower or plant which does not have any striking objective qualities of the seven categories mentioned previously. But he attends to it because of his own developed interest and knowledge. A hungry person may be attracted by anything that could be eaten. Such conditions which call for our attention are called subjective because they are dependent on our own mental make-up and training. They depend on their interest or general mood, their deeper affections, aspirations, etc. For example, a sleeping mother will not be disturbed by a whole lot of loud noise outside. But if her sick child raises even a faint cry, her attention may be caught at once, and she may wake up. When we are in a happy mood, we may notice things that are pleasant. But when we are in an unhappy mood, all sorts of small unpleasant things and mistakes of others will draw our attention.

Though for convenience we have stated the above factors under the two different headings, objective and subjective, in fact, at any one particular situations, such a sharp division may not be possible. Often the effectiveness of an objective condition itself may depend upon our subjective make-up. There can never be a condition which is purely subjective or purely objective. All the conditions under the two headings are dependent upon our psychological make-up. At any one particular time, much depends upon what may be called our 'set' or attitude. Because of the particular need of the moment, the whole body organism may be turned as it were like a radio to a particular thing. When one is attending to a very exciting football match, his whole self is tuned to it. When there is such a set, nothingelse will attract his attention according to the above-mentioned factors except under very extraordinary circumstances.

In this context, a few other problems related to this phenomenon of attention can be mentioned here.

a. Division of Attention

People have often wondered they can attend to more than one thing at a time. This problem is usually referred to as the division of attention. Laboratory experiments can be conducted to study this question. It is proved beyond doubt that we can attend to only one thing at a time. But we do come across people who can go on talking and at the same time do some other activity with their hands, such as knitting. This does not mean that they attend to two things at one and the same time. Often the knitting is not attended to at all. It has become an automatic activity needing no attention except when something goes wrong. At such a time, the talking or listening will be stopped. With some people of course, talking is habitual and mechanical without any thinking or attention. Sometimes, one may appear to be attending to more than one thing at a time, because of the fact that there is a rapid shifting from one to the other. You might have known people who can play three of four musical instruments at the same time. But it is not so. All these instruments will be unified towards one rhythm, and so actually, it is one composite unit that the individual is attending to. Laboratory experiments can be conducted with the help of a suitable apparatus to determine the extent to which attention can be divided between two physical tasks, between two mental tasks or between one physical and one mental task. This problem is called the division or divisibility of attention.

b. Shifting of Attention

Attention shifts from one things to another often very rapidly. The layman will think that one can attend to a particular thing for one or two hours. But in fact, we can attend to a thing continuously only for a few seconds. Continuous attention means continuity with plenty of shifting. Now and then, the attention will be diverted but will be immediately brought back. This is sometimes referred to as fluctuation of attention.

c. Span of Attention

Another interesting problem with reference to attention is what is called the span of attention. How many figures or letters can one notice in one act of attention? Surprisingly the total number that we can attend to in this manner is quite limited. This can be determined by the use of an apparatus called the Tachistascope. There are minor individual differences with regard to these, but usually four or five number or letters can be noticed at one glance. It will be noticed that the registration plate of a motor car contains usually (except some army vehicles) only four figures. Serial numbering will go up to 9999 but not 10000. This is because when a car runs fast, the traffic constable will not ordinarily be able to take note of more than four numbers. But for later cars, the letters are changed.

Methods of Arusing Attention, Factors and Conditions Favorable for Capturing Attention

One of the major problems in the field of education is that of capturing pupil's attention. How can they be made attentive to their tasks, so that they can achieve their desired objectives? A teacher for the success of his mission, should be acquainted with the means and methods of securing his pupil's attention. These are certain factors which produce and control the condition of attention in a person. These factors are classified as external (objective)—those that are found in the objects in one's environment and internal (subjective) those that lie within the person himself.

The methods of securing attention are, in fact, based upon these external and internal factors of attention. Let us try to understand these external and internal factors or conditions.

External Factors or Conditions

External factors or conditions are generally those characteristic of outside situations or stimuli which make the strongest bid for capturing our attention. Let us try to think of these characteristics.

A teacher should try to take care of both the internal and external factors for capturing attention of his students. He should see that his students possess a favorable bent of mind towards the topic going to be taught and can take genuine interest in it. For this purpose he may make use of proper teaching methods, techniques, devices and audiovisual aids that an appeal to the child's basic needs, drives and interest. He must emphasize the overall importance of the topic in hand and see the clear-cut aims and objectives of teaching it. He must make a judicious use of all the external as well as internal factors of securing attention. As far as possible the volitional attention should be more emphasized. For this purpose, personal, ambitions, and desires may be awakened and heightened in the students. They may be made to strive to achieve to desired motives and set goals. The factor of distraction (which will be discussed later in the present chapter) should be reduced to the minimum so that the students should not feel any inconvenience.

Sustained Attention

Mere capturing or attracting of the students is not enough. It is the beginning of a process and not the end. After capturing the attention, essential attempts should be made to hold it for a desirable long time. This needed task is named sustaining of attention. In the words of Woodworth "To sustain attention is to concentrate one's activity continuously upon some object or happening or problem". Thus, in the case of sustained attention, there is no wandering. The individual attention always remains on track and the activity proceeds systematically without any serious distraction.

To achieve the required objectives in a reasonable time, the habit of paying sustained attention is very helpful. One must be used to concentrate upon the activity which one is doing. The child who cannot keep his attention fixed for a reasonable period is sure to lag behind in his studies. An artist has to strive for the sustained attention so that he can finish his desired piece of art. A writer, a poet, a musician all have to care for the sustained attention. In holding the attention for long, there is a need of creating genuine interest of the external factors of getting attention can be helpful in this task. Therefore, a wise teacher should make use of them of sustaining the attention of his students.

He must exploit their basic needs, instincts and motives and make them conscious of the desired objective and purposes. He must bring desired modification in his methodology. Whenever needed the factors of novelty, change and contrast should be introduced, the use of effective devices and aids should be called for and the children should be given required freedom for encouraging their will. They must work with a zeal and enthusiasm and not under pressure. All the factors which create distraction and prove obstacles in the path of holding the attention long, should be removed. As far as possible, children should be made to work under most favorable environmental conditions and the causes which disturb them mentally and emotionally should be attended to carefully. Moreover the will power of the students should be developed and they should be made to struggle hard for acquiring their set objectives and higher ideals.

Importance of Attention in Education

In the process of education, attention plays a significant role. It is essential for the teachers to reach well and for the students to understand and learn well. An attentive class motivates, the teacher to put in his most valuable efforts. He can teach more efficiently and effectively. His energies are utilized fully when he perceives his students absorbed in his teaching. Not a single minute of his period gets wasted as he receives the responses immediately.

For the learner, attention is the most important key for the desired success. When one is attentive to the classroom activities one gests oneself completely ready and prepared. It puts one into a state of alertness. As soon as the teaching activities in the classroom begin or he is asked to perform certain activities, he finds himself physically, emotionally and mentally prepared. The various sense organs become specially prepared to receive stimulus. The muscles and organs of the body, the brain and nerves become specially prepared to act to the object of attention or to engage in the activity that is in the focus of attention. Such type of an all-round alertness help the learner to receive the knowledge given by the teacher.

Attention, in this way, is responsible for bringing efficiency in learning. It enables the students to learn properly within a short period of time. It also increases their abilities and develops the acquired skills. It also aids to their power of memorization and understanding. During attention, all energies are concentrated on a particular object or activity. This deep concentration on particular object or activity. This deep concentration and single aimness help the learner to achieve desired success in the focused activities or task. Moreover sustaining of attention has a psychological effect. It creates interest in a particular object or activity. It makes the students goal-directed. They try to strive hard with enthusiasm and proper bent to mind. In this way attention makes them able to achieve the required target within a short period and reasonable amount of efforts. Surely, the teaching earning process owes much to the process of attention and every system, of education should give it a proper place in the planning of its program say from MSP to MSZ or MSY and then continued, from one right upto 9999 again. One may ask what happens to these letters. It is an interesting capacity of the mind to organize the perceptual field into different units. The numbers go as one group containing four units and the three letters form a different group containing only three units. The limitation applies to the number of units within one group only. It is possible to have two or three groups each having four units within.

Distraction or Inattention

There is practically no such thing as inattention. Inattention simply means we are not attending to the specified thing but to somethingelse. We are attending always to something or other. What kind of things will distract us from our object of attention will depend upon the various conditions of attention referred to earlier. One interesting question has been studied by a large number of people with regard to the nature of distraction. Experiments have been carried out to determine the effect of distraction by all sorts of noise on intellectual tasks. For example, a group of people would be asked to memorize a poem or to do some arithmetical calculation. While they are working, noises like a pandemonium would be produced by bells, blow horns, sirens, hammering, etc. The people who are doing the mental work often complain that they feel disturbed and irritated. But the interesting result was that in most cases the total performances of the persons were little affected, and in some cases there was even considerable improvement. One might ask how can there be improvement when there is distraction. Probably in the attempt to fight against distraction, we put forth a great amount of extra energy to keep ourselves at our tasks. However, if one has to work continuously in the midst of heavy distractions, there may be fatigue in the long run.

Complaints of Losing Attentive Power

Quite a number of young people some time or other complain that they have lost their powers of attention and concentration. They mean by that, when they were younger, they were able to concentrate on things for much longer periods. But now they are not able to do so. From this, they come to the conclusion and develop a fear that they are losing their concentration power. In a few cases, the fear may grow to an abnormal extent and may produce a serious psychological disturbance. So a word of encouragement may be mentioned in such cases. Except in very severe cases of organic disease or decay affecting the central nervous system, power of concentration or ability to attend can never be lost. It does not decrease at all. What really happens in such cases is that now at the adolescent age, these people develop a larger number of interests, so much so, when they sit down to study or when they sit in the classroom, they are not able to attend to the book or the teacher. Their attention and their thoughts run to so many other things. It is quite a natural phenomenon for the adolescent age.

Conditions of Attention

As a selective act of the mind, attention depends upon several conditions. These conditions may be of two types—external or objective and internal or subjective. External or objective conditions are concerned with the environment. In the environment of the individual there are several stimuli, but he does not attend to all of them at the same time, because some stimuli are stronger than others. The factors making these stimuli stronger than others, are known as external determinants of attention. Besides the external conditions, the mental conditions, culture and heredity also influence attention. Owing to these internal conditions some objects attract our attention more than others. These internal factors are internal determinants of attention. The methods of achieving attention are based upon these external and internal determinants of attention.

External Determinants of Attention

The following are the most important external determinants of attention:

1. Nature of stimulus—Nature of stimulus means its types, i.e. whether it is visual, gustatory, auditory, olfactory or tactual stimulus. It has been found by experiments that in comparison with other sensations color and sound attract more attention. Among the pictures, those of human beings attract more attention than those of beautiful or objects. Among the pictures of human beings those of beautiful women attract more attention. Besides these, the colored pictures attract more attention than black and white. All these factors are important in advertisement. In the auditory stimulus, the melodious voice attracts more attention than other voices.

   All types of stimuli are not able to bring the same degree of attention. A picture attracts attention more readily than words. Among the pictures, the pictures of human beings capture more attention than those of animals or objects. Among the pictures of human beings those of beautiful woman or handsome men attract more attention. In this sense colored pictures are more forceful than colorless ones. In this way, an effective stimulus should always be chosen for capturing maximum attention.
2. Intensity of the stimulus—Intensity of the stimulus is a helpful condition in attention. In comparison with the weak stimuli the intense stimulus more attention of the organism. High sound, excessive pressure and acute pain attract our attention. In the

market there is always some buzzing sound and yet the pedestrians hear the horn of a motor car, since the sound of the horn is louder than other sounds. But it is not always necessary that one should attend to the intensity of stimulus. Sometimes while walking on the road, calling of our name attracts so much attention that we fail to hear even the loud sound of the horn. As a matter of fact the attraction of the attention does not depend on any single factor, but on several factors interconnected with each another. Hence it can be said that other things being the same, the more intense stimulus will attract more attention.

In comparison with the weak stimulus, the intense stimulus attracts more attention of an individual. Our attention becomes easily directed to a loud sound, a bright light or a strong smell. Similarly a large object in environment is more likely to catch our attention than a small object. A large building will be more readily attended to than the small ones. *Intensity:* Naturally our attention will be attracted towards a louder sound than a weaker one, a brighter color than a lighter shade and sharper pain in some part of the body than a light pain sensation in some other.

3. Size of stimulus—In the visual stimuli, the size of the stimulus is also a determinant of attention. As a general rule the bigger size attracts more attention, but a small advertisement on a very wide background also attracts attention. Thus the attraction of an object does not depend upon its size alone, but also on its background. To illustrate, a big black spot on a black face will not attract so much attention as a very small black spot on a white face. *Size:* Sometimes, the mere size also plays a part. A bigger patch of color will certainly draw our attention more easily that a small patch of the same color.
4. Location of the stimulus—The location of the stimulus also affects attention. In the visual stimuli, the most affective location is just in front of the eyes. The role of different pages in the newspapers or the magazine, and the different places on the same page, is important in advertisement. It has been found by experiments that advertisements given on the front page or on the upper half of any page attract more attention.
5. Contrast of the stimulus—The contrast of the stimulus is also an important determinant of attention, e.g. the presence of a woman among men and that of a man among women definitely attracts more attention.
   Contrast, change and variety—Change and variety strike attention more easily than sameness and absence of change. If we are talking to our students verbally, the use of maps and charts suddenly attracts their attention. We do not notice the ticking on the watch but it arrests our attention as soon as it stops. Any change in the stimulation to which we have become adapted immediately captures our attention. Actually the factor—contrast or change is highly responsible for capturing attention of the organism and contributes more than the intensity, size or nature of the stimulus. If all the LETTERS on this page were printed in capitalized word in this sentence would have no greater attention getting value than any other word. It is the contrast or change which makes it more forceful.
6. Change of the stimulus—Attention cannot be concentrated for a long time on some particular object. Hence the change of the stimulus also affects attention. Attention is sustained by change of the stimulus. The advertisers change their advertisements from time to time lest it may cease to be attractive.
   Change: We said earlier that repetition if continued beyond a point ceases to have attention value. But if there is a sudden change either in the intensity or in the size or

even by way of sudden stopping, then we at once attend to them. For example, the ticking of a clock in our room usually will not draw our attention because of this being repeated continuously. But if it suddenly stops, we may at once turn and remark 'Why has the clock stopped'? So, the stopping has attracted our attention. Similarly, any change in the physical characteristic of stimulus is able to attract our attention. Novelty also attracts attention. We are compelled to attend to anything that in novel. So it is always better to introduce the change or novelty for breaking monotony and securing attention.

Novelty: This factor needs no explanation. Anything new or strange or unusual, whether a sight or sound or any other sensation, invariable draws our attention.

7. Isolation of the stimulus—A man sitting alone in some corner of the park, hotel or club attracts more attention than other. A student sitting alone at the far corner of the class, is seen first. Thus isolation is an important external determinant of attention. This fact is based upon the reason that the isolated and hence seen separately in his own background. By experiments in advertisement it has been found that only the fact of isolation attracts 30 percent more attention. DE Berlyne (1951) pointed out the following principles based upon latest experiments:
   a. In comparison with the unchanged stimulus the stimulus changed in the near past has more possibility of attracting attention.
   b. The effect of change goes on diminishing with the passage of time.
   c. Whenever stimuli are changed together and one is left unchanged, the effect of change is not noticeable.
   d. If change goes on in the changed stimuli, the process of attention is rather permanent and strong.

   The modes of change also influence the process of attention. If there is an absolute change, it attracts more attention. While studying one does not hear the sound of the clock or that of electric fan but if either of these suddenly stops, one cannot fail to attend to it. Man becomes used to regular changes and does not pay much attention to them. But if some irregular change or any sudden change occurs, it at once draws attention.
8. Duration of the stimulus—As a general rule, the stimulus having more duration attracts more attention. Thus duration of the stimulus is an important determinant of attention. But sometimes the smallest flashing of a movement attracts more attention than the bigger stimuli, e.g. a sudden flash of light for several seconds will attract more attention in a dark night than the continuous burning lamp.
9. Repetition of the stimulus—Along with duration, repetition of the stimulus is also an important determinant of attention. It is a common place observation that when the teacher has to attract the attention of students towards a particular phenomenon, he repeats it several times. But sometimes man ceases to attend a phenomenon simply because it is repeated many times, e.g. if a man says something about him, we take interest in it once or twice, if we find that he always repeats the same thing, we cease to pay attention.

   Repetition is a factor of great importance in securing attention. We may ignore a stimulus at first instance but when it is repeated several time, it captures our attention. A mis-spelled word is more likely to be noticed if it occurs twice in the same paragraph than if it occurs only once. In the classroom also the particular point on which the teacher tries to draw the attention of the students is raised again and again. While giving the lecture the important aspects of the speech are often repeated, so that the attention of the audience can be easily directed to the valuable points. But this practice of repetition should be carefully used. Too much repetition of a stimulus may bring diminishing returns.

Repetition: Sometimes a stimulus even when it is not very intense or big in size may attract our attention because of the fact of its being repeated several times. If there is one gentle sound in the room where you are working, you may not notice. But if the sound continues then it is very likely to draw your attention. This shows that even at the first time, we became aware of it. It must have been in the field of consciousness, but in the outer fringe. Repetition brought it to the focus. It may be pointed out here that is the repetition goes on beyond a certain point and continues to be of a kind of permanent feature, it ceases to draw our attention. This is because of the negative adaptation which we have mentioned earlier.

10. Movement in the stimulus—In comparison with the static, the moving stimuli attract more attention. The position of a stimulus changes due to movements. An object lying in some corner of the room will not attract our attention, but even if there is some illusion of movement in it, we cannot help attending it. The influence of movement in stimulus is widely used by the shopkeepers and businessmen, who advertise through moving electric lights.

    A moving stimulus catches our attention more quickly than a stimulus that does not move. In other words we are more sensitive to objects that move in our field of vision. Most of the advertisers make use of this fact and try to capture the attention of people through moving electric lights.

    Movement by itself is able to direct our attention. Anything that moves, even if it is very small and does not satisfy the first two conditions mentioned above, is able to draw our attention. You must have noticed infants attending not only to movements of big animals or objects, but also to a small ant or any tiny insect that moves. Thus movement is an important condition.

Internal Determinants of Attention

Internal factors or condition. How much and in what way a person will attend to a stimulus depend not only upon the characteristics of that stimulus or the favorable environmental conditions but also upon his interest, motives, basic needs and urges, etc. Every person likes to do or to attend to those objects or activities that fulfils one's own desires or motives and suits his own nature, interest and aptitude. Let us try to see the part played by these inner factors in securing attention of a person.

The conditions of attention as described so far are the external determinants of attention. They can also be called external laws of attention. The presence of these conditions in the environment is helpful for attention. Besides these, internal conditions are also helpful in drawing attention. These conditions are related with motives. As a matter of fact the influence of external conditions depends on these internal conditions to a very great extent. A hungry man will attend to the form and stimuli of food. A man with full belly will not attend to food, however nice at might be. In the advertisements those demonstrating the naked organs of the woman have the maximum power of attraction of attention. Those interested in cinema look to the advertisement of cinema helpful in attention. Hence only the most important will be enumerated here:

1. Interest—Innate and acquired interest draw individuals attention to a particular object. Doctors, engineers, professors, all attend to the objects of their own interest. Even among the professors an object attracting the attention of a professor of Geology, need not attract the attention of a professor of Philosophy as well. Thus the innumerable differences in interests create innumerable distinctions of attention in different men. The stimuli influencing innate tendencies attract more attention than those influencing acquired interest.

   Interest is a very helpful factor in securing attention. We attend to objects in which we are interested and we do not attend to those in which we have no interest. If we go to the market to buy a book, our attention will be captured more by bookshops than by cloth and shoes shops, etc. A boy interested in Hockey will be more attractive in watching hockey match than the football or the volleyball matches played at the same time on the adjacent grounds. A wise teacher is able to secure the attention of his students if he tries or make his lesson interesting by connecting it with their basic needs, drives and interests.
2. Basic drives—Basic drives and impulses of the individual are also important in drawing his attention. An animal attends to particular stimulus when driven by the basic drives of hunger, thirst, sex, etc. A normal man motivated by sex will naturally attend to the individuals of opposite sex. We all know it by experience that when hungry we may attend to even a distasteful food, but while our belly is full, we may not attend to even the most tasteful one. Among the motives fear has got definite influence upon attention. All men who fear snake will attend to all things resembling snake. Like fear, curiosity also influences attention. We attend to event the smallest details of the object towards which we have curiosity.

   The basic drives and urges of the individual are very important in securing his attention. Thirst, hunger, sex, curiosity, fear are some of the important motives that exercise definite influence upon attention. A hungry person is sure to notice the smell of cooking food. The man who fears snake will definitely attend to all things resembling the snake. Sex drive occupies a unique place among the different drives. Even the most inattentive student in the class can be made to sit on the edge of his chair if the teacher announces that he is going to talk about the sex-practices of American Hippies. Nowadays in the world of advertisement sex is the drive that has been extremely exploited. We can see the shapely girls in bathing suits to sell such unrelated items as tyres, nut bolts and tractors.

   Innate need also is very important in attention. Normally the sexual need in human beings can be easily evoked. Hunger, thirst, etc. are felt occasionally and the means to satisfy them are also readily available, but neither the sexual need is ever fully satisfied nor the means of satisfying it are available to all persons all the times. Hence most of the advertisements draw attention by stimulating the sexual need in human beings.
3. Mental set—Mental set means the tendency or bent of the whole mind. A man will attend to those objects towards which his mind is set. In the days of examinations, the mental set of students is generally towards the examination and hence even the smallest thing concerning it will attract their attention.

   Mental set besides our interests and motives the mental set is important factor securing attentions. Mental set means the tendency or bent of the whole mind. A person always attends to those objects towards which his mind has set. A person waiting for the letter of his beloved can recognize her envelope among a huge lot of the envelopes. Similarly on the day of examination the slightest thing concerning the examination easily attracts the attention of the students. All this happens because persons concerned possess a definite bent of mind and consequently their attention is immediately directed towards the related objects.

4. Aim—Every man has some immediate and some ultimate aims, e.g. the immediate aim of a student is to pass the examination while his ultimate aim may be to get a job to earn living or anythingelse. The student whose aim is not to pass the examination will not be concerned with textbooks or notes, etc. but one who has the aim to pass the examination will at once attend to them.
5. Meaning—In comparison with meaningless things, meaningful things attract more attention. A man will not attend to a thing which has no meaning for him. One does not like to hear meaningless talk. If some persons are talking in Tamil, the Punjabi will not like to hear it since for him it has no meaning.
6. Habit—Habit is also an important determinant of attention. If a man is habituated to rising early and winding his clock early in the morning, he must attend to the clock as soon as he gets up. It has been rightly pointed out that man learns as to which object he should attend and which he should not and thus develops habits of attending and not attending to things. Thus habit two aspects in relation to attention. On the one hand men develop habits of attending to necessary and desirable things and on the other they develop the habits of not attending to unnecessary and undesirable things. Both these kinds of habits help man in following his daily routine.
7. Disposition and temperament—Both disposition and temperament are important internal and determinants of attention, e.g. a man having a religious disposition and spiritual temperament will attend to religious matters, while another person having a sexual disposition and criminal temperament will attend to matters concerning sex or crimes, etc.
8. Past experience—Past experience also affects attention. If we know by our past experience that a particular person is sincere to us, we shall pay attention to whatever he advises us. If our experience is contrary, we shall not attend even to his most serious advice.
9. Emotion—A mother seldom finds faults with her child. The lovers find the whole world singing and dancing and immersed in romance. It is a matter of everyday experience that we attend to even the smallest fault of a person whom we hate while we do not attend even to the greatest blunder of a person whom we love.
10. Social motives—Social motives are important determinants of attention. In advertisements the human figures attract more attention than figures of animals and things. News about altruism, bravery and saving other's life by putting onesell in danger attract our attention because we praise these qualities. Men attend to things concerning their duties for social motives.

Besides the conditions described above, many other factors influence attention. Heredity, education and training have a wide influence on attention. The family, school, club, class and society of which an individual is a member, do have some influence on his attention. The physical condition, desire, purpose of the person concerned also affect his attention. Thus all the factors influencing the personality of a man affect his attention as well. As a matter of fact it is difficult to describe all direct and indirect determinants of attention. The description given here, however, includes the most important of such factors.

Distraction

Distraction means the dividing of attention or some interference in attention. For example, when one is studying, the sound of a song or noise breaks in upon attention. The object which causes the distraction is called the distractor. In fact, broken attention is not the absence of attention because the distractor is associated with the activity, often though not always, and it no longer interferes with the activity.

When we are attending to an object to activity, there are things in the external environmental as well as inside ourselves that try to turn our attention away from that object or activity. These things are called distracters which interfere with our attention. Distraction, as a psychological term, has been defined HR Bhatia in the following way:

"Distraction may be defined as any stimulus whose presence interferes with the process of attention or draws away attention from the object to which we wish to attend."

The sources of distraction can be roughly divided into two parts—external and internal factors. Among the external or environmental factors the more common and prominent are noise, music, inadequate lightning, uncomfortable seats, unfavorable temperature, inadequate ventilation, defective methods of teaching, improper use of teaching aids, defective voice of the teacher and his improper behavior, etc. These sources of distraction are very much varied. They affect the individual according to his own mental set and personality characteristics. The conditions which cause distractions to an individual may prove helpful is sustaining attention to others.

Therefore, the common notion that the external unusual environmental conditions always hinder the progress of the work is misleading. People are found working better in a noisy environment. Many of us can concentrate better on the studies while radio is playing. Actually speaking, the source of distraction lies more commonly in the individual himself than in outside environmental conditions. Internal distractions such as emotional disturbances, ill-health, boredom, lack of motivation, feeling of fatigue or interesting thoughts unrelated to the matter in hand have more effect that the everyday external distracters. If one is keeping a normal health and does not suffer from unusual mental worries and emotional disturbances, then no power on earth can distract his attention in case he has determined with a strong will to proceed on his course. Most of us are in the habit of offering lame causes in the name of outside distraction, for our willingness and lack of determination. A teacher, from the very beginning, should realize the particular characteristic of his pupils, by all means, try to cultivate favorable mental attitude towards the subjects and activities.

But from this discussion, it should not be realized that external factors of distraction have little significance and should not be fared at all. Under the presence of external distraction, the individual has to struggle hard for overcoming it. He puts in greater energy to keep the object before his mind. Surely and certainly, there should not be such misutilization of energy which otherwise can be saved for achieving higher aims. Therefore great care should be taken to remove the environmental causes of distraction. The students should be provided with adequate rooms to sit in with proper ventilation, light and seating arrangement. The school building should be situated in a calm and quiet place. There must be a well-organized time table so that there may be no interference of different classes, sections, activities or teachers in each other's day-to-day work.

As far as the teaching facilities are concerned the school should be equipped with devoted, enthusiastic and expert teachers, an efficient headmaster and adequate aid material, playground, library, laboratory and recreational facilities. Students should be taught with modern progressive methods. They should get opportunity for self-education and self-expression. The teacher should inspire them for achieving higher aims and look after carefully about their physical, emotional and mental health. The essence is that children should be helped firstly in getting rid of the factors causing distraction; secondly, they should be helped in cultivating proper habits of paying attention and sustaining it for the required period in order to achieve success in the work in hand.

Thus, the notion that distraction invariably hinders work is misleading, it being seen, for example, that the laborer produces more when there is music. Some laborers, men and women, sing at work in view of this fact. Not a few people do their reading and writing while radio is playing. Some people work better in a noisy environment than in a peaceful one. Experiments conducted by Morgan indicated that at first distraction caused a drop in the speed of typewriting but constant pursuit of the work in the disturbed condition increased this speed, and it again dropped when the distraction was removed. But distraction, in some experiments by Weber, caused harm. Though it cannot be definitely said that distraction increases the speed of the work, it is possible, to say with some degree of confidence, that a decrease in speed due to distraction is not inevitable. Actually the effect of a distraction on some work depends in no small measure upon the capacity, interest, practice, skill and mental set of the worker. If the distraction is favorable the speed will be increased but if it is unsuitable the speed will drop.

Distraction can be divided into two forms:

1. Continuous distraction—As the name suggests, it is the continuous distraction of attention. Some examples of it are the sound of radio or gramophone played continuously the noise of the market place, etc. Experiments have led to the conclusion that adjustment to continuous distraction takes place quickly.
2. Discontinuous distraction—This type is irregular, being interspersed with intervals, e.g. the hearing of somebody's voice every now and then. It interferes with work because of the impossibility of adjustment.

Some major means of removing distraction are:

1. Being active in work—Work in distraction sometimes calls for more energy, so that one way of adjusting to it, or removing it, is to become more active in work.
2. Disregard of distraction—The presence of a distracting factor while a man works is no extraordinary condition, and so, the best way to remove this element is to disregard it. The distraction is effective only when attention is directed to it, so that in attention, even to the most serious distraction will keep the activity from being interfered within any way.
3. Making the distraction a part of the work—Distraction causes an obstacle only when it is distinct from or opposed to the activity since attention can be focused just on one subject at one time. Therefore another method of making a distraction ineffective is to make it a part of the work. Some people work better when listening to a song because they make it a part of their work. But it is very difficult to make an uninteresting and contradictory distraction a part of the work because in this the interests, nature and capacities of the person are involved.

Need of Attention for Nurses

The functions in the job of nursing involve a keen perception and total attention. In his routine services concerning the patient the Nurse has to keep record of his temperature and other physical symptoms, his progress and retardation and report it to the Doctor. If she is not a keen observer she will not be able to note some very critical or important symptoms with the result that sometimes the patient may die premature. Her job involves a total attention on the immediate task such a giving injection to the patient or attending his other needs. All types of distractions, false perceptions, illusions, and hallucinations should not scrupulously avoided by her. She should follow all the instructions given by the physician concerning the patient and keep watch on everything about him. Thus it is clear that a knowledge of the psychology of observation, sense perception and attention is necessary for every Nurse. This knowledge will enable her not only to keep her attention tied to her job but also to avoid distractions and false perceptions. She can use her knowledge concerning the sense organs for her sense training so that her eyes and ears may be trained for observations concerning her functions. She can use the psychology of attention for invoking not only voluntary but also involuntary attention to her job.

It is helpful that can the used one of the model for the assessing the attention in patients with neurological problems, i.e. brain damages client after coma as follows:

- Focused attention: Refers to the ability to respond discretely to specific visual, auditory, or tactile stimuli.
- Sustained attention: Refers to the ability to maintain a consistent behavioral response during continuous and repetitive activity.
- Selective attention: Refers to the capacity to maintain a behavioral or cognitive set in the face of distracting or competing stimuli.
- Alternating attention: Refers to the capacity for mental flexibility that allows individuals to shift their focus of attention and move between tasks having different cognitive requirement.
- Divided attention: Refers to the ability to respond simultaneously to multiple tasks or multiple task demands.

So attention helps the nurse in following ways:

- Helps to bring mental alertness and preparedness. Which nurses records mentally alert and tries to exercise their mental power effectively in taking care of clients.
- Helps to increase concentration by focusing on consciousness
- Helps to better perceptual organization for maximum clarify and understanding of client condition and status
- Helps to provide strength and ability to perform tasks of cognitive functioning in their career.

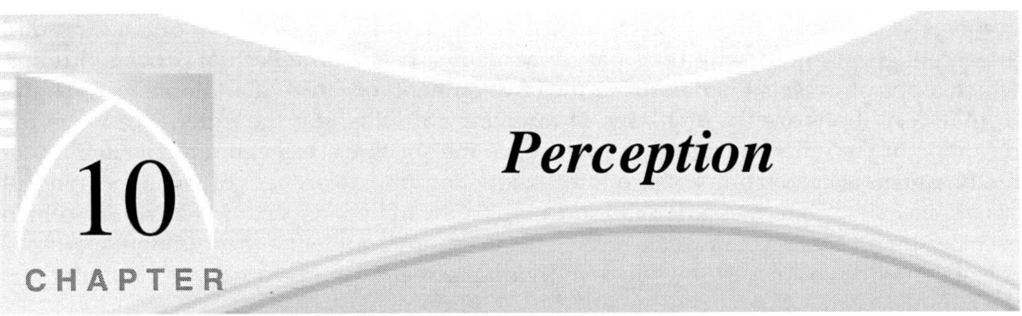

10 CHAPTER Perception

Introduction

The word 'perception' from the Latin 'perceipio' meaning 'receiving' collecting, action of taking possession, apprehension with the mind or senses. Perception is the process by which organisms interpret and organize sensations to produce a meaningful experience of the world perception in human beings describes the process whereby sensory stimulation is translated into organized experience. It is a complex process by which people select, organize, and interpret sensory stimulation into a meaningful picture of the world. As stated earlier it is concerned with the translation from the external physical world to the internal mental world, that each of us actually experiences.

Perception is the method by which people take all the sensations they experience at any given moment and interpret them in some meaningful fashion. Perception has some individually to it—no two people will perceive the world in exactly the same way. Two people might be looking at a cloud for example, and while one thinks it's shaped like a horse, the other thinks it's more like a cow. They both see the same cloud, but they perceive a different interpretation. As individual as perception might be, there are some rules for how people perceive the world around them. The following section discusses some of these basic principles.

Organism lives in an environment. It receives stimuli from the environment and reacts towards them. These responses can be internal as well as external, both of which are included in the term 'behavior'. This is the subject matter of psychology. As has been already explained, sensation is the first response of the organism to the environment. But sensation is never pure, it is always a part of perception. Hence in fact, the first response of the organism towards the environment is perception. It is here that all the activities of the organism begin. Thus, the knowledge of the processes and determinants of perception is important in the understanding of behavior.

Nature of Perception

Perception is the interpretation of the meanings of sensations. While seeing a rose, the various sensations of color, smell, touch, etc. are aroused. People are given to understand by these sensations that there is an object in front of them. They know from past experience that an object of this nature is a flower or a rose. Therefore, conclude that they are perceiving a rose. So perception in the selection, organization and interpretations of sensory input. It involves giving meaning to sensations. It is the activity of selecting, organizing and interpreting sensations with ones past experiences. It is an intellectual process through which a person selects the data from the environment, organize it and obtains meaning from it. Sensations are the first stage of receiving stimulus, it is the experience when the reception of the sense organs send impulses to the specific areas of brain. The activity of the organism is converting a sense impressions into the awareness of some meaningful situations called perception. It is an individuals awareness aspect of behavior in which each person processes the raw data receives from the environment into meaningful patterns. It is the intellectual process by which individual screens, selects, organizes and interpret the stimuli in order to give meaning to their environment.

Processes in Perception

Perception is a mental activity which acquaints us with the situation by giving us direct knowledge of it. The sensations are viewed as a whole, in perception. In it there is not just a perfunctory acquaintance with the object, there is a knowledge of it too. The sensation of color alone is not a sufficient proof of the identity of the object, and it is consequently, not possible to say on the basis of the color sensations that the pink object is a rose. The real meaning of the sensation is understood or revealed in perception. Only then as it known that the sensation originates from the rose. Accordingly, sensation precedes perception. When people speak of sensation they are thinking of stimuli and investigating the relationship of the individual experiences to various stimuli which reach his receptors; and when people speak of perception they are thinking of objects and are investigating how well the individuals experiences correspond with the objective facts". For example, when they see a certain object only some light sensations are actually experienced: e.g. when an individual see a ship at a distance, only some gray light sensations are experienced. Still he report that he see a ship. The various qualities and characteristics of a ship are not experienced through the senses at that moment. All these qualities are supplied by the mental process called 'perception', which depends on various factors. Whereas having a sensation is more a passive experience, perceiving something is an active process. Perception is a process by which the individual understands and establishes contact with the outside environment. The various factors which direct and determine this perpetual process under four heads: (i) Before perception can occur, there must be some sensation. In other words, the organism must have some sense organs with suitable mechanisms such as the nerve cells and receptor organs to record the stimuli that come from outside. This we have considered in the chapter dealing with the sense organs. (ii) The nervous system must be so structured that these outside stimuli yield various qualities such as different colors, different tones, etc. Unless we are able to differentiate these various kinds of qualities accurately, perception will not be possible. (iii) The influence of past experience: The few light sensations that come from a ship are interpreted as a ship because of our past experience with that particular object. Because of the past experience, we are able to supplement a number of characteristics that are not sensed at that particular moment. (iv) The set or mental attitude which the individual has at a given moment: for example, as an experimental measure, starve a few people for twelve hours and project on a screen certain irregular and vague shades. If the people are asked to report what they see, invariably the majority of them would say that they see some eatable objects, such as fruits or sweets. If these people are not hungry, they would have given completely different accounts.

Experiments of this type have been actually conducted and this principle has been sufficiently verified. When a person is angry, he perceives the mistakes of people around him more easily than when he is in a happy mood. When a person's attention is attracted towards a particular material, things relating to that material would be perceived more easily. Thus one's present set is an important factor in determining the activity of perceiving.

Perception being a complex process, reveals four processes, on analysis:

1. Receptor process—The first process in perception is the receptor process. The rose, by virtue of its presence, stimulates three different receptor cells thus activating three different receptor processes.
2. Unification process—This is the second step in the main process. For a perception of rose, a unification of the different sensations is necessary. Even if the flower were to be seen or rather experienced by the eye, a unification of all the sensations from the different parts of the flower is a must.
3. Symbolic process—This process is the next, the third process in perception. From our daily life, we know that most things have an experience attached to them. A rose reminds us of the friend who created in us the interest for roses. The flower symbolizes the friend. Thus, every time we perceive a rose, this symbolic process makes it much more than just a rose.
4. Affective process—This, too, is attached to perception, because a flower may also represent a happy memory of a friend or a feeling of sorrow at separation. Besides being pleasant or unpleasant, this process may also be indifferent.

The above detailed analysis of the processes of perception will make it clear that it is a complex process and not merely an aggregation of sensations. But even though it is a complex process involving many processes, its basic constituents are sensations and past experiences.

Characteristics of Perception

The main characteristics of perception are as follows:

1. Unity and continuity
2. Attention
3. Persistency with varied efforts
4. Free adaptation to varying conditions
5. Learning by experience
6. Reproduction in perception.

1. Unity and continuity—Perception is not possible if the sensation are scattered because they would, in that case, lack meaning. The perception of an orange includes the sensations of color, taste, smell, etc. which are unseparated. There is a unity and continuity in the sensations which enable us to perceive an orange.
2. Attention—Perception is the understanding of sensations. Thus the proximity of the sense organs and the object does not bring about perception, if there is no attention. You may not have noticed the building you pass by daily though it crossed your line of vision, because you never paid attention to it.
3. Persistency with varied efforts—The perceiver has to constantly change his efforts for complex perceptions. If, for example, a novel fruit, with which you are unfamiliar is placed upon your hand then you do not rest content with a mere glance at it but, rather,

you turn it over in your hand, smell it and, if it is innocuous, taste it. These changing perceptions have a unit and persistency.

4. Free adaptation to varying circumstances—In some cases of perception, the sensations are constantly changing. The wrestler keeps an eye on the trick of his opponent. In this perception, the sensations are changing behavior of his opponent.
5. Learning by experience—It is difficult to perceive an object with which one is totally unfamiliar. A person who has never seen a kite flying cannot make anything of the sensation of a path of color in the sky. Of course, if he once sees a kite, he will be able to recognize the sensation of color in the sky and identify it as a kite.
6. Recollection—The above example shows that there was recollection of past experiences concerning a kite and that the assimilation of present sensations and recollected past experience resulted in the perception of a kite. Recollection is thus, a characteristic as well as a sign of perception.

Factors Influencing Perception

Thus perception is an active process may be understood from the characteristic of this activity not only in selecting a particular stimulus at a particular time but also in the process of combining and grouping stimuli. This activity of combining and grouping enables us to perceive definite patterns or exact figures which have some meaning for us. This process of forming a pattern has been greatly emphasized as an important characteristics of the perceptual process by one school of Psychology called Gestalt School. One need not understand all the teachings of this school in order to appreciate this factor of grouping.

Perception is an active process, midway along a continuum from direct sensing to thinking, by which we organize and give meaning to the information we receive through our senses. Through perception we maintain the experience of a continuing, stable environment despite the constant changing of sensory stimuli. Perception is partly a process of filling in, enabling us to interpret a series of fragments as a whole when sensory data are incomplete. An illusion, or false perception, seems false only when we compare it with what we know to be true. Visual cliff experiments with infants indicate that there is some innate pattering of perception, although past learning usually plays a vital role.

Prof. Woodworth summarizes the various factors that go into the process of grouping or patterning under seven heads. He calls them the factors of advantage. We shall consider four of them here.

i. *Proximity or being near in space*. If there are some dots lying close together they will be seen together as one pattern. Dots that are separated in space may not be so easily included to form one group (Fig. 10.1).
ii. *Similarity*. Suppose there is a group of some dots and some other pattern say, small squares or triangles. If you just glance at such a picture, invariably you will perceive all the similar things, viz, all the dots as forming one group or one pattern. All the rectangles may similarly be seen together. Thus even if one rectangle and one dot are situated together, the factor of similarity may have a greater advantage over the factor of proximity.
iii. *Continuity*. Dots that lie along the same continuous line or if they are connected together by lines would be more readily seen as one group even though there. When the various factors of advantage are all present, there may be a sort of struggle and any one factor may supersede the other at a given moment.

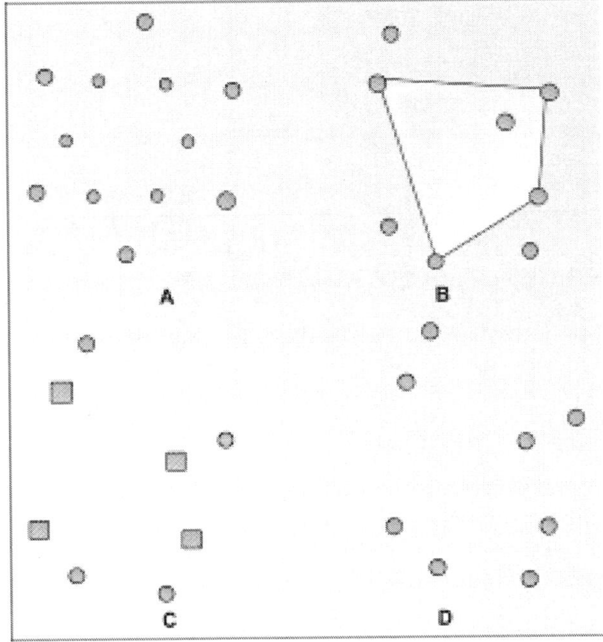

Fig. 10.1: The factors in grouping during the process of perception. (A) Inclusiveness (B) Continuity (C) Similarity (D) Proximity

iv. *Familiarity*. In some miscellaneous mass of dots or lines, the pattern of a familiar object or figure, say a circle, or a human figure will stand out more easily as one unit than others. In fact familiarity is a very strong factor of advantage.

Shifting of Perception (Fig. 10.2)

Another important characteristic of the perceptual process is that it often shifts from one aspect or one part of the stimuli to another. This shifting may be because of two principles which we have already considered.

i. When two or more factors of advantages mentioned above have equal strength, then something like a rivalry arises. For a few seconds, one grouping may be perceived, but soon another combination may get the better of the situation and push itself forward as it were. This makes the perceptual process to shift from one aspect to another. This is particularly noticeable in situations where an object is seen against a background but not where both the figure and the background have equal advantage for perception. This phenomenon is studied usually under the term 'figure and ground' under perception.
ii. While considering attention, we saw that attention shifts constantly because of fatigue and other reasons. Thus shifting of attention also results in shifting in perception.

In some other circumstances also, shifting of perception takes place particularly when we look at ambiguous or vague pictures, or even some type of geometrical designs. But all these can be brought under the two explanations given above.

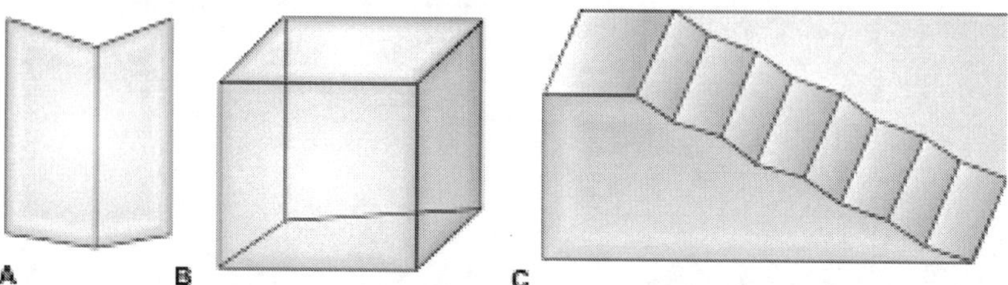

Fig. 10.2: Examples of the shifting of perception. (A) Looks like a book opened away from you and towards you. (B and C) Find out in how ways these two pictures appear

A number of factors operate to make us organize stimuli in a particular way. Some of these are characteristics of the stimulus object or situation—for example, the nearness of various elements to each other or their physical likeness, the inclusiveness of one perceptual pattern as opposed to another, the tendency to see a complete object (closure), and the context, or part whole relationships, of a situation. The way we perceive things—particularly in ambiguous situations—also depends upon such person factors as a tendency to create and maintain a stable structure, our particular past experience, our organic conditions, and our needs and values. Social and cultural factors encourage the development of others less likely. Zulus reared in round buildings, for example, are less subject to the trapezoidal illusion. Our deep rooted basic classifications of experience, which strongly influence perception, are also known as schemata. Success or failure may also affect perception. There is evidence of perceptual defense against stimuli with socially unacceptable connotations. Direct social suggestion can also influence what we see.

The accuracy of perception can only be inferred from an individuals report of what he has seen. Often perception is inaccurate, largely because of poor attention.

The senses interact, and stimulation in one sensory mode can change the perception in another. The tendency to have sensations in one sensory mode when another is stimulated is called synesthesia.

Psychologists have often considered the problem of perceiving space and time. The perception of space and time. The perception of space has been analyzed into various factors that help in giving us the idea of space. Some of these factors are the perception of movement, the perception of tactual stimuli on our body, perception of sounds of different intensity coming from different distances, factor of binocular perception mentioned earlier, the factors used by artists in painting landscapes, viz, by showing distant objects in smaller sizes and also by giving suitable color effects, etc. All these factors connected with our perceptual process help to give us an idea of space. But some psychologists have disagreed with this process of analysis and have pointed out that because of the very structure of the brain, the idea of space is directly given to all our perception and not inferred as a result of adding together several factors.

In the perception of depth and distance of objects in three dimensional space, we us cues provided by the stimulation of muscles in and around the eye (the principal cues to depth available for monocular vision), by the convergence of the eyes, and by retinal disparity. We also rely on cues from the stimulus pattern itself: distinctness, atmospheric perspective, linear perspective, texture, light and shadow, relative position, and known standards. In perceiving motion we use cues provided by the changing relationships between various objects and, in the case of radial motion, by the changes in the size of the retinal image.

When a sound comes from one side or the other, the sound waves stimulate the two ears differently and thus give us cues as to the direction of sound. We interpret the distance of sound by using cues of loudness and timber.

PERCEPTION OF TIME

Time perception is influenced by our sense of the sequence of events, our memory of the past, our feeling of how long it has been since a certain event occurred, and our orientation toward the future. Accuracy of time perception is affected by changes in body temperature, which affects rate of bodily activities. Accuracy increases with age, and subjective (felt) time is also influenced by motivation. Drugs may affect the apparent length of time.

How we learn to get an idea of time has been studied and investigated by many psychologist. Just like perception of space, perception of time also seems to be a complex process. It is not just a simple sensory perception. Obviously there is no one single sensation which is perceived as time. Various factors help us to get the experience of time. We all perceive change. Any perception of change naturally involves an experience of duration. We perceive movements of various objects. This also naturally gives us an idea of duration. We remember our experiences of the past, giving us the experience of something that has been; we also expect things to happen in the future which gives us an idea of 'not yet'. These experiences of 'has been' and 'not yet' naturally give us some idea of what we call time. Further, we experience the process of growth. We grow and we watch other people grow. There is an inner process of maturation and development going on in our organism. This developmental process will also be perceived against the concept of duration of time. Some psychologists have suggested that the human brain does not have to put together various experiences like these to get an idea of time, but that it is one of the functions of the brain to perceive time directly. They have suggested that the perception of space and movement are also similarly made possible by a direct action of the controversial points in the history of psychology. We need not go into the details of this controversy at present.

Reaction time, the speed with which we act in relation to a perceived situation, is measured by apparatus consisting of a stimulus key, a reaction key, and a device to check the accuracy of the timing mechanism, or chronoscope. In general, men have faster reaction times than women. Speed of reaction increases with age until about thirty, after which it decreases. Reaction time is influenced by the sense organs involved, the strength of the stimulus, the nature of the fore period, motivation to respond, the amount of practice we have had in responding, the complexity of the stimulus situation, and various special factors, such as body temperature or amount of radial or linear acceleration. In vigilance tasks the operator's accuracy soon falls far below his maximum but can be aided by brief rest period or by the presence of distracting stimuli (if the task is simple).

Experiments on sensory deprivation show that normal psychological functioning requires sensory stimulation. Low-level, ambiguous, or unstructured stimulation such as diffuse light produces more hallucination and is more difficult for subjects to endure than no stimulation at all. Hallucinations and perceptual distortions and past environment, as well as with the experimental setting. Recent research suggests that there is a need for dreaming, or at least for REM sleep, the kind of sleep during which dreaming occurs.

Research on extrasensory perception (ESP), which is said to comprise mental telepathy and clairvoyance, over a period of several decades has failed to produce clear-cut, universally accepted results. Most scientists do not regard ESP as a proved phenomenon.

ERRORS IN PERCEPTION

Psychology teaches us that we cannot always depend on our sense perception. This means that we cannot always believe our eyes or our ears. What we believe we see existing things in a distorted and mistaken form. Thus there are several possibilities of our perceptual process going wrong and misleading us. Such errors of perception are studied under two phenomena, viz, 'Illusions and Hallucinations'.

Illusions: An illusion is a wrong or mistaken perception. Here on individual get the sensory experience of a stimulus which has real existence. The perceptual process always involves an interpretation of the sensory experience in the light of our past experience, our present attitude and our organic needs. In some cases, this interpretation is done wrongly and so the stimulus is perceived wrongly. Such a phenomenon is called illusion. The classical example for this is our perception of a coil of rope as a snake in darkness. The stimulus is exactly like that coming from a snake and it is quite real and objective. Because of the similarity, we perceive the rope as a snake, guided mostly by our past experiences, our fear and the fact of darkness. Thus, when there is a well-defined and very similar stimulus, an error in its perception is called illusion. Psychologists have experimented with a number of geometrical designs to understand the phenomenon of illusion. Two of the well-known examples are the Muller-Lyer illusion and the horizontal vertical illusion (Figs 10.3 and 10.4). In this Muller-Lyer illusion there are two straight lines which are of equal length. One is bounded at the two ends by pairs of short lines opening outwards. The other is bounded by two pairs of short lines which are reversed and give the idea of closure. Though the two lines are equal in length invariably the latter is perceived to be shorter than the former. This of course is an illusion. In the horizontal vertical illusion there are two straight

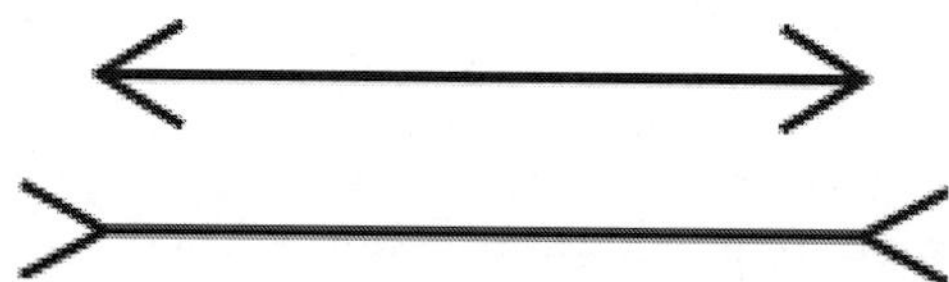

Fig. 10.3: Example of Muller-Lyer Illusion. Compare the length of the two lines

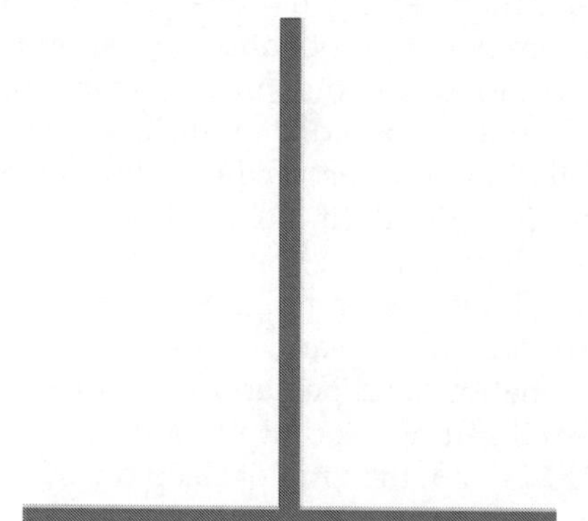

Fig. 10.4: Example of Horizontal—Vertical Illusion. Are these two lines equal?

lines—one horizontal and the other vertical. Both are of equal length. But invariably the horizontal line is perceived to be longer than the other.

The description of perception remains incomplete without the explanation of illusion. An illusion is a misinterpretation of the correct meaning of a perception. It is not a dream because the perceived object is present and it is not imagination because the object of perception is not a creation of the mind of the individual. An illusion is a wrong or false perception. A stick appears crooked when held partly under water. There is perception, of course, but not in keeping with the real form of the perceived object as it is falsified due to some reasons.

Hallucinations: Sometimes, people have another kind of experience which is different from that of having an illusion. They perceive a figure or an object purely because of our subjective conditions, when there is no stimulus at all. Such an error in perception which, has no basis in a real sensory stimulus is called 'Hallucination'. While illusion is wrong perception hallucination is false perception. If at night we see a ghost, when there is practically no stimulus in the form of a human figure or even anything resembling it, it will be an example of hallucination. But if some figure or even a scare-crow in the form of a human being is perceived as a ghost, then it will be an example of illusion. The phenomenon of hallucination raises a number of questions in psychology particularly in the field of abnormal psychology. Hallucination form a major symptom psychology in some of the psychological disorders. Such hallucination take place because of our inner fears and conflicts. Sometimes an intense wish or hope may also cause a hallucination. This is what happens in some cases of mirage. Hallucination is dissimilar to illusion. The vision of an oasis at a distance in a desert is a hallucination. Some people see a ghost in the dark. This is another example of a hallucination. Some people relate strange incidents of hallucination, e.g. a woman dressed in a white saree came at midnight and sat down on my bed and she massaged my feet, etc. These are examples of hallucinations.

Experiences like illusions and hallucinations naturally give us a caution. We have seen that even otherwise our perception depends to a large extent on factors like familiarity, our set or attitude, our inner needs, etc.

These needs point out that often actual sense experience may not be the determining factor. Realizing these possibilities of our perception being mostly determined by subjective conditions, one psychologist said 'We perceive things not as they are but as we are'. This statement is also true of many of our prejudicial ideas about other people. If we like a person for various other reasons, a particular action of his may appear to us to be very good, even though logically it may be just the other way. Similarly actions of people whom we dislike otherwise appear to be bad and blameworthy. It should be a mark of the student of psychology to be very careful in such matters, and develop a truly objective attitude which alone will lead him to truth.

There are the following distinctions between hallucinations and illusion:

1. In illusion, there is a distinct external stimulus, while in the case of hallucination the external stimulus is often absent, as it clear by the example of the white robed woman.
2. While illusion often happens to very ordinary people, hallucination befalls the lot of mentally afflicted, tired or intoxicated people.
3. In illusion the stimulation is usually external while the stimulations in hallucination are in the person himself, which makes the later a kind of subjective perception.

4. The perception of the same situation is identical to every person in the case of illusion. The stick in water appears bent to every observer. The illusion is, thus, a primitive organization. On the other hand, in a particular condition different people have different types of hallucinations due to diversified intoxications. Some people see ghosts, other snakes while still other people see giants with swords when in an uncommonly intoxicated condition.

THE VALUE OF PAST EXPERIENCES IN PERCEPTION

Sensation is not the only constituent of perception, it is caused by recognition based on past experiences. The perception of rose is a recognition of it, as such, by the perceiver. In this way, perception is an assimilation of recognition and sensation. Perception is the understanding of the sensory signs. This account should not create the impression that these processes of sensation and recognition take place step by step. In fact all the processes take place so much as a whole that there is no knowledge of these. It is sensed that the perception takes place immediately the flower enters the line of vision. As Ward very aptly and truthfully says—"Pure sensation is a psychological myth". Even the presence of sensation is known only upon an analysis of the perception. The understanding of sensation in perception does not depend exclusively upon past experience, muscular sensations and unconscious traces, all play an important part in the process.

PERCEPTION AND SENSATION

The distinction between sensation and perception is similar to the one between a whole and its part. Neither of the two is possible without the other. Sensations are the constituents and raw materials of perceptions. The perception of the external world depends upon the sensation of color, form, sound, taste, smell, heat, cold, density, amplitude, etc. Just as the whole cannot exist without its parts, in the same way perception is not possible in the absence of sensations. For example, the perception of rose involves the experience of the sensations of color, smell, touch, etc. To put the same more scientifically, the analysis of the perception of rose yields these sensations. Perception is a presentative process.

The second differences between sensation and perception is that while the former is a rudimentary and simple experience, the later includes a memory of past experiences too. For this reason perception has been termed a 'Presentative-representative process'. Sensation is the first or at least the first conscious response born of the stimuli. Perception is the second response to the sensation and only an indirect response to the physical stimulus. The order of events is stimulation, response of the specific sense organs and sensory nerve, first cortical response which is sensation, second cortical response which is perception. Using the old example, the sensory of rose first stimulates the specific sense organs. The sensory nerves convey this experience to areas of the cortex concerned. The third difference between the two is that sensation precedes perception.

ROLE OF PERCEPTION IN NURSING

There are a great many implications for nurse education in both clinical nursing and teaching. In clinical settings, students need to be taught about the factors that affect their perception of things, particularly the influence of 'top-down' processing, which might make them miss cues that patients might emit. Nurses need to recognize that patients perception may be altered by illness and must make the necessary allowance for this by giving more frequent explanations and reassurance, in case the patient may not have perceived the message.

Selective attention will operate in clinical areas where patients may be kept awake by jangling drug keys or the sound of a trolley. Some patients may become disoriented and so experience perceptual distortion, the nurse's role in this case is to reduce stimulation by maintaining a quite, dark environment.

In teaching, it is important to use methods that hold the attention of the student with, for example, bright visual aids and changes of activity at frequent intervals. The teacher should maintain his central position as 'figure' separate from the ground of background noise and distractions. He should teach for insight rather than always giving factual information, so that students experience penny-dropping when learning concepts.

Perception is essential to deal with the world around us as it influences our memory, thinking, reasoning, emotions and so on. The nurse needs to understand anything and interpret the whole environment and apply different perceptual skills to understand patients/clients. When caring for the sick, nurse needs to remember that the treatment of a part should not be attempted without treatment of the entity. For patients, hospital seem to be a grightening environment, since it is new and unfamiliar to them. Creates lot of anxieties, worries, etc. It may influence the thought, behavior and perceptual set of the patient. While perceiving patient promptly nurse can taking care of them properly by sharing the worries, fears, emotions of the sick person.

11 CHAPTER

Learning

Introduction

Cognition is the term given to those internal processes such as thinking, learning, problem solving, remembering and perceiving cognitive psychology is concerned with study of mental process involved in knowledge and can be defined as an approach to psychology defined by its commitment to modeling the internal process responsible for complex intelligence behavior.

Learning means modifying and changing one's behavior with reference to achieving a particular goal. Learning means establishing new relationship between a stimulus and a response. This would also include making a new neural connections. This is possible because of the existence of synapses. This means, that by learning individual are able to change the natural responses to certain stimuli made because of their innate structure.

Definitions

The term learning is one of those concepts whose meaning is crystal clear until one has to put it in actual words. Learning is when you learn something. Learning is learning how to do something. Learning is also a development of a method for dealing with problems. It is the development of a technique one learns how to deal with problem. The following are some definitions of learning which should make it clear:

1. In JP Guilford's opinion, We may define the term very broadly by saying that learning is any change in behavior, resulting from behavior. In this definition a distinction between change in behavior due to maturity and due to learning is not clear though both these activities occur simultaneously. In the words of Woodworth, typically at least learning consists in doing something new, provided this something new is retained by the individual and reappears in his later activities. So *Learning is change in behavior*.
2. According to Garrett, learning is that activity by virtue of which organize our responses with new habits. Thus the element of organization in learning is very much important. Guilford, too, maintains that learning involves organization of behavior. Thus in learning to ride a cycle we have to organize the activities of turning the pedal, balancing the handle, etc. in order to be reasonably safe with the vehicle. It is another matter that a person does not learn this organization at the outset and that he may take much longer time to learn to balance the handle than the time he may take to learn to turn the pedal.

But his learning of the activity of cycling will be complete only when he accomplishes this organization. So *Learning is an organization of behavior.*

3. RS Woodworth maintained that the learning of a new act is an addition to the person's store of experiences. Clarifying the statement further, Woodworth says that reinforcement, too, is an indispensable element in the act of learning because it helps forming only successful responses and weeding out the unsuccessful ones. To quote Woodworth, An activity may be called learning in so far as it develops the individual in any way, good or bad, and makes his environment and experiences different from what it would otherwise have been. So *Learning is the reinforcement of a new activity.*

The psychologists who stress external behavior consider learning to be a change of behavior while who lay emphasis on internal changes are convinced that learning is change in the perception of the individual. Combining these two views, Murphy writes, from this point of view it would be legitimate to regard learning as a modification both of behavior and of the way of perceiving. The following definition of learning given by Hilgard is an essence of all the foregoing definitions offered by other psychologists, Learning is the process by which an activity originates or is changed through reacting to an encountered situation, provided that the characteristics of the change in activity cannot be explained on the basis of native response tendencies, maturity or temporary status of the organism. Accordingly learning may be defined by different experts as given below:-

- Learning as a change in behavior resulting from repeated practice, where both the environment and the behavior interact to produce the learned change (**RS Woodworth**)
- Learning as a process by which the individual acquire various habits, knowledge and attitudes necessary to meet the demands of life in general (**Boaz 1984**).
- Learning as a process by which an activity originates or is changed through training procedures as is distinguished from changes by factors and attributable to training (**Hilgard**).
- A change in performance as a function of practice leading to a direction which satisfies the current motivating conditions of the individual (**McGoech**).
- Learning is that activity by virtue of which we organize our response with new habits (**Garrett**).
- Learning is defined as any relatively permanent change in behavior which occurs as a result of practice and experience (**Morgan and King 1978**).
- Learning is more or less permanent modification of an individuals activity in given situations, due to the practice in attempts to achieve some goal or solve some problem (**Bernhardt**).
- Learning is the process by which behavior is originated or change through practice or training (**Kingsley & Garry**).
- Learning is acquiring new activities or enhancing or improving the old activities (**Underwood**).

In above definitions of the term, Learning find that there is a common element, viz, effecting a change in one's response to a stimulus. If we observe this change closely, we would find that an attempt is always made to improve our relations with the environment. The changes are always made with reference to our relation with the environment. The learning is done so that we can react to the environment in more advantageous ways which would satisfy our needs. Taking this into consideration some psychologists prefer defining the term as effecting a change in behavior which produces an improvement in our relations to the environment.

A more useful definition is as that "learning is any relatively permanent change in behavior brought about by experience or practice". The "relatively permanent" part of the definition refers to the fact that when people learn anything, some part of their brain is physically changed to record what they have learned. This is actually a process of memory, for without the ability to remember what happens, people cannot learn anything. Although there is no conclusive proof as yet, research suggests strongly that once people learn something, it is always present somewhere in memory. They may be unable to "get" to it, but it's there. As for the part about experience or practice, think about the last time you did something that caused you a lot of pain. Are you going to do it again? Of course not. You don't want to experience that pain again, so you change your behavior to avoid the painful consequence. This is how children learn not to touch hot stoves. Of course, if a person does something that results in a very pleasurable consequence, that person is more likely to do that same thing again. This is another change in behavior. Think back of the prologue. Stephanie's experience with the doctor and the nurse changed her behavior from that of a friendly, outgoing infant to a frightened, screaming child whenever she saw anyone in a white coat coming near her.

It should be noted that not all change is accomplished through learning. Any kind of change in the way an organism behaves is learning. Changes like an increase in height or the size of the brain are another kind of change controlled by a genetic blueprint. This kind of change is called maturation, and it is not the same as learning. For example, children learn to walk when they do because their nervous systems, muscle strength, and sense of balance have reached the point where walking is possible for them—all factors controlled by maturation, not by how much practice those children have had in trying to walk. No amount of experience or practice will help that child walk before maturation makes it possible—in spite of what some eager parents might wish.

Learning is a permanent change in behavior that occurs as a result of practical experience. It is central to all our behavior as individual learn to speak, write, think and perceive. Individuals attitudes and emotional expressions also learned behavior. Learning brings change in behavior, that change takes place through practice or experience and not due to maturation. The change in behavior should be relatively permanent lasting for years, months and weeks.

Domain of Learning

Learning has following domains:

- ***Verbal learning:*** It helps to acquire verbal behavior resulting in speaking language and use of communication devices. Signs, pictures symbols, words, figures, sounds, voices, etc. are used by the individual. Motor learning: It includes learning motor skills such as walking, dancing, typing, swimming, etc. Acquiring various skills through such learning helps in speed and accuracy to perform the task with great ease and satisfaction.
- ***Affective learning:*** It deals with emotional learning such as learning of habits, interest attitudes, appreciation, etc. Acceptance and rejection are involved in emotion. The end products of this learning, i.e. attitudes, values and ideals determine the character of our motive power.
- ***Cognitive learning:*** In learning ideas, the learner acquires knowledge and information through which he forms concepts, sees relationships, and arrives at generalization. It includes learning of concepts, principles, problem solving, etc. Serial learning: When the learner is presented with type of learning that exhibits some sequential or serial

order. For example, children are expected to master lists of materials such as alphabet, multiplication tables, names of presidents in order or serial.

- ***Skill learning:*** It is carried out in conative or psychomotor domain. A skill is refined pattern of movement or performance based upon and integrated with perceived demands of the situation. The student nurse can learn the manner in which the movements are carried out, either by:
  - Listening to directions and explanations
  - Reading a description
  - Seeing a demonstration
  - Paying attention.

The practice is equally important that depends on attitude and will of the learner and eradication of mistakes.

Tennant's ASK

Tennant (1995) categorized learning as: ASK the acronym is as follow:

A represents "attitude" also known as affective learning. An example of this type of learning is a shift in attitude toward the academic abilities of students with disabilities.

S represents "skills" often called psychomotor or mutual learning. Learning to operate adaptive technology is an example of the development of skills. Practical skills are required in nursing.

K represents "knowledge". Cognitive learning is the formal term used for mental skills such as recall of information. An example of knowledge is information on available resources related to disability issues.

Modes of Learning

The principal modes of learning are: learning through imitation, learning through conditioned response, learning through trial and error and learning through insight. All these four forms are equally utilized by animals as well as human beings.

I. IMITATION

Learning through imitation is one of the most important forms of learning. The human child learns mostly through imitation. It is a common place observation that children imitate the behavior, habits, manners and ways of adults. In imitation the learner exactly copies the behavior of another person without understanding or thinking. Whenever this copying is observed, it is said that one has learned through imitation.

The main characteristics of learning through imitation are as follows:

1. The interior never does it before imitation, but performs the activity only after seeing it in another.
2. The imitator does not know earlier the activity to be imitated.
3. In imitation the learner exactly copies the activity performed before him.

In many of the experiments on animal learning, it was exactly seen that animals learn by imitation. In an experiment a particular instrument was used to observe imitation in monkeys. In this instrument there were two cages in which there were puzzle boxes placed in exactly the same positions. A monkey was put in each cage. The monkey who had not to imitate, was taught to open the puzzle box. The monkey who had to imitate was the other monkey opening the puzzle box which was also in its own cage. After seeing the act of opening the puzzle box, the imitator was given a chance to perform it, on his own puzzle box. If it does not do successfully within a minute, the experiment is held as unsuccessful. Now the monkey is given a new type of puzzle box, less complex that the older one and the same processes are repeated again. In such experiments it was found that out of 15 monkeys, one monkey could imitate the solution of 23 problems out of 24. Animals lower than the species of monkeys, e.g. dogs, cats, etc. do not show as much capacity for imitation.

Among the living beings man is the best imitator. In human learning, especially that of the human child, imitation has an important place. In an experiment, 42 children of 1st standard were selected. Two boxes were placed on two chairs in a room as shown in the figure given on next page. There was a bit of candy in one of the boxes. A place was fixed to start with. The leader of the boys was told which box was to be opened. As he opened the box, he found a piece of candy. Then another boy was asked to open either of the boxes. If this boy imitated the leader, he got the piece of candy. If he did not imitate he go no reward. In every experiment both boys were made to stand on the start. In the first experiment they were told that here are two boxes. There is a piece of candy in a box. You have to find the piece of candy. He will get first chance then you will get chance. If you could get it in the first chance, you will get another chance. The leader was always given first chance. The piece of candy was not always kept in the same box. 20 percent of the boys imitated in the first chance. The rest 80 percent boys did not imitate. These boys might have reasoned that because the leader has already taken out the piece of candy from the box, so it could not be there. On an average, in one out of 3 experiments every second boy imitated the first boy. When the situation was changed and four boxes were placed in the four corners of an imagined square, 75 percent of the children imitated. This shows that the tendency of imitation learned in the first situation was generalized or transferred into an individual direction. In other experiments the children were rewarded for not imitating the leader. This tendency of not imitating the leader was cent-percent transferred to new situation. It is important to note in this experiment that the children were asked to imitate an activity, which they could easily do, e.g. all of them could reach the box, open it and take out things from it. In the complex activities this point is even more important.

The process of imitation is very important in learning. The teachers make a wide use of this fact. Education becomes easier and more perfect by demonstration. In the teaching of dance, music, etc. demonstration is very important since imitation has an important role in them. The efficient teachers generally demonstrate whenever it is possible and encourage the students to learn by imitation. It is a well known fact that the students often imitate the manners, ways, methods and habits, etc. of the teachers. Thus by presenting good ideals himself, the teacher can easily create the same among the students.

II. CONDITIONED RESPONSE

The concept of conditioned reflex as proposed by Pavlov. Using this concept some people have attempted to explain all learning process as conditioned responses. According to them learning is nothing but making a new response to a particular stimulus. This learning of the new response is explained on the principle of conditioning. In the case of learning simple or complex motor activities and skills this explanation may work very well. But it will be stretching the point beyond its limits if we attempt to explain all our ideational learning such as learning the theory of relativity in physics as a process of conditioning. Those who explained all learning as the result of the conditioning process belong to the group of Thorndike. They do not believe in the possibility of insight playing any role in learning.

Conditioned response or conditioned reflex is one of the important processes of learning. It was Pavlov, the famous Russian physiologist who for the first time experimented upon the conditioned response in 1900. Pavlov operated upon a dog and removed its salivary system from the check in such a way so that the saliva could be gathered in a test tube and measured. The dog was made to stand before a window. In the experiment the food was given to the dog through the window. Before giving the food the bell used to be rung. As soon as the bell was rung, saliva began to flow from the glands of the dog, because the bell was taken as a sign of food. As the bell is not the natural object for the response of the flow of saliva so the response is a conditioned one. The saliva was collected in a glass pot which was graduated. As the saliva fell in the pot there was pressure due to which the lever was pressed. Due to pressure on the lever, the lines were drawn on the smoked screen. By these lines the experimenter could find out the number of the drops of saliva and regularity of its flow. From this experiment, Pavlov came to the conclusion that the response of the dog can be conditioned to a stimulus other than the natural one. In this form of learning the individual or animal learn to behave toward an object other than the natural one, because of its connection with it. Behaviorists claimed that all learning is conditioning.

Theory of Conditioned Reflexes

a. Classical/conditioning

Classical (also called respondent) conditioning results from the repeated pairing of a neural (conditioned) stimulus with one that evokes a response (unconditioned stimulus) such that the neutral stimulus eventually comes to evoke the response. In other words, a reflexive or automatic response transfers from one stimulus to another. For instance, a person who has had painful experiences at the dentist's office may become fearful at just the sight of the dentist's office building.

The Russian physiologist and Noble Prize winner *Ivan Petrovich Pavlov (1849-1936),* observed in his work on gastric secretion that a dog salivated not only, when food was placed in its mouth but also at the sound of footsteps of the person coming to feed it, even though the dog could not see or smell the food Pavlov analyzed these events and called the saliva flow that occurred with the sound of footsteps—a Conditioned Response (CR), a response produced under certain conditions by a particular stimulus.

Before conditioning

Food (UCS) → Salivation (UCR)

Bell (CS) with food (UCS) → Salivation (UCR)

After conditioning

Bell (CS) → Salivation (CR)

Because the food naturally produces salivation, it is referred to as an Unconditioned Stimulus (UCS). Salivation, a response that is reliably elicited by food (UCS). The bell, which was originally unable to evoke salivation but came to do so when paired with food, is referred to as a conditioned stimulus (CS). Classical conditioning is most often applied to responses mediated by the automatic nervous system.

The principles of classical conditioning are as follows:

- *Acquisition:* It is initial learning of the conditioned response, e.g. the dog learning to salivate at the sound of the bell. The factors that affect the speed of conditioning during this phase are order and timing of the stimuli. If delay, conditioning seldom occurs.
- *Extinction:* Once learned, a conditioned response is not necessarily permanent. This term is used to describe the elimination of the conditioned response by repeatedly presenting the conditioned stimulus without the unconditioned stimulus.
- *Generalization:* After an animal has learned a conditioned response to one stimulus, it may also respond to similar stimuli without further training. If a child is bitten by a large black dog, the child may fear not only that dog, but other large dogs.
- *Discrimination:* The opposite of generalization is discrimination in which an individual learns to produce a conditioned response to one stimulus that is similar, e.g. a child may show a fear response to freely roaming dogs, but may show no fear when a dog is on a leash or confined to a pen.

This view was not admitted by the modern psychologists since the other methods were found to be equally important in learning, e.g. the method of trial and error, the method of insight, the method of imitation, etc. Yet no one denies the importance of the conditioned response in learning in animals as well as among human beings.

The factors determining conditioned response are as given below:

- *The effect of the motives*—Motive has an important effect on the conditioned response. For the conditioning of the response, the stimulus must have the capacity to evoke the response. In Pavlov's experiment the dog was hungry; hence the associated the bell with the food and responded to it.
- *Time relation of the two stimuli*—The time relation between the two stimuli is important since conditioning of response depends upon their being associated with each other. It is necessary that before the response subsides the new stimulus must be perceived along with its natural sequence, that is to say, that first there should be new stimulus and then the old one. In Pavlov's experiment it was necessary to ring the bell before giving the food and the food must be given after ringing the bell, before the response had subsided. If there is too much interval or lapse of time between the two stimuli, it shall be difficult for the animal to find out the relation between the two. Suppose a dog is given food after an hour of ringing the bell, it will not find out any relation between the two stimuli. The learner links only those stimuli which are closely related in time.
- *Repetition of the stimuli*—In Pavlov's experiment the dog was given food after the bell was rung several times. If the dog is given food always after ringing the bell, the saliva begins to flow from the mouth as soon as the bell is rung. This repetition of the stimuli is necessary in the beginning.
- *Absence of the disturbing stimulus*—As the disturbing stimulus increases, conditioning will become difficult. In Pavlov's experiment the room used was without windows and sound-proof. If there is some other stimulus in between the two stimuli, the conditioning will be difficult because the learner will not be able to link the two.

As a general rule the higher the species of the animal, the more easily conditioning of response is achieved. Thus conditioning should be the easiest in the case of human beings. But man is a complex animal and hence the factors which distract his attention are larger in number than in the case of other animals. However, in spite of these distracting elements in conditioning of responses it certainly remains one of the most important methods of learning, especially in the case of children. In childhood many of the responses of the child are conditioned to particular objects and even when the individual becomes an adult, his conditioned response continues, e.g. if a man behaves wrongly with us, we develop a kind of fear, abhorrence or hatred with every person resembling him.

Applications of Classical Conditioning

Classical conditioning, is a basic form of learning that pervades many aspects of daily life. Fear and anxiety are examples of conditioned reflexes and it is easy to work out other the process as it affects any aspect of education. For example, a student nurse may fear examinations because in the past she has been humiliated by her school teachers when her performance has been poor, thus setting up a conditioned fear of examinations. Even though such an experience may have been long ago, the student may still find it is a very powerful learned emotion. It should be remembered, though, that conditioned reflexes occur for positive feeling as well as negative, and the learned associations between pleasurable events and feeling can serve to make students enjoy the experience of learning.

There are two main ways in which the nurse teacher can use classical conditioning with students. Firstly, the teacher may have to deal with a student who has learned a conditioned response to some aspect of education, such as participating in small-group discussion or leading a seminar. The technique that may be appropriate here is 'systematic desensitization', a commonly used technique for treating phobias such as fear of spiders or heights. The principle is that the subject should be taught relaxation to counter the effects of anxiety and then the particular stimulus that is causing the fear is presented in a hierarchy of contact. In our example, the student would first be taught relaxation and then go through the problem situation in a series of small steps, beginning with discussions with one or two other students only, gradually building up to a full group size.

The second way in which students may be helped by classical conditioning is by prevention of those negative conditioning situations in the first place. Hence, when a student nurse is first introduced to clinical setting, a concerted effort should be made to get her to associate the visit with such positive events as a warm welcome, a sense of *esprit de corps* and a general air of interest and helpfulness.

It should be remembered that classical conditioning is a very basic form of learning, which is confined to lower-order learning and quite unrepresentative or ordinary classroom learning in a school of nursing or college of nursing.

The principles of classical conditioning can be used in the following areas of animal and human learning.

- *Developing good habits:* Good habits like cleanliness, respect for elders, punctuality, etc.
- *Breaking of bad habits and elimination of conditioned fears:* All learning is acquired in the social environment, e.g. deconditioning anxiety and fear in maladjusted children.
- *Training of animals:* Animal trainers have been using for long without being much aware of underlying mechanism.
- *Developing attitude:* It helps to develop favorable attitude towards learning.
- *Use in psychotherapy:* To treat phobias and other unwanted behaviors, such as alcoholism and addiction.

As has been pointed out earlier, modern psychology does not admit the view that all learning is conditioning, but no psychologist denies that conditioned response is an important method of learning both in the case of animals as well as of human beings. A person can find hundreds of examples of conditioning of response in his daily life. In the case of the tamed animals the conditioning process is very much used to teach so many activities. The conditioning of response as it's established can also be extinguished. In the establishment of the conditioning the stimuli has to be repeated while in its extinction the stimuli is not repeated. Thus in the example of Pavlov's dog, if the dog's response has been conditioned by the ringing of the bell, it will be deconditioned if food is not served in spite of the ringing of the bell or food is served without ringing the bell. Similar examples of deconditioning process can be found in the case of human beings. Suppose a person is used to get out for a walk to bridge with a certain friend, he will always remember his friend when he is absent. The sight of the bridge will make him recall his friend, because the always used to come with him to bridge. Thus the bridge and the presence of his friend have been linked. Now if the friend is absent and returns after a long time and the man has to go alone for a walk, he will forget his friend gradually and the sight of the bridge will no more awake the memory of him. In this example, one finds deconditioning of a certain response to a particular stimulus. Just as a response can be deconditioned, it is also re-conditioned. Conditioning, deconditioning and reconditioning of the response are governed by the same fundamental principles.

b. Operant Conditioning

BF Skinner (1904-1990) developed a theory of learning and behavior known as operant conditioning. It involves increasing a behavior by following it with a reward, or decreasing a behavior by following it with punishment. For example, if a mother starts giving a boy his favorite snack everyday that he clean up his room, before long the boy may spend time each day cleaning his room in anticipation of the snack. The boy's room-cleaning behavior increases it is followed by a reward or reinforce. Unlike classical conditioning, in which the conditioned and unconditioned stimuli are presented regardless of what the learner does, operant conditioning requires action on the part of the learner. That boy in the example will not get his snack unless he first cleans up his room. The term operant conditioning refers to the fact that the learner must operate or perform a certain behavior, before receiving a reward or punishment.

BF Skinner has made an important contribution to the study of learning by his work on another form of conditioning called operant or instrumental conditioning. As we saw in the last section, classical conditioning has little relevance for the kinds of learning with which education is concerned. This is because the conditioned response can have no effect on the environment, which means the animal cannot control the events that occur. For example, the dog in Pavlov's experiments made a conditioned response of salivation, but this response in no way affected the speed of delivery of the food. Operant conditioning, on the other hand, by definition, operates on the environment and the learned behavior is instrumental in controlling events.

He placed a rat inside a glass box (skinner box) containing a lever and food tray. The animal was free to explore the box whenever the lever in the box was pressed, automatically a pellet of food was dropped on the tray. Pressing of lever was the response to be learned (the operant response) and the food was stimulus consequence (reinforcement).

Principles of operant conditioning includes the follows:

- *Reinforcement:* It refers to any process that strengthens a particular behavior—i.e. increases the chances that the behavior will occur again.

Positive reinforcers include material possessions, money, friendship, love, praise, attention and success in one's career. Negative reinforcement is a method of strengthening a behavior by following it with the removal (avoidance) or omission (escape) of an unpleasant stimulus.

- *Reinforcement schedule:* It is a rule that specifies the timing and frequency of reinforcers. In his early experiments, Skinner rewarded animals with food every time they made the desired response—a schedule known as continuous reinforcement. Skinner soon tried rewarding only some instances of the desired response and not others a schedule known as partial reinforcement. He found that animals should entirely different behavior patterns.
- *Punishment:* Whereas reinforcement strengthens behavior, punishment weakens it, reducing the chances that the behavior will occur again. Positive punishment involves reducing a behavior by delivering an unpleasant stimulus if the behavior occurs like parents spank, scold or shout at children for bad behavior, fine, imprison, etc. Negative punishment or omission involves reducing a behavior by removing a pleasant stimulus if the behavior occurs, e.g. parents take away various privileges due to bad behavior.
- *Shaping:* It is a reinforcement technique that is used to teach animals or people behaviors that they have never performed before, e.g. teacher begins by reinforcing a response the learner performs easily, and then gradually requires more and more difficult responses.
- *Extinction:* It is elimination of a learned behavior by discontinuing the reinforcer of that behavior. For instance, parents often reinforce temper tantrums in young children by giving them attention. If parents simply ignore the child's tantrums rather than reward them with attention, the number of tantrums should gradually decrease.
- *Generalization and Discrimination:* These occur much the same way as in classical conditioning. In generalization, people perform a behavior learned in one situation in other similar situations. For instance, a man who is rewarded with laughter when he tells certain jokes at a bar, may tell the same jokes at restaurants, parties or wedding receptions. Discrimination is learning that a behavior will be reinforced in one situation but not in another. For example, the man may learn that telling his jokes in church or at a serious business meeting will not make people laugh.

Applications of Operant Conditioning

Operant conditioning has practical importance in many areas of human life. That is behavior modification, for example:

- Parents can reinforce their children's appropriate behaviors and punish inappropriate ones. One must analyse how complex the desired behavior is
- Teachers reinforce good academic performance with small rewards of privileges
- Behavior therapists use the learning principles of operant conditioning to treat children or adults with behavior problems or psychological disorders.

Usually the stimulus- response or behaviorist theories of learning can be applied to nurse education in a number of ways.

Reinforcement is a fundamental principle and can be used as feedback on learner performance. Knowledge of success is said to act as a reinforce of behavior, so it is important to give immediate feedback on performance, in both clinical and theoretical situations. The use of praise is also reinforcing.

Since it acts as a reward, but it is important to vary the type of reinforcement given, so that the behavior is maintained. This is more difficult that it sounds, for the teacher may appear insincere if he thinks too much about the way he is responding, for example smiling, nodding, and praising and the like.

We saw earlier that the variable-ratio type of reinforcement produces the highest rates of responding, so this is the schedule that should be most effective. When learning a new response, the learner should be given reinforcement at frequent intervals and as performance improves, it is reinforced less frequently, so that eventually only really good performance are reinforced.

A fixed-interval schedule of reinforcement can be effective when it is given following such things as a weekly test in the school, or feedback during the daily ward report.

Behavior modification is a well-tried technique in clinical psychology, where selective reinforcement is used to shape acceptable behaviors in patients with mental handicap. It has been suggested that teachers may use it in class to encourage acceptable behaviors and to discourage negative ones. If the nurse teacher wishes to shape a student nurse to answer questions in class, he may praise her each time she answers a question, regardless of whether or not it is correct. Gradually the teacher will begin to praise the student only when she gets the answer correct.

Extinction can be applied to unwanted behavior such as dominating a lesson or discussion, or coming into class late. If the teacher ignores these behaviors, they may undergo extinction, rather than being reinforced by having attention drawn to them. The concept of programmed learning is outline; this notion was Skinner's and it was an attempt to apply the theories of shaping of behavior to the process of education. Skinner devised the linear type of program, in which material is presented in an orderly, logical succession of small steps. Each step requires the learner to make a response and if this is correct, she is said to receive reinforcement from providing such a response. Linear programs can be obtained in book form, or in a roll that can be inserted into a teaching machine. In the latter type, the learner presses a button to indicate her response and the program moves on automatically. As indicated earlier, there is evidence to suggest that reinforcement is not necessary in order for learning to take place and it may be that programmed instruction is successful because the objectives are carefully devised and the sequence logical.

III. TRIAL AND ERROR

One of the most important methods in learning is known as trial and error. It was Thorndike who for the first time declared that all learning is trial and error. Thorndike was interested in finding out how the animals learn. He placed a hungry cat in a puzzle cage and put some food outside the cage. The cat was hungry and so she tried to come out of the cage. There was a particular device to come out of the cage. As the cat did not know the device, so she tried haphazardly, sometimes striking here and sometimes there. Thus trying for a period of time she somehow pressed the button and came out the cage. She was put in the cage again, she tried several times to come out of it and finally came out by pressing the button. When this was repeated several times, the cat learned to come out of the cage by pressing the button. In the experiment, Thorndike found that the cat learnt the trick to open the cage by trial and error. Thorndike experimented on many other animals also and concluded that all learning is trial and error.

During our growth process, a good deal of motor activities and motor skills are learned. Perhaps this kind of motor learning is the simplest form of learning. On the other hand, there are also other forms of learning called 'ideational or conceptual learning'. Motor learning is mostly effected through the method of trial and error. Take swimming for example. Many wrong and movements and strokes are tried and discarded one by one till after some months of practice correct movements are established. Throughout this period, the trial and error process has been going on. The discarding of the wrong movements and establishment of the correct ones are done according to certain laws.

Law of effect: The most important law is known as the 'Law of effect'. If the activity gives us the satisfaction of success, then that activity is fixed in and established. On the other hand, when a particular movement does not yield the desired result, a feeling of disappointment and dissatisfaction helps towards discarding that particular movement. In other words, it is governed by the effect that such a movement produces. That is why this law is called 'the law of effect'.

Law of frequency: When any activity is repeated a certain number of times, there is a tendency for the same to be permanently established. This is called "the Law of frequency". Anything repeated gathers a certain amount of strength in its favor, by which it would be easier to repeat it again. Again, the time factor also plays an important part.

Law of recency: An activity which has just recently been undertaken has an advantage of being repeated once again, for the simple reason that it is fresh in the experience of the organism. This principle is called 'the Law of recency'.

Thus these three laws of effect, frequency and recency govern the process of learning by the trial and error method. The question has often been raised whether all learning involves this trial and error method. Certainly animals learn mostly by this method of trial and error. Human beings also learn most of the simple motor skills by this method. But a good deal of learning is done by human beings using other methods as well involving an ideational planning, ideational foresight of the possible results of a particular activity, etc. This method is called 'The method of insightful learning'.

The chief characteristic of trial and error method of learning is the gradual decrease in the number of errors committed and the gradual decrease in the time taken to complete the task.

Thorndike's contribution to learning theory stems from this concept of reinforcement, in which he sees the reward acting as a positive reinforce for the association between stimulus and response. This is now seen as a form of conditioning, which was also independently by BF Skinner.

Trial and error theory of learning: This was first scientific study of learning by American Psychologist EL Thorndike (1874-1949), considered as the father of educational psychology, conducted series of experiments on animals learning and came out with conclusion that animals have no rational faculty in learning. They do not learn by reasoning but by trial and error. Animals go on hitting the target by impulse or learn out of "hit and miss", known as trial and error learning.

Experiment: A hungry cat was put inside a puzzle box. A piece of food (motivation) was kept outside the box at the little distance so that the cat cannot reach it unless she opens the door of the puzzle box. The cat had to press the lever by pulling the loop of the chord to open the door and to get the food. At first, the cat tried a number of ways, made lots of unnecessary movements to open the door. In this way, after trying several hit and miss random acts, making enough struggle accidently, the loop was pulled and the door opened. Finally, the animal reached its goal. After several trials like this, the cat learnt to go straight to the lever, press it, open the door and reach the food. Comparison of the time and unnecessary movements from the first to the last showed gradual decrease in time taken to reach the food. In this case, the cat learns through errors.

Edward L Thorndike (1874-1949) was also concerned with animal learning and in 1989 he formulated his law of effect. This was based on his work with cats in a 'puzzle box'. He confined a hungry cat in a puzzle box and placed food outside the box so that it was clearly visible to the animal. It was possible for the cat to escape from the box by clawing at a cord which released the door. Thorndike observed its behavior and in particular, the length of time taken to escape. Initially, the cat made various movements in an apparently random fashion, such as scratching at the door, until it succeeded by chance in escaping. It was allowed to eat the food and was then put back in the puzzle box and Thorndike observed that over a period of trials, the animal's movements became less and less random. It managed to open the door in a successively shorter time in each trial, until it eventually opened the door immediately it was placed inside. The *law of effect* states that behavior that results in success or reward is more likely to be repeated than behavior that does not. Thorndike explained the importance of what he termed the satisfier in reinforcing behavior. In the puzzle box, the cat was rewarded for the responses that led to escape, because those responses enabled it to obtain the food, whereas responses which did not lead to escape were gradually phased out. Thorndike also formulated another law, called the law of exercise, which states that knowledge of results must occur before the behavior can be reinforced.

Application of Trial and Error

The method of trial and error is used in the following circumstances:

1. The method is used when the learner is completely motivated and can see the goal clearly. If the cat is not hungry she will not to try to come out of the cage or leave the attempt after trying it without success for some time. The cat tries to come out of the cage simply because she is hungry and knows that there is food outside the cage. In the absence of the food outside the cage the cat will not try to come out of it. Thus it is clear that motivation as well as the presence of the goal is necessary for awakening the response of learning through trial and error.
2. The method of trial and error is used when perception alone or learned activities are not sufficient. If the cat could come out of the cage by merely moving in some direction, there was hardly any need of several trials and errors.
3. The method of trial and error is used when the learner fails to find the solution of the problem. In Thorndike experiment the cat trial and error method simply because she did not know how to come out of the cage. In the case of human beings in such situations, if the subject knows the solution of the problem, there is hardly any question of trial and error. It is only when he fails to find out the solution of the problem that he proceeds blindly, tries in various directions, commits errors, eliminates them and finally arrives at the successful response.

Thus the method of trial and error is widely used both by animals as well as by human beings. In the case of human beings, however, this process is somewhat different, because man has better powers of perception, understanding, intelligence and language, etc. Man uses the method of trial and error, but he also takes the help of language and other instruments in the process of learning. This method is used when:

- The learner is completely motivated and sees the goal clearly. As the rat is hungry (motive) and knows the food (goal) is there.
- When perception or learned activities are alone not sufficient.
- When learner fails to find the solution to the problem through perception, understanding, intelligence and language. Then, he proceeds blindly, tries in various directions, commits errors, eliminates them and finally arrives at the correct response.

IV. INSIGHT

Cognitive theories of learning: Cognitive learning theories focus on the role of understanding. Cognition implies understanding the connection between cause and effect, between action and the consequences of the action. The learner forms a cognitive and structure in memory which organizes information into relationships and meanings without any known reinforcement.

a. Insight theory of learning: It was developed by a group of Gestalt psychologists Kurt Koffka, Wolfgang Kohler and Max Wertheimer who concluded that the individual learns by his ability known as insight and not by blind trial and error. It explains that a person can deduce the solution by insight if he perceives the situations as a whole. The situation viewed as a whole will definitely look different from that viewed through its parts. Sum total of the parts may create a new situation in a complete form known as Gestalt. First, the stimulus is observed as a whole, then it is analyzed part by part that will produce an insight into the problem in an individual.

Insight is an important constituent in the solution of problems, and is found in the higher class of animals and human beings. It is the best method among the methods of learning.

According to Gestalt psychologists, a person can deduce the solution by insight if he perceives the situation as a whole. A German Gestaltist, Kohler, prepared some simple problems for experiments with dogs, hens, monkeys, and chimpanzees. In an experiment, a hungry animal was released from the house while some food was place behind the fence adjoining the wall. Both the dog and the hen trotted around in the vicinity of the wall but as soon as they found the way out they made their exit and reached the food. This perception of the change in the meaning of the wall is insight. Before the insight the wall was an insuperable obstacle, but after insight it was no longer an obstacle but an object necessitating circumvention. The result of insight is the understanding of new relations, the discovery of new patterns and the formation of new organizations.

Kohler's experiment: The most famous experiments conducted by Kohler in relation to insight were those that were carried out on chimpanzees. Some bananas were placed outside the cage of a chimp called Sultan, who was then given two sticks so constructed that they could be fitted together. Sultan tried to pull the bananas with the sticks, an effort which he kept up for an hour, but he got tired of the attempt and gave it up for playing. While playing he brought the two ends together and suddenly he got an idea which resulted in his fitting the smaller stick in the hole of the bigger one. He then used the two together to draw the banana inward. The two sticks disintegrated but he fitted them together again. He then pulled in everything within reach as if he were trying out his discovery. The next day he took far less time to fit the two together. It is a peculiarity of insight that once the solution is learnt, it is not forgotten though its memory may become hazy with the passage of time.

Experiment conducted by Kohler in relation to insight on a chimpanzee called *Sultan*. Some bananas were placed inside the cage of Sultan who was given two sticks so constructed that they could be fitted together. The hungry Sultan tried to get bananas by extending out his hands. Then, he took up one of sticks and tried to pull the bananas, an effort which he kept up for an hour. Then, he tried and started to play with the sticks. Meanwhile, one end of one stick got incidentally fastened into the ring fixed on the end of the other stick with the result that both the sticks were joined together. Now, Sultan used this joined stick to pull in the bananas and succeeded.

The above experiments make it quite obvious that learning by insight has certain characteristics of its own. They are briefly as follows:

1. Insight is sudden.
2. Insight alters perception.
3. Old objects appear in new patterns and organization by virtue of insight.
4. Insight is relative to the intellectual level. The higher species of animals including human beings have more insight than the members of lower species.
5. In insight understanding is more useful than dexterity of hands.
6. In Woodworth's opinion, insight is sometimes hindsight and at others it is foresight. Foresight is seeing the way to the goal before taking it or perceiving the uselessness of a certain lead without buying it and hindsight is observing that a lead is good or bad after trying it. When the whole situation is clear and above-board, there is a good chance for foresight, but when important characteristics of the situation have to be discovered by exploration and manipulation, hindsight is the best we can expect.
7. Previous experience is of assistance in insight, though its excess does not necessarily increase insight because organized perception too is an essential factor in learning
8. Maturity also affects insight as evidenced by the smoother working of insight in older age than in adolescence.
9. If the pieces essential for the solution of the puzzle are present together when perceived, insight comes about earlier.
10. Some psychologists say that learning by insight is associative learning. Insight appears suddenly after the manipulation of thoughts or objects for a small though significant length of time.
11. The insight gained in particular circumstances is of assistance in other circumstances. A verbal formula is generally extracted by people learning by insight and this formula is capable of facile application to other circumstances.

The above mentioned characteristics of learning through insight apply both to human and animal learning. The solitary difference is the fact that a human being by virtue of his superior capacities of experiencing and understanding, observes relation between various objects quickly and sees the patterns concealed in them with alacrity. He is assisted in this by language. As a matter of fact insight occurs only when the learner perceives the related link hidden in the activity. The learning curve is altered suddenly problem, because familiarity is very necessary for insight. A student of literature will have no insight in any scientific problem because he does not know even the a b c of science. When the subject of study becomes a part of life, insight becomes easier. History can be made alive by exhibitions, Geography travelling and Arithmetic by shop accounts. Familiarity is also important besides the theoretical study.

One example of human learning by insight will suffice. A student of arithmetic tries hard to solve a difficult problem of arithmetic. He tries many methods but fails to secure a solution. He gives up and lays it aside or goes to sleep. After some time suddenly or when he is awakened the solution suggests itself and he notes it down in his notebook. When he is confronted with similar problems in the future, he will have no difficult in solving them. The insight method is superior to imitation or conditioned response because both the latter methods take more time. It is superior to trial and error in the following respects:

1. Trial and error emphasizes the acquisition of motor skill but in insight mental effort is stressed upon.
2. While insight depends upon perception, trial and error depends upon sensory motor coordination.
3. The person keeps an eye on the goal, in trial and error and all activity is goal-directed but in insight it is the unconscious mind which exerts the most while the conscious activities are either very few and or aimless.
4. Every new problem has to be tackled from the very beginning if the trial and error method is used. On the other hand, both generalization and differentiation are present in insight, which adds to the possibilities of transfer of learning and the use of old insight in the solution of novel problems.

Against this position of Thorndike came Wolfgang Kohler with his experiments on monkeys and a different theory of learning. He found in his experiments that the method of learning used depends on the problem. He explained that the problem set by Thorndike was too difficult for the animal. The latch was not at all in an obvious position. Naturally the cat could use only the trial and error method. Under similar circumstances even man will use only the method of trial and error. Suppose a man is locked up in a room and there is a concealed electric switch which if pressed will open the door. Let us suppose that this man is not told anything about this switch or about the means by which he could come out. It is certain that this man will use only this method of trial and error. He will naturally try various possibilities one after another, till at last he succeeds. There is very little for him to think about. Thus Kohler accused Thorndike of setting too difficult a problem to these animals.

Students will be permanently helped by the use of the insight method of learning in place of the trial and error method in their study and other daily activities. They will also be able to conserve their energy. Suppose that a person has to arrange furniture in a room. An average person will determine the position of the table by using the trial and error method and shifting the table from place to place. An intelligent person will take up a position from where the whole room is visible, and imagine all the possible positions of the pieces of furniture in an imagined framework of the room and then place the respective pieces accordingly. But this does not mean that trial and error method is not meant for the intelligent. By no means is this so. In many novel situations progress is not possible without it. An intelligent person should use both these methods according to the needs of the situation.

b. Sign theory of learning: According to Tolman (1930), learning is a total process, takes place by cognition. Cognition includes concepts like knowledge, thinking, planning, inference and purpose. The learner recognizes some cues or signs through his experience and then relationships with goals. Learning consists in the recognition of signs and their meanings in relation to goals. The individual follows certain signs and clues, forms a mental map, learn their significance and meanings and finally reaches at goal.

c. **Social learning theory:** It relies on role modeling, identification and human interactions. A student nurse can learn by imitating/observing the behavior of another nurse, but personal factors are involved. When a person dislikes a role model, imitative behavior is unlikely.

Social learning or observational learning occurs when an individual learns something by observing another person doing it, in other words it is learning by modeling. According to social learning theory, behavior is seen as a two-way interaction between an individual and his environment, that is, 'Both people and their environments are reciprocal determinants of each other' (Bandura, 1977). Exponents of this theory view the behavioristic approach to learning as one that limits the idea of the potential of an individual and his influence over his own behavior. According to social learning theory, an individual possesses no inherent behavior patterns at birth other than reflexes, so must learn everythingelse. Such learning occurs as a result of observing the behavior of other people, which allows complex patterns to be acquired in a more efficient way than trial and error. Indeed, some behaviors such as language can only be learned, according to Bandura by observation of human models, as it is highly unlikely that mere reinforcement of random vocalization would lead to the complex use of speech that forms the everybody language of an individual. Learning, then, is envisaged as behavior that is acquired by observation of modeling stimuli, providing the learner with a symbolic image of such behavior, which may serve as a guide. Bandura identifies four processes involved in the observational learning situation.

- **Attentional processes:** These processes are concerned with the characteristics of the model and of the observer. In the former, some of the factors which influence learning are variables such as interpersonal attraction between the model and the observer, the usefulness of the observed behavior and the distinctiveness, complexity and frequency of contact with the modeled stimuli. Observer characteristics comprise the level of arousal, capacity to process information, the perceptual set and amount of previous reinforcement.
- **Retention processes:** It is obviously important to remember the modeled behavior if one is to learn from it, so the role of such strategies as rehearsal is crucial. Jeffrey (1974) found that the highest level of learning was achieved when the modeled behavior was first organized and symbolically rehearsed before actually performing the behavior.
- **Motor reproduction processes:** The learner must be capable of actually carrying out the observed behavior and of evaluating it in terms of accuracy.
- **Motivational processes:** Modeled stimuli are more likely to be learned if the observer sees some value in them, but the role of reinforcement is social learning theory is one of facilitation rather than necessity. It may take the form of external reward such as money, or self-reinforcement, where the learner rewards herself with something when a predetermined behavior has been achieved. For example, she may set herself a number of objectives to achieve for a course and having attained them may reward herself by going out to dinner. The likelihood of the modeled behavior being learned is increased when the observer sees the model being reinforced for performing that behavior. This is termed vicarious reinforcement.

Information can be transmitted by the model in a variety of ways, such as an actual physical demonstration, by pictures, words and the mass media. Abstract modeling is the term used for the process whereby the observer elicits the principles of behavior from a variety of modeled stimuli and applies them to a situation that is similar to the ones which were observed. For example, observation of various models performing a surgical dressing would allow the observer to learn the rules of the procedure and these could then be applied to similar situations. How does social learning theory explain the development of novel or creative responses? Bandura sees the novel response as a utilization of the qualities of many models, to produce a new creative behavior. There are a number of characteristic of both the model and the observer that make learning more likely. Experiments indicate that persons who possess status, prestige and power are more effective models for those kind of behaviors. Individuals who are lacking in self-esteem and confidence and those who are dependent tend to be more easily influenced by the behaviors of models who are obviously successful. However, one needs to interpret such results with caution, as many confident people readily adopt behavior of those whose actions are seen to be of value.

Bandura's experiment: Albert Bandura and other researchers conducted a classic set of experiments that demonstrated the power of observational learning. A preschool child worked on a drawing while on a television set showed an adult behaving aggressively toward a large inflated 'Bobo doll/a clown doll that bounces back up when knocked down. The adult pummeled the doll with a mallet, kicked it, flung it in the air, sat on it and beat it on the face while yelling remarks. The child was then left in another room filled with interesting toys, including a 'Bobo doll". Compared with children who witnessed a nonviolent adult model and those not exposed to any model, the children who witnessed the aggressive display were much more likely to show aggressive behaviors toward the Bobo doll, and they often imitated the model's exact behaviors and hostile words.

Application of Social Learning Theory to Nurse Education

Observational learning can be a powerful tool for the nurse teacher in a wide range of applications. One of the important early aspects of nursing the new student must acquire is that of the professional role and this can be fostered by allowing the student to observe a prestigious trained nurse going about her daily work. The student will be able to observe not only clinical skills, but interactions with patients and other members of the health-care team, thus learning about professional attitudes as well as techniques. This strategy has been used in nursing with some success; Kramer (1972) took students into the clinical areas and had them work in the vicinity, but not actually attached to her. The students thus had the opportunity to see her interacting with patients and giving care and she acted as a model for their observational learning. In a British study in an elderly care setting. Raichura and Riley (1985) used modeling as a strategy for teaching trained staff about care of the elderly.

The nurse teacher must also act as a professional model when he is with students, showing enthusiasm about nursing and the ability to do the job skillfully. A good role model must also be a good practitioner if students are to learn the correct roles. It is a useful idea when working with student groups to pair the students so that the weaker ones are working with the more able students and learning by observation. The teacher should ensure that the more able students are given responsibility, since these high-status students are more likely to serve as models for the others. The main used of social learning theory includes the following.

- Both children and adults learn a great deal through observation and imitation. Young children learn language, social skills, habits, fears and many other everyday behaviors by observing their parents and older children.
- Many people learn academic, athletic and musical skills by observing and then imitating a teacher.
- It plays an important role in a child's personality development.
- Fearful children become less fearful when they watch other children acting fearlessly in the same situation.
- Demonstrating fearless approach to a phobic situation may be useful to motivate a patients approach to the feared object or situations.
- Modeling is also used in weight reduction and smoking cessation programs.

Humanistic Psychology

There is no single theory that represents the humanistic approach, but all theories share a common view that this approach involves the study the man as a human being, with his thoughts, feelings and experiences. This is in direct contrast to the stimulus—response theorist, who study man from the point of view of his overt behavior, disregarding his inner feelings and experiences. Humanistic differs from cognitive theory also, in that the latter is concerned with the thinking aspects of man's behavior, with little emphasis on the affective components. Exponents of humanistic theory claim that the other two theories omit some of the most significant aspects of human existence, namely feelings, attitudes and values. Humanistic theory is closely related to the philosophical approach called phenomenology, which asserts that reality lies in a person's perception of an event and not in the event itself. The humanistic viewpoint is summarized by Hamachek (1977) as follows:

It is a psychological stance that focuses not so much on persons biological drives, but on their goals; not so much on stimuli impinging on them, but on their desires to be or to do something; not so much on their past experiences, but on their current circumstances, not so much on life conditions *per se*, but on the subjective qualities of human experience, the personal meaning of an experience to persons, rather than on their objective, observable responses.

Humanistic theory, then, is concerned with human growth, individual fulfillment and self-actualization and it is claimed that this approach is 'intuitively right', as it agrees with the ideas most people have about what is uniquely human. However, the behaviorists approach is not considered to be wrong, but humanistic theory prefers to emphasize the affective aspects of man as being of equal importance to the cognitive and psychomotor elements.

There are two main principles that apply to the humanistic approach to learning and teaching, namely teacher-student relationships and the classroom climate. The former stresses the importance of the interpersonal relationships between learner and teacher as major variable affecting learning and this in turn affects the climate of the classroom. The presence or absence of conflict and tension will depend largely on the quality of relationships within the classroom setting.

Maslow and 'third force' psychology: Abraham H Maslow (1908-70) was a major exponent of the humanistic approach to psychology, and has also made a significant contribution to motivation theory with his theory of a hierarchy of needs. He coined the term 'third force' psychology because he considered the first force to be Freudian psychotherapy and the second to be the stimulus—response school. The latter school, he felt, had little relevance to the human personality. These extensive books on the psychology of learning are of no consequence, at least to the human center, to the human soul, to the human essence (Maslow 1971). One of the key concepts he defined was that of 'self-actualization' and he studied the behavior of people whom he classified as self-actualisers. Maslow stated eight ways in which an individual self-actualizes, and these include 'experiencing fully, vividly, selflessly, with full concentration and total absorption.' He mentions the 'peak experience', which is an ecstatic moment that can be brought on by such experiences as classical music and religious experiences. For the humanist, the goal of education is to assist the individual to achieve self-actualization, or, as Maslow puts it, 'to help the person to become the best that he is able to become'. This intrinsic approach is in contrast to the extrinsic educational ethic, in which the transmissions of factual knowledge is seen to be more important than the development of an individual. The ideal college, according to Maslow, would be eon in which the main objectives would be the discovery of one's identity and the destiny or vocation for each person.

Rogers and student-centered learning: Carl R Rogers made his reputation as a psychotherapist, developing a new approach that he called client-centered therapy (Rogers, 1951). This involves the therapist in a nondirective role in which the client is encouraged to develop a deeper understanding of himself. The role of the therapist is to provide a non-critical atmosphere, in which there is no attempt to interpret for the client, but simply a reflecting back of his statements in order to assist him in developing self-awareness.

This concept of client-centered therapy led Rogers to formulate his student-centered approach to learning, which is contained in his most important work on the subject (Rogers, 1969). In this work, he states a number of principles of learning:

1. Human beings have a natural potentiality for learning.
2. Significant learning takes place when the subject matter is perceived by the student as having relevance for his own purposes.
3. Learning which involves a change in self-organization is threatening and tends to be resisted.
4. Those elements of learning which are threatening to the self are more easily perceived and assimilated when external threats are at a minimum.
5. When threat to the self is low, experience can be perceived in differentiated fashion, and learning can proceed.
6. Much significant learning is acquired through doing.
7. Learning is facilitated when the student participates responsibly in the learning process.
8. Self-initiated learning, which involves the whole person of the learner—feelings as well as intellect—is the most lasting and pervasive.
9. Independence, creativity and self-reliance are all facilitated when self-criticism and self-evaluation are basic and evaluation by others is of secondary importance.
10. The most socially useful learning in the modern world is the learning of the process of learning, a continuing openness to experience and incorporation into oneself of the process of change.

These ten principles illustrate Rogers approach to learning and his emphasis on relevance, student participation and involvement, self-evaluation and the absence of threat in the classroom.

Rogers sees the teacher as a facilitator of learning; a provider of resources for learning, and someone who shares his feelings as well as his knowledge with the students. Thus the prerequisites of an effective facilitator of learning are awareness of self, being oneself in the classroom, acceptance and trust of the students and understanding and empathy.

Rogers has further articulated his approach to education in his book Freedom to Learn for the 80s (Rogers 1983). He sees learning as being a continuum, with much meaningless material at one end and significant or experiential learning at the other. The former could describe many curricula, which are seen as virtually meaningless by the student for whom they are intended. Experiential learning, on the other hand, has a number of qualities such as personal involvement, self-initiation, pervasiveness, self-evaluation and meaningfulness. He contrasts the kind of learning that is concerned solely with cognitive functioning with that involving the whole person. Teaching, according to Rogers, is a highly overated activity, in contrast to the notion of facilitation. Teaching by giving knowledge does not meet the requirements of today's changing world. What is required is the facilitation of learning and change and this calls for a different set of qualities in the facilitator. The most important factor is the relationship that exists between facilitator and learner and Rogers suggests a number of qualities that are required for this:

1. Genuineness, i.e. the facilitator comes across as a real person rather than as some kind of ideal model. Hence, it is important that he shows normal reactions to the students so that they accept him as a real person.
2. Trust and acceptance, i.e. acceptance of the student as a person in her own right as a person who is worthy of respect and care.
3. Empathic understanding, i.e. putting oneself in the students shoes in order to see and understand things from her perspective.

Rogers suggests that it is possible for the teacher to build into a program the freedom to learn, which students require. This can be done by using students own experience and problems so that relevance is obvious and by providing resources for the students in the form of both material and human resources. He also recommends the use of learning contracts that help to make the students have autonomy over their own learning. The goal of education that of the student becoming a fully functioning person.

Applications of Humanistic Psychology to Nurse Education

The humanistic approach to education centers on the relationships between teachers and learners, each learner being considered as individuals. The use of forenames between teacher and learner can increase the feeling of identity for the learner and help to reduce barriers to communication. Involvement in decision making is a further step in helping the learners develop a sense of personal value and worth. While it is impossible to involve each learner in major planning decisions, it is quite simple to have elected representatives from each set to contribute ideas and suggestions from the group. I have used this strategy to involve learners in the process of education, by inviting the representative of a set to attend a planning meeting for a forthcoming module. Such issues as the day on which an examination should fall can be decided by the learners in consultation with the teachers, leading to a feeling of participation.

Most teachers are aware of the individual differences between learners prior to commencing training, but many are not so sensitive to the fact that they will still have learners are individuals, even though they have been exposed to a common training program and to encourage them to maintain their unique attitudes and values, rather than aiming for a conformist, homogenous end product. The role of the teacher is seen by the humanistic approach as being that of helper and facilitator, rather than a conveyor of information. In other words, the teacher becomes another learning resource for the learner.

In order to perform his role satisfactorily, the teacher must fully understand himself, and be flexible in his approach to teaching. The classroom climate is seen to be of major importance and should be an environment where psychological safety exists and where the learners feel at ease. Some of the barriers between teacher and learner may be lessened by the rearrangement of the seating and the use of small-group techniques. These also facilitate the discussion of feelings and values, an aspect that is considered crucial in the humanistic approach and which is often given too little attention in nurse education.

One of the specific applications of humanistic psychology is in the use of learning contracts, which give the student the opportunity to take responsibility for her own learning. Learning contracts are discussed. Since Rogers approach to education is derived from his work in psychotherapy it is hardly surprising that nurse teacher in mental-illness nursing have tended to adopt a humanistic approach to students for many years. In that specialism, the rigid hierarchy of authority, which is characteristic of general nursing, seems largely absent, with staff mixing freely in hospital social clubs, regardless of seniority.

One of the most serious criticisms of this approach is that it is lacking in empirical evidence to support its claims, relying upon observations and assumptions of human behavior. In addition, there is concern that this approach may lead to the teacher becoming an amateur psychotherapist with all the attendant dangers of this. Many observers equate this approach with one of total freedom for the student, as exemplified by the Suffolk school, Summerhill. This was the brainchild of AS Neill and the students were given considerable freedom of choice with regard to attendance at lessons.

Transfer of Learning

It is a matter of common experience that we are facilitated in the learning of something new by some previous learning. The son of a businessman is proficient in the arithmetic class because of his learning in accountancy at the shop.

Transfer of learning is the carry-over of habits of thinking, feeling or working of knowledge or skills, from one learning area to another.

Transfer refers to the transfer of knowledge, training and habits acquired in one situation to another situation.

Transfer is a process by which some influence is exercised over our new learning or performance by our previous learning or training.

Types of Transfer of Learning

Commonly, there are two types of transfer of learning. These are as follows:

1. **Positive transfer of learning:** In this type of transfer, the effect of the training on the new type of learning is favorable or positive and learning is enhanced. For example, one group was taught Latin while another was not. Both the groups were constituted of students possessing similar interests and intelligence. Now, they were taught English

for equal lengths of time together and the result was that the group equipped with the knowledge of Latin took less time and gained comparatively more skill. The reason for this is the positive transfer of the training in Latin to the learning of English.

2. **Negative transfer of learning:** The training received in the learning of one thing hiders the learning of a new thing and it is accordingly classified as negative. For example, wrestlers are weak in studies because wrestling consumes too much of their energy to leave any for studying. Thus, wrestling is a hindrance in studying.
3. **Zero transfer of learning:** In case, the previous learning makes no difference at all to the performance or learning in a new situation, there is said to be zero transfer from the previous situation to the new one.

Theories of Transfer of Learning

1. **Theory of identical elements or components** propagated by Thorndike, the transfer-positive or negative from one situation to another is possible to the extent that there are common or identical elements in the situations. For example, in the case of learning cycling and driving a car, the transfer does take place on account of the presence of common elements like steering movements, knowledge of the rules of road, necessity of having proper visual perspective by looking ahead, etc. The presence of these common elements in the situations may bring either type of transfer-positive or negative. In this, the presence of common elements help us to make an association in such a way that learning in one situation helps the other, the transfer is positive. But in case the association so formed brings interference with the new learning, the transfer is negative.
2. **Theory of generalization** put forth by Charles Judd advocates the transfer of generalizations in the new situations in place of identical elements as suggested by Thorndike. This theory says that as a result of certain experiences, an individual may arrive at some conclusions or generalizations in the form of general rules, laws or principles like 'The green or unripe fruits are sour or bitter in taste". In these generalizations, principles or rules that are put to use (through the transfer process) by the individual in the coming new situations.
3. **Theory of ideals** is put forward by WC Bagley. According to this theory, transfer of learning or training takes place in the form of ideals. The experience we have, the generalizations or conclusions we arrive at, all do transfer if they are imbibed as ideals of some value or desirable by the individual. For instance, the ideal of 'tolerance for other's opinion developed on the basis of qualities of a nurse laid on things with tolerance on ward duty is likely to be transferred in performing all other activities in a similar behavior in other situations.

None of these theories is able to explain transfer in its total aspects. However, an elective view of all these theories may help us in this direction.

Applications of Transfer of Training

- Transfer of training has a lot of educative value. Along with its influence in the classroom learning in our day-to-day life, many of our habits, attitudes, social values and acquired traits develop due to transfer, e.g. a child hating his friend in playground because he is poor, he will also hate his parents, friends, books and even his beloved puppy.
- Many of our values, social and personal habits, likes and dislikes are due to transfer, e.g. if you don't like milk, you may not like all milk products. If you like fish very much, any type of fish may satisfy you.

For a long time the educational program in schools and colleges has been based on a behalf in what is called "transfer of training". In western educational methods (which we have copied to a large extent), it was believed that if a student learned Latin, it improved his memory power. Studying such subjects for the sake of training and improving his mind was called "formal discipline". The main principle behind education was this idea of formal discipline by which the training obtained could be transferred to other activities of the mind. In recent years, however, psychologists began to test this hypothesis experimentally. William James of America started the first experimental work on this problem. He wanted to find out whether practice at memorizing really improved memorizing ability. He conducted the experiment on himself. First he learned about 150 lines from one of the works of Victor Hugo. He noted the time taken. Then he committed to memory Milton's "Paradise Lost". This took about a month. When he had mastered this "Paradise Lost", he came back to the same work of Victor Hugo and tried to memorize another portion of the same number of lines. He found that this book more time than for learning the first portion. From this he concluded that the practice he had in learning Milton's "Paradise Lost" had not improved his memorizing ability because in the second attempt at Victor Hugo's book, he took more time. He used different passages of the same book so that the style and the difficulty would be more or less the same. Still it may be pointed out that one is not absolutely sure that both passages were of the same difficulty.

The educational psychologist, Thorndike, conducted many experiments under more scientific laboratory conditions. His experiments also proved that there is no such transfer by which a mental activity would gain an advantage from formal discipline. Many others also have come to the same conclusion. The positive conclusion of these were common elements or common ideas, or common forms of expression, then a certain amount of transfer took place. In other words, if the second task is similar to the first task, the second task become easier to learn because of having learnt the first. This perhaps is easy for us to understand.

Many offer simpler experiments on transfer of training have also been conducted. Many of these experiments have taken the form of experiments with the right and left hands. If we learn a motor activity with the right hand, it has been found that it is easier for us to learn the activity using the left hand. The number of trials with the left hand would be more if we did not at first learn the activity with the right hand. This definitely shows that there is a transfer of training from the right hand to the left hand. This kind of transfer is usually called "bilateral transfer".

Though the experiments have disproved some of the aspects of transfer of training, the value of formal discipline in various school subjects needs not be completely discarded. A particular subject that we study in school or college may not be of direct value and use to us in daily life. It is also possible that it would be have increased certain abilities of ours such as memorizing or even reasoning have increased certain abilities of ours such as memorizing or even reasoning. But during the process of study, we do acquire certain habits such as collecting data, methods of working, a certain discipline, etc. This will always be useful to us in tackling other problems that face us in real life. Thus it would be wrong to dismiss formal discipline as absolutely useless.

Applications of Learning Theories in Nursing

Theories about how and why people learn can be traced to the 17th century. Three main theoretical constructs are behaviorism, cognitivism and humanism.

Behaviorism was originally advanced by Edward Thorndike, whose major contribution applicable to teaching is that learning should based on the learners behavior. In addition to Thorndike, major behaviorist theorists include I Pavlov, BF Skinner and A Bandura.

In the behaviorist school of thought, an act is called a response when it can be traced to the effects of a stimulus. Behaviorists closely observe responses and then manipulate the environment to bring about the intended change. Thus, to modify a person's attitude and response, a behaviorist would either alter the stimulus condition in the environment or change what happens after a response occurs.

Skinner's and Pavlov's work focused on conditioning behavioral responses to a stimulus that causes the response or behavior. To increase the probability of a response, Skinner introduced the importance of **positive reinforcement** (e.g. a pleasant experience such as praise and encouragement) in fostering repetition of an action. Bandura, however, claims that most learning comes from observational learning and instruction rather than from overt trial and error behavior. Bandura's research focuses on **imitation**, the process by which individuals copy or reproduce what they have observed, and **modeling**, the process by which a person learn by observing the behavior of others.

Cognitivism: Cognitivism depicts learning as a complex cognitive activity. In other words, learning is largely a mental or intellectual or thinking process. The learner structures and processes information. Perceptions are selectively chosen by the individual and personal characteristics have an impact on how a cue is perceived. Cognitivists also emphasize the importance of social, emotional, and physical contexts in which learning occurs, such as the teacher-learner relationship and environment. Developmental readiness and individual readiness (expressed as motivation) are other key factors associated with cognitive approaches.

Major cognitive theorists include J Piaget, K Lewin, and B Bloom. Piaget's five major phases of cognitive development include the sensorimotor phase, the preconceptual phase, the intuitive phase, the concrete operation phase, and the formal operations phase. Each phase is discussed in Chapter 21. Lewin states that learning involves four different types of changes: change in cognitive structure, change in motivation, change in one's sense of belonging to the group and gain in voluntary muscle control. His widely known theory of change has three basic stages: unfreezing, moving, and refreezing. These stages are discussed in detail in Chapter 26.

Bloom (1956) has identified three domains or areas of learning; cognitive, affective and psychomotor. The cognitive domain, the "thinking" domain, includes six intellectual abilities and thinking processes beginning with knowing, comprehending and applying to analysis, synthesis and evaluation. The affective domain, known as the "feeling" of a "person's depth of emotional response to tasks". It includes feelings, emotions, interests, attitudes and appreciations. The psychomotor domain, the "skill" domain, includes motor skills such as giving an injection.

Nurses should include each of Bloom's three domains in client teaching plans. For example, teaching a client how to irrigate a colostomy is in the psychomotor domain. But an important part of a teaching plan for a client with a colostomy is to teach why a specific amount of fluid is used and when the irrigation should be carried out; this is in the cognitive domain. Helping the client accept the colostomy and maintain self-esteem is in the affective domain.

Humanism: Humanistic learning theory focuses on both cognitive and affective qualities of the learner. Prominent members of this school of thought include Abraham Maslow and Carl Rogers. According to humanistic theory, learning is believed to be self-motivated, self-initiated, and self-evaluated. Each individual is viewed as a unique composite of biologic, psychologic, social, cultural and spiritual factors. Learning focuses on self-development and achieving full potential; it is best when it is relevant to the learner. Autonomy and self-determination are important; the learner identifies the learning needs and takes the initiative to meet these needs. The learner is thus an active participant and takes responsibility for meeting individual learning needs.

The major attributes of the behaviorist theory include the careful identification of what is to be taught and the immediate identification of and reward for correct responses. However, the theory is not easily applied to complex learning situations and is limiting in terms of the learner's role in the teaching process. Nurses applying behavioristic theory will:

- Provide sufficient practice time and both immediate and repeat testing and redemonstration.
- Provide opportunities for learners to solve problems by trial and error.
- Select teaching strategies that avoid distracting information and that evoke the desired response.
- Praise the learner for correct behavior and provide positive feedback at intervals throughout the learning experience.
- Provide role models of desired behavior.

The major attributes of cognitive theory are its recognition of developmental levels of learners and acknowledgements of learners motivation and environment. However, some or many of the motivational and environmental factors may be beyond the teachers control. Nurses applying cognitive theory will:

- Provide a social, emotional, and physical environment conducive to learning.
- Encourage a positive teacher-learner relationship.
- Select multisensory teaching strategies since perception is influenced by the senses.
- Recognize that personal characteristics have an impact on how cues are perceived and develop appropriate teaching approaches to target different learning styles.
- Assess a persons developmental and individual readiness to learn and adapt teaching strategies to the learners developmental level.
- Select behavioral objectives and teaching strategies that encompass the cognitive, affective and psychomotor domains of learning.

The major attributes of humanism are its focus on the feelings and attitudes of learners, on the importance of the individual in identifying learning needs and in taking responsibility for them, and on the self-motivation of the learners to work toward self-reliance and independence. Nurses applying cognitive theory will:

- Convey empathy in the nurse-client relationship.
- Encourage the learners to establish goals and promote self-directed learning.
- Encourage active learning by serving as a facilitator, mentor or resource for the learner.
- Expose the learner to new relevant information and ask appropriate questions to encourage the learner to seek answers.

Learning depends upon three main factors. The nurse has to look into the following factors:

1. Nature of the learner.
2. Nature of the learning material or task to be learned.
3. Nature of the learning situation or learning methods.

1. Nature of the learner

- **Age:** Age can influence upon the capability of learning. A child cannot learn the things what elders can learn and an aged person will have difficulty to learn modern ways of knowledge.
- **Intelligence:** Intelligence effects very much on learning, if subject/individual has maximum level of intelligence he can learn more and easily at maximum level.
- **Attention:** If a person does not pay attention towards how to learn specific knowledge, skill or experience, he cannot learn easily. But if the individual pays attention, the results are *vice versa*.
- **Interest and motivation:** Subject has intelligence and can also pay attention towards but he does not have interest in how to learn a specific knowledge, skill or experience. Therefore, level or process of learning would be very slow.
- **Mental and physical health:** If an individual does not have mental health or physical one, the subject can fulfill the demands of the process of learning due to his weak and physical capabilities.
- **Fatigue and rest:** If an individual is tired, he cannot pay full attention to learn something. So, take rest in between your studies.

2. Nature of learning materials

If the knowledge is interesting in nature, meaningful, clearly printed and written in easy understandable language and pattern, etc. any individual can learn it more efficiently.

3. Nature of learning method

a. **Definite goal:** It enhances motivation if clear goals are written or in mind.
b. **Recitation:** It is more effective tool of learning, if an individual recites something louder he can learn more effectively.
c. **Exercise and repetition:** Single act is learnt in single trial but complex acts require repeated trials. If a material is difficult to learn, it can be learnt through exercises or repeated trials.
d. **By parts learning:** If the material is so long, it can be divided into small parts, so individual can learn specific knowledge, skill, etc. more effectively.
e. **Reward and punishment:** The presence of reward or punishment can affect learning. Generally, reward is more effective in promoting learning than punishment. Punishment does have some effects on learning. It tends to repress a desired response than to extinguish it.
f. **Knowledge of results or psychological feedback:** Frequent and regular review of the amount of progress being made towards the goal, acts as a strong motive to promote continuing effort on the part of the learner.

Factors Affecting Learning in Nursing

Many factors can facilitate or hinder learning by a client. The nurse should be aware of these factors, particularly when available teaching time is limited.

Motivation: Motivation to learn is the desire to learn. It greatly influences how quickly and how much a person learns. Motivation is generally greatest when a person recognizes a need and believes the need will be met through learning. It is not enough for the need to be identified and verbalized by the nurse; it must be experienced by the client. Often the nurse's task is to help the client personally work through the problem and identify the need. Sometimes clients or support people need help identifying information relevant to their situation before they can see a need. For instance, clients with heart disease may need to know the effects the smoking before they recognize the need to stop smoking. Or adolescents may need to know the consequences of an untreated sexually transmitted disease before they see the need for treatment.

There is no doubt that motivated individual learns faster than an unmotivated one. In any aspect of life the motivation of people is central to any form of behavior. Human motivation is characterized by basic needs directed towards achieving certain desirable goals. *A few of the determinants of motivation at work are hierarchies of need. Frustration, attitude, conflict, group relation, etc.* these factors further interact in some manner with many other factors such as personal experiences, emotions, likes, dislikes, fears, etc. to form a motivational base for each individual. In addition to this another very important factor is the set of values and beliefs of individual relating to his job.

The motive is defined as the conditions of the organism to direct the organization towards a goal. Motives are generally of two types:

i. Internal
ii. External.

The intrinsic motivate is related to the task and there is a definite relationship between task and goal of the learner. Extrinsic motivation is independent of the task. The intrinsic motivation provides the trainee with a job interest even after completion of training.

In all the experiments, it was found that the animals learn more efficiently and quickly if there is strong motive. In experiments, the biological needs such as food, water, protecting the young ones and sex are usually used as motives. It was found that if the animal was not hungry at all and the food was kept at the goal end of the puzzle box or the maze, the animal took a long time to learn. It was not sufficiently motivated. On the other hand, if it was hungry it learned quicker. If the animal was thirsty and water was kept at the goal-end it learned to run the maze very quickly. Similarly if a young one was kept outside the cage, the mother animal was strongly motivated. As additional information from these experiments we are also able to compare the strength of these various biological needs. For this purpose the following experiment could be conducted. Suppose the animal is in a box. It can come out of the box only through a metallic grill. We can pass an electric current through this grill and give a fairly strong shock to the animal when it attempts to come out. If the animal is not motivated say by being hungry it will not take the trouble of undergoing the shock to reach the food. So its willingness to put up with the shock will depend upon the strength of its motivation. With this principle we can study the comparative strength of different motives by varying the strength of the shock. If the motive is very strong the animal will run the risk of getting even a very severe shock. Actual experiments have been conducted on these liens and it has been found that in many animals such as rats, thirst is the strongest motive. It is stronger than food, sex and the desire to protect the young. Perhaps, with some other animals, giving protection to the young may be the strongest.

Educational psychologists have been very much interested in experiments studying the effect of motivation in learning. They have generally attempted to find out whether reward or punishment serves as a better incentive to learn. It has been found that punishment has some effect within limits as a motivation to learn. But all experiments showed that reward and praise and congratulations is the most effective way of motivating him to learn. Another interesting result of these experiments is the fact that if one is neglected and indifference is shown to him he learns much less than the one who is at least punished.

The usual motives in the case of human beings are:

1. Praise and approval by society.
2. Competition.
3. Indirect satisfaction of biological needs such as food and sex through preparing oneself for a job.
4. Pure enjoyment resulting from a sense of success and achievement.

Any nurses or nurse teacher should make use of these following incentives in a planned and balanced manner.

Readiness: Readiness to learn is the demonstration of behaviors or cues that reflect the learner's motivation to learn at a specific time. Readiness reflects not only the desire or willingness to learn but also the ability to learn at a specific time. For example, a client may want to learn self-care during a dressing change, but if the client experiences pain or discomfort she may not be able to learn. The nurse can provide pain medication to make the client more comfortable so that she is more able to learn. The nurse's role is often to encourage the development of readiness.

Active involvement: When the learner is actively involved in the process of learning, learning becomes more meaningful. If the learner actively participates in planning and discussion, learning is faster and retention is better. Active learning promotes critical thinking, enabling learners to problem solve more effectively. Clients who are actively involved in learning about their health care may be more able to apply the learning to their own situation. For example, clients who are actively involved in learning about their therapeutic diets may be more able to apply the principles being taught to their cultural food preferences and their usual eating habits. Passive learning, such as listening to a lecture or watching a film, does not foster optimal learning.

Relevance: The knowledge or skill to be learned must be personally relevant to the learner. Clients learn more easily if they can connect the new knowledge to that which they already know or have experienced. For example, if a client is diagnosed with hypertension, is overweight, and has symptoms of headaches and fatigue, he is more likely to understand the need to lose weight if he remembers having more energy when he weighed less. The nurse needs to validate the relevance of learning with the client throughout the learning process.

Feedback: Feedback is information relating a person's performance to a desired goal. It has to be meaningful to the learner. Feedback that accompanies the practice of psychomotor skills helps the person to learn those skills. Support of desired behavior through praise, positively worded corrections, and suggestions of alternative feedback such as ridicule, anger, or sarcasm can lead people to withdraw from learning. Such feedback, viewed as a type of punishment, may cause the client to avoid the teacher in order to avoid punishment.

Nonjudgmental support: People learn best when they believe they are accepted and will not be judged. The person who expects to be judged as a "poor" or "good" client will not learn as well as the person who feels no such threat. Once learners have succeeded in accomplishing a task or understanding a concept, they gain self-confidence in their ability to learn. This reduces their anxiety about failure and can motivate greater learning. Successful learners have increased confidence with which to accept failure.

Simple to complex: Learning is facilitated by material that is logically organized and proceeds from the simple to the complex. Such organization enables the learner to comprehend new information, assimilate it with previous learning, and form new understandings. Of course, simple and complex are relative terms, depending on the level at which the person is learning. What is simple for one person may be complex for another.

Repetition: Repetition of key concepts and facts facilities retention of newly learned material. Practice of psychomotor skills, particularly with feedback from the nurse, improves performance of those skills and facilitates their transfer to another setting.

Timing: People retain information and psychomotor skills best when the time between learning and active use of the learning its short; the longer the time interval, the more learning is forgotten. For example, a woman who is only shown literature and videotapes about administering insulin but is not permitted to administer her own insulin until discharge from the hospital is unlikely to remember what she learned. However, if she is allowed to give her own injections while in the hospital, her learning will be enhanced.

Environment: An optimal learning environment facilitates learning by reducing distraction and providing physical and psychologic comfort. It has adequate lighting that is free from glare, a comfortable room temperature, and good ventilation. Most students know what it is like try to learn in a hot, stuffy room; the consequent drowsiness interferes with concentration. Noise can also distract the student and interfere with listening and thinking. To facilitate learning in a hospital setting, nurses should choose a time when no visitors are present and interruptions are unlikely.

Privacy is essential for some learning. For example, when a client is learning to irrigate a colostomy, the presence of others can be embarrassing and thus interfere with learning. However, when a client is particularly anxious, having a support person present may give the client confidence.

Learning and Maturation

Learning changes behavior and so does maturation. Thus sometimes it becomes difficult to say definitely as to which of the subject's activities are the results of learning and which are the consequences of maturation. Automatic activity, random acts, reflexes and instincts and sudden expression of emotion can be accepted as unlearned actions and the result of maturation, but in most of the activities of human beings it is difficult to decide whether these activities result from maturation or learning. In fact, these activities develop both due to learning and maturation. Take the example of learning a language. It is true, of course, that a child is manifestly incapable of learning a language until he reaches a certain stage in maturation, but it is also equally true that he does not learn the language just because he attains that stage. The language is taught to him.

An experiment on co-twins indicates the extent of the changes in behavior caused by maturation and the extent to which changes may be affected by learning. The purpose of the experiment was to measure the extent of advantage of learning in such activities as climbing the stairs. Two twins were chosen for the experiment because due to the similarity in heredity, the speed of maturation is the same and any changes which may occur may be attributed to learning. One of the twins 'S' was not given the opportunity of climbing stairs for 53 weeks while the other twin 'T' was taught to climb the stairs from her forty sixth week. On examination this twin 'T' failed to climb at all the age of 46 weeks and had to be aided up all the 5 stairs. In the space of four weeks she climbed all the stairs in 26 seconds.

When 'S'; was placed on the stairs at the age of 53 weeks she climbed all the five stairs unaided but it took her some 45 seconds. After two weeks of practice 'S', at the age of 55 weeks, traversed the distance in 10 seconds. In this way, at this age 'S' was ahead of 'T', who, at a younger age, had practiced three times as much. 'S' was three older than 'T'. Thus in spite of all kinds of learning, 'T' was left behind, due to a lack of maturity.

The experiment proves that learning plays an insignificant part in reflex and other physiological activities peculiar to one's species. Those activities which appear in all human beings at a certain age, are due to maturity. Those activities which do not inevitably appear in every person are affected by maturation to the extent that they can be learnt with ease at the age maturity. Some examples of this type of activities are swimming; horse riding, facile by motor, sensory and neural maturation.

The above exposition on the relation of learning and maturation provides some very practical suggestions for learning and training. It is not useful to make an attempt to teach a child forcibly before he matures. Many parents try to precipitate their children into higher classes with the help of coaching, at a young age. This coaching cannot have a lasting or permanent effect and the children become weak in senior classes. The teaching of the proper job at a specific age depends on many factors two of which are the child's mental and physiological development. But a general age for the beginning of teaching of various subjects can be established. For example, it is comparatively easier to study Algebra at 15 to 16 than it is at 11 or 12. This relation between maturation and training justifies the suggestion for the fixing of a minimum age limit for admission to universities.

Maturation and Learning

We know that the physiological system is the basic equipment with which the organism learns and expresses itself. So, the process by which the physiological system develops and becomes mature has an important reference to learning. This could be illustrated by a simple example. However much we practice a six month old child with walking exercise, the child cannot learn to walk. The muscles of the child have not matured enough for it to learn to walk. This particular learning is possible only when the nerves and the muscles have attained a particular stage of maturity and development. Similarly most of our learned activities depend upon the stages of growth reached by the central nervous system and the muscular system.

Woodworth mentions an interesting experiment conducted on chicks. It is based on the observation that chicks do have to learn in the initial stages to peck at grains correctly. Some chicks were hatched in the dark and were kept in a darkroom. To prevent them from doing any pecking they were hand-fed for 2 to 5 days. After that period, they were brought into the light and given a chance to peck at grains. Their success on the first day in the light was not better than that of a normal newly hatched chick. But they improved very rapidly with practice and very soon caught up with the normal chick. The normal chick which is given the freedom of ordinary practice begins with a poor performance on the first day and gradually improves day by day with practice.

This experiment draws our attention to two facts:

1. A maturation process was going on in the experimental chick which was reared in darkness. This process of maturation helped the chick to learn much quicker.
2. Even with maturation, some learning and practice are necessary for any activity.

Another interesting experiment with children has been conducted by one psychologist by name Arnold Gesell. The experiment was conducted on a pair of infant girls who were twins. One of the two was trained at 46 weeks of age to climb stairs. Day by day she was given practice for a number of weeks and the child learned to climb the stairs well. Seven weeks later her sister, the other child, started on the same training. By now this child was seven weeks older and hence more mature in its muscles and nerves. The result showed that the second girl soon reached the same standard as that of the first child. What the first child learned in several weeks was learned by the second child in two weeks.

These experiments which emphasize the part played by maturation in the process of learning, have a practical bearing for some of us. In our country many parents attempt to cut short the number of years that a child has to be in school. They give high pressure tuition at home it is suited for by way of physical and emotional development. Psychology teaches us that such an attempt does not really pay in the long run. It may even injure the child severely.

Some Interesting Experiments with Animals

Numerous experiments on animal learning have been conducted all over the world. They are not all repetitors of the same type. Different psychologists have studied any number of different aspects of the learning process as seen in animals. Some of these have given us valuable information regarding learning process in general. Some experiments have given us valuable information regarding the nature of animal mind. We will quote here a few experiments just to indicate the scope of this kind of study. One type of experiment is called the 'Discrimination experiment'. The purpose is to find out whether the animal can discriminate between different types of stimuli.

The usual laboratory experiments deal with discriminating between right side and left side, between having a signal such as a light and not having one, and between different degrees of brightness in color. A rat is placed in front of a compartment which has two doors. The two doors are side by side, the door on the right side admits the rat to a box which contains food. The door on the left side leads the animal only to a blind alley. In the actual experiment the rat learns to discriminate the correct door very quickly. Now the experiment is made more complicated. The apparatus is made in such a way that the door which leads to the food box may be changed at the will of the experimenter. The correct door is indicated by a light signal over it. The experimenter changes this in a random order. In actual experiment it has been found that the rat still learns to notice the signal and go to the correct door. But it is found that it requires several hundred attempts before learning to make this discrimination.

A modified form of this experiment has also been conducted quite often. In this particular form, the experiment is called the 'brightness discrimination experiment'. Two patches of color (by way of colored lights if necessary, one brighter than the other) are placed as signals above the doors. The brighter for example indicates the correct door which leads to the food box. Here again the lights can be changed at random, but the brighter always indicating the correct door. Here again, it has been found that the rat and in fact, several other animals, learn to make this discrimination. But they fail if the difference in brightness between the two colors is less than a certain degree.

We now come to a different type of experiment. This is called 'the delayed reaction experiment'. This experiment introduces a new problem in animal behavior. Take the second experiment, for example, where the rat learns to notice a light signal over the correct door. In this experiment, after the rat has thoroughly learnt this trick, give the stimulus by putting on the once. The light is put out and the rat is held back for some time and then released to go. This is an attempt to find out for how long the rat can 'remember' the signal. In an actual experiment with three doors side by side, the maximum duration for the 'memory image' was 10 seconds for rats and 5 minutes for dogs. If the interval was longer, the animal could not go straight to the correct door. Similar experiments have also been tried in modified forms with monkeys. With monkeys it has been found that this interval could extend upto several hours.

These experiments have also raised a number of other problems which are beyond the scope of this book.

Animal Learning and Human Learning

From what has been said above a few important differences between animal and human learning can be observed. For most of the simple necessities of life the animals are provided with innate mechanisms commonly called instincts. They do not have to learn many things in life by way of getting food, building nests, mating, rearing the young, etc. All these are carried on as unlearned activities. Man, on the other hand, has to learn almost everything, even with regard to the maintenance of his biological existence. In addition to this he has to learn a host of things to fulfill his responsibilities and maintain his place as a member of society. Thus man has to learn many more things than animals. For this purpose nature endowed him with more intelligence. In addition, though some animals have an extra-ordinary power of retention, on the whole man excels the animals in his power of retention and recall. Further, because of man's intelligence and his capacity for forming concepts and ideas he has developed language as a means of communication which helps him a great deal.

Thus, the following main differences between animal and human learning emerge from the superior intelligence of man:

1. Man uses more insight in his learning process.
2. Because of his superior memory he makes more effective use of past experience in the solving of a present problem so that there is a minimum of wastage of time and energy.
3. Because of his capacity for ideational thinking man develops the process of reasoning and much of the trial and error is done on the imaginary level. Animals on the other hand must carry out every activity and then learn from it.
4. Because of his capacity to use language man learns more quickly, helped by reading other people's experiences and instructions.
5. The human child is also found to be much better than the animal in learning by imitation.

Some of the higher apes are found to have this capacity to imitate, but within very narrow limits. The capacity to imitate is a great help in the case of human beings to learn more efficiently.

Factors inhibit learning: Some of the most common barriers to learning are described in Table 11.1.

Table 11.1: Barriers to learning		
Barrier	*Explanation*	*Nursing Implications*
Acute illness	Client requires all resources and energy to cope with illness	Defer teaching until client is less ill
Pain	Pain decreases ability to concentrate	Conduct pain assessment before teaching
Prognosis	Client can be preoccupied with illness and unable to concentrate on new information	Defer teaching to a better time
Biorhythms	Mental and physical performances have a circadian rhythm	Adapt time of teaching to suit client
Emotion (e.g. anxiety, denial, depression, grief)	Emotions requires energy and distract from learning	Deal with emotions and possible misinformation first
Age • Elders • Children	Vision, hearing, and motor control can be impaired in elders Children have a shorter attention span and vocabulary differences	Consider sensory and motor deficits and adapt in teaching plan Plan shorter and more active learning episodes
Culture/religion	There may be cultural or religious restrictions on certain types of knowledge, for example, birth control information	Assess the client's cultural/religious needs when planning learning activities
Physical disability	Visual, hearing, sensory, or motor impairments may interfere with a clients ability to learn	Plan teaching activities appropriate to learner's physical abilities. For example, provide audio learning tools for the client who is blind, or large print materials for the client whose vision is impaired
Mental disability	Impaired cognitive ability may affect the clients capacity for learning	Assess clients capacity for learning and plan teaching activities to complement the clients ability while planning more complex learning for the clients caregivers

Emotions: Emotions such as fear, anger, and depression can impede learning. A high level of anxiety resulting in agitation and the inability to focus or concentrate can also inhibit learning. Clients or families who are experiencing extreme emotional states may not hear spoken words or may retain only part of the communication. Emotional responses such as fear and anxiety may be lessened by information that relieves uncertainty. Medications may be prescribed for extremely distraught clients or families to reduce their anxiety and put them in an emotional state in which understanding or learning can occur.

Physiologic events: Learning can be inhibited by physiologic events such as a critical illness, pain or sensory deficits. Because the client cannot concentrate and apply energy to learning, the learning itself is impaired. The nurse should try to reduce the physiologic barriers to learning as much as possible before teaching. For example, providing analgesics and rest before teaching is often helpful.

Cultural aspects: There are also cultural barriers to learning, such as language or values. Obviously the client who does not understand the nurse's language will learn little. Western medicine may conflict with a clients cultural healing and practices. To be effective, nurses must deal directly with this conflict; otherwise the client may be partially or totally noncompliant with recommended treatments. Another impediment to learning is differing values held by the client and the health team. For example, a client who comes from a culture that does not value slimness may have difficulty learning about a reducing diet.

Psychomotor ability: It is important that the nurse be aware of a clients psychomotor skills when planning teaching. Psychomotor skills can be affected by health. For example, an older client who has severe osteoarthritis of the hands may not be able to tie a bandage. The following physical abilities are important for learning psychomotor skills:

i. *Muscle strength:* For example, an older client who cannot rise from a chair because of insufficient leg and muscle strength cannot be expected to learn to lift herself out of a bathtub.
ii. *Motor coordination:* Gross motor coordination is required for movements such as walking and fine motor coordination is needed when using utensils such as a fork for eating. For example, a client who has advanced amyotrophic lateral sclerosis (ALS) involving the lower limbs will probably be unable to use a walker.
iii. *Energy:* Energy is required for most psychomotor skills, and learning these skills uses more energy. People who are ill or elderly often have limited energy resources; learning and carrying out these skills must be timed for when the client's energy sources are not depleted.
iv. *Sensory acuity:* Sight is used for most learning (i.e. walking with crutches, changing a dressing, drawing a medication into a syringe). Clients who have a visual impairment often need the assistance of a support person to carry out such tasks.

It may be defined as the sum total of behavioral changes resulting from experience at training. Learning is said to have occurred if there is a change in the individual behavior. The entire process of learning is based on understanding and remembering. Many channels are functioning at the time of learning. The learning during a general education involves seeing (75%), hearing (13%), smelling (3%), testing (6%). While "On the Job" Training utilizes the sensory channel of feeling to the extent of 60 percent, hearing 10 percent, seeing 20 percent, smelling and testing 5 percent.

Learning Pattern

Nurse Managers need some understanding or the pattern in which new skills are learnt by the trainees. The 'learning curve' is shown in Figure 11.1.

In any learning process, after a certain level of proficiency, a span of time arrives in which no improvement takes place in the trainee. This period is later on followed by the increase in skill if the supervisor handles the situation intelligently. The period during which very little or no improvement takes place is known as 'plateau'. The plateau in the learning curve can be eliminated by improved methods of instruction.

The learning curve shows that when the trainee first begins to learn a new skill, he is likely to find himself unusually clumsy. During the early stage, the learner needs the trainer's encouragement. The duration of the first stage, will depend upon the complexity and newness of the skill being learnt. After this period the typical learning rate is raid. This is the stage of increasing returns, in which small additional amounts of practice by the trainee produce substantial increases in job proficiency. During this period, the trainee's confidence and satisfaction rises.

After more training time has elapsed, a plateau develops. Now additional training time does not result in significant increases in proficiency. At this stage the trainee begins to feel that there is nothing further to learn now at the place of his training. But this is only an illusion created by the plateau in the trainees learning curve. In order to push the curve of learning further up, what is needed is motivation to make renewed and vigorous efforts. This is where the trainees ability to learn on his own is really put to test. Therefore, a trainee should not be taken away by his phenomenon and should go ahead with renewed zeal.

The plateau in the training curve seems to be the result of two factors (i) loss of motivation because of the fact that further progress becomes more difficult and (ii) the trainee need for substantial blocks of time to develop new and improved skills. At the beginning the trainee may be forced to learn a new skill in segments, but a great deal of practice is required before a real breakthrough takes place which permits these separate parts to become merged and the motions to be joined into a single coordinated sequence of actions. To break away the plateau and to establish high level of proficiency some sort of motivation in the form of financial and nonfinancial incentives is required. Such motivation produces great concentration effort and a new attitude toward the job by which trainee can coordinate the elements of the job in a new way expressed as a whole.

One the trainee has achieved higher skill, he should be asked to continuously repeat the training so that over-learning takes place in the near future. *An experience swimmer can refrain from swimming for six months or even six years and still he will be able to swim when it is required.* This is largely the result of over-learning which reduces the likelihood of forgetting the skill. The rate of forgetting varies with the type of information, the extent to which it was originally learnt and the nature of individual. The relearning of material takes much less time than the original learning.

Conditions Favorable for Learning

Psychologists have experimented widely on different subjects of learning and prescribed the different factors favorable to each of them individually. Different conditions are ideal for different subjects of learning, in the presence of which learning is quicker, more efficient and permanent and it is desirable to pay close attention to these conditions. Learning may be accepted to be of three types:

1. Cognitive learning perceptual and conceptual
2. Motor learning
3. Affective learning conative.

a. Conditions Favorable for Cognitive Learning Perceptual and Conceptual

The cognitive perceptual and conceptual type of learning is made more effective by the following conditions:

1. *Beginning the Work with Enthusiasm*—The absence of enthusiasm is a detrimental factor because while it prevails no perceptual or conceptual learning can be carried into effect. Learning is an acting process and one which demands effort; the more enthusiastic a start, the more success is likely to attend the learning. Mere perception is inadequate for the understating of a perceptual subject while personal application gives better results and this is the reason for the importance given to experiments in the study of psychology. The slow speed in learning is due, largely, not to lack of intelligence but to the absence of enthusiasm.

2. *Distribution of the Time of Study*—It is better to learn a subject by introducing intervals in the time of study than to study uninterrupted for any length of time. The study of any subject should always be conducted on the interval pattern of time distribution. Spaced learning is better than unspaced learning.
3. *Presence of Assisting Factors*— The presence of assisting factors is of advantage in both perceptual and conceptual types of learning. The assistant factors in conceptual learning are—dictionary, tables and graphs, preparing an outline, writing a précis, taking notes, etc. for perceptual learning, the use of laboratory instruments in perceptual learning, the use of laboratory instruments in perception is desirable.
4. *Whole or Part Learning According to the Material to be Learnt*— The approach to learning, whether as a whole or part, depends upon the capacity of the learner and the quantity of the subject to be learnt. The whole method is good for intelligent learners and is shorter subjects while the part method is used with advantage by the intellectually weaker learners and in large subjects. Suppose we have to memorize a poem. Now, if we read the whole poem at once, the relation between the various lines will become clear and assist in the learning of it. If, on the other hand, the poem is difficult and lengthy, it would be better to divide it into parts than to study it as a whole. A student used to the part method of study finds the whole method inflexible and cumbersome. As a matter of fact, as far as the matter of studying books is concerned, it is better if the student first reads the whole book and then studies the chapters individually.
5. *Assistant Habits*—These too are of some importance in learning. To succeed, the student should form the habits of consulting the dictionary, making a fixed time table for study, not working when exhausted, using sketches, illustrations, and briefs, studying alone in the morning and evening, repeating the lesson, preparing according to plan and with regularity, minimizing lip movement and reading silently and concentrating the mind, etc.
6. *Other Assisting Conditions*—Besides the conditions mentioned above the following conditions also assist in study—absence of fatigue and boredom, presence of average brain, mental capacities and active attention, no nervous or emotional tension, absence of economic worries, absence of worry about personal and family problems.

b. Conditions Favorable to Motor Learning

The above mentioned conditions are also applicable to motor learning as much as they are applicable to cognitive learning. Practice is of great importance in motor learning, because it is the only way of obtaining skill. Reward is preferable to punishment but in some cases punishment may prove efficacious. Health rivalry also effects progress in motor as well as other learning but it should not be allowed to assume harmful proportions. The knowledge of results favors motor learning and it is an important condition because motor learning is not possible without it. In an experiment, ten students were made aware of the results while they were being trained. After some time, the light was switched off so that they no longer received any knowledge of the results. Consequently their learning curve steadily declined.

c. Conditions Favorable to Affective/Conative Learning

Those conditions which assist mental learning also assist, to no small degree, the Conative affective learning. This type of learning can also make considerable use of practice. The training of emotion is also significant in these kinds of learning. In affective Conative learning as in all others, punishment is of consequence in the cessation of mistakes while the making permanent of a response or the encouragement of effort is helped by reward. The elimination of the various types of tensions is also useful because they interrupt learning.

Meeting of Learning Needs of Clients by Nurses

Modern nursing is a complicated job. It requires a constant learning on the part of the nurse as newer techniques are always being discovered and invented in medical science. Thus knowledge of the learning process is helpful to the nurse not only while she is a student but throughout her career. The more she is prepared to receive new ideas, make new adjustments and learn new techniques, the more she will be successful in her profession. Learning is essential for development and modification of behavior, so the knowledge of learning process is useful when applied to clinical situations and academic events. The principles and process of learning helps the nurses to modify their own behavior which in turn to help in modifications of behavior of clients. But nurse must have well-defined purpose and goal in all learning situations.

Every patient, admitted in the hospital, has something unique about him. He cannot be treated as bed number so and so, the nurse should learn all possible things about him. This will lead to better adjustment and an early cure.

Like all people, clients have a variety of learning needs. A learning need is a desire or a requirement to know something that is presently unknown to the learner. Learning needs include new intellectual knowledge but can also include a new or different skill or physical ability, or a new behavior or a need to change an old behavior. Learning is a change in human disposition or capability that persists and that cannot be solely accounted for by growth. Learning is represented by a change in behavior.

Teaching: Client care for attributes of learning as mentioned below:

Learning is:

- An experience that occurs inside the learner
- The discovery of the personal meaning and relevance of ideas
- A consequence of experience
- A collaborative and cooperative process
- An evolutionary process
- A process that is both intellectual and emotional.

An important aspect of learning is the individual's desire to learn and to act on the learning, referred to as *compliance*. In the health care context, compliance is the extent to which a person's behavior coincides with medical or health advice. Compliance is best illustrated when the person recognizes and accepts the need to learn, and then follows through with the appropriate behaviors that reflect the learning. For example, a person diagnosed as having diabetes willingly learns about the special diet needed and then plans and follows the learned diet. The term compliance, however, is viewed in a negative perspective by many people because the term implies the learner is submissive and this is in conflict with the learners right to determine his or her own health care decisions rather than be told what to do by a health care professional.

Another term that is seen in health care literature is adherence, which is commitment or attachment to a regimen. Bastable (2003) explains that both compliance and adherence refer to the "ability to maintain health-promoting regimens, which are determined largely by a health care provider".

Andragogy is the art and science of teaching adults, in contrast to pedagogy, the discipline concerned with helping children learn. Geragogy is the term used to describe the process involved in stimulating and helping elders to learn.

Nurses can use the following andragogic concepts about adult learners as a guide for client teaching.

- As people mature, they move from dependence to independence
- An adults previous experiences can be used as a resource for learning
- An adults readiness to learn is often related to a developmental task or social role
- An adult is more oriented to learning when the material is useful immediately, not sometime in the future.

While meeting learning needs of clients nurses should teach them on the basis of type of learners. As given below:

- **Visual learners (learn through seeing):** These learners need to see the teacher's body language, hand gestures, eye contact and facial expression to fully understand the content of a lesson. They tend to prefer sitting at the front of the classroom to avoid visual obstruction. For example, if a visual learner is only presented with verbal information they will absorb and retain less information than if the verbal instructions were combined with visual materials. Tools used are books, videos, computers, posters.
- **Auditory learners (learn through listening):** They learn best through, verbal lectures, discussions, talking things through and listening to what others have to say. They interpret the underlying meanings of speech through listening to tone of voice, pitch, speed and other nuances. Tools used are talks, discussions, and debates.
- **Tactile/kinesthetic learners (learn through moving, doing and touching):** These learners learn best through a hands on approach, actively exploring the physical world around them. They may find it hard to sit still for long periods and may become distracted by their need for activity and exploration. The tools used are skits, drama and art.

Some diseases leave the patient crippled in one way or another and he has to learn news ways and techniques to substitute the function of the crippled organ. This requires knowledge of the learning process by the patient as well as by the nurse. This knowledge gives them hope and confidence and ultimately success. This knowledge is equally useful during the period of convalescence. Both the patient and the nurse should be prepared to learn new ways and techniques discovered by medical scientists. Knowledge of the psychology of learning, therefore, is a prerequisite for the nurse.

Use of Principles of Learning

The learning principles which should be taken into account in designing, a training program can be summarized as follows:

a. The learner should be motivated to learn.
b. The response should be meaningfully related to each other and to the motives which the learner brings with him into the situation.
c. The new responses should be reinforced by some reward or information that the response has been made correctly.
d. The new responses to be learnt should not be in conflict with old response. If they do, the training should provide an opportunity for the old responses. If they do, the training

should provide an opportunity for the old responses to be unlearnt before the new response are learnt.

e. The learner should be an active participant in the learning process.
f. The learning situation provides opportunities to practice the new responses and allows for 'plateau' periods of little improvement which often precede marked improvements.
g. The new responses to be learnt should be broken down into learnable units and presented in an appropriately placed sequence.
h. Coaching should be available to help the learner develop new responses.
i. The learning situation should allow for individual differences in the speed of learning, the depth of learning and should be designed as per individual requirements.

Whole *versus* Part Learning

This refers to the amount of the training content that are presented to the trainees. Whether the whole or the part training is superior depends upon the particular situation. Thus in the development of training but rather particular practice should be used which seems appropriate to specific situation. Following factors are important in one or more situations of whole versus part learning:

i. For the more intelligent subject the whole method of learning should be used.
ii. The advantages of whole method increases with practice.
iii. The meaningful material favor the whole method.
iv. Part method of learning requires the need of connecting the separately learnt parts.
v. Very short and very long passage call for the whole method of learning while in between favor part learning.

Knowledge of Results

There are two ways in which the principle of knowledge of results can have an effect upon learning:

i. In providing the basis for correcting one's errors.
ii. In making the task more interesting and meaningful to the learner.

An operator would have trouble in learning to manipulate the controls of an equipment unless he knew how the equipment respond to his control action. W Stockbride and B Chambers in 'Aiming Transfer Learning and knowledge of results' dealt with rifle practice. The situation was one in which men fired rifles at moving targets in a simulated rifle range where 'knowledge of results' was furnished to the subjects.

The subjects were divided into two equal groups, one receiving the feedback which other did not receive any feedback of results. The figures shows that the second group leveled off in its performance while the first group continued to improve.

In providing feedback or knowledge to trainees, following are some considerations which should be kept in mind:

i. Knowledge about the trainees' performance to the feedback should specific rather than general.
ii. Trainees should not be overburdened with information. Only the necessary information should be presented which is appropriate for the proficiency of the trainees.
iii. Feedback about the trainee's performance should be immediate otherwise its impact is lost.

Being an educator or teacher is an important and primary role for the nurse. Clients and families have the right to health education in order to make informed decisions about their health. The nurse is in a position to promote healthy lifestyles through the application of health knowledge, the change process, learning theories, and the nursing and teaching process when teaching clients and their families.

- Learning is represented by a change in behavior.
- Three main theories of learning are behaviorism, cognitivism, and humanism.
- Bloom has identified three learning domains, cognitive, affective and psychomotor.
- A number of factors affect learning, including motivation, readiness, active involvement, relevance, feedback, nonjudgmental support, repetition, timing, environment, emotions, physiologic events, psychomotor ability and cultural aspects.
- Teaching, like the nursing process, consists of six activities: assessing the learner, diagnosing learning needs, developing a teaching plan, implementing the plan, evaluating learning outcomes and teaching effectiveness, and documenting instructional activities.
- Teaching strategies chosen by the nurse should be suited to the client and to the material to be learned.
- A teaching plan is a written plan consisting of learning outcomes, content to teach, and strategies to use in teaching the content. The plan must be revised when the client's needs change or the teaching strategies prove ineffective.
- Evaluating the teaching-learning process is both an ongoing and a final process in which the client, nurse and support people determine what has been learned.
- Documentation of client teaching is essential to communicate the teaching to other health professionals and to provide a record for legal and accreditation purposes.

The trends in nursing explains how the nursing as a profession has improved. More detailed, complex studies, researchers, new medical instruments and equipments and specialization and superspecialization in nursing are all in dire need of well-qualified and practically efficient nurse. The student nurse must have clear goals for learning. She has to learn theoretical as well as practical knowledge of nursing. She must update her knowledge and learn new equipments and techniques for better patient care.

In the hospital, she should have good understanding and learn more about each patient. Involving the patient and relatives in performing nursing procedures and health education, the student nurse requires the knowledge of learning process. She learns through observation limitation, reinforcement and punishment, practice, assignments, presentations and so on.

Teaching Client Education

Teaching client education is a major aspect of nursing practice and an important independent nursing function. A patients bill of rights mandating client education as a right of all clients. In addition, legislation related to nursing frequently has included client teaching as a function of nursing, thereby making teaching a legal and professional responsibility.

Client education is multifaceted, involving promoting, protecting and maintaining health. It involves teaching about reducing health risk factors, increasing a person's level of wellness and taking specific protective health measures.

Areas of Client Education

i. Promotion of Health

- Increasing a person's level of wellness
- Growth and development topics
- Fertility control
- Hygiene
- Exercise
- Nutrition
- Stress management
- Lifestyle modification
- Resources within the community.

ii. Prevention of Illness/Injury

- Health screening (e.g. blood glucose levels, blood pressure, blood cholesterol, Pap test, mammograms, vision, hearing, routine physical examinations)
- Reducing health risk factors (e.g. lowering cholesterol level)
- Specific protective health measures (e.g. immunizations, use of condoms, use of sunscreen, use of medication, umbilical cord care)
- First aid
- Safety (e.g. using seat belts, helmets, walkers).

iii. Restoration of Health

- Information about tests, diagnosis, treatment, medications
- Self-care skills or skills needed to care for family member
- Resources within health care setting and community.

iv. Adopting to Altered Health and Function

- Adaptation in lifestyle
- Problem-solving skills
- Adaptation to changing health status
- Strategies to deal with current problems (e.g. home IV skills, medications, diet, activity limits, prostheses)
- Strategies to deal with future problems (e.g. fear of pain with terminal cancer, future surgeries, or treatments)
- Information about treatments and likely outcomes
- Referrals to other health care facilities or services
- Facilitation of strong self-image
- Grief and bereavement counseling.

Teaching is a system of activities intended to produce learning. The teaching process is intentionally designed to produce specific learning.

The teaching-learning process involves dynamic interaction between teacher and learner. Each participant in the process communicates informations, emotions, perceptions, and attitudes to the other. The teaching process and the nursing process are much alike.

Nurses teach a variety of learners in various settings. They teach clients and their families or significant others in the hospital, the home, or in assisted living and long-term care facilities. Nurses teach large and small groups of learners in community health education programs.

Nurses also teach professional colleagues and other health care personnel in academic institutions such as vocational schools, colleges, and universities, and in health care facilities such as hospitals or nursing homes.

Teaching Clients and Their Families

Nurses may teach individual clients in one-to-one teaching episodes. For example, the nurse may teach about wound care while changing a client's dressing or may teach about diet, exercise, and other lifestyle behaviors that minimize the risk of a heart attack for a client who has a cardiac problem. The nurse may also be involved in teaching family members or other support people who are caring for the client. Nurses working in obstetric and pediatric areas teach parents and sometimes grandparents how to care for children.

Because of decreased length of hospital stays, time constraints on client education may occur. Nurses need to provide client education that will ensure the client's safe transition from one level of care to another and make appropriate plans for follow-up education in the client's home. Discharge plans must include both information about what the client has been taught before transfer or discharge and what remains for the client to learn to perform self-care in the home or other residence. Nurses using nursing process in taking care of client and providing education for the client and families by using teaching process. The comparison for both processes shown in Table 11.2.

Teaching in the community: Nurses are often involved in community health education programs. Such teaching activities may be voluntary as part of the nurse's involvement in an organization such as the Red Cross or Planed Parenthood, or they may be compensated as part of the nurse's work role. Community teaching activities my be aimed at large groups of people who have an interest in some aspect of health, such as nutrition classes, CPR or cardiac risk factor reduction classes, and bicycle or swimming safety programs. Community education programs can also be designed for small groups or individual learners, such as childbirth classes or family planning classes.

Teaching health personnel: Nurses are also involved in the instruction of professional colleagues. Nurses in nursing practice settings are often involved in the clinical instruction of nursing students. Experienced nurses may function as preceptors for new graduate nurses or for newly employed nurses. Nurses with specialized knowledge and experience may share that knowledge and experience with nurses who are new to that practice area.

Table 11.2: Comparison of the teaching process and the nursing process

Step	*Teaching Process*	*Nursing Process*
1	Collect data; analyze client's learning strengths and deficits.	Collect data; analyze client's strengths and deficits
2	Make educational diagnoses	Make nursing diagnoses
3	Preparing teaching outcomes • Write learning outcomes • Select content and time frame • Select teaching strategies	Plan nursing goals/desired outcomes and select interventions
4	Implement teaching plan	Implement nursing strategies
5	Evaluate client learning based on achievement of learning outcomes	Evaluate client outcomes based on achievement of goal criteria

Such specialized courses include acute care nursing, perioperative nursing, and quality improvement/quality assurance.

Nurses may also be involved in teaching other health professionals. Nurses may participate in the education of medical students or allied health students. In this capacity, the nurse educator is often clarifying the role of the nurse for other health professionals or how the nurse can assist them in their care of the client. The nurse may also teach health care colleagues knowledge or skills that are considered the domain of nursing, such as nonpharmaceutical comfort measures.

Reward versus Punishment

The experience has shown that punishment is less effective in learning that reward. The punishment can fix the undesirable behavior but it cannot eliminate altogether and it may have some undesirable side effects such as disliking of the punishing person. In fact the mild punishment executed immediately following the undesirable behavior and suitably placed the efficiency of learning is more.

Spacing of Learning Periods

In most of the learning situations the length and spacing of learning periods are important factor for carrying out efficient training. Learning is more effective when it is split into periods rather than being continuous. The length and spacing of the material depends to a great extent on the material to able learnt if the learning is split into more steps, there are fewer mistakes. Efficiency of learning is more.

Role of Learner

Management can only provide facility and help for individual development and development cannot be a substitute for individual responsibility for self-development. As such each individuals should be made to realize that he provide a climate where an individual should be able to develop himself according to his own need and desire. The employee will make efforts for self-development if there is a:

i. Desire for development
ii. Right climate
iii. Proper encouragement
iv. Proper reward.

To introduce the above, the training specialist must interview the experienced employees and should get their ideas on training needs, goals, and appropriate techniques to satisfy them.

Transfer theory of learning: It refers to the popular concept that man should be given training in a general way which includes language, mathematics and classics. This training in these areas is transferred positively to various walks of life. It is found that formal education is transferred to various life situations and vocations. Hence, it is also called "theory of identical elements".

The laws of effective learning are dealt in Chapter 12.

12 CHAPTER

Habits, Skills and Interest

Introduction

Habit can be described as an automatic behavior as all work activated by habit takes place without thinking or volition. Some of our activities like dressing, sitting or eating take place casually everyday due to habits. Habits may either take place casually every day due to habits. Habits may either be good or bad. Some habits like early rising, regular study, less eating, etc., are classified as good habits while drinking, lying and abusing are categorized as bad habits. Every one is desirous of forming good habits, though it is difficult to know how to go about doing it. It has been found that number of activities performed by other persons that seem to be quite easy and mechanical though initially they were quite difficult and tiresome. Our walking, talking, dressing, eating, writing, smoking, typing, driving, swimming are all such acts. All these learned activities are commonly known by the term 'habit'. A number of attempts have been made to define the term 'habit' in a suitable way. Let us have a look at them.

1. "Habit is the name given to behavior so often repeated as to be automatic".—Garrett
2. "By strict definition, those acts are habitual which are performed with little or no thought and always in approximately the same way".—Sturt and Oakden
3. A habitual action "is the result of many repetitions of the act in approximately the same way. It is done without conscious thought, performed smoothly and with the maximum speed required".—Ryburn

Characteristics of Habit

These definitions point out that habits are the product of experiences and practice. Initially what we do, think or feel, may require a voluntary and deliberate attention and strenuous efforts on our part. But when this particular action is repeated several times, almost in the same way under the similar circumstances, it does not require voluntary attention and efforts and tends to become quite automatic like reflex-action. It is now termed as habitual action and thus a habit is established.

In addition to the above discussion the following characteristics of habitual behavior may also throw light on the nature of habits.

1. Acquired dispositions: Habits are acquired dispositions. They are not innate and inherited.

2. Uniformity: Habitual actions are uniform actions. They are performed every time in the same way.
3. Promptness: Habitual actions are performed with promptness. This action is so quick and speedy that it resembles reflex action.
4. Ease and facility: Habitual actions are performed with great ease and facility. In the beginning one may feel difficulty in performing some task but once habit is established it is performed smoothly with great ease and facility.
5. Accuracy: Habit brings accuracy in the action. We see an Accountant adding columns of figures all day without a single mistake. Similarly a typist can be able to type with great accuracy only due to his developed habit.
6. Reducing the need of paying attention: Habitual acts are performed with least attention or no attention. Women do their knitting, almost paying no attention to the work. Similarly the person playing on harmonium or violin places his fingers on the required place with no careful attention on his part.
7. Diminishing fatigue: Habit diminishes fatigue. Due to habit formation, the work that is too difficult and tiresome in the beginning becomes to simple and spontaneous engagement for hours. The fact can be easily verified when we observe a driver driving the bus on a long route for hours. Actually with the habit of driving he learns to make the fewest and simplest movements and thus does not become the victim of fatigue easily.
8. Resistance to modifications: Habitual actions possess a strong tendency of resisting any modification or change. Once a habit, good or bad, is formed, it is difficult to give it up or bring changes in this functioning. A habitual smoker or gambler finds it difficult to give up his habit of smoking or gambling. On the other hand a man who is not accustomed to accept bribe cannot be allowed to accept bribe and thus change his habit.
9. Nervous system is the base of habits: The nervous system is the principal factor information of habits. The role played by nervous system has been described beautifully by Ryburn, in the following words:
   "Nerves carry messages to and from the brain. When approximately the same message is taken to the brain, and the same answer comes back, for the same action to result, a kind of track is worn. So that the answer to the message carried to the brain becomes more and more automatic. It becomes more and more difficult for any other answer to come to the in-going message than the one that one has been given again and again in response to what is approximately the same message. Thus the basis of habit is this groove, as it were, which is born in the nerves".
10. Habits have a large field of operation: Habits do not confine themselves to conative acts alone. We may have habits of thoughts as well as of feelings.
11. Habits are useful as well as harmful: In general, habits are divided into two groups—good habits and bad habits. Good habits like speaking the truth, punctuality, proper habits of work, etc. are considered useful for the welfare of the individual as well as of the society whereas bad habits like smoking, gambling, telling lies, etc. are considered harmful to both the individual and the society.

Habits, instincts and reflex actions are many times confused with one another as all of them are automatic and mechanical. They do not need any voluntary attention. They have similar characteristics marked by uniformity, accuracy, promptness, ease and facility. But there are so many points of difference which makes them quite different from one another. They are—

i. Instincts as well as reflex actions are universal and are found in all the members of any one species. But habits are individual and specific.
ii. Reflex actions are thoroughly mechanical. We sneeze almost in the same way as our remote ancestors did. They are incapable of any modification or change. But instinctive and habitual actions are capable of modification and change.
iii. Instincts as well as reflex actions are innate and inborn while the habitual action are acquired and learned.
iv. Reflex actions are regarded as somatic or physiological phenomenon while the habitual and instinctive actions are considered physical or mental.

Importance of Habits

Habits play an important role in one's life. If we analyze our day-to-day behavior and activities, we would find that a major portion of them is dominated by our habits. Our acts like sleeping, walking, talking, writing are nothing but the spontaneous, mechanical habitual actions. Through habit formation it is impossible to do more than one thing at a time. Women knit, spin and cook while they talk. Thus, habit brings great economy in our life. As a result we can save out energy and time for the more important things of life. Absence of habits hampers the progress of an individual as James observes, there is no miserable human being them one in whom nothing in habitual but indecision, and for whom the lighting of every cigar, the drinking of every cup, the time of rising and going to bed everyday and the beginning of every bit of work are subjects of express volitional deliberations. Full half of the time of such a man goes to the deciding, or matters which ought to be so ingrained in him as practically not to exist for his consciousness at all.

The man is known by his habits as his personality is clothed in habits. All the personality traits—good or bad are reflected through one's habits. Man in fact, is a creature of habits. He tends to become what he repeatedly practices. One who is habitual of gambling, smoking, eve-teasing, stealing, etc. is sure to develop into a socially undesirable, unscrupulous person while the one who practices honesty, regularity, generosity, industriousness will become a useful and productive member of society. Not only our actions but our interests, aptitudes, attitudes, beliefs, prejudices, opinions, faiths, feelings, emotions and sentiments are influenced and controlled by our habits. Therefore, in short what a man is, has been or will be, is decided by his habits of thoughts, actions and feelings.

In the field of education too, habits exercise a strong impact. Good habits help acquiring, learning and knowing of so many things with great ease and facility. The student who is habitual of concentrating on his studies for hours in school as well as at home is not easily overcome by fatigue. Similarly habits of efficient writing, reading and conversation help them a lot. Habits of proper reasoning, thinking, making judgments, punctuality, regularity, neatness, cooperativeness, honesty—all help them in their proper adjustments as well as in acquiring and learning all the essential knowledge and skills in a short time with great facility.

Thus in all walks of one's life and sphere of activities, habits tend to play a decisive role in making or marring one's present and future depending upon their nature—good or bad. While good habits are responsible to infuse in an individual what is good from social and moral angles, the bad habits create obstacles in the path of his proper development, bring bad name to him and prove dangers to the society.

It is, therefore, essential that proper care should be taken to develop desirable habits of work, though and feeling in children from the very beginning. They should not be allowed to pick up undesirable or bad habits. In case if they are found to develop any evil habit they should be helped to get rid of them. In the following pages we would try to pay attention over these aspects.

Formation of Habits

Formation of a habit is an important aspect of the learning process. When we first learn an activity it takes a certain amount of time, energy and will power. We have to plan the activity and make deliberate efforts to do it. When we have repeated this a large number of times, and when it has become a habit, it becomes so easy to do it. There is no necessity for deliberate effort to do it. The will power plays practically no part. The time factor is very much reduced. The activity becomes very easy to perform. It becomes almost an automatic activity without any conscious deliberation, almost like a reflex action. Since there is an economy of energy and time, formation of good habits is necessary to increase our efficiency. But they can be formed only after patient and sustained practice. In the initial stages, there will be difficulty and inertia. Unless we determine to break through these difficulties and persist in our efforts, the habit cannot be formed.

Breaking a bad habit is of equal interest to us. Whereas good habits help us to be more efficient, bad habits pull us down. Often, we struggle to break our bad habits. Through ignorance and carelessness and because of various other reasons, we might have formed some bad habits. Later, we realize they are bad habits, and wish to break those habits. Often we find it very difficult to do so. Psychology has a few simple suggestions to offer to anyone who wants to break a bad habit.

1. If that particular activity can be associated with some painful or disgusting experience, then the "law of effect" operates, and it may be easier for us to break that habit.
2. A psychologist, Dunlap by name, has demonstrated the value of particular method to break certain kinds of habits. Suppose someone has a bad habit of biting his nails, and he wants to get rid of that habit. He could go before a mirror and deliberately bite the nails several times. This could be repeated two or three times everyday. It is important, however, that while doing so, he should silently repeat to himself that he is biting his nails deliberately. If the habit is not complicated by being connected to some deep-seated unconscious complex, it is quite possible that after a few days, the activity, we make it a conscious one. As a habit, it is more or less unconscious, and so, we have no control over it. When we make it into a conscious deliberate activity, then we will be able to exert control over it. Thus in the course of time, the conscious mind gets mastery over the habit and we are able to break the habit.

Just as in the case of the formation of a habit, in the attempt to break one also, we must be consistent, fully determined and allow no exceptions to occur. There should be a proper motivation to break the habit. We must fully believe in the undesirable consequences of the habit. The gains from breaking the habit should be properly related to our main philosophy of life and aspirations in life. Unless there is such a strong motivation, it may not be easy to break a habit.

The following general rules are found to be useful in the task of habit formation:

1. To start in the earlier age. The early years of childhood are very important from the point of view of habit formation. Younger age is marked with too much plasticity and receptivity. It is the most impressionable or formative period of life. Most of our habits,

good or bad are the product of this age. Therefore, it is proper to keep an eye over the youngsters. They should be provided with congenial environment for developing proper habits. The inculcation of right habits in children should be started as early as possible so that they may be saved from picking up wrong habits and modes of action, thoughts and feelings.

2. Firm determination and initiative. Firm determination and powerful initiative help much in the acquisition of desirable habits. It is said where there is a will there is a way. If you decide that you would like to get up early in the morning, decide it with all the firmness and launch the new habit with all the initiative of which you are capable. A public announcement or pledge, that you would get up early or attend the playground regularly from such and such date, can prove a powerful initiative to start with. It provides a strong emotional stimulus and ego involvement and thus provides the most appropriate environment for launching the new habit.
3. Setting up definite specification for the new habit. It is of no use to declare that from tomorrow I will be good boy or I will work hard with my studies. Such vague resolutions do not materialize. If one really intends to study harder he should chalk out a definite schedule of hours and subjects and stick to it.
4. Seizing the very first opportunity to act. It is of no use to make resolution after resolution not to put even a single of them into action. It is not proper to wait for the future. Tomorrow never comes. When you determine to develop a habit, it is better not to postpone it for the next day and so on.
5. Starting along the right track. In an attempt to form a new habit, one should start in the right direction from the very first time. The initial mistakes are very costly. It is difficult to unlearn the wrong practices and improper habit. Therefore early stages of habit formation must be watched over very carefully and every precaution should be taken to make the students learn the things rightly.
6. Sufficient practice and repetition. For the habit formation it is essential that action should be repeated frequently in the same way under similar circumstances. Therefore, sufficient opportunities for practice and repetition should be provided to the students for the formation of desirable habits. It requires great patience on their part. They must be made to make persistent efforts in practicing a particular mode of behavior (action, through or feeling) until it is established into a habit.
7. Allowing no exception in the persistent efforts. It is not enough to get a right start along the right track in the information of habits. In making persistent efforts for the repetition and practice of a particular mode of behavior (which is established as a habit) it is kept in mind that no exceptions are made to it. Every exception to the habit permitted helps to defeat our purpose. If one tries to reach school in time, one can never do it by reaching in time for two days and then going late on the third day.
8 Due appreciation and encouragement. Pleasure giving and satisfying behavior or response tends to be repeated. Therefore, the good behavior and conduct of the students should get proper appreciation and encouragement. Public praise and reward work as a great motivating force to children. They do not only help in developing good habits among those who are rewarded but also stimulate others to pick up the desirable habit.

Psychologists have come across many laws in their search for ways of forming or breaking habits, some of the important elements being mentioned below:

1. *As enthusiastic a start in the work as is possible:* The original enthusiasm in the breaking of habits is of importance because it helps to contradict the old habits. There is a well

known English proverb 'Well begun is half one' which means that if some work is started properly half of the work is almost done. This proverb means that a new work should be started with enthusiasm.

2. *Voluntary repetition of new work:* The application of will power in the formation of new habits is essential. Voluntary repetition of the new habits is essential. If we want to make a habit of getting up at four in the morning, we should go to sleep after having made up our mind to get up at four in the morning. This determination should be voluntary. After we become used to getting up at four in the morning the necessity of making an effort is eliminated.
3. *Absence of exception:* Another important principle in the formation of habits is the absence or avoidance of any exception in the process of formation. If, for example, a student decides to from the habit of regular study and accordingly makes a timetable to which he address enthusiastically and strictly for about days, but on the fifth he decides to leave it off and enjoy life for a bit, not realizing the harm in this practice, he will never form the habit he wants to. He will, instead, form the habit of putting off his work, because this tendency gradually gains strength and in the process, weakens his will power. In fact, the most difficult step in the formation of a habit is not its inception but rather the avoidance of any exceptions which may threaten to break its habit. Many people take to physical exercise, but how many see it through? The failure to take exercise one day puts you back six days in the direction of the formation of the habit. Thus, using this as an example, if you want to form some habit, do not interrupt it no matter what the pain, laziness, necessity, because if you once succumb to any allurement no extent of effort on occasions will make up for it and you will never succeed in your attempt.
4. *Use of negative adaptation:* The application of negative adaptation to the formation or breaking of habits is very important. It means learning not to repeat the habitual response. If an adult mouse is given an electric shock every time he comes near females, he will gradually avoid them. If a drunkard is given adulterated wine which causes him to vomit violently he will run away from wine.

The formation or breaking of habits represents two facets of the same process. If one wants to form the habit of early rising, he will have to give up the habit of late rising. The habit of daily exercise involves the riddance of the habit of abstaining from exercise. Thus to break a habit, it is necessary to form the opposite habit. Hence the same three laws of the formation of habits prove efficacious in the breaking of habits as well.

If a habitual drunkard wants to give up his habit of drinking he is well-advised to make an enthusiastic beginning and to avoid drinking inconsiderate of any distractions whatsoever. If a regular smoker finds himself unable to think of any discrepancy in smoking one more cigarettes, he will never give it up, even if he were anxious to do so. One intending to give up a habit should close the door to it like Suryaji, a prominent general of Shivaji. He once entered the castle of an enemy by climbing up a wall with the help of a rope. When the fight started some less determined soldiers in his group beat a hasty retreat to the only means of escape, the rope. Suryaji did not approve of this, and, not intending to put up with this show of cowardice, he cut the rope so that there may be no way to escape. Now the soldiers fought gallantly and won the battle.

Bad habits are harmful to the individual as well as to the society. Therefore, it is needless to say that they should not be allowed to grow. But as we usually find evils and vices are more easily caught and spread than goodness and virtues, so the bad habits also are easily picked up. They are the blots on the personality of an individual. Therefore, every attempt should be made to get rid of them. The following suggestions can be found fruitful in breaking bad habits:

1. Firm determination and strong will power. First of all one should realize the necessity of setting oneself free from the pawn of a bad habit. Then one should have a firm determination to break it. Thus there is a need of strong will power so that the temptations, however powerful they may be, should be over-come. Exceptions should never be allowed as a single action of the repetition of a bad habit may bring back the individual on the starting point.
2. Strong initiative with quick action. Bad habits are like powerful and dangerous enemy. Therefore, the initial attack should be well-planned. One should leave nothing to chance public declarations and pledges help much in this direction as they give sufficient emotional strength to an individual. One who declares publically that one would not smoke from such and such date, receives an inner strength to give up his bad habit. But mere declaration and resolution do not suffice. They should be followed by actions.
3. Use of voluntary practice. Many improper habitual actions can be rectified by the use of voluntary practice. Incorrect spellings, mispronunciation, improper way of performing certain skilled work, etc. can be corrected and improved by adopting and practicing the right way of performing these acts.
4. Substitution of bad habits by the appropriate socially approved behavior. One of the convenient approaches in removing the bad habits is to replace them by socially desirable habits. These socially desirable habits gradually make the bad habits die their natural death. That is why the person who wishes to give up his habit of smoking is often advised to take cough drops or betel nuts, when the urge to smoke is strong. Similarly bad habits like telling lies, negligence, improper eating habits, etc. can be replaced by truth telling, care and proper eating habits for making them neutralized in a course of time.
5. To hit on the root causes of the bad habits. The root causes of the bad habits should be discovered and attempts should be made to remove these causes. If we try to analyze the genesis of bad habits we can find that many habits are developed due to so many varying reasons. Sometimes they are formed due to certain complexes, inner conflicts, or emotional disturbances. Nervous habits like nail biting, pen-chewing, and nose picking belongs to this category. No direct measure is useful in removing such habits. The emotional factor which causes such habits should be taken into consideration and children should be indirectly told to give up such undesirable habits.

Physical defects also sometimes cause bad habits. Proper medical care and treatment in such cases should be arranged. Bad company and uncongenial atmosphere at home and the school also contribute in developing bad habits. In this way, bad habits are developed on account of so many personal and environmental causes. The roots of all such causes should be discovered and attempts should be made to remove all such causes.

In the end we can say, that teacher should try to seek an active cooperation of the parents digging out the root causes. It is the duty of the parents, elder members of the society and teachers to make their best attempts to provide good and congenial environment to children. They must not do what they intend not to be done by the youngsters. Their own behavior should be a model for the inculcation of good habits among the children. It will help not only in checking the growth of bad habits but will provide strong stimulation of the development of desirable habits among the youngsters.

Some of the important facts connected with this subject are given below:

1. *Breaking of habits by voluntary practice:* To make a practice of making a mistake willfully is a good way of getting rid of it. Mistakes in typewriting can be conclusively eliminated by their willful repetition. If a person persists in spelling 'the' as 'the' he should commit the mistake knowingly in order that he may get rid of it. If we knowingly spell it that way time and again we become used to it and are in a position to control it and eliminate it. We are unable to control many habits like wrinkling the nose, making faces, coughing uselessly because we do not know their causes. Conscious repetition tends to give us a control over them, thus facilitating their cessation at will.
2. *The formation of a contradictory habit to break it:* It is sometimes possible to break a habit by the formation of a contradictory habit. People frightened of a mob can be cured of it by being forced to attend. If a person has fallen into the bad habit of remaining dumb in company, he should force himself to speak wherever people get together. Thus he will get rid of this habit.
3. *Breaking of habit by doing it to excess:* Some habits are broken by doing them excessively. If a drunkard drinks too much and makes himself ill, the bitter experience may break his propensity towards drink. This, however, depends very much on the effect the illness has on the individual and the strength of his habit. And this makes it clear that all habits cannot be broken by bitter experience and loss of interest.
4. *Formation of other habits:* Some people desirous of breaking a habit adopt the unpsychological method of struggling with the habit, taking oaths ever so often of giving it up and concentrating upon it. This method is rarely, if at all, successful. If a habit has to be broken, it does not pay to struggle with it, but to form some new habit contradictory to the previous one, to forget about it and substitute some other work for it. If we, for example, want to give up smoking, it will serve no purpose to swear about it and to get excited. One should become indifferent towards cigarettes, interest oneself in some work and put some chewing gum or lemon drops in the mouth whenever there is a desire to smoke.
5. *Meditating on the evil of aspect of the habit:* Indian psychologists have laid great importance upon meditation on the evil aspect of habit in the breaking of a bad habit. One should not run from a cigarette but analyze and contemplate the harms involved. It makes the breaking of habit easier.

Habits and the Nurse

Habits are time saving and energy saving techniques. However difficult a task may be in the beginning, and whatever hard work it may involve, if the nurse develops a habit of doing it cheerfully and accurately, it becomes easy for her. Habits are not only mental but also physical since they require control and coordination of muscles and correct reaction time. The profession of a nurse requires both these. For example, patients are constantly coming in and going out of the hospital, their nursing has to be regularly requires regular habits in the nurses. James Maxims, a pioneer in psychology of habits, has underlined the following Maxims for forming correct habits:

i. In order to form a habit, we should make a strong start. We should launch ourselves with as strong and decided an initiative as possible. We should start with determination and must feel the strong need of making the new habit a part of our mental equipment.

ii. We should not allow any exception to occur till the new habit is firmly rooted in our life. Lapses should not be allowed to occur. Postponement of practice and permission of exceptions hinder the building of a new habit.
iii. We should seize all the possible opportunities that help in the formation of a habit and avoid those which do not help. For example, to form the habit of getting up early in the morning I should start immediately and try to be in the company of students who have formed this habit. I should decline all midweek invitations if I want to form the habit of studying in the evening and get down to study promptly after dinner.
iv. We should practice the new habit. Mere resolution or determination will not be sufficient. We need faithful, persistent, day-by-day practice until the desired goal has been achieved.

Habit formation, however, is only one side of the picture. While we know the advantages of habit formation, we are also aware of the tyranny of wrong habits. The nurse should, therefore, also remember the laws for breaking wrong habits. Forming correct habit and breaking a wrong habit are the two aspects of the same process.

Development of Study Habits in Nursing

The student nurse should

1. Study with a definite purpose in mind
2. Evaluate immediate and remote goals
3. Provide a definite place for study
4. See that physical conditions are conducive to study
5. Plan and follow a definite time schedule
6. Look for the main ideas in the reading material
7. Cultivate the habit of reading rapidly and carefully
8. Outline the study material
9. Make brief, well-organized notes in your own language
10. Evaluate the difficulty of the material
11. While reading, raise significant question on the material to be learned; then answer them
12. Study with intent to recall
13. Attend carefully to all illustrative material
14. Complete all study assignments
15. Let active study and rest period be interspersed with each other
16. Try to learn the unit or the lesson as a 'whole' when possible
17. Concentrate on what you are studying at the time
18. Shut out all emotional distractions
19. Over learn sufficiently so that delayed recall is possible
20. Learn to summarize and review what you have learned or read
21. Be alert to ideas emphasized by the teacher
22. Think over the statements made by the author and try to challenge them
23. Find out the several authorities say about a topic or an idea
24. Make intelligent use of the dictionary.

Learning starts from the moment of birth and continues till death. For successful adjustment with life, he has to acquire knowledge about many things, change his behavior according to the needs of the situation. The child starts to understand the world around him through learning.

The language development, development of basic values, knowledge regarding various aspects of life all come through learning or training. The process of learning has, therefore, tremendous importance for the human beings and for some animals to live and exist. Without learning, life becomes completely meaningless, capacity to adjust becomes nil.

Skills and the Nurse

In the words of Boring, Langfeld and Weld *"When we acquire through learning a coordinated series of responses which are performed with proficiency, we speak of the accomplishment as skill".*

In this way, skills are the efficient ways of performing certain tasks. We try to acquire proficiency in performing some activities or task with the help of learning some skills. Successfully and efficiently performing the tasks like speaking, typing, driving a car, flying a plane, playing a piano, reciting a poem, playing badminton and hitting a moving target, drawing a geometrical design, adding and multiplying long digits, performing experiments and handling various instruments are all skills. Learning a particular skill helps an individual to acquire speed and accuracy in the field of operation of that skill and creates a sort of confidence in him to perform the task with great ease and satisfaction. In this way learning of skills is indispensable for us in case if we aim to lead an effective and fruitful life.

Nursing is a skilled profession. That is why it requires a long training running into years not months. According to Munn, a skill is proficiency in the performance of a task. This proficiency has to be learnt by constant practice and a sound knowledge of the principles of the profession. Besides, it requires a keen interest and a strong desire, a clear and definite idea and instructions from those who and sometimes even demonstrations by the instructors and teachers. In order to develop skill for her profession the Nurse should remember the following suggestions:

1. Read as much literature concerning your profession as you can.
2. Develop a keen interest and strong desire for your profession since unless there is sufficient motivation, one does not become skilled in a job.
3. Do not allow any gaps in your learning. Avoid exceptions as far as possible.
4. Practice the different functions involved in your job for a sufficiently long time so that they may become a second nature.
5. Get instructions about specialized functions from specialized instructors. If you have an occasion to observe a demonstration, observe it keenly and remove your doubts if you are allowed to do so.
6. Avoid all emotions and conflicts in your profession. Try to develop a cool and detached mind so that your job may be facilitated.
7. Use all your intelligence and skill already given to you in your present profession.
8. Do not avoid any job which you come across in your professions but try to do it however difficult it may appear at first sight. Do not look for help on all the occasions but try to do maximum work yourself.
9. Develop a habit of introspection and self-criticism so that you may yourself understand your difficulties and pitfalls. Remember that if you are not prepared to improve, none else can improve you. An intention for improvement is a must in the mastery of all skills.

Some life skills may be used to for promotion of positive health, and these skills should be taught to every individual to maintain positive mental health includes problem-solving, decision making, creative thinking, critical thinking, effective communication, interpersonal relationship, self-awareness, coping, cropathy and so on.

Developing or Improving Skills

Every skill, whatever it may be, requires a series of organized actions or responses that have to be learned and get fixed for acquiring desired proficiency. All the learning principles and theories discussed in the chapter can help a lot in devising methods and techniques of acquiring desired skills. Therefore, a wise teacher must try to exploit all of these learning methods and techniques for developing the required skills in his pupils. However, the following points may prove more beneficial to him in guiding his students towards the development of a skill in a special area:

1. *Readiness to acquire a skill:* Unless or until one is ready for the acquisition of a certain skill one cannot be made to learn or acquire that skill. Therefore the first step in guiding a learner towards the development of any skill is to make him ready to learn that skill. He must be given adequate incentive or sufficient motivation to start the learning of skill with great enthusiasm and efforts.
2. *Securing positive transfer of skills:* Phenomenon of transfer of learning may help a lot in learning new skills. A person who has learnt a wide variety of skills is able to learn new skills with greater case. Therefore, by securing the help of positive transfer, the teacher should guide the students to acquire new skills.
3. *Concentrating on the actual task to be learned:* It should be kept in mind while securing help from the transfer that training by transfer from a similar skill always gives performance inferior to direct practice. Therefore, as far as possible learning should be directed to the actual skills, we want to learn. No attempt should be made to practice tennis by playing badminton as the old habits may interfere with the new.
4. *Demonstration and illustration of the right way of learning skills:* Skills cannot be acquired by merely reading or learning techniques or ways of performing the tasks. They are better learned by observing the demonstrations or the actual performance of the experienced and skilled persons. Therefore, attempts should be made to arrange demonstrations and exhibiting models for acquiring skills.
5. *Practice correct performance from the start:* Learning of skills requires consistent practice. Therefore, sufficient opportunities and encouragement should be provided for practicing the activities involved in performing a task skillfully. But it should be also seen that mere practice is not enough. Practice makes a man perfect only when practice is restricted to the correct performance. Therefore, the correct responses should be given to the students to acquire a skill to the level or extent over learning so that there may be a smooth flawless coordination of responses.
6. *Learning in natural units (to keep balance between whole v/s part method):* The unit of practice as Boring, Langfeld and Weld advocate "must involve the entire sequence—a pattern which is essential for correct performance. Neither the learner should involve him in peace-meals learning or concentrate on minute details, nor he should choose very large units for practicing. In all situations he should try to keep a proper balance between the whole and part methods of learning.
7. *Using spaced or distributed practice in learning:* In place of continued or massed practice, the distributed practice should be adopted. It is better to practice a skill for 10 days by giving one hour than to devote 5 hours daily for two days.

8. *Maintaining a proper balance between speed and accuracy:* Speed as well as accuracy both are important for the proper learning of a skill. Which one of them should be given main importance is a difficult question to be answered. Many opinion that opinion, both are equally important as they add to the proficiency and competency of a person in a specific area. Therefore, both should be given equal weightage in learning a skill.
9. *Giving adequate guidance:* The students should be given adequate amount of guidance at the proper time in learning a skill. Too much help makes the students dependent and kills their originality and imitative while denial of guidance discourages them in learning further. There, an intermediate principle should be followed. They should be given help when they need it but cultivate self-reliance in their learning.
10. *The knowledge of the results:* There must be a continuous appraisal of the skill learned so that the learner may be acquainted with the pitfalls in his learning. This can give additional incentive to keep him on the track and help him to learn correct response in place of incorrect ones.

In addition to these things mentioned above, these are other factors like suitability of learning environment, the moods, temperament and other internal factors of the learner, that should be kept in mind while guiding the students to learn a skill. Much depends upon the will and determination of the learner. If he wishes no power can check him to acquire desired proficiency in any skill he desires to learn.

Tips for Effective Learning in Nursing

The society respects and honors those who succeed in their tasks. A job well done is indeed its own reward. But in order to succeed one must be efficient in action and devoted to one's goal. The goal of a student nurse is to learn maximum during her training and become skilled in nursing. In order to be skilled one must be well-informed and know all the relevant facts regarding useful if it is effective, that is, if it results in sound learning. The student nurse must learn rudiments of a number of subjects. She must know how to read quickly and absorb learning by referring to Encyclopedias and reference works. In order to make best use of her training she must know the basic principles of effective studies. Forgetting is a natural process. But by the study prosecuted after the knowledge of psychological principles of memory, retention, etc. the forgetting can be reduced. An intelligent study is useful because one can make suitable variations in the changed contexts whereas learning without interest is useless save in a limited field. The principles and techniques of effective study yield effective learning without interest is useless save in a limited field. The principles and techniques of effective study yield effective learning and this is essential because only by intelligent application of her learning. She can meet the variety of situations and challenges she is bound to encounter. A parrot like learning will prove counter productive to a nurse because she has to deal with human beings whose reactions and behavior are unpredictable.

Nature of effective learning is accomplished by single-mindedness and concentration on the topic to be learned. One must be intelligent in picking things up. This is best achieved if one has definite goals and is dedicated to these. Recognition of goals and a desire to achieve them produced in one spontaneous interest and zest for learning. A learning of the anatomical details and of certain physiological processes is of little value unless one knows when, where and how they are to be applied. Therefore one must remind oneself constantly as to what for a particular topic is being learnt and think of its possible uses and application. In short one must attend to the details but at the same time remember the general features.

Effective learning requires cultivation of certain habits and techniques. Effective study, according to psychologists, presumes following traits and attitudes in the student:

a. Interest in subject of study and an awareness of its value and importance for the nurse
b. The nurse should have the requisite skills and abilities. These imply (i) ability for fast reading with adequate grasp (slow reading does not facilitate understanding as is generally believed); (ii) capacity for observation and learning from experience (This implies lack of strong likes and dislikes); (iii) facility of expression; (iv) capacity for cogent thinking and perceiving relations (one should be able to compare and discern).

Above all the nurse should be hardworking and observe regular hours of study daily. She must not procrastinate; to perform rightly at the right moment and in the right way is the golden rule of success. The exchange of ideas is a good way to stimulate the mind.

Learning is essentially changed behavior due to experience and that certain elements must be presented for learning to take place. The elements of learning process are:

- *Goal or goals* related to the motivation
- *Stimulus* the response is produced by the type of stimuli
- *Perceptions* the person learn things by visual, auditory or kinesthetic learning
- *Consequences* practice/skill should be able to produce change in behavior
- *Integration* association of new behavior with previously learned behaviors is related to transfer of learning.

As stated earlier, there are three major laws of learning. These are:

Law of readiness: This law is indicative of the learner's state of mind to participate in the learning process. If a person is ready to act, acting gives him satisfaction. If he is not ready to act, it is annoying him to act. Some sort of preparatory attitude or the mind set is necessary. The right moments concerning the learning situation and the learners state of mind should be recognized and maximum use should be made. In order to make learning effective, a person should show willingness to learn. This willingness prepares him to face learning readily. Readiness gives him stimulation.

Law of exercise or practice: We learn what we practice, we do not learn what don't practice. Learning takes place through exercise and repetition. It supports the law of use and disuse. We learn skills in games, music, crafts or nursing care through constant exercise and practice.

Law of effect: Learning can be set to have taken place properly when it results in satisfaction and the learner derives pleasure from it. The connection between stimuli and responses becomes stronger when we drive or get satisfaction. These responses remain weak or are not formed at all when we get annoyance. This law brings the importance of feeling in the process of learning repetition and practice but without satisfaction is of no use. Activities which are accompanied by a feeling of pleasure or satisfaction are more readily and effectively learned than activities which are implemented and annoying.

Law of attitude: Learning is guided by total attitude of the organism. The student nurse performs the nursing procedure properly if she has developed a healthy attitude towards the task.

Law of analogy: An individual responds to a new situation on the basis of responses made by him in similar situations in the past. He makes responses by comparison of analogy.

Law of association: The learner learns/responds of which he is capable, associated with any situation to which he is sensitive.

Law of multiple response or varied reactions: The law implies that when an individual is confronted with a new situation he responds in a variety of ways before arriving at correct response.

Methods of Effective Learning

The various laws and theories explained in the foregoing pages suggest various methods of effective learning. These methods can be summarized as under:

i. Learning by doing (practice method or experimentation)
ii. Recitation method
iii. Learning through association
iv. Learning by observation
v. Learning by imitation
vi. Learning by mixed (whole and part) method
vii. Learning through spaced and unspaced method (distributed and massed practice)
viii. Learning through the use of insight.

Please see the chapter memory and forgetting for the discussion of these methods).

Based on such principles as well as methods of learning the Educationists have given birth to so many efficient methods (individual as well as collective) of teaching and learning. These methods are –

i. Heuristic method
ii. Laboratory method
iii. Observation method
iv. Project method
v. Problem solving method
vi. Analytic-synthetic method
vii. Inductive-deductive method
viii. Question answer method
ix. Discussion method
x. Dalton method, and basic method, etc.

Which of the above methods will be suitable in a given learning situation depends upon so many factors described earlier. A wise teacher should try to choose a proper method for carrying out the learning process effectively.

Obstructing Factors in Study

The lack of motivation is the biggest handicap in study. If you are indifferent to goals, you can have no interest and feel no joy in what you do. The lack of interest can be due to poor health, emotional instability, compulsion, conflicting desires or inflexible habits and attitudes of mind. Some nurses consider that nursing is an art and that book learning is of no consequence. They do not believe that the study can improve their skill. This is a faulty attitude.

The remarks and reactions given in Brown's 'Managing the Class Room' are typical of the difficulties of the students. These are as follows:

a. I did not know we were to have that today. I lent my book to so and so and he did not return it to me to study, for my lesson
b. Talking a great deal and asking impertinent questions
c. You study a little, look round for a while, turn, stretch and start to study again for a while and repeat this behavior
d. Memorizing the words of the text
e. Delay in starting your work and often complaining of being sick
f. You are generally afraid of being questioned on any subject in the class, and often fail to bring to the class the material you will need for the period
g. Showing evidence of distraction and poor adjustment to work conditions
h. Feeling sleepy and sluggish
i. A new idea or a new word keeps you from doing anything that day
j. You cannot make the practical use of class in your daily life
k. Putting much time in the activities you enjoy, and giving little or no time to the activities you dislike
l. You often pity yourself and make excuse when caught in a fault.

But if you are well-motivated and feel an active interest in your activities because you are convinced of the worthiness of your goal, you will not display reactions enumerated above. It is well known that lack of interest is the main cause of boredom, lethargy and fatigue. If you are mentally distracted you may feel fatigue even after a whole night sleep. You must plan your studies and make adequate preparations before hand. All the books and reference works must be at your disposal. It is better not to study at times when for some reason you cannot concentrate. The study made when mind is haunted by other ideas will yield no learning. It will be sheer waste of effort. Play while you play and work while you work is a golden rule. There must be a time for study and a time for recreation. Above all cultivate interest in what you are doing and relate it to practical life.

The Rules of Effective Learning

Psychologists have studied thoroughly processes of learning, memory, retention, recall and forgetting. They have examined the various methods of learning, by conditioning, trial and error and insight. When applied to the problem of study they reveal the following characteristics of the learning process which are the basis of most of the principles and techniques of study:

1. *Initiative:* The real learning is an active process. The learning must be mentally and physically alert for learning to take place. For this learning must be self-indicated. The student nurse must herself take the initiative for the learning.
2. *Goal-Directed:* The student nurse must know clearly for what purpose she is studying. Why has she chosen to become a nurse. That is, she must perceive clearly her goals of life and the place of this study in her scheme of things.
3. *Meaningful:* The intelligent learning is meaningful learning. Learning must be understood in all its interrelations. The use of the study of anatomy and physiology must be clearly visualized. For example, when a nurse deals with a cardiac patient she must know about the sensitiveness and hypochondriac behavior of these patients.

Techniques of Effective Learning

There are a number of things which must be borne in mind by the nursing student so that their learning be effective. These are as follows:

1. *Self-prepared uses:* The need of sound health, good eye sight, emotional stability and freedom from physical and mental aberrations are the prerequisites of undertaking any fruitful activity. This is equally true of good study. A person suffering from observations or one who has unduly pessimistic outlook cannot prosecute studies with profit. Besides the student nurse should have capacity for hard work; be able to stand for long hours; must be free from visual defects. Moreover she should not tire easily.
   It is advisable to cultivate the habit of fast reading. It is a myth that slow reading leads to better grasp. As a matter of fact slow reader is liable to be distracted. The reading should be silent and there must not be lip movements while reading.
2. *Wholeness:* It is better to have a general idea or a bird eye-view before detailed study. The idea of whole subject before going into details is very useful. The survey of the whole subject will give the nurse a bird-eye view of the whole assignment and will enable you to perceive the whole context; skimming is a good exercise for this purpose. Dr. Buchanan recommends that the entire course outlines should be skimmed in order to select main ideas of the whole course and to find the parts which deserve close study. The experiments in psychology of learning have proved that whole learning is better than learning by parts. Of course this rule must be applied with discretion. If the assignment is so big that it cannot be studied as whole in reasonable time, it is preferable to break it into parts.
3. *Planning and organization:* The student nurse should have a time-table for the whole day in which definite periods for study should be set apart. The time to study should be such when the chance of disturbance is minimum.
4. *Clarity of purpose:* If the student nurse knows what she is to do at any particular time it will be very useful. For example when she goes to library she must know what book she wishes to study and avoid fiddling with other books. It is the definiteness of purpose and goal that create interest in the work. The problem, solving attitude is the best of effective learning. The work in hand should be associated with as many issues as possible. She must ask herself what can she do with this particular bit of learning. The nurse should not do work in order to please the tutor but understand its worthwhileness and the uses it has for her in her life. In particular she must know the place of what she is learning in her career. For example in learning psychology she must observe the behavior of persons around her and see if it helps her to understand them better.
5. *Prompt start:* When one has to study one should get down to it without delay and should not waste time in trivia. If the hours of study are regular, the place of study is fixed and it has sober surroundings, clean and adequately lit, one easily gets into mood for study. The best formula for avoiding waste of time is to forget easily the personal hurts and unpleasant episodes. A happy and cheerful frame of mind is very helpful in studying.
6. *Search for essentials in an assignment:* The student must always look for the basic facts of the subject under study. She should not be carried away by the style of the writing but try to grasp the central ideas and facts. The basic facts are more important to know than to remember beautiful quotations. Of course beauty of style is a great qualification but this should not be at the expense of facts. The style should not be

used to cover one's ignorance of facts. Besides facts, general principles should be appreciated. Unrelated facts will take us no where. Therefore we must learn the general principles as well as details.

7. *Note-taking:* Students should cultivate the habit of taking notes while studying. Note-taking lends seriousness to the study and helps the student to think and reason. If you don't take notes the study may become mechanical. But, at the same time, note-taking can also become mechanical if you jot down lines after lines verbatim. The note-taking must be intelligent. First you must understand and then make notes. As far as possible notes must be in your own language. Notes help to review and revise the subject and also to retain it. Good notes imply analysis and rational appraisal of what has been read. The notes should be brief and to the point. They should concentrate on the vital ideas and leave out the details. Notes must be well-organized and follow some definite order. One exercise book should be used for one subject. It is not good practice to jumble notes from various books or on different subjects in the same exercise book.
8. *Review and overlearn:* The rate of forgetting is far in excess of what is retained. Therefore constant review is required to retain the essentials of any subject. Besides one must learn more than what is necessary. It is advisable to read one topic from many books. After finishing the lesson an attempt should be made to recall what has been learned. If the recall is unsatisfactory the lesson should be revised. Experiments of Ebbinghaus on learning indicate that we forget most of what we learn on the first day. Therefore periodical review of the same topic is a must. One must also overlearn in order to be able to retain enough to answer examination papers. Overlearning, according to Crow and Crow, means the continuation of study beyond the point of single correct reproduction. Overlearning is helped by repetition and recitation.
9. *Paying attention to words, charts, tables, formulas and questions:* Whenever you study you must be armed with a good dictionary. As and when any new word occurs it must be checked up in the dictionary. It is better to note down the new words and write down their meanings. This helps review and is by itself a technique to effective learning. The students must be able to study the charts and tables well. They are pictorial summary and let us know things at a glance. It is good if you study the possible questions which can be framed and study the chapter in the light of those questions.
10. *Proper physical surroundings:* The physical environs in which a student studies must be clean, hygienic and tidy. The importance of physical surroundings is little realized, but infact it is immense. The place of study should be sober, free from noise and must be adequately illuminated. It is harmful to study in poor light and the noise distracts. The place of study must not be very cold nor very hot. Poor light, bad ventilation, extreme cold and heat reduce efficiency in learning. Since it is difficult to find physical surroundings ideal for study it is desirable that the student should learn to put up with small irritations such as noise, heat and cold. It is better to work at a fixed seat. A little of bodily tension is good for intellectual work. Therefore the place of study should not be stuffed with luxury outfits.
11. *Interrelationship:* A fact conductive to effective learning is the habit of discovering interrelationship or correlation between various subjects. In nursing one must have the knowledge of anatomy, physiology, chemistry, etc. But mere knowledge is not enough. One must also know how these subjects would help in dealing with the new.

Examination as Tool for Effective Learning

Examinations evaluate how effective one's learning is. They help us know our abilities and test our achievements in various subjects. Examinations are like mirrors wherein we can see what we are and what we expect to be. Thus they provide us with incentives to improve our performance and tell our teachers how best this can be done. The teacher will point out our strong and weak points and how to make amends. Thus they make both learning and teaching effective. We should look upon examinations hopefully and as true friends, and we should not be apprehensive and nervous about them. In the absence of examination we will not know whether our learning is real and effective or just a make believe. When we will appreciate the true value of examinations we will cease to be afraid of them and will not regard them as ordeals that have to be faced. Therefore when you study for examination your attitude should be positive and thinking hopeful. All nervousness should be avoided and it is better not to study on the previous night. The lack of sleep and nervous exhaustion their low grades though they believe they had done rather well. The psychologists believe that all night session prior to an examination seldom serves any constructive purpose. It leads to confusion in mind and distorts the judgment. Above all cramming should be avoided. In cramming there is no intelligent learning or grasp. It is mechanical. It is like a long chain, and even if a single link slips off the mind the entire chain is broken. Useful study consists of constant review and reflective analysis.

The following 25 suggestions listed by Crow, Crow and Skinner may be of practical value to the nurses in the development of the habits of effective study:

1. Study with a definite purpose in hand
2. Evaluate immediate and remote goals
3. Provide a definite place for study
4. See that physical conditions are conducive to study
5. Plan and follow a definite time schedule
6. Look for the main ideas of reading material
7. Cultivate the habit of reading rapidly and carefully
8. Outline the study material
9. Take brief, well-organized notes in your own language
10. Evaluate the difficulty of the material
11. While reading, raise significant questions on the material to be learned, then answer them
12. Study with intent to recall
13. Attend carefully to all illustrative material
14. Complete all study assignment
15. Let active study and rest period be interspersed with each other
16. Try to learn the unit or the lesson as a 'whole' when possible
17. Concentrate on what you are studying at the time
18. Shut out all emotional distractions
19. Overlearn sufficiently so that delayed recall is possible
20. Learn to summarize and review what you have learned or read
21. Be alert to ideas emphasized by the teacher
22. Think over the statements made by the author and try to challenge them
23. Find out what the several authorities say about a topic or an idea
24. Apply subject-matter learned in as many practical situations as possible
25. Make intelligent use of the dictionary.

Meaning and Definitions of Interest

Interest is the central force that drives the whole machinery of teaching-learning process. All our best attempts are aimed to make our studies interested in the learning experiences given to them. Interest as a driving force not only helps children to acquire certain learning experiences but also color and fashion their attitudes, aptitudes and other personality traits. It thus directs the course of their growth and development and individualizes their personalities. Visualizing such many sided importance of interest, it is proper to know actually what they are. Many psychologists and thinkers have tried to explain the meaning of this term. Let us have a look at a few of these explanations.

1. Crow and Crow states that Interest may refer to the motivating force that impels us to attend to a person, a thing, or an activity or it may be the effective experience that has been stimulated by the activity itself. In other words, interest can be the cause of an activity and the result of participation in the activity.
2. Ross states that A thing that interests us is just something that concerns or matters to us.
3. Bhatia states that Interest means making a difference. We are interested in objects because they make a difference to us, because they concern us.
4. BN Jha states that Interest is that enduring mental system which sustains conation and continues the activity called attention.

Nature and Characteristics of Interests

The definitions given above and the studies and experiments carried out by the psychologists give enough grounds to know more about the nature and characteristics of interests as given below:

1. Our interests are very much linked with our wants, motives, drives and basic needs.
2. Interest is a great motivating force that persuades an individual to engage in a cognitive, conative or affective behavior.
3. Interest and attention are closely related to each other. Commenting on their relationship, McDougall writes—"Interest is latent attention, and attention is interest in action". This observation is true. Interest is the mother of attention. We attend to those objects in which we are interested and thus interest prepares us mentally to pay attention towards an object, person or a thing. While attention always implies the activity, what we have in our mental structure in the form of an interest which is given practical shape in the form of some activity, i.e. making one attend.
4. Interests are innate as well as acquired dispositions.
5. Interests is the personal meaning that a thing has for us. This meaning colors all the aspects of our vision. Interested in a thing, we interpret everything in line with the interest.
6. Pursuit of one's interest is always satisfying. If helps an individual to realize the goals and aims set by him.
7. Interest helps in overcoming unusual or early arrival or frequent repetition of plateaus in learning. They also give sufficient strength to an individual to resist fatigue and avoid failure.
8. Interests and attitudes although, have close similarly on the ground that both represent mental readiness or preparation for a particular behavior pattern, yet there is a clear-cut distinction between the two. The individual usually like the things in which he is interested and the thing interests also activity sought. Attitudes on the other hand, may

orient and individual either favorably or uniformably towards certain objects, places, ideas, etc. Also they are comparatively passive. A person may possess attitudes but may do nothing about them.

9. Interests are not permanent and fixed. They get changed as a result of maturation, learning and other internal as well as environmental conditions and factors.

Need for Interest

As a matter of fact our innate or inborn tendencies are basically responsible for our peculiar interests. We are interested in the things which give satisfaction to our innate desires and urges. From the early childhood it can be easily seen that the instinctive drives (like curiosity, constructiveness, acquisition, self-assertion, etc.) play a great role in making children interested in one thing or the other.

As one grows older, one's instinctive urges get developed and modified. Now in which manner and to what extent these urges get developed depends upon so many environmental factors. Environmental forces are responsible for giving a particular shape to the inborn or innate urges and basic drives. As a result the interests do not remain innate or inherited qualities, but get changed into acquired tendencies or characteristics.

Moreover, instinctive behavior, as we grow older, gives birth to sentiments and complexes which in turn bring ideals and purposes in life. We began to pay attention to things connected with our sentiments and complexes. Our attitudes, temperament and other personality traits also begin to influence our interest patterns. Such striving and struggle tries to give a new form to our interest patterns and as a result new interests are developed or acquired by us.

It is therefore, not proper to consider interests purely as inborn or inherited characteristics. They are actually acquired dispositions or characteristics and the result of constant interaction between the instinctive behavior of the organism and the peculiar environmental forces. Both internal or personal factors affect the interest patterns of an individual in the course of his growth and development. We can sum up these factors as below.

Personal factors

i. His physical health and physical development
ii. His mental health and mental development
iii. His social development
iv. His age and sex
v. His emotions, sentiments and complexes
vi. His wishes, ideals, motives and goals of life
vii. His attitudes
viii. His own patterns of instinctive behavior.

Environmental factors

i. Socioeconomic status of his family
ii. His culture and social environment
iii. His education and training
iv. Opportunities available to him for exploring the potential interests.

Ways to Improve Interest

The key of the success of a teacher in his task lies in arousing and maintaining interest of his pupils. Therefore, most of their strenuous efforts are always directed in making their students interested in some or the other, learning activities. All the factors involved in teaching learning process namely the learner, learning material, learning environment, learning methods and teacher, have to be controlled and designed is such a way that all of them may contribute significantly toward the maintenance of proper interest in a learning activity at a particular time. Therefore, the task requires a multidimensional attack. However, for the general guidance of teachers, the following points may be proved fruitful.

1. **Setting the proper aims and objectives:** Before learning a lesson or engaging children in a learning activity they should be told about the need and importance of learning that activity. The aims and objectives of teaching a particular lesson or unit should be clearly defined and the students be made to set definite goals and purposes.
2. **Proper selection and organization of learning experiences:** The unsuitability of the content makes children disinterested in a particular lesson. Therefore, the teacher should select and organize the contents to be taught or the matter to be delivered in a suitable way by keeping in view all the psychological principles.
3. **Use of appropriate methods and teaching aids:** Most of the time it is the teaching method that makes a particular learning most interested or distasteful. The teacher should adopt efficient and effective methods of teaching for the delivery of his lesson and use suitable audiovisual aids.
4. **Exploitation of various instincts of children:** The interests of children are controlled and guided by their instincts. Therefore, a wise teacher should try to exploit the basic drives like curiosity, constructiveness, acquisition, self-assertion and sex, etc. for making his students interested in a learning activity.
5. **Make proper use of sentiments and ideals:** Sentiments and ideals also control and direct children interest. Therefore, they should be harnessed for creating and maintaining interest.
6. **Arranging proper learning situations or environment:** Learning situation or environment plays a great role in making children interested or get bored and tired. Therefore, the teacher should take care of the suitability of learning environment. The classroom furniture, seating-arrangement, lighting and ventilation, the scheduled time-table for learning a particular subject or activity, general atmosphere, physical and mental state of the pupils as well as teacher, group-climate, etc.—all should be properly considered while making attempt for arousing and maintaining interest of the pupils in a learning activity.
7. **Teacher's personality and determination:** Teacher's personality and his determined bid to make the students interested in the teaching count much in this direction. A good teacher with his proper behavior and personality traits can motivate, inspire and make the students almost lost in his teaching. Therefore, a teacher should try to imbibe the desirable personality traits and characteristics. He should bring honesty and sincerity in his thinking, doing and feeling and make the best possible efforts on his part to take his students along with his teaching by making them interested in his teaching.

13 CHAPTER Memory and Forgetting

Introduction

Memory is a neurochemical process mediated by the brain that accounts for the capacity to retain and retrieve information. Memory is a key cognitive ability to exercise judgment, make decisions, or even be oriented to time and place, a person must remember past experiences.

Memory is defined as the ability of an organism to store, retain and subsequently retrieve the information (either the total body of information or specific items of information). So *Memory*—is special ability of our mind to conserve or store what has been previously experienced or acquired through learning and *Memory*—is a complex process which involves factors like learning, retention, recall and recognition. The process of memory begins with learning or experiencing something and ends with its revival and reproduction. Therefore, memory is said to involve four stages: learning or experiencing something, its retention and finally its recognition and recall.

Three brain structures are critical to the formation of memories, the medial temporal lobe, certain diencephalic nuclei and the basal forebrain.

1. *The medial temporal lobe:* It houses the hippocampus, an elongated, highly repetitive network. Animal studies have defined a hippocampal place code, a pattern of cellular activation in the hippocampus that corresponds to the animal location in space. When the animal is introduced to a novel environment, the hippocampus is broadly activated. As the animal explores and roams, the firing of certain hippocampal regions begins to correspond to specific locations in the environment. In about one hour, a highly detailed internal representation of the external space (a "cognitive map") appears in the form of specific firing patterns of the hippocampal cells. If the animal is manually paced in a certain part of a familiar space, only the hippocampal regions show intense neural activity. If the animal is removed from the environment for several days and then returned, the previously registered hippocampal place code is immediately reactivated.

   The amygdala is adjacent to the anterior end of the hippocampus. It has been suggested to rate the emotional importance of an experience and to activate the level of hippocampal activity accordingly. Thus, an emotionally intense experience is etched in memory, but indifferent stimuli are quickly disregarded.
2. *Certain diencephalic nuclei:* Within the diencephalon, the dorsal medial nucleus of the thalamus and mammillary bodies necessary for memory formation. These two structures are damaged in thiamine deficiency states usually seen in chronic alcoholics, and their inactivation is associated with Korsakoff's syndrome.

3. *The basal forebrain:* The motor cortex within the cortex receives directives from the association areas. The performance of a noval act requires constant feedback from the sensory and association areas for completion and functional neuroimaging studies have demonstrated widespread activation of the cortex during unskilled acts. Memorized motor acts initially require activation of the medial temporal lobe. With practice, however, the performance of ever-larger segments of an act necessary to achieve a goal becomes encoded within the discrete areas of the premotor and parietal cortices, particularly the left parietal cortex, with the result that a much more limited activation of the cortex, is seen during highly skilled acts and the medial temporal lobe is bypassed. This process is called the corticalization of motor commands. In lay terms, the process suggest a neuroanatomical basis for the saying "practice makes perfect".

There are three main functions of mind: Cognition, conation (psychomotor activity) and affect (mood). Cognition refers to the processes through which information coming from the senses is "transformed, reduced, elaborated, recovered and used".

Information refers to sensory input from the events occurring in environment.

Cognitive processes are the mental processes involved in knowing, i.e. they are important in perception, attention, thinking, problems solving and memory.

Cognitive psychology is that which deals with cognitive processes (including memory).

Theories about Memory

i. **Theory of general memory functions:** There are three distinct processes of memory:- *encoding* (the process of receiving sensory input and transforming it into a form, or code, which can be stored and retrieved); storage (the process of actually putting codes information into memory) and *retrieval* (the processes of gaining access to stored, coded information whenever required. Fault in any of the three components resulting faulty memory. Memory is seldom an accurate record of what has been experienced.

   The first step in the memory system is to get sensory information (sight, sound, etc.) into a form that the brain can use, a process called **encoding**. Encoding is the set of mental operations that people perform on sensory information to convert that information into a form that is usable in the brain's storage systems. For example, when people hear a sound, their ears turn the vibrations in the air into neural messages from the auditory nerve, which makes it possible for the brain to interpret that sound. The next step in memory is to hold on to the information for some period of time, a process called **storage**. This period of time will actually be of different lengths, depending on the stage of memory being used. For example, in one stage of memory people hold on to information just long enough to work with it, about 20 seconds or so. In another stage of memory, people hold on to information more or less permanently.

   The biggest problem may people have is retrieval, getting the information they know they have out of storage. Have you ever handed in an essay test and then remembered several other things you could have said?

II. **Information-processing theories:** (Multistore theory). These theories compare the memory processes to a digital computer that takes items of information in processes them in steps or stages; and produces an output. There are various information processing theories, out of these some prominent are—*Richard Atkinson and Richard*

Shiffrin's (1968) theory. According to it, memory starts with a sensory input from the environment. This input is very brief (for several seconds at most) in a sensory register (It is the storage functions of sensory channels). Information that is attended to and recognized in the sensory register may be passed onto short-term memory (STM) (This is held for about 20-30 sec). Some of the information reaching short-term memory is processed by being rehearsed and may then be passed along to long-term memory or may be lost. One convert sentences to units of meaning called propositions (It is a unit of meaning that expresses a unitary idea and is composed of abstract concepts rather than words).

III. Levels of processing theories: This is theory of memory (proposed by Craik and Lockhart) that portrays processing beyond the sensory register as accomplished by a single memory system, and retention and subsequent retrieval of information as dependent on the depth or elaboration of encoding. According to this model, incoming information can be worked on at different levels on analysis, the deeper the analysis goes, the better the memory. The different depths of analysis are perception, first level (is what gives us immediate awareness of the environment); structural analysis is somewhat deeper level of analysis; and finally at the deepest level of processing, the meaning of the input is analyzed. Analysis to the deep level of meaning gives the best memory. Many of the routine happening of daily life are not processed deeply.

In the initial version of the model, retention of information depends on whether initial processing is shallow or deep. In the revised model, it is not only depth but spread or elaboration of encoding, that results in better learning (Elaboration involves making associations between a new item of information and old ones that have already been stored or among several new items to be stored. It also involves analyzing the various features of a particular item). The greater is the elaboration at the level of processing of the meaning, the best is the memory. Vivid detailed recollections of the circumstances in which one learned of or perceived some significant or surprising event are flashbulb memories.

Memory Process

Memory is defined as the capacity to retain and retrieve information. It also refers to the mental structure or structures that accounts for this capacity and to the material that is retained (either the total body of information or specific items of information). Memory both preserves the past and guides the future. Memory can be defined as an active system that achieves information from the senses, organizes and alters it as it stores it away, and then retrieves the information from storage.

The three processes are encoding, storage and retrieval.

Memory process can be divided into stages for the purpose of understanding (Figure 13.1).

- **Sensory input:** Memory starts with the sensory input or stimulus from the environment. The input is received through sensory channels such as vision, hearing or touch and is held briefly (seconds) in a sensory register.
- **Short-term memory:** The information is passed through sensory register to short-term memory store where it is held for 20-30 seconds. Some part of the information from STM is further processed as rehearsal buffer, i.e. information is repeated and in some way linked with other information already stored in memory.

- **Long-term memory (LTM):** From the rehearsal buffer, processed information is passed on to long-term memory store where it is organized in categories and stored for years. The information not so processed, is forgotten. This process can be compared with your day-to-day experiences. To learn new technical words, or names, you have to rehearse several times.

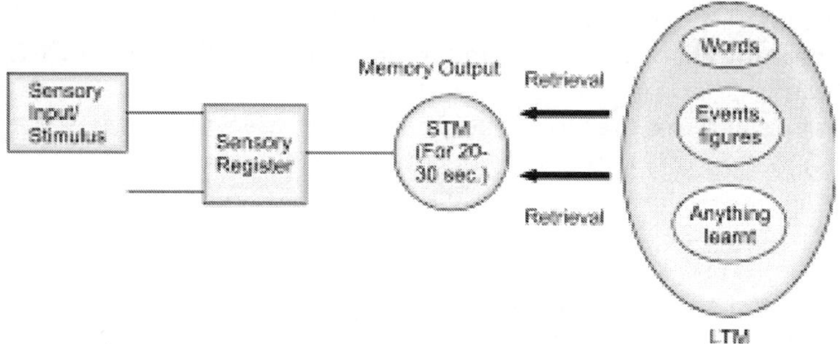

Fig. 13.1: Memory process

Long-term memory is the system in which memories that are to be kept more or less permanently are stored and is unlimited in capacity and relatively permanent in duration. Information that is more deeply processed, or processed according to meaning, will be retained and retrieved more efficiently.

Procedural memories are memories for skills, habits and conditioned responses. Declarative memories are memories for general facts and personal experiences and include both semantic memories and episodic memories.

Implicit memories are difficult to bring into conscious awareness', whereas explicit memories are those that a person is aware of processing.

LTM is organized in the form of semantic network, or nodes of related information spreading out from a central piece of knowledge.

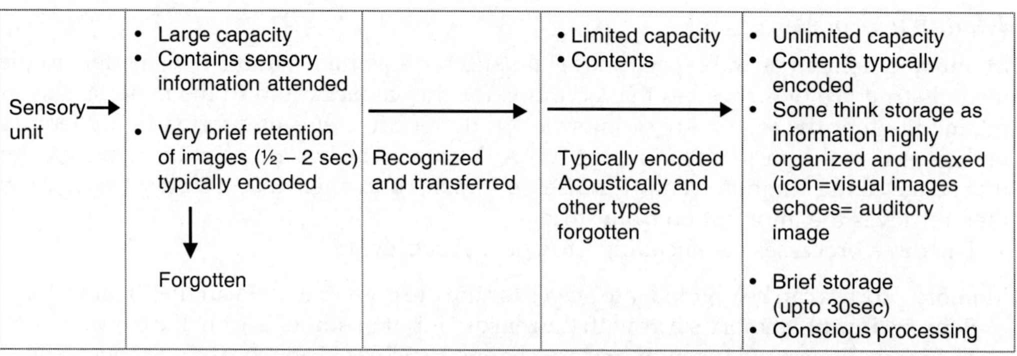

Sensory→ unit	• Large capacity • Contains sensory information attended • Very brief retention of images (½ – 2 sec) typically encoded ↓ Forgotten	→ Recognized and transferred	• Limited capacity • Contents → Typically encoded Acoustically and other types forgotten	• Unlimited capacity • Contents typically encoded • Some think storage as information highly organized and indexed (icon=visual images echoes= auditory image • Brief storage (upto 30sec) • Conscious processing

Free-Recall commonly used to test the short-term memory (STM) may be influenced by the serial position effect (i.e. role of serial position in free recall); Primary effect (i.e. better recall at the end of the list). The storage capacity of short-term memory (STM) may be increased by a process called Chunking, i.e. several times are combined into a chunk" (A Chunk is a meaningful unit of information; may be comprised of matter units).

	Sensory Register	Short-term Memory	Long-term Memory
Approximate duration	For vision, upto about 1 second, for hearing; upto about 5 seconds.	Upto about 30 seconds but it varies, depending on a number of factors.	Days, months, years, on lifetime
Capacity	Relatively large – upto at least 16 items, but probably much more	Relatively small-up to about 7 items or chunks under most conditions	Very large-no known limit
Transfer processes	Attention and recognition. Items attended to and recognized move to short-term memory	Rehearsal items appropriately rehearsed move to long-term memory	—
Type of information stored	Copy of input	Sounds, visual images, words, and sentences	Primarily meaningful sentences, life events and concepts, some images, semantic and episodic memory
Major reason information is lost	Decay of trace	Displacement of old information by incoming information	Faulty organization or inappropriate retrieval (search) strategy, interference

The process of rehearsal consists of items of information in the center of attention perhaps by repeating them; silently or aloud.

This helps in training transferring information from STM to LTM (long-term memory). Just going over and over what is to be remembered (called maintenance rehearsal) does not necessarily, succeed in transferring information to LTM.

Elaborative rehearsal involves giving the material organization and meaning as it is being rehearsed. It is an active process and helpful in transferring information to LTM. According to multistore model, rehearsal is the key of transferring material from STM to LTM.

Long-term memory (LTM) contains words, sentences, ideas, concepts and the life experiences. It consists of semantic memory (semantic meaning) containing meanings of words and concepts and the rules for using them in language; procedural memory (internal representations of personally experienced events). Tip-of-the-tongue (TOT) state is the subjective certainty that information is available in long-term memory even though one is having difficulty retrieving it (The TOT phenomenon indicates the information is organized in long-term memory. The organization of information and imagery helps in promoting is organized in long-term memory. The organization of information and imagery helps in promoting retention. The paired associate learning and constructive processes in encoding information help in improving information. Retrieval cues or reminders help in reading out information. Reconstruction (sometimes called confabulation) is the modification of already stored input.

Retrieval cues are words, meanings, sounds, and other stimuli that are encoded at the same time as a new memory.

Encoding specificity occurs when physical surrounding become encoded as retrieval cues for specific memories.

State-dependent learning occurs when physiological or psychological states become encoded as retrieval cues for memories formed while in those states.

Recall is a type of memory retrieval in which the information to be retrieved must be "pulled" out of memory with few or no cues, whereas recognition involves matching information with stored images or facts.

The serial position effect, or primacy or recency effect, occurs when the first items and the last items in a list of information are recalled more efficiently than items in the middle of the list.

Memory is viewed by cognitive theorist as an attempt to isolate some of the processes that act between the input of the stimulus and the response output. Memory is divided into four stages—attention, encoding, storage, and retrieval.

Attention and selection: The first process of memory is attention. There is such more information in our environment than we can process at any one time. Thus, we must make choices (conscious and unconscious) regarding the stimuli to which we will attend.

Encoding

Once something is attended to, it must be encoded to be remembered. Basically, encoding refers to translating incoming information into the mental representation that can be in memory. For example, one can encode information according to its sound (acoustic code), what it looks like (visual code), or what it means (semantic code).

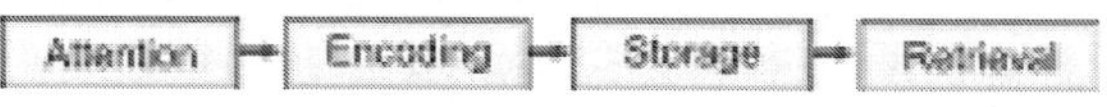

Fig. 13.2: Memory process

Storage: It is the process of holding information in memory. It can occur neither in short-term memory or long-term memory or from short-term memory to long-term memory.

Retrieval/recall: It is the process of actually remembering something when you want to. If you think about tip-of-the tongue experiences, when you know a word or name but just can't seem to recall it, you will understand how retrieval is different process related to encoding and storage. For example, if you encoded something visually, but are trying to retrieve it acoustically, you will have difficulty remembering. Like encoding, information can be retrieved through visualizing it, thinking about the meaning or imagining the sound, etc. (Figure 13.2)

Modern psychology will deal with "remembering. Just as mentioned that perception is an active process, memory also is a process in which a good deal of organized effort is brought into play by the individual. This does not merely mean the activity that takes place while memorizing. But this also means that even retaining is an active process. This will be made clear as we proceed further.

Memory plays an important part in our daily life. It makes our life more pleasant though sometimes, of course, remembering painful experiences of the past will depress us. Yet on the whole, it is because of this ability to remember that people are able to learn more about their environment and become more efficient in their different professions. Particularly for the students, memory is an important aid. A student has to answer an examination paper, but also because only by remembering what has been learnt is it possible to learn more. Thus for a student who wants to learn more and more and increase his knowledge, remembering is very important. Remembering is different from thinking. In the former, individuals just reproduce what has been previously learnt. In the latter, we attempt to do new things with the help of past experience. But practically no thinking is possible without memory. Thus to progress in learning and to develop one's constructive thinking, memory becomes an absolute necessity. Therefore it is important for any student to know the psychological principles of this process of remembering.

The process of remembering may be studied under four different aspects—learning, retaining, recalling and recognizing. All these four aspects are so much interrelated that they really from one single activity. Each aspect involves one or more of the other aspects.

Conditioning of Memorizing

Before anything can be remembered, it must be learnt. Learning in this context means memorizing. Ever since psychology became an experimental science, a number of experiments and investigations have been carried out to determine the laws of memory. These experiments attempted to find out the most efficient methods of learning or memorizing that would yield the best results from the point of view of remembering effectively for a long time. These may be called the 'conditions of memorizing'. Some of these conditions which have been established by experiments are:

i. **Meaningful learning:** Paying attention to the meaning of a whole passage that has to be memorized helps the process of memorizing. This is called meaningful learning with understanding. If a poem or a long passage has to be memorized it is much better to read through the whole assignment and get its general meaning fairly clear in the mind. In getting the meaning, it may be advantageous to find out the relationships between the different parts of the passage. This can be easily proved by making subjects memorize a list of meaningless syllables and another list of meaningful words or a poem of a few lines. Keeping other things constant, it would be found that the meaningful passage always has an advantage over the other.

   Memorizing is usually done by using the method of repetition. This is called rote learning. In learning meaningless syllables, only the method of brutal rote learning is used. There is no chance of understanding and acquiring meaning. On the other hand, if repetition is done with an active understanding of the meaning, memorizing becomes easier and quicker. Mere rote learning also does the trick, but it has its limitation. Wt has been learnt by mere tore learning may not be our best advantage. We will not be able to make use of such material to further our intellectual development.

ii. **Spaced and unspaced repetition.** When a fairly long assignment has to be memorized, what is the best method to be adopted? Is it better to sit at it till it is mastered? Or is it better to take it up at intervals? It has been shown by experiments that there is a definite advantage in favor of the method of spaced repetition. This method just like the method of making the assignment meaningful has the advantage of helping us to remember what has been learnt for a much longer time. When there are intervals between the attempts at memorizing, the learning process that has been initiated at first goes on working beneath the threshold of awareness and thus fixing more durably whatever has been learnt. Most of us forget the things that we prepare for the examinations. This happens with many students because they try to memorize a whole lot of things continuously, a short while before the examination. Often this attempt may be successful in that we may be able to answer the questions in the examinations. But as a process of real learning, it will have no value at all. What was thus learnt would be soon forgotten.

iii. **Whole versus part learning.** Experiments have been conducted to find out whether it is better to memorize a lesson as a whole or it is better to divide it into parts and master each part separately. The answer to this question depends upon certain other variable factors also. If the assignment is too long, certainly a division into subgroups will become an absolute necessity. On the other hand, if the assignment is quite small and manageable it would be obviously better to study it as a whole. But what happens with assignments of a size in between the above the two categories? The general principle, that studying a lesson as a whole is more advantageous, has been proved in all such cases. In general, it is more economical and efficient to learn a whole lesson as one unit. This is particularly because, and then only it becomes more meaningful. The first advantage which we mentioned is made use of. Even when it is of definite advantage to divide the assignment into parts, care must be taken that the division is made in such a manner that each part by itself will become one composite continuous meaningful whole.

iv. a. *Repetition and Recitation.* It has been already assumed that repetition is necessary for most of us. There may be some brilliant exceptions where one is able to learn and remember a particular assignment even after attending to it just once or twice. This may be because such a person has a very strong capacity for imagery or it may be because of some special ability developed by that person. Such cases are very rare. Most of us will have to repeat our lessons before we can fix them up in our minds. It must be done taking into account the factors mentioned above. From the point of view of permanence of retention, it has been found by experiment that the more we repeat, the better it is. Repetition carried on even after mastering the assignment has great value from the point of view of retention. Such extra amount of repetition is usually called "over learning". Over learning gradually reduces the forgetting that would ordinarily take place. Thus it is always useful to practice the material to a definite degree of over learning. It is particularly necessary to remember this because, ordinarily, we find it difficult to continue our study after getting a feeling of knowing the subject. This is the natural tendency of any student. Therefore students have to be convinced of the advantage of doing some over learning.

Sometimes, students wonder whether it is advisable to read aloud or to read silently. No definite answer has been found for this question on experimental basis. But if one has the capacity for strong auditory image reading aloud may have some definite advantage. However, with some people at least, reading aloud may help them to maintain concentration and overcome distraction. On the other hand, if reading loudly is done over a fairly long period of time, extra energy is spent and fatigue may result. Perhaps it actually depends on the habits formed by a particular individual.

b. *Recitation or Reviewing.* A student must always be encouraged to review or to recite to himself the material learnt. After reading a lesson a few times, the student must try to review the whole thing without the help of a book. When there are difficulties he could of course check up. It has been found by experiment that this method has a great advantage for efficient learning. This not only economies the energy to be applied but also helps towards permanent retention. Repetition must be done with reviewing in between. The method of reviewing helps the student to gain confidence because of the awareness that he has managed to master portions of the assignment. Further, the method of recitation helps him to focus his attention on portions that require special effort.

v. **The will to remember.** In one sense, the learning that we have been dealing with concerns intentional or willful learning. We are dealing with the factors involved when the student wants to learn something. But this factor of wanting to learn or as it is sometimes called "the will to learn" needs some emphasis. Along with the will to learn, the strong "will to remember" must be learn. An interesting classroom experiment to show the importance of will to learn is as follows:

Give the class a list of paired words such as the following:

Karnataka—Kannada
Judge—High court
Beach—Goa
Mountain—Tree
Apple—Health, etc.
Nurse-Patient

Ask the students to learn the second word of each pair, so that they could give it when the first word is mentioned. Allow the class sufficient time to master this. When they have mastered this, suddenly change the question. Ask them to say which pair comes below a particular pair. Many in the class may not be able to answer. They may even protest that it is an unfair question. They never meant to learn that. They were only connecting the words in each pair and not one pair with another. In other words, they did not intend to learn in that manner, and hence do not know it. Thus we find that an intention to learn is essential.

It is equally important to develop a strong intention to remember. Many students do very well in the examination and soon after the examination, almost everything they had is forgotten. This may be explained by the fact that when they study, their intention was only to remember it for the examination and it was successfully done. Since they did not intend to remember it more permanently, the whole thing was forgotten seen. Hence, it is very important that everyone should constantly remind himself of this principle particularly when one has to learn things of permanent value.

Retention

What was said regarding the process of learning, was towards ensuring retention or a permanence of what was learnt. When memory is essential for the learning process and for the development of our intellect in general, it mean remembering retaining. So this aspect of retention or retaining is important for the consideration of the learning process as much. When we are learning, we are active. But retaining does not mean the continuation of that activity. It is more passive. It is just retained in mind. It is retained when we are not at all thinking in mind. Even in sleep it is retained. But at the time, another kind of activity has been going on. We would consider this along with forgetting.

The question has often been asked what exactly is the mechanism of retention. It has been suggested by many that the learning process procedures certain structural modifications in the cerebral cortex. These structural modifications are referred to as 'memory traces'. These memory traces are retained. We may compare these memory traces to impressions or marks that we make on a plastic substance. Under what conditions these traces may disappear or get mutilated can be seen when we consider the process of forgetting.

Measuring retention Psychologists have developed certain methods for measuring the amount of retention of a material that has been learnt. This experiment would also serve as evidence for retention, partial or full. Three of the common methods are: (a) relearning method, (b) recall method, and (c) recognition method.

a. *Relearning method:* If we master an assignment, it may happen that after six months, we may be able to recall a portion of it or nothing at all. These two possibilities are there. Suppose it took us one hour or 20 repetitions to learn that matter during the first time. Now after a week's time, we attempt again to master the same. Suppose we now take only thirty minutes or only ten repetitors in order to master the same matter. This would mean that there has been a saving or gain during this second period of learning. This saving must have been due to the retention of what was learnt first. There has been a saving of fifty percent in the effort made to relearn it. We may safely assume that fifty percent of what was learnt before was retained at the end of six months.
b. *Method of recall:* We all know that we can recall a particular subject matter only if we have retained it. So this is a very direct method of testing retention. This method is used in the ordinary type of examinations where the question is asked in such way that the student has to write everything that he knows about it. In other words, his retention is tested by his ability to recall and reproduce.
c. *Recognition method:* In recent years, particularly in schools, the method of testing retention by the recognition method is becoming more popular. The modern types of tests are based on this method of recognition. The student has to recognize the correct answer from a wrong one. Either in the 'true-false' type of questions, or in the 'multiple choice' types of questions, the principle is the same. By his ability to recognize the correct answer, his retention of the subject studied is measured. This certainly puts less strain on the student during the examination time.

The retention curve: One of the earliest experiments in psychology was conducted by a psychologist named Ebbing-Haus as early as 1885 on this aspect of memory. His chief aim was to determine the rate of forgetting as time lapsed. He used lists of nonsense syllables and to measure retention he used the relearning method. The relearning was done after specified intervals to find out how forgetting increased or retention got weaker. The results were plotted in a curve (Fig. 13.3). This curve came to be called "curve of forgetting" or "curve of retention". From this graphic representation of the curve, certain characteristics

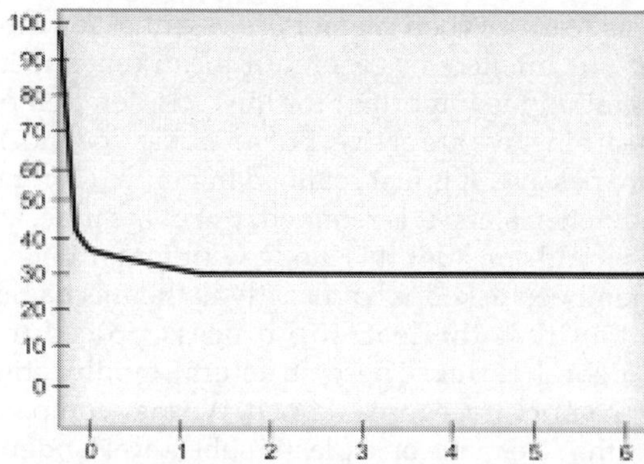

Fig.13.3: A common shape of the retention curve—Notice the rapid falling within the first twenty-four hours

of this process of retaining became obvious. It can be readily seen that at first forgetting is rapid and as time lapses, the rate of forgetting becomes slower and slower. Many experiments have been done on this problem. They have all shown similar results. It has also been observed that there are individual differences in this matter of forgetting. Also, this retention would depend upon the extent to which the advantageous factors in learning have been observed. A striking example of the fact of overlearning on retention is mentioned by Woodworth in his book "Psychology". He says that a student who had practiced on a typewriter for 200 hours and then dropped it entirely for a year, recovered all the lost ground in less than an hour of fresh practice, thus showing a retention of over 99 percent.

Recall

The third aspect of the process of remembering is recall. It is not a technical term and we all know what the word means. We learn things in order to recall them when we need. If we are not able to recall things which we had learnt when the necessity arises, our learning has not been efficient. So the ability to recall at will is essential. Failure to recall need not necessarily mean that there has been no retention. We would have experienced our failure to recall a particular name or date when required, but suddenly remember that name or date some time later. Of course we feel very bad about it because our memory has let us down. But the fact that we are able to remember later shows that there was retention. Sometimes, there is what is called partial or incorrect recall. A certain part of the fact may be recalled correctly but it gets mixed up with other unwanted things. We get a vague feeling of being wrong and we struggle against it often with no use. These are some of the questions to be studied under recall. Why is there no recall even when there is retention and why does such incorrect recalling occur?

When there is no recall, we say we have forgotten. When a student says he has forgotten a thing and he is not able to answer a question put to him, it is important to determine the nature of this forgetting, viz. whether it was simply an inability to recall even though there was retention or whether the retention itself was very poor. Failure to recall with retention intact, is usually referred to as "recall amnesia". When the retention itself is poor it is referred to as "retention amnesia". If it is retention amnesia, further learning should be done in order to strengthen the retention. If it is recall amnesia what is needed is more of encouragement or even just dropping that matter at that particular time.

Recall amnesia usually takes place because of a blocking in the process of recalling. This blocking is often caused by emotional disturbances such as fear, anxiety or self-consciousness. We would all be familiar with the experience of a stage fright under which one is not able to recall what he knows perfectly well. Many a student may fail to answer a question in the class because of such emotional disturbances. It would be wrong in such cases to scold him or to take him to task. This would only increase his emotional disturbance and make recall more difficult.

There can also be another reason for failure to recall. This reason is usually said to be interference. In interference, some other experience of the past is also interference, some other experience of the past is also aroused by the question, by the process of association and there is a kind of conflict between two lines of associative process. This makes the required recall difficult and impossible. When we want to recall a particular name, some other name having some association with it comes to the mind and makes it impossible to recall the correct one. This associative blocking can be best dealt with by simply is to drop the whole thing and try to recall the wanted fact at a later time.

Recall is also affected adversely or in a helpful manner by our set or attitude at that time. The will to recall is important and the whole attentive process should also be directed towards the details relevant to the fact wanted.

If we want to find out whether a student knows the names of the rivers of the India, two kinds of questions can be framed. We can put the question in the form asking him to name the rivers that are in India or we can give the names of a few rivers as Ganges, Godavari, Krishna, Cauvery, etc. and ask the student to say in which country they are. We can add to this list a few rivers that are not in India. Admittedly, the latter form is easier to answer, and puts less strain on the student. In the first form of the question, unnecessary interference in the recall may arise in the mind of the student because he knows the names of a number of rivers both in India and in other countries. Thus the recalling process is made more difficult. The modern types of achievement tests with which we are familiar are based on this principle.

Sometimes recall is partially correct. But it gets mixed up with some other facts not wanted at that time. This getting mixed up with some other part is a very important and interesting phenomenon in the psychology of forgetting. When we recall only a portion, it somehow does not satisfy the mind. And a sense of completeness is given by adding on to it a part of another. We will consider this in more detail presently with reference to the process of forgetting.

Recognition

Recall and recognition are closely related. Recognition is the act of indicating that such and such a thing has been seen or experienced before. It is a kind of feeling of being familiar. When we meet a person, we may feel that his face is familiar to us which means we recognize him as having seen before. Recognition is more a passive behavior than an active process like recall.

Experiments to study the process of recognition usually take the form of presenting to the subjects a series of pictures of objects or people for a short period of time, say 15 seconds and then after some time, presenting these pictures with many more pictures and asking the students to recognize the pictures which had seen.

If we do this experiment and observe carefully with the help of introspection, we may be able to analyze certain experiences which are related to this process of recognizing. The first thing we would notice is that we put ourselves in a particular set, tune ourselves in some relevant way that would make us recognize the pictures seen before. We collect in our minds the necessary images and keep our attention in a kind of expectant manner in readiness to recognize the required object. We may also notice that sometimes while actually looking over the pictures the second time, hesitation occurs in our minds. This shows that the process of recognition is not always easy, and it is not always passive. Sometimes, we get a feeling of familiarity even with a picture which was not presented to us at first. Sometimes, the picture seen already completely eludes us by not evoking any feeling of familiarity. Sometimes we may just hesitate between an act of recognizing and not recognizing. We then come to a decision, though the possibility of going wrong is always there.

If we do the actual experiment we would find that in certain cases the recognition was confidently done not because we recognize the whole picture, but because we were able to recognize a small but significant part of it. This kind of experience which makes use of a "reduce cue" is common to all learning experiences. It is made up of on the stage for making people remember their speeches. The prompter stays behind the screen and gives out a word here and there as a clue. Reacting to a reduced cue is made possible because of the association we have built up between the various parts of the assignments to be learnt. In fact, all students who have learnt a lesson should find out and establish striking relationships within the various parts of the lesson. This would make it easy for the students to recall or to recognize. Recognition is closely connected with the learning process and the process of recall. What has been learnt well will also be recognized easily.

An experiment conducted by an American student of psychology by name Seeleman has brought out another interesting fact regarding this process of recognizing. He presented pictures of Negro students and White students. For the second presentation, he included pictures of more Negro students and more White students. From the students to whom these pictures were presented for experiment, he had previously collected data regarding their general attitudes and approach towards the Negros. In the recognition experiment, it was found that those students who were favorably disposed towards the Negroes were able to recognize more of the Negro faces. Those who had racial or other prejudices against Negroes were found to be poor in recognizing the faces of the Negro students first seen. This experiment indicates that motives and emotional prejudices play an important part in directing the process of recognition. This may be related to the more general fact that on the whole pleasant experiences are remembered more easily than unpleasant experiences. (This is true only within certain limits. An extremely painful experience may be remembered very well and long).

Classification of Memory (Fig. 13.4)

Memory is the ability to access information in the mind relating to past events or experiences. It is further divided into:

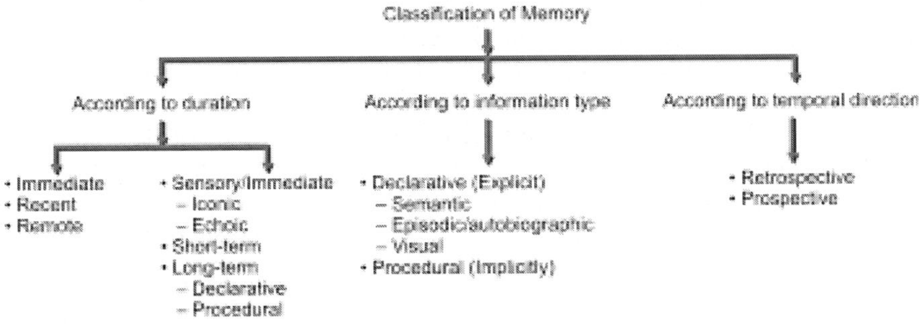

Fig. 13.4: Classification of memory

1. **According to duration:** A basic and generally accepted classification of memory is based on the duration of memory retention and identifies three distinct types of memory.
   a. **Sensory or immediate memory:** It remains the sensory image for only a small part of a second, just long enough to develop a perception. It corresponds approximately to the initial 200-500 milliseconds after an item is perceived. The ability to look at an item, and remember what it looked like with just a second of observation, or memorization, is an example of sensory memory. Because this form of memory

degrades so quickly, an individual see the display, but be able or unable to report all the items. This cannot be prolonged via rehearsal. It can be of two types (Fig. 13.4).

Iconic memory: A form of sensory memory that holds visual information for almost quarter of a second or more. It makes visual world appear smooth and continuous despite frequent blinks and an eye movements.

Echoic memory: A momentary sensory memory of auditory stimulus; if attention is elsewhere, sounds and words can still be recalled within 3-4 seconds. It would playback auditory information and gives you time to recognize sounds as words.

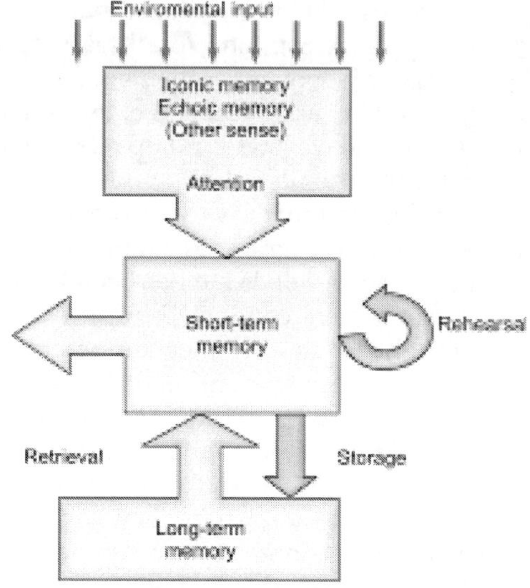

Fig. 13.5: Memory model

b. **Short-term memory (STM) or working memory:** Some of the information in sensory memory is then transferred to short-term memory. It allows one to recall something from several seconds to as long as a minute without rehearsal. Its capacity is also very limited. Modern estimates of the capacity of STM are lower, typically on the order of 4-5 items and we know that memory capacity can be increased through a process called 'chunking'.

For example, if presented with the string 'FBIPHDTWAIBM', people are able to remember only a few items. However, if the same information is presented with 'FBIPHDTWAIBM', people can remember a great deal more letters. This is because they are able to chunk the information into meaningful groups of letters.

This type of information stored consists of sounds, images, words or sentences. The information is lost from STM may be transferred to LTM through either maintenance or elaborative rehearsal. If you pay attention by rehearing the information such as humming the song you heard or taking the notes of a lecture, the information will be encoded for storage in LTM. Recalling the instructor's words for long-term memory depends partly on how it is encoded. Good encoding makes new association which increases the chances of recall.

c. **Long-term memory (LTM):** The storage in sensory memory and short-term memory generally have a strictly limited capacity and duration, which means that information is available for a certain period of time, but it is not retained indefinitely. By contrast, long-term memory can store much large quantities of information for potentially unlimited duration (sometimes a whole life span). For example, remembering telephone numbers for many years through repetition is said to be stored in LTM.

2. Accordingly information type

(A) Declarative (Explicit) memory: It requires conscious recall, in which some conscious process must call back the information. It is subdivided into.

i. **Semantic memory:** It is the accumulation of facts and experience gained over a lifetime. Semantic memory is used for remembering everyday types of facts and information. It is also called knowledge. Unlike other forms of memory, you usually do not remember where or when you learned the information in semantic memory. For example, you may have known that Paris is the capital of France, but you may not have known where or when you learned that. It means concerning facts taken independent of context.

— In what city is the Eiffel Tower located?
— Is this animal diurnal or nocturnal?
— What does this symbol indicate?

Effects of ageing on semantic memory: It is related to experience. As people grow older, semantic memory typically remains stable or even improves. To keep your semantic memory, there are some simple things you can do, like reading, crosswords and puzzles.

ii. **Episodic memory:** It concerns information specific to a particular context, such as a time and place. It is used for more personal memories such as sensations, emotions and personal associations of a particular place or time. It is a record of what has happened to us, our remembrances of past things. It is less organized and hence will be forgotten faster.

Autographical memory is mentor for particular events within one's own life is generally viewed as either equivalent to, or a subset of episodic memory.

iii. **Visual memory:** It is part of memory preserving some characteristics of our senses pertaining to visual experience. We are able to place in memory information that resembles objects, places, animals or people in sort of a mental image.

(B) Procedural (Implicit) Memory

It is not based on the conscious recall of information. It is primarily employed in learning motor skills and should be considered a subset of implicit memory. It is revealed when we do better in a given task due only to repetition—no new explicit memories have been formed, but we are unconsciously accessing aspects of previous experiences. Procedural memory involved in motor learning depends on the cerebellum and basal ganglia.

Memory can also be classified in terms of duration as:

1. **Immediate memory:** It is ability to remember a small amount of information over a few seconds, e.g.
   - Dialing a phone number I was jut told
   - Copying a figure I have just seen
   - Solving this equation $\frac{2+2+6}{10}$ in may head.

Immediate memory is an important type of memory for making sense of what is going on around you. For instance, it is used when reading to recall what happens sentence by sentence, or when recalling a phone number just looked up in the phone book. There is a limit to how much can be stored in immediate memory. Unlike other forms of memory, information in immediate memory fades very quickly (lasts only a few seconds).

Immediate memory is not affected much by age. At any age, people can usually store 5 to 7 pieces of information in immediate memory.

Tips to maintain or improve immediate memory:

- Keep your mind active. Participate in activities that require you to think and learn, such as playing cards or attending a lecture.
- *Exercising*. There is some evidence to suggest that physical exercise contributes to memory retention.

2. **Recent memory:** It is the ability to remember information from minutes, hours, or days ago. For example, do you remember the title of this website? What did you have for breakfast today? What was the name of someone you met for the fist time last week?

   When people say, "My memory is not what it used to be", they are most likely referring to their recent memory under normal conditions, recent memory changes gradually over time. It is not something that happens quickly or overnight. Thus, abrupt changes in memory capacity may be a result of other factors. Recent memory declines with age. Older people have more difficulty recalling information from recent memory.

   Tips to maintain or even improve recent memory:
   - *Keeping your mind active.* Studies indicate that engaging or intellectual pursuits (reading, problem solving, etc.) helps memory retention.
   - *Keeping your body active.* Studies indicate that there may be correlation between physical activity and memory retention, i.e. exercise helps memory.
3. **Remote memory:** It is the ability to remember things that happened years ago. Remote memory is difficult to study because it is hard to validate whether old memories (personal ones) are accurate or not. The research on remote memory and normal ageing is somewhat contradictory. As an example, old people can often clearly remember an emotional event from years past and often tell the story. It is unclear whether this is due to remote memory or whether it is a result of telling the story over and over again. Remote memory in older people is similar to that in younger people.

   Tips to maintain or even improve remote memory:
   - Socializing with friends and family and talking nostalgia
   - Writing your emotions
   - Reading old letters and clippings you have saved and asking why you saved these.

3. **Other memory classification by temporal direction is:**

Retrospective memory: It is the ability to remember the content happened in the past. It includes semantic memory and episodic/autobiographical memory.

Prospective memory: It is the ability to remember the content happened in the future, or remembering to remember. It can be further broken down into event-and time-based prospective remembering. Event-based prospective memories are intentions triggered by cues, such as remembering to post a letter (action) after seeing a mailbox (cue).

Factors that may Affect Memory

1. **Personal characteristics**

- **Age:** The cognitive development occurs from birth as he grows. But the old age influences the memory.
- **Gender differences:** Studies show that sex and prenatal hormones affect cognitive performance, e.g. estrogen combines with stress to impair memory. Memory problems at menopause. There are greater differences in brain, frontal lobe neuron density.
- **Development:** Prenatal factors (exposure to cocaine, air pollutants, solvents, lead, etc.) alcohol exposures, influence the memory of an individual.

2. **Food and supplements**

- Healthy diet news reports improvement in cognitive performance
- Vegetables, omega-3, antioxidant-rich diets boost memory

- Dietary supplements like vitamin D, long-term β carotene, vitamin B_{12}, folate, folic acid, zinc supplements, may help to prevent cognitive decline.
- Natural supplements like gingko biloba may act as memory enhancer in patients with multiple sclerosis.

3. Drugs and chemicals

Hormone therapy, alcohol, nicotine, ecstasy, other illegal drugs (e.g. cannabis, amphetamine, marijuana, cocaine) and metals (lead, solvents, mercury, chemicals in clear plastics) may cause cognitive problems in adults.

4. Exercise

Physical activity, aerobic exercise, lifestyle changes, fitness are associated with mental processes.

5. Emotion

Emotion provoking situations immediately before or immediately after learning have got obliterating effect on memory, e.g. stress.

6. Environment

Nuisance distractions can impair learning ability. Aircraft noise may affect children's reading and memory. It can be a place, person or time which influence one's memory.

7. Clinical conditions

Epilepsy, chronic pain, migraine, repeated common infections, high BP, AIDS, cancer, multiple sclerosis, head injury, diabetes, PTSD, autism are linked to poor memory.

Forgetting

Forgetting has positive and negative values in life. It is a great blessing to mankind. Life would have been very tragic and miserable if memory for all painful events would have been preserved in our mind. The process of forgetting washes away sad and shocking experiences from the mind.

Individual might think that normal forgetting is a very passive process quietly taking place with the passing of time. But experiments have shown that it is not always so. Suppose we hear a new story that it is not always such as names of people, of places, dates, events, etc. After a month or so we naturally forget many of these details (if we have not reviewed or relearned the story in the meantime). Later, if there is a necessity to recall the story, we do not simply admit that we have forgotten certain details. Without any conscious desire on our part, certain extra details are substituted in the places where we have forgotten. So we actually will repeat a full and complete story, only some of the details are not the same as in the original. Some names may be different. Either completely or partially some dates also may be different and so on. At the time of repeating we do not become aware that we give wrong details. We have a definite feeling that we are recollecting exactly as we several psychologists have conducted experiments on this phenomenon.

This unconscious effort at filling the gaps which are produced by forgetting has been studied along two lines.

a. It is viewed as a process of distortion taking place unconsciously. According to this view there is a tendency to distort, even during the process of learning, some of the incidents to suit our inner prejudices and subjective conditions (just like what happens during the process of perception). Even as we learned the story the perception of some of the details was not quite correct. The impression made by some details even at that time was more determined and directed by subjective conditions other than the actual facts. Or just by association, some other facts or details might have been suggested to the mind which made a stronger impression even at the time of learning the story. Therefore the substitute details get fixed in the mind. This suggestion is certainly possible and such a process may take place in many cases.

b. Another slightly different suggestion is made to explain this filling in of gaps. This is based on a particular view of our minds. From various other considerations it is generally agreed that our minds do not feel happy with anything that is incomplete or incoherent. There is always a desire to make things complete. With children this desire may also take the form of making things dramatic and striking. This being so, when we forget some of the details of the story the mind is not satisfied with that. There is an active process of filling those gaps with some other details which may sometimes be more dramatic and more appealing. Thus finally a complete and finished story (though different from the original) is produced. Professor Bartlett of the Cambridge University has established this point on the basis of several experiments conducted by him. Suppose we learned a figure. After some times some of the parts of the figure are forgotten with the result that only unconnected and meaningless bits are remembered. If we are asked to reproduce the figure, the mind without any conscious awareness fills in some details and produces a connected and complete picture though very different from the original. Professor Bartlett has even demonstrated the stage by stage working of this active process of filling the gaps.

Perhaps both these ways of looking at this process are true. Both phenomena may be working together or separately. In actual practical life, this principle of active forgetting is evident in two forms of our experiences.

1. *Giving testimony:* Suppose we saw a severe fight on the road between two people. We stood there and watched everything, thus becoming first-hand eye-witnesses. All of us would have carefully noticed the most significant fact of one person hitting or stabbing the other. But there are also so many other details connected with the main incidents. These may or may not be significant. These include details such as which direction each was facing, what dress they were wearing, the height and the appearance of the persons, whether there was anybody else nearby, whether there was a cycle parked behind the one, etc. All of us would have had a general glance at all these details. But we would not have noticed all of them with equal attention. The result would be that a few days later we might forget many of these details. But one things we know. We were eye-witnesses to the incident. So if we are asked to give evidence to this incident, a clever lawyer may put a number of question regarding the details. But we have already forgotten some of these details. The tendency of the mind, without any conscious attempt to do so, is to fill up these gaps with other possible details. To our utter surprise the lawyer may prove that all these statements of ours are wrong, thus proving us to be false witnesses. Such an interesting experience often happens.

   As a classroom experiment we can try something similar to this. We can arrange some striking incident in the classroom and then ask the entire class to write a report of what they saw. The deviations obtained would be very interesting indeed.

2. *Rumor:* All know about rumors. Sometimes how different a rumors is in its final form from the way it started. A small incident that takes place somewhere is passed on from mouth-to-mouth until at last it takes a form which is completely different from the

original. Names of new people come in, things get exaggerated and the whole thing is given a very dramatic and significant form. Here also the same principles of distorting and active forgetting are at work. The student of psychology should all the more be careful in accepting and passing on of rumors.

Humans have been preoccupied to store and process information for a very long time. Any learning is effective when we can remember it for a long duration. It allows humans to use the experience of the postgenerations and that of the others. The memory of each person defines him/her. Losing memory is like losing past and future, living in a continual present.

Learning is very important in our daily life. Without it we can't move forward to perform the task. Whatever we have learnt, it must retain in our mind, stored up somehow, to be used when the need arises.

In psychology, an organism's ability to store, retain and subsequently retrieve information is known as 'Memory'. In recent decades, it has become one of the principal pillars of a branch of science called *cognitive neuroscience,* an interdisciplinary link between cognitive psychology and neuroscience.

From the negative aspect, forgetting is a very important practical problem in our everybody life, e.g. you have given book to your friend and searching it at home, a patient forgets to carry his medicine and has problem on the way. Such other problems pose great botheration for us. So forgetting is defined as the permanent or temporary loss of the ability to recall or recognize something learned earlier. —Munn (1967).

FORGETTING AS A PROCESS

A great deal about forgetting has already been implied in the previous sections. Still it is better to consider this process of forgetting separately. Forgetting need not always be to our disadvantage. Indeed when we consider the number of experiences that we have everyday, and a good part of them unpleasant, forgetting is a great blessing to the human being. Imagine our minds being crowded with all kinds of experiences, everything that has taken place in the past! Our life would surely be miserable. Further, there are several things which we should not forget. Hence it is important to understand what exactly happens when we forget and why we forget. As is already mentioned, forgetting may be retention amnesia or recall amnesia. The latter has already been discussed. In this section we will consider problems connected with the retention amnesia, partial or full.

As a process, forgetting can be studied under two categories, the division being on the basis of the causes that lead to forgetting. They are: (1) Normal forgetting and (2) abnormal or pathological forgetting.

NORMAL FORGETTING

It takes place because of three causes. (a) Atrophy through disuse; (b) interference and (c) retroactive inhibition.

a. ***Atrophy through disuse is easy to understand:*** If not performed for a long time and kept in disuse, a skill is liable to be forgotten. A geometrical theorem however well it was mastered, might be forgotten in the course of time if never in the meanwhile. If on the other hand, periodically some problem was attempted using that theorem, then the problem itself would not be forgotten. Occasional reviewing of what has been learnt and applying the general principles once understood, will greatly aid retention. Atrophy through disuse takes place mostly with the passage of time.

Interference we said that retention is made possible because of certain impressions or memory traces made on the brain structure. Any experience and everything that we learn will thus be making its own impression. It is indeed wonderful how a small object like the human brain could retain all these traces. Still, commonsense would tell us that if too many traces are made, perhaps, one over the other, the traces may tend to be disfigured and destroyed. The fact of interference gives us a warning that we should not try to learn too many things at one and the same time. Selection and a slow pace would yield much better results in the long run. Trying to finish the syllabus just before the examination in a frantic hurry will not produce any real learning. Even if by chance we are able to answer some questions in the examination, we can be sure that there will be no real learning achieved through such as effort. By interference we mean here different memory traces overlapping and disturbing each other.

Interference in memory: Some forgetting occurs because similar items of information interface with each other. This occurs both in STM and LTM and is especially common when one has to recall isolated events. The different types of interferences in memory are:

Retroactive Interference: Forgetting that occurs when recently learned material interfers with the ability to remember similar material stored previously.

Proactive Interference: Forgetting that occurs when previously stored material interferes with the ability to remember similar, more recently learned material.

Motivated Forgetting: Forgetting due to a conscious or unconscious desire to eliminate awareness of painful or unpleasant experience or information.

Cue-dependent Forgetting: The inability to retrieve information stored in memory because of insufficient internally or externally generated cues.

State-dependent Memory: The tendency to remember something when one is in the same physiological or emotional state as during the original learning or experience. Without it, the person has difficulty in retrieval.

Autobiographical Memory: It is the memory which gives each of us a sense of identify.

***b. Retroactive inhibition*:** It has been noticed another interesting phenomenon known as retroactive inhibition. In the ordinary law of cause and effect, the effect always follows the cause. It cannot precede it. In retroactive inhibition, curiously enough, just opposite takes place. What we learn now effects and disturbs what was learnt earlier. In other words, what we learn now has an effect on what was done before. The effect of the present activity is thrown back upon an earlier activity. That is what the term retroactive literally means. Inhibition means withholding. Applied to the process of remembering, retroactive inhibition means that sometimes, what we learn at the present moment may make us forget what has been learnt immediately earlier.

The effect of retroactive inhibition and the fact that rest immediately after learning helps retention have suggested to some people a theory regarding the formation of memory trace. It is quite possible that when we learn something, the memory traces that are formed take some time to get fixed. Some time is needed for the traces to get mature, as it were, before they can be well-established. It is compared to the process of hatching. So this process is technically called 'incubation'. Thus according to the incubation theory anything that has been learnt requires some time before it is properly strengthened for purposes of retention. Any activity during this time of incubation disturbs what was learnt. Therefore rest is necessary and it is because of this reason that retroactive inhibition also takes place. This process of memory traces getting established is also referred to as the process of 'consolidation'.

This fact suggests that a period of intense learning activity should not be immediately followed by another period of equally intense learning activity. This would certainly have a bearing on the arrangement of our daily time-table in our classroom. It has been shown by a number of experiments that a short period of rest or sleep after learning activity helps towards the better retention of what has been learned. In some experiments retention has been disturbed by over fifty percent because of retrospective inhibition. We may incidentally mention here that it has been experimentally determined that forgetting is slow during sleep. This of course is understandable because during the period of rest or sleep no additional memory traces are formed which might disturb the memory traces already established.

The precautions that could be taken against this normal cause of forgetting are all implied in the methods recommended for efficient learning. Here we have added only one more factor, viz. a short period of rest immediately after a period of learning activity.

ABNORMAL OR PATHOLOGICAL FORGETTING

Abnormal forgetting does not depend upon the time factor. It happens because of certain unusual and striking circumstances. It has no relation to the factors of advantage considered earlier. It has nothing to do with the factor of interest, meaningful learning, over learning and reviewing, etc. It invariably happens immediately after an experience. The causes of this abnormal forgetting are usually two: *Exogenic and Endogenic.* 'Exogenic' means 'arising from outside causes'. A severe injury to the brain such as a shock resulting from a fall, etc. could disturb the memory process badly. This is more neurological and such a case would need medical attention. The psychologist cannot do much to help such a case.

'Endogenic' means 'causes from within'. Ever since Freud brought out the importance of the unconscious part of our mind and its working, it has been accepted by all that many experiences of ours are just completely forgotten in the flash of a second. This is because of the operation of a particular phenomenon technically called 'repression'. The experience is just drawn into the unconscious mind. The person will not be aware of the fact that it has been drawn within. After repression has taken place, he will have complete recall amnesia. This happens because of emotional conflicts leading to conditions of psychopathology. They can be brought out only by technical methods such as psycho-analysis, dream analysis and hypnosis. Dealing with such phenomena is the job of the psychotherapist.

Freud reports a number of interesting examples taken from his life and from the experience of others to illustrate this phenomenon of abnormal forgetting caused by repression. They can also be viewed as intentional forgetting or convenient forgetting. But the intention is not a conscious one.

One psychologist relates the case of a lady who forgot to keep her appointment with the dress-maker to try on her bridal gown the day before the wedding, recollecting it only at 8 in the evening. One must suppose that her whole was not in the marriage and, in fact, she has since been divorced.

Causes of Forgetting

The factors responsible for forgetting may be divided into two clear-cut parts:

1. Factors operating at the time of learning

a. *Strength of original learning:* It has been found experimentally that when the original learning is weaker, the neural traces formed in the brain are fainter and hence are properly retained. But the amount of retention cannot increase indefinitely as a function of the degree of overlearning. A point of diminishing return is to be reached. However, overlearning is always preferable than undertaking.

b. *Nature of material:* It is found that the meaningful and rhythmic material decrease the rate of forgetting. Ebbinghaus found that any material with an associative value decreases forgetting. The meaningless materials or nonsense syllables need to relate with some meaning or association to these quick remembering.

c. *Method of learning:* Various methods are used for learning and memorizing as given under memories mnemonics technique.

d. *Learning under abnormal conditions:* It is one of the major causes of forgetting at the time of learning. Some unpleasant experiences are more quickly forgotten than pleasant ones.

e. *Speed of learning:* Speed of learning also determines the degree of forgetting. According to Underwood, "When learning is rapid, forgetting will be slow and vice-versa".

2. Factors operating after learning: These are the factors which operate between learning and retention test; and at the time of recall. This is explained on the basis of theories of forgetting.

a. *Decay/trace decay/disuse theory:* It tries to explain why forgetting increases with time. The neural traces which are formed in the brain at the time of learning are decayed due to lack of use. Thus, they grow fainter and fainter with passage of time. Such fading or decay could be the result of normal metabolic processes of the brain. If we do not use a particular memory trace, it becomes out of use and fades away. It is argued by the disuse theorists that many skills, mathematical formula, poems that have been learnt in the past and not used for a long time are forgotten. By relearning these memory traces are strengthened and hence do not fade away.

b. *Displacement theory:* It is given by Waugh and Norman (1965). It explains that in a limited capacity STM system, forgetting may occur through displacement. When the system is "full", the oldest material in it would be displaced (pushed out) by incoming new material.

c. *Retrieval: Failure theory and cue-dependent forgetting:* According to retrieval failure theory, memories can't be recalled because the correct retrieval cues are not being used. The role of retrieval cue is demonstrated by the tip-of-the-tongue phenomenon, in which we know something but can't retrieve it at that particular moment in time (Brown and McNeil, 1966).

d. *Interference theory:* According to this, forgetting is influenced more by what we do before or after learning than by the mere passage of time. It determines the course of forgetting, what we do in the interval between learning and recall. Experimental studies have shown that learning new things interferers with memory of what is learned earlier and prior learning interferes with memory of things learned later.

   i. *Retroactive inhibition:* This is a technical name for new learning that may interfere with material previously learned. This has been demonstrated in experiments as following:

Groups	Activity		
	I	II	III
Experimental	Learn A	Learn B	Recall A
Control	Learn A	Unrelated activity	Recall A

As an example you may learn one chapter of physiology in activity I, then learn one chapter of Anatomy in activity II, then try to recall what you had learned in physiology. The amount of information you forget would be due to interference caused by learning anatomy. Compared to this, if you learn a chapter from physiology, rest for sometime then recall physiology you would find that your recall is better than that of the previous chapter.

ii. *Proactive Inhibition:* When prior learning interferes with the learning and recall of new material, it is called proactive inhibition. To demonstrate this type of interference experiment is designed as following:

Groups	Activity		
	I	II	III
Experimental	Learn A	Learn B	Recall A
Control	Rest or Unrelated activity	Learn B	Recall B

Supposing you learn English, then French and recall French, you would find that study of English interferes with your recall of French. Here what you learned earlier, interferes with the subsequent memory.

e. **Motivated forgetting/Repression theory:** Emotional factors also play an important role in forgetting. If we encode information while in one emotional state and try to recall it. While in another, our recall suffers. Many lapses of people we do not like. Repression theory holds that we forget because the retrieval of memories would be painful or unacceptable in some way to the person. Freud, in his book "The Psychopathology of Everyday Life" had illustrated many examples of repression in forgetting. Repression includes, retrieval failure for the associations of the threatening, anxiety-provoking information.

Amnesia—Forgetting During Sickness

Amnesia refers to loss of memory due to disease. It is of two types:

- **Biological Amnesias:** Forgetting could be due to any of the following reasons—diseases of the brain like senile dementia, Korsakoff syndrome, concussion from blows on head, brain damage, brain infections, tumor, stroke, temporary disturbances in the blood supply or effect of high dose of alcohol and drug abuse.

Biological Amnesias

- Transient global amnesia is a profound memory problem with no loss of amnesia. It can be retrograde and anterograde.
- ***Drugs:*** Marijuana and alcohol have a limited short-lived effect on the encoding, storage and retrieval of information. Alcohol induced amnesia is an example of state-dependent memory.
- ***Disease of the brain:*** Infections, e.g. neurosyphilis, strokes, brain tumors, disorders of brain metabolism, head injury, multiple sclerosis, etc. can result in amnesias. Senile

dementia is characterized by deficits in many intellectual abilities, memory, attention, judgement and abstract thought, *Senile forgetfulness* (characterized by difficulty in storage of relatively recent events) cannot be classified as amnesia, primary degenerative dementia, like senile dementia, can result in anterograde as well as retrograde amnesias.
- **Psychological amnesia:** These types of amnesia occur due to psychiatric diseases where the person has his identity also.

Childhood amnesia is due to the differences in the ways young children and older people encode and store information. *Defensive amnesia* is when people forget their names, where they have come from, who their spouses are, and many other important details of their past lives. It is called defensive because this is usually considered to be a way of protecting oneself from the guilt or anxiety that can result from intense, intolerable life situations and conflicts. It is thus an extreme of repression.
- ***Amnesia.*** The amnesia refers to loss of memory. It is profound memory deficit due to either the loss of what has been stored or to the inability to form new memories. Types of amnesia are psychological amnesia and biological amnesia. ***Psychological amnesia are:***
  i. *Childhood amnesia:* Forbidden guilt arousing sexual and aggressive urges are forgotten, especially through repression.
  ii. *Dream amnesia:* It is an example of state-dependent amnesia. Dreams seen many times during each night are not all remembered.
  iii. *Defensive amnesia:* This type protests oneself from guilt or anxiety that can result from intense intolerable life situations and conflicts. Amnesia episodes can last for weeks, months or years.

  Normal ageing has its problems too, but the typical forgetness of old age is hardly severe enough to be called amnesia. The memory problem centers largely on the storage of relatively recent events; it is anterograde in nature.

Methods to Improve Memory

TECHNIQUES TO IMPROVE MEMORY

Following memory techniques and strategies can help you to improve your memory.
1. **Pulling it all together:** Organizing and ordering information can significantly improve memory. As learning a large amount of unconnected and unorganized information from various classes can be very challenging. By organizing and adding meaning to the material prior to learning it, you can facilitate both storage and retrieval. In other words, you can learn it better and recall it easier, e.g. organizing material on paper such as when you make an outline or idea web, or simply organizing material in your memory, such as learning it in a particular order or making intentional associations between ideas.
2. **The Funnel approach:** This means learning general concepts before moving on to specific details. When you understand the general concepts first, the details make more sense. Many textbook chapters are organized in a "general to specific" format.
3. **Organizing through meaning and association:** When learning, a person continually makes associations. We make association between what we are learning and the environment we are in, between the information and our mental states, and between

the information and our stream of thoughts. When things are associated in memory, thinking of one helps bring the other to mind.

a. Deep processing relating the material to yourself: One way to process information more deeply, and also to create meaningful associations, is to think about how the information can be personally meaningful, e.g. relating new material to your life, your experience or your goals.

b. Grouping: It means organizing material by grouping similar concepts of or related ideas together. Arranging the material into related groups helps your memory by organizing the information, e.g. grouping all sports into one of following categories—winter sports, track and field sports using a ball and so on.

4. **Vivid association:** When learning something new and unfamiliar, try pairing it with something you know very well. Such as images, puns, music, etc. The association does not have to make logical sense. For example, remembering Robert Green by picturing Robert playing golf (on the green), wearing green clothes, or covered in green paint.
5. **Active learning:** Active learning facilitates your memory by helping you attend to and process information. All of the memory techniques (already discussed) require active learning. Even if you attend every lecture and read every assignment, there is no guarantee that you will learn and remember the information. Thus, you always attend to and think about what you are learning.
6. **Visual memory:** Some people remember information best when it is encoded visually, include charts, cartoons, diagrams, tables, outlines, pictures or any other visual material.
7. **Talk it out:** Repeat ideas verbatim (when you need to do rote memorization), repeat the ideas in your own words (indicates true understanding of information). Repeating information aloud can help you encode the information (auditory encoding) and identify how well you have learned it.
8. **Visualize yourself teaching the material:** An effective way to enhance recall and understanding of dense material is to teach it to an imaginary audience. By doing so, you are forced to organize the material in a way that makes sense to you and to anticipate potential questions that may be asked to your students.

   Mnemonics: Organization of materials is extremely important to improve memory. The term 'mnemonics' is derived from the Greek word which means 'to remember'. The mnemonics are short, verbal devices that encode a long series of facts by associating them with familiar and previously encoded informations in the recent past. If materials lack natural organizations, artificial organization are necessary to be used by the learner for better memory, e.g. colors of rainbow are associated with 'VIBGYOR'.

The following mnemonic devices are used to improve memory.

a. Method of loci: Loci is the plural of Latin word 'locus' which means 'place'. The method of loci says that visualize a scene and fit the items to be remembered in that scene. The scene can be a street, a building with rooms, the layout of a college campus, a kitchen or just about anything that can be visualized clearly and contains a number of discrete items in specific locations to serve as memory pegs. Supposing you want to remember for examination 'classical conditioning'. Then start by imagining a dog, experimental room, food, bell and any person as an experimenter. Rehearse this image over and over until it is well-established in your mind. After you have formed your image, associate the events like stimulus substitutions, extinction with this. This trick is to make associations with as many concepts as needed.

b. Rhyming: Like the method of loci, number and letterpeg systems is to establish, main idea in your long-term memory, a well-organized set of images of which the to-be remembered items can be linked. In number systems, you form an image with each number. For instance, a rhyming system can be used for the number 1 through 10. For letter systems, you can establish mnemonic pegs by forming strong distinctive images of words that start with the sounds of the letter of the alphabet, e.g. number and letter pegs.

One is fan	Six is a disc
Two is a shoe	Seven is a pen
Three is a tree	Eight is a light
Four is a door	Nine is a fine
Five is a knife	Ten is men and so on

c. Narrative stories: You can make a story and in that you can fit the facts, like you read in elaborate rehearsal. The important thing for good memory is your motivation and ability to organize the material. One strategy in remembering things well is to organize, or arrange, the input so that it fits into existing long-term memory categories, is grouped in some logical manner, or is arranged in some other way that makes sense. The organizational encoding may be inherent in the input itself or it may be supplied by individuals as they learn and remember new things.

d. Chunking: This mnemonic technique illustrates systematic ways of encoding information. If you want to remember a long list of digits, e.g. 20061506080 you can break the numbers into chunks. The first four digits could be remembered as the year of your engagement or associate with any significant things that happened in that year. Next four digits could be taken as someone's birthday and last three digits as someone's weight. Like this, chunks can be associated with some important thing for lasting memory.

Other ways to improve memory are:
- Keep an active brain
- Make associations: Creating mental link between the things you already knew and new information
- Visualize and observe: Create a mental picture of what you are interested in
- Repeat things; Practice makes it perfect
- Meditation and exercise: Improves blood circulation throughout your body, be more alert and relaxed
- Eating and sleeping: Keeps brain healthier
- Organize your life
- Reduce stress.

Testing Memory

Wechsler memory scale: The Wechsler Memory Scale—Revised (WMS—R) is the most widely used memory test battery for adults. It is a composite of verbal paired associate and paragraph retention, visual memory for designs, orientation, digit span, rote recall of the alphabet, and counting backward. The scale yields a Memory Quotient (MQ), which is corrected for age and generally approximates the Wechsler Adult Intelligence Scale Intelligence Quotient (WAIS IQ); amnestic conditions, such as Korsakoff's syndrome, are characterized by a disproportionately low MQ but a relatively preserved IQ.

Benton visual retention test: It is sensitive to short-term memory loss.

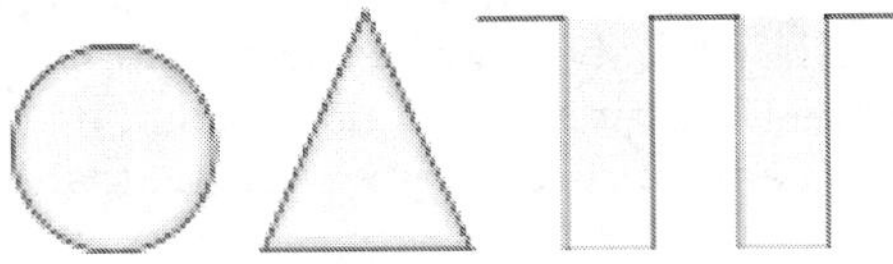

The most frequently used testing condition involves the presentation of each geometric figure for 10 seconds, after which the patient attempts to draw the figure from memory.

- Memories are reconstructed from the various bits and pieces of information that have been stored away in different places at the time of encoding in a process called constructive processing.
- Hindsight bias occurs when people falsely believe that they knew the outcome of some event because they have included knowledge of the events true outcome into their memories of the event itself.
- People experience when trying to remember something stored in the long-term memory.
- The misinformation effect refers to the tendency of people who are asked misleading questions or given misleading information to incorporate that information into their memories for a particular event.
- False memory syndrome refers to rather than improving retrieval, hypnosis makes the creation of false memories more likely.
- False memory syndrome, is the creation of false or inaccurate memories through suggestions, especially while hypnotized.
- Pezdek and colleagues assert that false memories are more likely to be formed for plausible false events than for implausible ones.

Forgetting

- Ebbinghaus found that information is mostly lost within one hour after learning and then gradually fades away. This is shown as the curve of forgetting.
- A failure to encode information will not produce a memory.
- Memory trace decay theory assumed the presence of a physical memory trace that decays with disuse over time.
- Forgetting in LTM is most likely due to proactive or retroactive interference.

It is the apparent loss of information already encoded and stored in long-term memory. Much of what we have forgotten does not really qualify as forgotten "because it was never encoded and stored." Due to lack of attention, it may not have reached STM from sensory register due to inadequate encoding and rehearsal; it may not have been transferred from STM to LTM. Forgetting occurs most rapidly shortly after learning and faulty remembering is not forgetting.

Decay theory of forgetting: is the theory that information in memory eventually disappears if it is not reactivated; it appears to be more plausible for STM than LTM. Like remembering, a certain degree of forgetting contributes to our survival and sanity. Adoptive forgetting (and not disrupture forgetting) is healthy and helpful Sigmund Freud called the unconscious willing of forgetfulness "repression".

Improvement of Memory in Student

Students, particularly when they come to their higher classes or when they enter college often complain that their memory power has become weak. They would say that in spite of studying well they were not able to remember. In most of these cases, the difficulty will lie only with the method of learning. The most important things would be to make sure that they are really interested in what they study. For developing the interest, they should employ the methods of efficient learning mentioned earlier. It should be understood that the capacity to retain cannot be improved in any intrinsic manner. Only the methods of learning could be improved.

A different kind of complaint would often be made by students particularly around the adolescent period. This complaint would take the form that they had once very good memory, but somehow they had lost it. They should be told straightway that memory power or properly speaking, the capacity to remember can never be lost or reduced (except in serious neurological disorders). When these people were younger they had limited interests and they were able to attend to their studies with more interest and hence with greater concentration. Naturally, they were able to remember what they studied. During the adolescent period, their interest widen and because of the developing sex interest and urges, all sorts of psychological problems also crop up. These disturb them, sometimes producing emotional conflicts and sometimes a sense of guilt. Their minds get occupied with these personal problems with the result when they attempt to study, they are not able to pay sufficient attention to their work. Consequently they do not remember as efficiently as they did before. To make matters worse, they now develop a fear that they are losing their memory power. Things are made worse. A vicious circle sets in. The only way to break this vicious circle is to convince people that their memory power is absolutely intact and only they are passing through a stage in their developmental process when various kinds of interests claim their attention. Thus they should be encouraged and helped to get over this period without developing any fear or depression. Regaining confidence is the only way of meeting such a situation.

Sometimes, people take to commercial courses offered for the training of memory. The only way to train memory is to develop proper habits of observing and helpful method of learning. They may also be helped to regain and maintain their confidence in themselves. In no other way is memory training possible. Some people may complain that they are weak in remembering certain things such as faces, dates, etc. We would have come across people who say "I have a very good memory except for remembering dates". Here it should be remembered that just like in other psychological phenomena, there are wide individual differences. But the actual difference comes from the habits and interests one has developed. If we take a genuine interest in the people whom we meet we will seldom forget their names or faces. But sometimes when someone is introduced to us we may not take any interest in him. We would have just mechanically wished him without paying any attention to any information connected with him. Some people by temperament and by cultivated habits would always take an interest in some social facts connected with the people they meet. In such cases, it would be easy to remember names or faces. The same is the case with the other details also. To a large extent, our capacity to remember such details can be improved if we deliberately cultivate the habit of taking an interest in those details.

Some tips for improving memory as given below:

1. *Mnemonic devices:* Some Mnemonic devices are easily memorized rhymes whereas others use visual images or verbal associations.
2. *Mental stroll method* ("Method of Loci"): A favorite method is to remember a list of items by talking a mental stroll through one's items by taking a mental stroll through

one's house, forming a visual image of each item at a particular location (the method of loci).

3. *Pay attention:* Attention is important for encoding. Impairment in attention, e.g. in depression may result in impaired encoding causing pseudodementia.
4. *Encode information in more than one way:* The more elaborate the encoding of information, the more memorable it is. Elaboration can be in many forms, e.g. remembering a telephone number by sound of the individual digits.
5. *Add meaning:* The more meaning material is, the more likely it is to link up with information already in long-term memory. Meaningfulness also reduces the number of chunks of information one has to learn.
6. *Use visual memory:* Memory for pictures is often better than the memory for words.
7. *Take your time:* If one has to remember large amounts of verbal material, leisurely learning spread out over several sessions will produce better results than rapid cramming.
8. *Take time out:* If possible, minimize interference by using study breaks for rest or recreation. Sleep is the ultimate way to reduce interference.
9. *Overlearn:* Overlearing—Studying information even after you think you know it is one of thc best way to remember it.
10. *Planning to learn:* Plan a study schedule, regular rehearsal, subjective organization and retrieval cues, testing oneself (feedback) and review help in memorizing (i.e. "PRO"- Planning, Rehearsal, Organization and "FRO"- Feedback, Review and Over-learning).
11. *Avoiding use of drugs:* Alcohol, benzodiazepines, antihistaminic and other CNS depressants may impair the memorizing process. *Nootropics (Brain tonics) are not useful in normal persons.*

14 CHAPTER

Imagination, Thinking and Reasoning

Imagination

Image refers to a representation of the external form of a person or a thing in art. Images as mental picture consist of personal experiences of objects, persons or scenes once actually seen, heard or felt. These mind pictures symbolize actual objects, experiences and activities. In thinking individual usually manipulate the images instead of actual objects experiences or activities. Image is a general impression that a person, organization or products presents to the public.

Thinking also includes more than just a kind of verbal stream of consciousness when people think they often have images as well as words in their minds. Mental images are one of several tools used in the thought process. Imagination may be defined conveniently as "mental manipulation". This process involves the recall of past experiences in the form of mental images and arranging them in patterns that are already familiar, or sometimes in rearranging them in new and strange ways to produce new combinations. A familiar example is the image of a mermaid (Mermaid, a mythical sea creature with the head and trunk of a woman and the tail of a fish), which has become so common in our literature. This image of a mermaid is composed of the images of a woman and a fish both of which are obtained from our familiar experiences. In this manner, person can imagine numerous things which might be real or unreal.

This process of imagining is very useful because with the help of this, man is able to invent new things, produce fine works of art, create entertaining stories, write novels, etc. These things which amuse or enrich our knowledge and thus make our life better are made possible because of our ability to imagine. Even the child makes use of this process for a good deal of its play and amusement. It is by imagination that the child is able to put itself into situations which really do not exist and thus make its play more complicated and enjoyable. What people usually call creative art depends greatly on one's ability to do constructive imagination. This kind of constructive or productive imagination is sometimes contrasted with mere reproductive imagination which simply recalls actual images experienced in the past.

MEANING OF IMAGINATION

Imagination is mental manipulation. Suppose that a person has to decorate a room with furniture. One way of doing it is to move every individual piece of furniture all over the room and to find a suitable place for it. This will only mean a wastage of a lot of time, and there is little possibility of success because the correct place for a piece of furniture can be defined only in the background of the rest of furniture. Individual does not know the most suitable place for a chair in an empty room. The question of its most suitable position arises only when other pieces of furniture have also to be placed. Decoration by physical manipulation is bound to be tedious and it is, therefore, better to turn to imagination. If now the person takes up a strategic position in the room, from where the whole room is visible, he can picture the room in his mind and decide the location of the various pieces of furniture by moving them around in his mind. This involves mental manipulation as a substitute for physical manipulation. It is thus an example of imagination.

This ability to imagine is also helpful in the processes called thinking and reasoning. To find the sum of two and two, if a child takes two marbles and then again adds two more marbles and then counts them, one, two, three, four, it is said to be using the method of motor manipulation. But if the child uses a mental image of two things twice over and does the accounting mentally then it is using the process of imagination. We can see here that motor manipulation as a method of solving our problems cannot lead us very far. It has serious limitations. Only because of our ability to imagine we are able to develop our thinking and reasoning processes and improve our intellect. As states earlier, the artist, the sculptor, the architect, the inventor, the poet and the novelist are able to contribute their share to the richness of life only because of their special abilities in imagination. At the same time it is because of this imaginative process that we ourselves are able to appreciate and enjoy the creation of these artists and inventors.

IMAGES

Imagination is made possible because of our capacity to form images. Images are mental pictures. They may be either exact reproduction of a past percept or they may be new and strange combinations of various bits of past experiences. When you are sitting in the classroom you can imagine the face of your mother and form a mental picture of her. This mental picture is an image. You also have a mental picture of your mother when she is actually standing before you and you are looking at her. That mental picture is not called an image. It is called a percept, because you have the required sensations and the object, viz, the mother, actually presented to your eyes. But when we do not have the actual sensation but depend upon our memory to recall a picture of an object we call that an image. It is also called a memory image.

Individual can have memory images of all sorts of things relating to the different kinds of sensations. We can imagine the shape and form of an object, the voice of a person, the smell of a flower, the taste of a particular substance, the feeling of the muscles when tired, etc. Thus there are different kinds of memory images, such as the visual image, the auditory image, the olfactory image, the kinesthetic image, etc. Naturally the memory image will not ordinarily be as strong and clear as the percept. Individuals differ in their capacity to form memory images. Even the same individual may not be equally good in forming memory images belonging to the different kinds of sense experiences. One may be very good in having visual memory images but not so good in the field of smell. Musicians usually have a strong auditory memory image. Artists usually have a strong visual image. Some psychologists have tried to devise tests to measure the strength of imagery in different people. The well-known among these tests is one by Francis Galton as given below:

Directions: Sit quiet and *imagine* to yourself the following objects or situations and grade them for their vividness or *clearness*, on the given scale:

	Marks
a. Absolutely no imagery at all	0
b. Very vague and dim	1
c. Sketchy in outline but clear in parts, appearing now and again	2
d. Fairly clear in general but details rather misty, and apt to disappear soon	3
e. Very vivid and clear-cut both in outline and details, appearing for a fairly long time	4

Types of Images

Visual Images—
1. Fifty paisa
2. The front of the house you live in
3. A railway engine
4. The face of your mother or wife
5. An elephant or a giraffe.

Auditory or Sound Images –
1. The barking of a dog
2. The voice of your best friend
3. The howling of wind
4. The sound of your own voice.

Kinesthetic or Muscular Images—
1. The feeling of kicking a football or other object
2. The feeling of running very fast
3. The feeling of lifting some very heavy weight
4. The feeling of pricking while taking injection.

There are also images other than memory images. Some children especially are known to have a peculiar ability to form a clear and exact photographic image of a complicated scene or picture, which they have seen. If you show them the picture of a complicated scene and then remove it and ask them to mention the details they have seen they will be able to form in their minds the exact copy of the picture and correctly reproduce every detail. Such an image which they form in their minds is called 'eidetic image'. All children do not have this ability. Also adults are not known to possess the capacity for eidetic images.

- After images: Yet another type of image is called after image. Perhaps, really speaking after images are not images in the real sense. To is better to call them as after sensations. After images are of tow kinds positive and negative.
  Positive after image: Suppose one keeps staring at a green square patch and them shifts his vision to a neutral gray background. The green sensation continues for some time even though the individual is not actually looking at the green patch. This continued sensory experience even after the removal of the actual stimulus is called an after image.

An after image is thus, continuation of a sensory experience even after the removal of the actual stimulus. An after image have the same color and other characteristics of the original sensation.

Negative after image: In the above example if the person still goes on looking at the neutral gray background, the positive after image suddenly changes into a reddish image. This changed sensory experience which follows the positive after image is called the negative after image. Negative after images is take on a complementary hue (color). If the original sensation was green the positive after image will be green but the negative after image will be red, red being complementary to green. Similarly for a blue sensation the negative after image will be yellow. After images are results of brain processes.

Classification of Imagination (Fig. 14.1)

Imagination has been classified in a number of ways, the most general classification being reproductive and creative.

Reproductive imagination—Reproductive imagination is directed by external suggestions. Students of history, to take a common example, are able to imagine incidents which took place some thousands of years ago. The vividness of this imagination will be more less according to the vividness or otherwise of the description. Similarly, when a person loses himself in some novel which he is reading, he feels, for some time at least, that he is seeing everything with his own eyes. Even when people are moving around in historical places, incidents related to them present themselves to the spectators through their imagination. In all these examples, the basis of imagination is external, the imagination being a mere reproduction of external objects and not an individual or original construction. These are, therefore, examples of reproductive imagination.

Creative imagination—But, if some person writes a story, poem or drama, it is not merely a reproduction of external happenings but it has an additional element of original imagination. Creation is not the same thing as reproduction. The difference between creative and reproductive imagination is the same as that between an author and his reader. The poet, author, artist and the like depict their emotions and feelings through the medium of creative imagination.

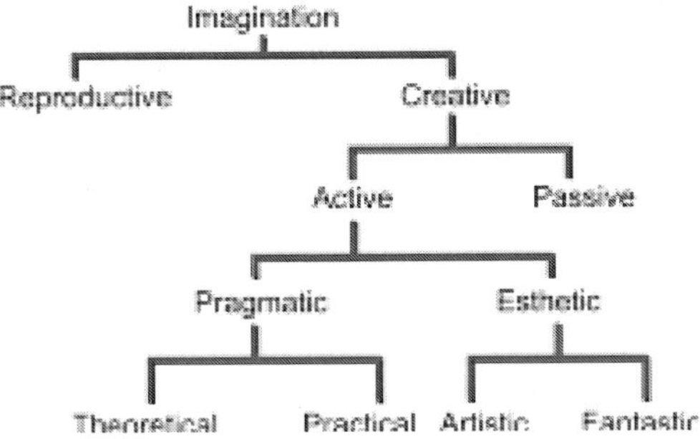

Fig. 14.1: Classification of imagination

1. *Passive creative imagination*—Sometimes and as a matter of fact quite often, when a person's brain in unoccupied, imaginative ideas flit through the mind one after the other. The person has to make no effort in their coming or going. This is called passive

creative imagination because in this state the mind is passive. Among instances of passive imagination are included dreams, day-dreams and other imaginations of the type. Some sports are also included in this class, due to the passivity of imagination in their case, but most of the other organized games cannot be classified under this heading. Now chess, for example, calls for active imagination. Imagination is passive in dreams and day-dreams. The aim of day-dream is the fulfillment of desires through the imagination instead of effort. The person imagines himself to be the hero of his day-dream. The conquering hero fulfills his desires through victory while the suffering hero does the same through suffering. Adler attributes these desires to power while Freud considers them to be related to sex. These day-dreams are useful to man in as much that they fulfill unfulfilled desires and restore a balance in personality. In fact, every person day-dreams some time or the other but if it becomes abnormal and an excuse to escape from the realities of life, it causes grave harm to the individual. The dream, too, is a similar passive creative imagination. Freud maintains that dreams fulfill unsatisfied sex desires. According to other psychologists external physiological factors also influence dreams.

2. *Active creative imagination*—In the case of active creative imagination the subject imaging various things has predetermined goal in view. The reality and reasoning are not disregarded. From the view point of aim or goal, active creative imagination can be classified as (a) Pragmatic, and (b) Esthetic Imagination.
   a. *Pragmatic imagination* — The making of a plan for a big bridge or canal, deducing of a mathematical theory or the exercise of the faculty of imagination for an invention are all examples of pragmatic imagination. In these cases imagination was guided by some particular object in view. Pragmatic imagination, as is implied in the name, has a particular end in view. Pragmatic imagination, in its turn, can be divided into two classes, as follows:
      i. *Theoretical imagination*—Imagination which helps in the proof or classification of some theory is theoretical imagination. This is the type of imagination employed in scientific theories.
      ii. *Practical imagination*—The construction of a plan for a bridge or a canal are examples of this type of imagination. Practical imagination is the imagination which helps us in constructing something useful and not to prove some theory.
      iii. *Esthetic imagination*—On the one hand, the aim of the pragmatic imagination is to find something advantageous while on the other, esthetic imagination aims simply at the creation of beauty. This is the type of imagination employed in literature, music and art. A poem, created by a poet, aims only at the creation of beauty and not any other practical aim. It is not necessary to include all literature, music and art in the class but it is undoubtedly true that these are the creation of beauty. Esthetic imagination is of two types—artistic and fantastic.
      - *Artistic imagination*—In the artistic esthetic imagination, beauty has a specific pattern and its description in literature or painting is attempted. Thus, even though artistic esthetic imagination is as free from the limitations of the external world as possible, it is directed towards the fulfillment of some predetermined aim of the artist. In the writing of a story the imagination of the author does create beauty but even then some aim and pattern is concealed in it. It works within a predetermined framework.
      - *Fantastic imagination*—As opposed to artistic imagination, fantastic imagination has no direction, pattern or aim and everything depends on the fantasy of the individual. Fairy tales and fantastic poems are examples of this type of imagination.

Though this, too, results in some advantage to the society or the individual yet as in the case of artistic imagination fantastic imagination has no predetermined framework.

IMAGINATION AND THINKING

Though both thinking and imagination are mental activities, they are not identical. Thinking is mental exploration. It starts with some problem and its solution is searched for, the search being mental and not physical. If, for example, the problem is one of arranging furniture in the room there is nothing to be explored. Thus, what is needed is imagination and not thinking. But if, for some reason, the person is incapable of setting the furniture, the problem of finding someone will arise. He will have to find someone, and if this hunt is mental, it is the activity of thinking. Many doubts arise in his mind, as to who will bring the furniture and in order to come to some decision the examines the merits and demerits of every such person. While coming to the conclusion he is compelled to use not only his imagination but also perceptions, signs, language, concept, etc.

Thus imagination is mental manipulation, while thinking is mental experiments, and both have dissimilar instruments and uses. Imagination is free while thinking is a controlled mental activity. Imagination results from a free association of thoughts and images but this association is controlled in the activity of thinking. Thinking is the search for solutions of problems.

TESTS OF IMAGINATION

Various normal forms of imagination are helpful phenomena for intellectual growth and development. So, sometimes it is possible to measure one's intellectual vigor and strength by means of studying one's imagination. If one is able to have a rich and fertile imagination that would necessarily show that he is having quite a vigorous and active mind. Strength of imagination will show one's ability to organize past experiences and put them to use for new situations and problems. This process is studied as 'fertility of imagination'.

Whipple, a psychologist proposed a test for measuring one's fertility of imagination. He used a series of ink-blots which were presented to the subject and ideas suggested to him by the picture in a given short period of time. Such blots will be rather vague in outline and form, so that each blot may suggest several things, such as an animal, a bird, a landscape, a geographical continent, etc. The blots have to be vague because if they actually represent one definite concrete object there will be no scope for our imagination. If an accurate picture of a dog is presented everybody will see only a dog and no other objects or animals could be imagined on the basis of that picture. Therefore, all these ink-blots in such experiments will have to be vague. Naturally one, who has a very rich imagination and also is quick at using his past experiences, will be able to give many more responses than one whose imaginative process is poor and low. By counting the total number of discrete and definite responses we measure one's fertility of imagination.

Sometimes a variation of this test is used to measure what is called one's 'verbal imagination'. Since ease and readiness with which one can use words is very important in the matter of one's education and general efficiency, it is very desirable to have a test to measure the capacity for verbal imagination. The test is very simple. Six letters, such as E, A, P, L, R, I, are given and the subject is asked to form as many words as possible by using at least three or four of these letters in each word. It is not enough to have a good vocabulary to do this test well. One must be able to imagine quickly various combinations and then use his own store of vocabulary.

Similar tests of imagination are nowadays used for an entirely different purpose also. A very well-known test is what is called Rorschach's ink-blot test. This is used for testing one's personality traits.

Day-dreams as Imagination

Imagination is not always directed to a particular goal, viz, of producing some work of imagination. With most of us it is often just a form of play. When we are not doing anything in particular and when we are not attending to what is happening around us, our imagination goes on like a continuous chain working out various themes of stories in which we may play the central part. This sort of free imagination is called day-dreaming. Day-dreams may often appear to us as meaningless rambling of the mind. They may be considered purely as idle thoughts. But this is not so. If we study them carefully we would always find some definite theme and definite motives connected with our own deeper aspirations, hopes and experiences of life. Thus they are not mere idle meaningless thoughts. To the student of psychology they are full of meaning and significance. A study of one's day-dreams would reveal a good deal of his mental make-up and his problems in life. How many of us have not at some time or other lost ourselves in building castles in the air and imagining ourselves doing wonderful feats in sports or in studies or in scientific invention. Day-dreams are usually divided into three kinds:

1. *Winning hero type:* Often day-dreams consist in a hero doing wonderful things, winning victory over all sorts of obstacles or, in other words, getting on the top of the world. Often the hero will be the dreamer himself. The particular theme may vary according to the age. A small child may be imagining a whole story where he gets everything that he wants and flies about like a fairy. An older child may imagine that he is driving the train or in modern days flying an aeroplane. An adolescent boy may be imagining that he is successfully carrying out all sorts of adventures, fighting, creating world records in sports, etc. An adolescent girl may imagine, particularly in these days, that she is growing into a beautiful glamorous well-dressed screen star or that she is appreciated and sought after by all the best young men of that place. We all know the story of the milkmaid in its various forms. All such day-dreams are characterized by the mastery that we achiever over our environment. So they are called the mastery day-dreams of the conquering hero type. These dreams usually arise because of a consciousness of our weakness and inability and at the same time our natural desire to achieve great things. Since this goal cannot be achieved in reality we seek a satisfaction of achieving them at least in imagination. Thus these day-dreams play the part of substitutes for our weakness. In other words, such as day-dream is a mechanism for compensating our actual inferiority.
2. *Suffering hero type:* There is also another kind of day-dream called the "suffering hero type". Here instead of imagining oneself to be reaching the top of the world one imagines himself to be ill-treated by everybody, or having all sorts of misfortunes, or failing in everything because of bad luck and being betrayed by other people, etc. In this process slight disappointments or injuries actually received are exaggerated upto a point where one would be very naturally sympathized with by other people. So here again we see the same kind of motive at work. This also is another indirect way of satisfying our desire for importance and recognition at the hands of others.

3. *Worrying hero type:* There is a third type of day-dreams which is different from the above two kinds. In this the individuals just imagines himself to be in all sorts of difficulties and also imagines that all kinds of calamities may happen to him or to somebody connected with him. This is merely an organized worrying. We all occasionally worry about something or other. But some individuals because of abnormal reasons develop a habit of entertaining day-dreams of the worrying type. Why this happens is an interesting study in abnormal psychology. We would presently consider some simple facts about the unconscious part of our mind, the contents of which often come out in the form of day-dreams and dreams in various shapes and forms.

On the whole, day-dreams play an important part in our growth and development. Through such dreams only we can plan our future. By day-dreaming we can plan for improving our achievements in life. But to be able to use our day-dreams to such positive and beneficial ends we must support our day-dreams with relevant actions. One should not be content to live in the world of imagination alone. If real acts are set in motion as a result of our imagination and day-dreams then, it would be all the better for us. But if day-dreams are used merely as substitute gratifications, without any attempt to connect them with real facts of life, then we would be developing ourselves into poor specimens of human beings.

IMAGINATION AND UNCONSCIOUS MIND

Imaginative process controlled by past experiences and often contents of the unconscious mind in griding and directing the imaginative process. Understanding of unconscious mind and other related contents discussed as given below:

- **The unconscious mind:** The common man will mean by mind only that part of which he is conscious. But according to modern psychology mind consists of regions other than the conscious part. It consists of three areas or three levels of working. We should not think that these are spatial divisions. The psychologist Sigmund Freud has greatly contributed to our knowledge of the different levels of mental working.

At any given time we are aware only of a narrow range of our environment. We may be attending to one particular thing. Yet a few more things also will be in our conscious mind. For example, when we are listening to the lectures the center of attention is the teacher. Yet we are aware of a number of other things such as the existence of our classmates, the breeze, the singing of the bird outside, the dress of someone sitting before us, etc. All these put together cover the conscious area of our mind.

Just below this level there are a host of things which we are not aware of at that moment, but which could be brought to the conscious mind if we wanted to, e.g. a friend whom we met that morning, the picnic which we enjoyed the previous month, a festival which we attended some years ago and countless other experiences of the immediate and remote past. These things have not been forgotten. They are in some area of the mind from where they can be easily beckoned at our will. Obviously this area is much vaster than the area covered by the conscious part of the mind. This area is technically called the preconscious or the foreconscious part of the mind. Some people also use the term subconscious mind but it is better to avoid this term.

Below this second level there is still another vast region called the unconscious. We are not at all aware of the contents of this area. Neither can we bring to the conscious level the contents of this at our will. In other words we cannot recall anything from this area. We are really unconscious of this region. The question may arise how then do we know that such a things exists. Modern abnormal psychology has taught us various ways by which we could recognize most of the contents of this unconscious mind. The unconscious mind is not controlled by our will. But the contents of that region do not remain dead and buried. Many experiences of the past particularly those connected with emotional conflicts, unpleasant events, that brought us shame, feelings of guilt, etc. form the major part of the contents of this unconscious mind. They are not actually forgotten according to the normal laws of forgetting. But they have been taken away from the conscious mind by a process technically called repression. Now, these experiences do not simply lie quiet in the unconscious mind. They all try to come out. But because of the peculiar nature of the unconscious mind these contents are not allowed to come out directly. They come out in various indirect and disguised forms. The boundary between the unconscious mind and the foreconscious mind is heavily protected by some psychological mechanism. To escape these guarding phenomena the contents of the unconscious mind are forced to come out only indirectly.

Further this unconscious mind often indirectly motivates our behavior, though we would not be aware of this real motive. For example, someone to whom you are an apparent friend makes an engagement with you. For all conscious purpose you seriously and sincerely promise to go. But when the actual time comes you forget. Later you come to remember this and perhaps send an apology saying that you forgot. Here you do not tell a lie at any stage. But on proper psychological enquiry it may turn out that you forgot because your unconscious mind wanted you not to keep that appointment. So the forgetting was caused purposefully. This is what we sometimes call convenient forgetting. It is actually a trick played on us by the unconscious mind. We not know that most of our psychological diseases like hysteria, phobias, obsessions, etc. are produced by the contents of the unconscious mind. Therefore modern treatment of these disorders depends on an analysis of the contents of the unconscious mind.

The unconscious mind has a great hold over all of us. It is very powerful and always active. Most of our behavior is directed by this mind rather than by the conscious rational part. The unconscious mind does not very much respect the principles of logical reasoning. So it is sometimes said to be blind. Neither does the unconscious mind very much care for the various accepted moral principles. All our moral principles are based on rational thinking and social living. The unconscious does not care for any of these. It works blindly in its own way. This does not mean that the unconscious is immoral or that it necessarily makes us do wrong things. On the other hand it is simply nonmoral or amoral.

Freud has shown that almost all our lapses of memory, slips of the tongue and pen, mistaking one name for another, etc. are all because of the interference of the unconscious mind. In other words, what we would explain as a mere accident, say if we meant one name and wrote down another name, has now been shown to be a deliberately motivated activity of the unconscious mind. With good training in abnormal psychology it is possible to analyse the contents of one's unconscious mind and its ways of working by the use of the technical method known as psychoanalysis. In this analysis two major methods are used, viz, free association and dream analysis.

- **Complexes:** All come across the term 'complex' in some connection or other. Though it is a technical term in psychology, the layman uses this term quite often rightly or wrongly. Common literature often uses the term Inferiority Complex. If a person is rather timid and feels that he is no good in his studies or in some other task, the layman ordinarily explains this as the result of an inferiority complex. Such as usage of this term complex is wrong.

As started earlier that many of our past experiences are drawn into the unconscious mind under certain circumstances. This happens mostly with strong emotional experiences such as anger, moral conflict, shame, guilt, fear, etc. When these experiences are drawn into the unconscious mind they are organized into different systems. Experiences of similar nature organize themselves into a cluster or group around one strong experience. These clusters constantly try to come out to the surface. But they do so only in disguise. Such organized groups of the contents of the unconscious are called complexes. No person can detect his own complex except through proper analysis. Since complexes come out only in disguised and indirect ways the person himself will be unable to see or recognize his own complex. Thus one cannot complain that he is suffering from an inferiority complex on the basis of his timidity and difference, of which he is fully conscious. Since he is fully conscious of his inferiority he can only say that he is suffering from inferiority feeling and not complex. In fact the conscious inferiority feeling may be the indirect expression of a superiority complex of which the individual himself will have no awareness at all. In abnormal psychology one would learn about a number of major complexes that are common to many individuals. These are the complexes that are often responsible for abnormal behavior and psychological disorders. Hence, detection of complexes is an important part of the treatment of psychological disorders. Two different complexes have been believed to be the most important and basic by two leading psychologists. According to Freud, 'Oedipus complex' connected with the development of the sex urge in the child is the basic complex in all human beings. According to Adler, another great original thinker, inferiority complex is the most basic.

- **Free association** is a very common phenomenon with which we may all be familiar. This simply means that one idea suggests another idea almost automatically because of being associated together in our past experiences. If one utters the word 'chair' most probably the idea of 'table' may be suggested at once along with it. This is because most of us have seen table and chair always together. If we hear the word 'father' perhaps the word 'mother' may occur to our minds along with it. Thus if we begin with any one word and go on uttering it. Thus if we begin with any one word and go on uttering or writing down all the words and ideas that are suggested one after another, it will make a whole series of connected and unconnected ideas. We may begin with the word 'chair' but may end up after five minutes in any word or idea. No two people will have the same train of thought or the same association of ideas. This letting off of the mind on a free rambling without any conscious and deliberate control is called free association.

But this free association is not really free in the sense that the connected ideas are suggested merely by accident. Always there are some principles working underneath determining what comes next. Sometimes two apparently unconnected ideas may be uttered together. It is such examples that are interesting for the purpose of analysis. For example, if a man responds with; the word 'mother' to the word 'father' there is nothing strange. It is quite normal and natural and does not reveal anything special about the deeper workings of his mind. But if he responds, say, with the word 'belt' then we stop and wonder as to what exactly is the connection between 'father' and 'belt'. It is possible that his father was fond of a particular type of belt. Or it is also possible that something unpleasant happened between himself and the father with reference to a belt. This association of belt was actually given by a patient of mine and on further enquiry it turned out that when he was a young boy the father in extreme anger had one day beaten him with a belt that was lying near. In spite of apparent love and devotion for the father this boy was carrying deep down in his mind a strong grudge against his father. Thus we see that by a simple application of the free association method something which was hiding in the mind of this young man came to light.

All instances may not be so simple as this. Sometimes one may fail to give any association word at all even to a simple harmless word. Or there may be a blocking and disturbance in the man and he may take an abnormally long time to give a response. The boy who gives instantaneous responses one after another in a series, stops after a particular word, say "Motor Car". It is possible that on further enquiry we would find that this boy had experience of an accident or in some other way has a strong fear of motor car.

This principle of free association is sometimes adopted in a particular form called word-association. Here the individual is not asked to go on at a tangent giving a chain of associated words or ideas, but is asked to respond one after another to a list of words that we have proposed. But the underlying principle is the same. Thus we see that in the process of free association actually there is no real freedom. Our imaginative process in controlled by our past experiences, particularly by experiences which have great emotional significance to us. Often contents of the unconscious mind also express themselves by guiding and directing this imaginative process. So this method is used to understand one's unconscious mind.

As started the unconscious mind expresses itself in various indirect ways. It expresses itself in our slips and mistakes, by controlling our associative process and by producing psychological disorders. Another important phenomenon by which the unconscious mind expresses itself is the dream. In fact one of the best ways of analyzing one's unconscious mind is to analyse his dreams. Dreams give such an insight into the deeper workings of one's mind that they are often referred to as "the royal road to the unconscious". How the dreams are formed, what exactly are their nature and how dreams are to be interpreted

are all very interesting problems in modern abnormal psychology. Our scientific understanding of the dreams is perhaps completely different from the ideas of the layman about them.

The common man believes that dreams foretell events that are going to take place in the future. Most people have even definite charts or tables by which a dream is interpreted. Some people believe that if one dreams of smallpox he will soon get a lot of money. Many believe that in dreams divine begins or their dead ancestors come and speak to them. Some believe that in dreams our soul leaves our body and takes a journey in the spirit-world. Thus dreams have been understood by people in various ways.

All knew that most of our dreams are determined by our past experiences. Some dreams are merely the working out of ideas and experiences in the preconscious part of our mind. For example, A, was carrying on an interesting conversation with his friend B. When he was just in the middle of saying something interesting C dropped in and broke their conversation and then they talked about other things. It is quite possible that after a few days or even that night A may continue the original interesting conversation in his dream. The original experience was not completed and it was interrupted in the middle. It was not forgotten either. Such expression which are actually held in the preconscious may come out in the dreams. Dreaming about friends, relatives, lovers, etc are mostly of this type.

On the other hand, let us take the following example. A particular person when he was a small boy at school was one day badly treated by his teacher. He was ridiculed, and let us say, even beaten in the class. This boy felt very badly about this incident. At that moment strong feelings of anger, helplessness and shame came to his mind. He was very angry with the teacher and would have like to give a good kick back. But he was helpless because he was smaller in size and also because the teacher had power and authority. He was deeply ashamed because he thought he was made very small in the eyes of his class-mates. Naturally he could not do anything. There was a severe conflict in his mind. Being unable to do anything the whole incident was just "forgotten". It was removed completely from his memory. But actually it was not forgotten in the sense in which we use the term 'forget'. It went down into the unconscious and there this experience has been very active wanting to take some vengeance and thus give an expression to the anger. It is quite possible that after some years this boy may one day-dream of a rat fighting successfully with a cat and actually managing to kill it. Apparently it is silly dream and nobody will take it seriously. It sounds absurd because a rat ordinarily cannot kill a cat. But we know that many of our dreams appear actually absurd and far-fetched like this. In this example, the rat which comes in the dream is actually the person himself. The cat stands for the teacher. Since in the original experience the teacher was big and powerful and boy was small and helpless, in the dream the boy becomes the rat and the teacher becomes the cat and the desire to win over the teacher is directly expressed in the dream.

This is exactly what happens in most of our dreams. By some processes a kind of transformation takes place by which people and objects appear the dream in different forms and in different guises. This process is called symbolization. In other words, the characters in our dreams are mostly symbols for real people, objects and ideas about whom we had experiences in the past. Such dreams on analysis will give an idea into one's unconscious mind. These dreams are motivated and produced by the unconscious mind. It effects various forms of disguise, works out dramatic themes and then actually a story is produced when we are asleep. Therefore to understand the dream we must get behind the apparent meaning to the real meaning which lies hidden behind symbols and other disguise. Interpreting a dream naturally requires good experiences and knowledge of abnormal psychology.

According to Freud, all our dreams refer to our wishes and longings of the past that were not satisfied. Thus he explains dreams as the substitute satisfaction for those unfulfilled desires. He goes one step further and says that these wishes which are satisfied in the dreams refer to our sex urge. However, this theory is not universally accepted.

Thinking

Thinking is a mental activity that goes on in the brain when a person in processing information—organizing it and communicating it to others. Thinking includes memory, but it is much more. When people think, they are not only aware of the information in the brain but also are making decision about it, comparing it to other information and using it to solve problem.

The quality of human life and the welfare and progress of the human race depend to a large extent on our capacity to think. As stated earlier that because of the ability to imagine we have inventors, artists and authors. But, perhaps, we should add that all these intellectual achievements have been possible because of a particular kind of imagination. Free and fertile imagination there must be; but mere rambling and wandering of the mind does not lead us very far. Imagination has to be systematized and directed to some purpose. This kind of imagination is called thinking. Whenever there is a problem to be solved we begin to think. The problem may be a practical and simple one such as, how best arrange the furniture in a room. Or the problem might arise from a curiosity to know how exactly a plane flies; or it may be an arithmetical problem. In all these cases we begin to think in order to get the answer. In this process we certainly use our past experiences, the knowledge that we already have and, of course, also imagine new relationships and new ways of combining. Scientific discovery and inventions are the results of the best forms of thinking. While thinking, we imagine various possible alternatives and discard the unnecessary or the wrong ones, without actually trying them out. This naturally means that thinking helps us to save a good deal to time and energy. When we get involved in serious thinking, sometimes we suddenly see some new clues and new relationships between the various parts of the problem. Such an experience is called insight. Insight is certainly very good to have but it seldom comes without a good deal of trial and error manipulation in our thinking. This fact is perhaps best expressed in the dictum 'there is no inspiration without perspiration'. The best inventions are usually made at the level of insightful thinking. A psychologist by name Kohler demonstrated with the help of experiments that chimpanzees also can think at the level of simple insight.

MEANING OF THINKING

In the words of *Correct*, thinking is behavior which is often implicit and hidden and in which symbols, i.e. images, ideas and concepts are ordinarily employed. *Climer* states that thinking is a problem-solving process in which people use symbols in place of overt activity. Whittaker opined that thinking is a carier cognitive forms of behavior which occurs only at relatively advanced stage of development, when singular or more direct methods of dealing with environment have proved ineffective and singular memory is adequate to solve problems.

Thinking which is a complex mental activity, cannot be easily separated from learning, memorizing, etc. As Warren puts it, "Thinking is an activity concerning ideas. It is symbolic in character, initiated by a problem or task which the individual is facing, involving some trial and error but under the directing influence of that problem and ultimately leading to a conclusion or solution of the problem". Thus, the activity of thinking originates from some problem and involves the response of the individual to this problem. The solution of the problem takes place internally and not in the form of external activities. Thinking continues till the person becomes fatigued by this effort. There cannot be any thinking in the absence of some problem. Problems in human life come in an incessant stream and they have to be solved by thinking. No general rule not identical or even similar. One situation may appear problematic to one person while a number of other persons may find nothing of the nature of a problem in it. The problems of different persons like philosophers, scientists, and religious minded persons are dissimilar. The problems of a logician appear meaningless to the uninitiated but the logician is immersed day and night, in a search for their solutions. Some problems are theoretical while others are practical. The problems of study in B. A are practical but the problems of the logician are theoretical. The solution of practical problems assists day-to-day life while the solution of the practical problems leads to the satisfaction of curiosity.

NATURE OF THINKING

Thinking is an activity concerning ideas. Symbolic in character initiated by a problem or task which the individual is facing, involving some trial and error but under the directing influence of that problem and ultimately leading to a conclusion or solution of the problem.

- Thinking is the organization and reorganization of current learning in the present circumstances with the help of learning and past experiences.

- Thinking is the perceptual relationship which provides for the solution of the problem.
- Thinking is a higher mental process involving symbols, images concepts and ideas that mediates or goes between stimuli and responses.

  Therefore,

  Thinking is a cognitive activity.
  Thinking is the form of information processing.
  Thinking is a problem solving behavior.
  Thinking is goal directed.
  Thinking is a process of mental exploration.
  Thinking process involves the use of symbols, concepts and images.

Thinking, the mental solution of problems, requires the use of the symbols of objects. Thinking involves the solution of problems by employing the trial and error method. There is a kind of flow in the activity of thinking, one problem leading to the thinking of another by reminding the person of that other problem. Thus many things come to the thinker's mind when he is thinking. The instrument of thinking, images, imagination, signs, indications and such like are also internal. Thinking continues to be an internal activity unless and until it takes the form of verbal thinking. The aim of purposeful thinking may be discovery, either a solution to it is found or, instead some new idea is found. This process involves both analysis and synthesis. There is foresight in thinking because the remotest possibilities of the future are thought of in advance. Hind sight is also an element of thinking because it involves use of material collected from past experiences. Thinking is done with the help of abstract signs of real objects, which adds to thinking the element of abstraction.

CONDITIONS FAVORABLE FOR THINKING

Valid thinking is faultless and logical thinking. It needs the introduction of correct methods of thinking besides the elimination of faulty methods. Many conditions are useful in valid thinking. The major favorable conditions are as follows:

1. *Interest and attention*—Both interest and attention favor thinking. Conclusive or authoritative thinking is extremely difficult if not impossible when the subject is such as does not interest us. Attention, too, is difficult in the absence of any interest. On the contrary, both attention and thinking are natural in a subject which interests us. If for example, we find arithmetical problems interesting, we enjoy thinking about them and we find no difficulty either in attending to them or doing some deep thinking.
2. *Strong motivation*—Strong motivation is needed in valid thinking, the latter being impossible in the absence of motivation. Organized and controlled thinking needs strong motivation. Thinking involves the solution of problems. The effort of the mind in thinking corresponds to the strength of motivation for the solution of problems. Motivation maintains enthusiasm and postpones fatigue. Necessary mobilization of energy for thinking is made easier by motivation in keeping with the saying that "where there is a will, there is a way". The extent for motivation determines the amount of thinking in the search for the solution and an individual will not rest content until a solution is found.
3. *Alertness and flexibility*—Alertness and flexibility also favor valid thinking because they serve to keep external faults from contaminating. Alertness checks mistakes and fallacies from creeping into thinking. Flexibility keeps thinking free from conservatism and blind belief. An alert person keeps new methods and ways in view and whenever necessary

makes use of them in thinking. In this way, he immediately understands the meanings of assisting signs and formulae in thinking and makes use of them. Thinking aims at the solution of problems, and it is necessary, therefore, that there should be no mistakes and omissions of details, the latter requiring alertness. If one solution or possibility in thinking does not serve the purposes it has to be discarded and another one taken in its place. This needs flexibility. Thus both alertness and flexibility serve useful purposes in thinking, and at the same time, make themselves essential.

4. *Time limit should not be rigid*—When a solution to some problem is being sought, the time limit provided should not be too rigid because if it is so, then normal thinking is hampered. Very inflexible and short time limit cannot admit of valid thinking. Time limit for any interesting problem is superfluous because as it is every person exerts himself to the maximum. But if the subject is uninteresting a time limit which is not rigid may be imposed upon.
5. *Wide range of wisdom*—The wide range of wisdom is also a favorable factor in thinking. Thinking needs insight, which is constituted of hindsight and foresight. A proper development of capacities of the mind is essential for these activities. If a solution is to be evolved it is essential to keep an eye on the various aspects of the problem and their mutual relationships and this, too, needs a developed and mature range of intelligence.
6. *Incubation*—Another factor which favors thinking is incubation. If the solution of some problem proves elusive despite strenuous and persistent effort, it is advisable to lay aside the problem and to busy oneself in some other activity. While one is engaged in this other work, the mind ponders over the earlier problem and just as eggs are hatched by incubation, a solution is evolved through pondering. Nothing definite is known so far about the process of incubation, but it is common experience that if the problem is left in this way, the solution often comes suddenly or, at least, its solution is facilitated when it is taken up again. But incubation proves advantageous only when the problem is set aside after it has been fully thought over, with all energy. Incubation does not imply running away from the problem of abstaining from collecting adequate material for the problem, because in this case incubation is useless.

Besides the favorable conditions detailed above, it would be helpful if some other favorable factor in thinking are kept in mind. Thinking should be free from bias, prejudice and emotion. Suggestions should be attended to only when the whole problem is in view, because appropriate suggestions will assist thinking but wrong suggestions will be a hindrance. The various stages of the conclusion should be clearly understood because if this is not done, the solution will not be understood in its complexity. Thus after the solution has been evolved, every logical step should be gone over in order to eliminate any possibility of fallacy.

Factors which Hinders Thinking

Thinking is a mental process which needs alertness, flexibility and motivation besides a wide range of intelligence. There should be voluntary and independent reasoning in this process. If these factors are absent or if the opposite conditions are present, thinking will be adversely effected or hindered. The following are the main factors which hinder thinking.

1. *Emotion*—Emotion hinders thinking because strong emotion disturbs the mental equilibrium and thereby obstructs thinking. Even if thinking is pursued in an emotional state, it will be extremely one sided and biased. It is no uncommon experience that

people cannot think when they are excited by emotions like anger, sexual passions, fear, hatred, love, etc. If the emotion is mild, the speed of thinking will be augmented instead of being hindered. But, for correct thinking it is better to have control over the emotions.

2. *Suggestions*—Suggestion also obstructs thinking because it makes it one sided. Thinking moves along the path suggested. If, for example, some one is told that he will not live long, his thinking will be very adversely effected, making him a pessimist. But it is not essential that suggestions be invariably harmful to thinking because healthy suggestions assist thinking. Self-control strengthens self-confidence and assists in thinking out the solutions of problems. The absence of suggestions is however, considered desirable in pure thinking.
3. *Supervision*—Supervision is just as harmful as prejudice. It contradicts reasoning. Superstition is belief in something without any thinking or reasoning. It is unreasoned belief, for example, if we superstitiously believe some theory, opinion, or person, we will always think in favor of him and never see his faults. The people who believe superstitiously in a certain religion believer mutually contradictory things but never reason them out. Due to superstition people attribute any cause to anything. If success in something is not achieved some Hindus attribute it to some cat's crossing their path. Similarly, various difficulties and troubles are supposed to be the result of different ill omens but no enquiry is under taken to discover the real cause.
4. *Prejudice*—Prejudice, like the two aforesaid factors, has a detrimental effect on thinking, the only point of distinction being the extent of damage, which is more in this case than in the two cases discussed earlier. The word 'prejudice' suggests the meaning namely some preconceived idea. If we are going to start thinking on some problem with an inclination in a particular direction all our thinking will be colored by our bias and will not be impartial. If we have already accepted some particular person as our benefactor, any harm that he may inflict upon us will be attributed to some other person without casting any doubt on this person. The same applies to prejudices which we may have about some occupations because even if they are suitable we don't spare a thought for them when we are confronted with the choice of those professions because we shall ignore their advantages and consider only disadvantages. It is obvious from these examples that when prejudiced, thinking becomes partial and incorrect. Valid thinking requires the elimination of all prejudices in thinking.

Besides the hindering factors detailed above, there may be many other allied factors such as ignorance about the laws of logical thinking and defect in personality. If a person is to think he should have qualities of the mind besides the absence of these hindering elements.

Types of Thinking

1. Perceptual or concrete thinking.
2. Conceptual or abstract thinking.
3. Creative thinking.
4. Logical thinking/reasoning.
5. Problem solving.
6. Convergent *Vs* Divergent thinking.

Perceptual or Concrete Thinking

It is based on perception. Perception is the process of interpretation of sensation according to one's experience. It is also called concrete thinking as it is carried over the perception of actual or concrete objects and events.

It is one-dimensional and literal thinking which has limited use of metaphor without understanding nuances of meaning. Being the simplest form of thinking, small children are mostly benefitted by this type of thinking.

Conceptual or Abstract Thinking

It does not require the perception of actual objects or events. It is also called abstract thinking as it makes the use of concepts or abstract ideas. It is superior to perceptual thinking as it economizes efforts in understanding and helps in discovery and invention.

Concepts: In the process of thinking we have a good deal of what is called ideation. This simply means dealing with mental images and abstractions. As against concrete and motor manipulation, thinking involves ideational working and manipulation. This process of ideation and abstraction is possible because of our ability to form concepts. A concept is a generalized image which need not necessarily be based on any actual experience. It is general idea which stands for all our experiences with regard to a particular object. We can have, for example, the concept of a human being. This concept is derived from our knowledge of human beings we have met. Still, the concept itself is not the actual picture or image of any particular individual. It is a generalized picture which more or less is formed out of the general characterizes that all people do have. This ability to form concepts is gradually learned and developed by the child as its grows. In this process language and development of vocabulary also play a part. The child gradually learns to abstract the common features of different objects and then to combine them into one idea. But for this process of concept formation, thinking will not be possible at the highly efficient level which we are all capable of.

It is ability to appreciate nuances of meaning. It is multidimensional thinking with ability to use metaphors and hypotheses appropriately. Language plays an important part in conceptual thinking.

Creative Thinking

It refers to the ability for original thinking, to create or discover something new. It is the ability to integrate the various elements of the situation into a harmonious whole to create work refers to creative thinking. Creative thinkers are great boons to the society as they enrich the knowledge of mankind.

In creative thinking, there is general freedom from rigid thought patterns, i.e. freedom from 'the old beaten track'. The creative thinkers tries to achieve something new, to produce something original and something unique.

There are some common stages of critical thinking, are:

i. Preparation
ii. Incubation
iii. Inspiration or illumination
iv. Evaluation
v. Verification or revision.

- *Preparation* of means whole preparation of a person for creative work. It can be general preparation and specific preparation for specific problems. It involves formulation of a problem, collection of information, survey of relevant work in the area, preliminary knowledge of the subject, trial and error, all are essential for creative thinking.
- *Incubation* occurs when the individual is unable to find a solution in spite of long and concentrate efforts. The ideas which were interfering with the solution of a problem tend to fade away. What he learns and experience in the meantime may give clues to solution.
- *Illumination/Inspiration:* The creative ideas, the solution of the problem comes to the mind all of a sudden, in a sudden flash. It provides a specific direction towards the goal and it makes the person to think in that direction.
- *Evaluation:* The thinker finds out if the solution which has come to his mind is correct or not verification/revision: if the solution is found to be correct, it is accepted. If it is wrong or does not suit the assumption of creative thinker, he has to again start from the beginning. In certain cases, some modification or revision may be necessary.
- *Verification or revision:* The thinker will verify the above stages and revise if needed.

Logical Thinking or Reasoning

When thinking process is guided by some logical principles will be called as logical thinking or reasoning. It is a step-wise thinking and it is highly purposeful, controlled and selective thinking. *Skinner* states that reasoning in the word used to describe the mental recognition of cause and effect relationships. It may be the prediction of an event from an observed cause or the inference of a cause from observed event.

Man's life is an endless stream of problems, situations for which the individual has no readymade formula or solution. Being unequipped with the proper solution, he requires to think and reason before he can solve the problem. Reasoning is the highest form of thinking that needs a well-organized brain. The process of reasoning requires two conditions—first that the person's mind should have completely formed concepts and the second that he should be endowed with the power of reaching decisions. It is because the children lack these two faculties that they are not able to reason. In the process of reasoning, the individual reasons from the past known circumstances to the present or further unknown conditions on the basis of past experience. In this manner, reasoning helps to reach certain conclusions concerning the future without anything having been achieved in actual practice. Evidently, such an application needs some imagination as an essential part. To see an object lying on the table is to perceive it, when we think of it we are thinking, but if we try to know how that particular object came to be on the table at all, we fall into the process of reasoning.

It is cognitive process of looking for reasons for beliefs, conclusions, actions or feelings. It is the process of drawing conclusions based on evidence. It is a form of controlled thinking in which the thought process is directed consciously towards the solutions of a problem.

It is rather difficult to differentiate clearly reasoning from thinking. When we think, this process is guided by certain logical principles. An application of such principles is called reasoning. Good thinking involves reasoning and good reasoning helps the thinking process to be efficient and to reach correct solutions. Reasoning is mostly directed towards getting at certain conclusions and definite affirmatives based on facts. These facts are put together according to logical principles of reasoning.

Reasoning may go wrong if all the relevant data were not taken note of. It may also go wrong if the data were not properly combined and grouped. It may also go wrong if proper laws of logical reasoning were not applied. For example, suppose we have the following two statements such as:

All men are mortal
Socrates is a man.

By our reasoning process we put these two statements together and conclude that Socrates is mortal. This is a particular kind of reasoning. Logic teaches us several other kinds of reasoning.

Reasoning is combining past experiences in order to solve problems, it is genuine thinking that involves a definite goal or purpose. It also an implicit act involves problem solving behavior.

Reasoning is the highest form of thinking to find out cause and predict effects. An individual tries to solve a problem by incorporating two or more aspects of his past experience. It is classified into:

Inductive reasoning: This is process of reasoning from parts to the whole, from examples to generalizations. It is carried out generally within the field known as informal logic is described as "the science of deduction."

Deductive reasoning: This moves from the whole to parts, from generalizations to underlying concepts to examples. Formal logic is described as "the science of deduction."

Adbuctive reasoning: It is cognitive process often involves both inductive and deductive arguments.

Problem Solving

Problem solving is a process of overcoming difficulties that appear to interfere with the attainment of a goal. It is a procedure of making adjustment inspite of interferences. Problem-solving behavior occurs in novel or difficult situations in which a solution is not obtainable by habitual method of applying concepts and principles derived from past experiences in very familiar situations.

Convergent and Divergent Thinking

The ability to produce responses that are based primarily on knowledge and logic.

Convergent thinking is cognitive processing of information around a common point, an attempt to bring thoughts from different directions into a union for common conclusions.

Divergent thinking starts from a common point and moves outward into a variety of perspectives. For example, teachers use the content as a vehicles to prompt divers or unique thinking among students rather than a common view.

Training in Rational Thinking

For this, it is needed that the thinker possesses a scientific attitude, self-confidence and patience. The teacher himself must be capable of scientific and unbiased reasoning, as he cannot otherwise teach his students to reason with clarity. In training the children to think rationally in school, it is necessary to keep the following things in mind:

1. *Acquaintance with problems of daily life*—In order to acquaint the child with the problem, the subjects that he is taught should be related to real life. It is only when the illustrative

examples in study are taken from day-to-day life that the child can think of the problems with any facility.

2. *Development of necessary qualities*—Rational thinking requires experience, intellect, determination and other qualities such as persistence and application. And of these, with the exception of intelligence, all the others can be developed through effort. Hence, efforts should be made to develop these in the child.
3. *Solution of problems of practical utility*—Children should be asked to solve problems of practical utility. One such problem could be the following—the nine spots in such a manner as to create three lines, each of which contains three spots, and, without lifting the pencil from the chart draw lines that connect all the spots. Ability to solve such problems can be developed. In addition to this, children should be made cognizant of the problems that occur in daily life, and inspired to solve them.
4. *Knowledge of special subjects*—Solution of specific kinds of problems inevitably requires skill in the appropriate subjects. Hence, the teacher should pace problems before the students only after they have gained adequate knowledge of such subjects.
5. *Acquaintance with the environment*—Problems on which the student is required to cognitive should bear relation to his life. And for this it is essential that he be acquainted with this environment. Knowledge of the individuals, associations, institutions, and processes that occur around him will make it possible for him to comprehend their problems, and he will himself be inclined to reason out a solution be corrected by their teachers. Students devise all kinds of arguments when concerned in a debate to prove their point. The sensible teacher can, after the debate is over, individually or collectively, bring to the notice of the students the fallacy in their reasoning.
6. *Knowledge of logic*—A study of the general principles of logic will be especially beneficial to a training in reasoning. The teacher himself should be acquainted with the general rules of logic, and he should impart them to the student. Lacking knowledge of these principles, even some really well-educated persons are seen reasoning incorrectly and illogically.

Briefly, then, there are two main elements in training in reasoning-knowledge of the subjects concerned with the problem, and knowledge of the rules of logic or reasoning. In addition to this when the students get adequate opportunities of reasoning and arguing, they develop good reasoning ability that stands them in good stead in life.

ERRORS IN THINKING

While so many errors might occur in our thinking we should make a special note of two forms of thinking which not only result in errors but are also responsible for a good deal of strife and misunderstanding in social relationships.

1. **Autistic thinking:** If we observe children carefully we could notice that often in their thinking they assume the existence of everything according to their own advantage. But this actually may not be so. Yet they will refuse to take into account anything that is of disadvantage to them. On this assumption they proceed to think. Naturally the end result of that thinking will lead them to difficulties. Such as form of thinking, where the main consideration is one's own satisfaction, which includes only favorable factors is called autistic thinking. It is also called wishful thinking. Strictly speaking the term thinking should not studied his lessons fully and properly. He begins to think that questions will appear only on the portions that he knows. He even begins to argue out that those

are the most important questions and finally he satisfies himself with the conclusion that he is bound to pass. Such a piece of thinking is nothing but wishful thinking.

2. **Prejudiced thinking:** In the next chapter, we would see another aspect of the human mind, viz, and the emotions. Of course, we are all familiar with experiences of anger, fear, hatred, etc. These are some of the emotions. It has been found that often our thinking is influenced by these emotions more than by principles of logic. When we do not like a person and if we are very angry with him we think and believe a number of uncomplimentary things about him which may not be really true. Because of some actual experience we might hate one individual who belongs to a particular community. Guided by this hatred we form a hasty generalization and condemn the whole community to which he belongs. All such thinking are examples of prejudiced thinking. An educated man should try as far as possible to avoid such forms of prejudiced thinking guided by emotions. We must learn to behave like rational beings, guided by proper reasoning. All sorts of petty prejudices, misunderstandings, superstitions, etc. should not be allowed to influence our thinking. Our lives could be made much happier and more efficient if we would take care to avoid this type of prejudiced thinking.

To sum up, the following precautions may be mentioned to ensure correct thinking:

(1) Wide and alert observations. (2) Before reaching any conclusions one must be sure that all the relevant data has been taken note of. (3) One must be sure that in collecting the data prejudices have not influenced. (4) Hasty generalizations should be avoided. (5) Exaggeration in statements should be avoided. (6) Judgment must be fair and accurate.

TOOLS/ELEMENTS OF THINKING

Thinking process uses various tools:

1. Percept
2. Images
3. Concept
4. Language
5. Decision making and judgment.

1. **Percept:** The object or stimulus which is perceived is called the percept. The percept stimulates thinking. When the percept is absent, it may come in the form of image.
2. **Images:** These are mental pictures of actual sensory, experiences. People usually make a 'visual map' to solve their problem. Some psychologists assumed that thinking requires the use of images, but other stated that images are not necessary for thinking.
3. **Concept:** A concept is important language symbol used in thinking. A concept is a symbolic construction that represents some common and general feature (S) of many objects or events. For instance, the concept of hospitals represents different kinds of hospitals, viz, small, large, city, rural, general and specialized one.
4. **Language:** A language is a dynamic set of visual, auditory or tactile symbols of communication and the elements used to manipulate them. It is best medium of thinking. It provides the most useful and common kinds of symbols in human behavior. Language is extremely important for thinking because it allows new learning to be communicated to others and stored for future generations.
5. **Decision making and judgment:** Decision making is a kind of problem solving in which we are presented with several alternatives among which we much choose. Decision making involves complicated judgments.

The steps of decision making process are:
- Identifying and understanding of the problem.
- Defining and clarifying goals.
- Alternative goals.
- Analyzing the anticipated consequences of each alternative.
- Selecting a course of action.

The decision making process and the nursing process share similarities and the nurse uses decision making in all steps of the nursing process. Table 14.1 compares these processes.

Table 14.1: Comparison between the nursing process and the decision making process

Nursing process	*Decision making process*
Assess	Identify the purpose
Diagnose	
Plan	Set the criteria Weight the criteria Seek alternatives Project
Implement	Implement
Evaluate	Evaluate the outcome

How to Improve Thinking

Here are five quick ways to improve the quality of thinking.

1. **Keep yourself only with current project:** Clutter creates confusion. Get organized and work with a fresh canvas. On an average, we spend about 45 minutes a day looking for things, e.g. Where are my keys? Keep only the current project you are working on in front of you.
2. **Dedicate an hour of focus time to your most important task:** multitasking is highly over-rated and cause a loss of upto 40 percent efficiency. Get yourself one hour of focused seclusion to work on your most important task. It will increases both productivity, creativity and morale.
3. **Stir up your visual senses and creating talents with exposure to the arts:** Go to a gallery, pick up an art book or spend time with nature.
4. **Learn how to 'mind map':** This is a best practice that allows you to visualize and map your projects, and strategies. It is also a life-saving memory device that will help you remember more and organize your thinking.
5. **Finally, on the hour........stop thinking:** When you have been working on something for more than an hour, you start loosing concentration and focus. So, stop, get up and walk around and then go back to your work.

Alterations in Thinking

Thought process is the 'how' of the patient's self-expression. A patient's thought process if observed through speech.

- **Psychosis:** It is a mental disorder in which reality testing is not intact; behavior may violate gross social norms. It is just opposite to neurosis in which reality testing is intact and behavior may not violate social norms. Many psychiatric disorders such as schizophrenia, mania, depression, etc. come under psychosis. It includes various disturbances in thinking.

- **Delusion:** It is false, persistent, irrational belief not shared by persons of same age, race, education standard which cannot be altered by logical arguments. Delusions are classified into.
  - **Persecutory delusions:** The individuals feel interfered discriminated against, threatened or mistreated, e.g. the patient says, "My family members want to kill me."
  - **Delusion of reference:** The individual feels that others are talking about him, other's remarks/actions have special significance for him.
  - **Delusion of influence/passivity:** the individual believes that he is influenced by and controlled by others. For example, "the cardiologist puts transmitter near heart that controls my feeling and thoughts".
  - **Delusion of sin and guilt:** The individual has a belief that he has committed unforgiveable sin/some wickedness in past leads to calamity to others. So, he is evil and worthless.
  - **Hypochondrical delusions:** These are delusions of some bodily disease.
  - **Nihilistic delusions**: The individual has a false idea that he self, a part of the self, others, or the world in nonexistent.
  - **Delusions of grandeur:** The individual has an exaggerated feeling of importance, power, knowledge or identity, e.g. "I am King of Mysore."

Implication of Thinking in Nursing

The job of a Nurse is not mechanical. It requires a lot of thinking. As thinking has been defined as problem solving, she has to learn its process so that she may be able to solve the problems of the patients. In this type of thinking she will get help from her observation of the symptoms in the patient as well as her discussions with the patient, his relatives and friends. A knowledge of the psychology of the process of thinking as well as the technique to improve it, is therefore very much helpful to the Nurse. In her book *Aids to Psychology for Nurses,* Mackenzie has described six situations in the life of a Nurse which require the use of reasoning and thinking. Firstly, she requires it for solving the practical problems such as planning a holiday or arranging the room of the hospital, etc. Secondly, the diagnosis of the disease being hypothetical she requires thinking for verifying a hypothesis put before her. Thirdly, she requires others. Fourthly, she has to use reasoning to explain things simply and clearly to others. Fifthly, she requires reasoning, deductive and inductive, to arrive at certain reasoning, deductive and inductive, to arrive at certain conclusions, from general to particular and particular to general. Sixthly, she requires reasoning to check on quick or unwise actions in her everyday life.

In order to be able to think clearly and reason out properly the Nurse should cultivate a habit of correct thinking and reasoning. She should create a detached outlook, and ability to gather facts and arrive at inductive generalizations. In her book Psychology for Nurses Cunningham has made certain recommendations for students Nurses in order to think correctly and reason out properly. These recommendations are as follows:

1. Gather a wealth of factual material with which to think
2. Form the habit of looking for relationships
3. Practice generalizing from facts

4. Distinguish between facts and opinion
5. Consider the source
6. Look for a central problem
7. Size up the whole situation
8. Recognize that differing viewpoints resulting in differing interpretations
9. Avoid prejudices and look for new meanings
10. Be attentive to important details
11. Meet problems directly instead of evading them or shifting responsibility to another person
12. Avoid hasty generalizations; form judgments slowly; be tolerant of solutions proposed by others
13. Regard conclusions as tentative until they have been checked; keep an open mind; question yourself as well as others.

The above recommendations will undoubtedly help the Nurse to develop a habit of correct thinking and reasoning. This positive approach however, has a negative aspect. The Nurse has not only to develop the positive habit of correct thinking and reasoning, she should also be on her guard against wrong and incorrect thinking. She should know the fallacies likely to creep in her thinking. She should know the fallacies of deductive and inductive logic so that she may avoid wrong reasoning. Since correct reasoning and thinking is a result of correct observations, perceptions, beliefs, meanings and techniques, the Nurse should take care that these should be correct, otherwise she may incur wrong thinking and arrive at wrong conclusions. Verification of results is a common practice for checking the validity of conclusions. Some verifications are possible through observation of facts and comparison with data. Other conclusions may not be so easily verifiable since they do not depend upon factual data. These conclusions can be verified by principles of logic. The following points should be remembered in order to avoid incorrect thinking.

Gather complete and correct information

1. Do not allow emotions to enter your judgment
2. Have no prejudices or preconceptions
3. Keep your eye on as many details as possible and do not ignore even the most insignificant fact
4. Remember the rules of logic in deductive and inductive reasonings
5. Never become egocentric but always pay attention to the suggestions and views of other who know
6. Do not indulge in wishful thinking or childish imagination. Always keep a control on yourself.

If the Nurse wisely utilizes the above instructions to avoid wrong thinking and creates a habit of correct thinking and sound reasoning she will be more successful in her job.

Critical Thinking and Nurse

Critical thinking is "the intellectually disciplined process of actively and skillfully conceptualizing, applying, analyzing, synthesizing, and/or evaluating information gathered from, or generated by, observation, experience, reflection, reasoning, or communication, as a guide to belief and action". Nurses are expected to use critical thinking to solve client problems and make better decisions. Thus critical thinking, problem solving, and decision making are interrelated processes, with creativity enhancing the result.

Critical thinking is essential to safe, competent, skillful nursing practice. The amount of knowledge that nurses must use and the continuing rapid growth of this knowledge prevent nurses from being effective practitioners if they attempt to function with only the information acquired in school or outlined in books. Decisions that nurses must make about client care and about the distribution of limited resources force them to think and act in areas where there are neither clear answer no standard procedures and where conflicting forces turn decision making into a complex process. Nurses therefore need to embrace the attitudes that promote critical thinking and master critical-thinking skills in order to process and evaluate both previously learned and new information.

Nurses use critical thinking skills in a variety of ways:

- Nurses use knowledge from other subjects and fields. Because nurses deal holistically with human responses, they must draw meaningful information from other subject areas (i.e. make interdisciplinary connections) in order to understand the meaning of client data and to plan effective interventions. Nursing students take courses in the biologic and social sciences and in the humanities so that they can acquire a strong foundation on which to build their nursing knowledge and skill. For example, the nurse might use knowledge form nutrient, physiology, and physics to promote wound healing and prevent further injury to a client with a pressure ulcer.
- Nurses deal with change in stressful environments. Nurses work in rapidly changing situations. Treatments, medications and technology change constantly, and a clients condition may change from minute to minute. Routine actions may therefore not be adequate to deal with the situation at hand. Familiarity with the routine for giving medications, for example, does not help the nurse deal with a client who is frightened of injections or with one who does not wish to take a medication. When unexpected situations arise, critical thinking enables the nurse to recognize important cues, respond quickly, and adapt interventions to meet specific client needs.
- Nurses make important decisions. During the course of a workday, nurses make vital decision of many kinds. These decisions often determine the well-being of clients and even their very survival, so it is important that the decisions be sound. Nurses use critical thinking to collect and interpret the information needed to make decisions. Nurses must, for example, use good judgment to decide which observation must be reported to the physician immediately and which can be noted in the client record for the physician to address later, during a routine visit with the client.

Creativity is a major component of critical thinking. When nurses incorporate creativity into their thinking, they are able to find unique solutions to unique problems. Creativity is thinking that results in the development of new ideas and products. Creativity in problem solving and decision making is the ability to develop and implement new and better solutions.

Characteristics of a Creative Person

- Curious
- Seeks problem
- Enjoys challenges
- Optimistic
- Able to suspend judgment
- Comfortable with imagination

- Seeks problems as opportunities
- Seeks problems as interesting
- Problems are emotionally acceptable
- Challenges assumptions
- Does not give up easily: Preserves, works hard.

Positive Attitude for Creativity

1. **Curiosity:** Creative people want to know things—all kinds of things. In addition to knowing, creative people want to know why, what are the reasons behind decisions, problems solutions, events, facts and so forth? Why this way and not another? And why not try this or that?
2. **Challenge:** Curious people like to identify and challenge the assumptions behind ideas, proposals, problems, beliefs and statements. Assumptions, often come as a new ideas, a new path, a new solution.
3. **Constructive discontent:** It is ability to see a need for improvement and to propose a method of making that improvement and to propose a method of making that improvement. It is a positive, enthusiastic discontent, reflecting 'hey , I known a way to make that better.'
4. **A belief that most problems can be solved:** By faith at first and by experience later on, the creative thinker believers that something can always be done to eliminate or help alleviate almost every problem.
5. **The ability to suspend judgment and criticism:** The creative thinker should suspend judgment when new ideas are arriving, to have an optimistic attitude towards ideas in general, and to avoid condemning them, e.g. "That will never work ; that's no good; what an idiotic idea; that's impossible,' and so forth.
6. **Seeing the good in the bad:** Creative thinkers, when faced with poor solutions, don't cast them away. Instead, they ask, "what's good about it"?
7. **Problems lead to improvements:** The attitude of constructive discontent searches for problems and possible areas of improvement, but many times problems arrive on their own.
8. **A problem can also be a solution:** One person describes a fact as a problem can sometimes be a solution for someone else.
9. **Problems are interesting and emotionally acceptable:** Problem solving is fun, educational, rewarding, ego building, helpful to society.
10. **A belief that mistakes are welcome:** Make sure you make a reasonable number of mistakes. Mistakes are educational and can lead to success because they mean you are doing something.

Negative attitudes that block creativity:

- Oh no, a problem!
- It can't be done
- I can't do it/there's nothing I can do
- But I' am not creative
- That's childish
- What will people think?
- I might fail.

Creativity is required when the nurse encounters a new situation or a client situation in which traditional interventions are not effective. For example, Ned Rodriguez, a pediatric home health nurse, is caring for 9-year-old Pauline, who has ineffective respirations following abdominal surgery. The physician has ordered incentive spirometry (a treatment device that promotes alveolar expansion). Pauline is frightened by the equipment and tries quickly during the treatments. Ned offers Pauline a bottle of blow bubble sand a blowing wand. Pauline is delighted with blowing bubbles. Ned knows that the respiratory effort in blowing bubbles will promote alveolar expansion and suggests that Pauline blow bubbles between incentive spirometry treatments.

Creative thinkers must have knowledge of the problem. They must have assessed the present problem and be knowledgeable about the underlying facts and principles that apply. For example, in the previous situation, Ned knows the anatomy and physiology of respiratory function and is aware of the purpose of incentive spirometry. He also understands pediatric growth and development. In trying to assist Pauline, he builds on his knowledge and comes up with a creative solution. Using creativity, nurses—

- Generate many ideas rapidly
- Are generally flexible and natural, that is, they are able to change viewpoints or directions in thinking rapidly and easily
- Create original solutions to problems
- Tend to be independent and self-confident, even when under pressure
- Demonstrate individuality.

Skills in Critical Thinking

Complex mental processes such as analysis, problem solving and decision making require the use of cognitive critical-thinking skills. These skills include critical analysis, inductive and deductive reasoning, making valid inferences, differentiating facts from opinions, evaluating the credibility of information sources, clarifying concepts, and recognizing assumptions.

Critical analysis is the application of a set of questions to a particular situation or idea to determine essential information and ideas and discard superfluous information and ideas. The questions are not sequential steps; rather, they are a set of criteria for judging an idea. Not all question will need to be applied to every situation, but one should be aware of all the questions in order to choose those questions appropriate to a given situations. Socrates was a Greek Philosopher who developed the Socratic method of posing a question and seeking an answer. Table 14.1 lists Socratic questions to use in critical analysis. Socratic questioning is a technique one can use to look beneath the surface recognize and examine assumptions, search for inconsistencies, examine multiple points of view, and differentiate what one knows from what one merely believes. Nurses should employ Socratic questioning when listening to an end-of-shift report, reviewing a history or progress notes, planning care, or discussing a clients care with colleagues.

Two other critical thinking skills are inductive and deductive reasoning. In inductive reasoning, generalizations are formed from a set of facts or observations. When viewed together, certain bits of information suggest a particular interpretation. For example, the nurse who observes that a client has dry skin, poor turgor, sunken eyes, and dark amber urine may make the generalization that the client appears dehydrated. Deductive reasoning, by contrast, is reasoning from the general to the specific. The nurse starts with a conceptual

Table 14.1: Socratic questions

Questions about the question (or Problem)
- Is the question clear, understandable, and correctly identified?
- Is this question important?
- Could this question be broken down into smaller parts?
- How might – state this question?

Question about Assumptions
- You seem to be assuming __________; is that so?
- What could you assume instead? Why?
- Does this assumption always hold true?

Questions about Point of View
- Your seem to be using the perspective of ____. Why?
- What would someone who disagrees with your perspective say?
- Can you see this any other way?

Questions about Evidence and Reasons
1. What evidence do you have for that?
2. Is there any reason to doubt that evidence?
3. How do you know?
4. What would change your mind?

Questions about Implications and Consequences
- What effect would that have?
- What is the probability that will actually happen?
- What are the alternatives?
- What are the implications of that?

Table 14.2: Differentiating types of statements

Statement	*Description*	*Example*
Facts	Can be verified through investigation	Blood pressure is affected by blood volume
Inferences	Conclusions drawn from the facts, going beyond facts to make a statement about something not currently known	If blood volume is decreased (e.g. in hemorrhagic shock), the blood pressure will drop
Judgments	Evaluation of facts or information that reflect values or other criteria; a type of opinion	It is harmful to the clients health if the blood pressure drops too low
Opinions	Beliefs formed over time and include judgments that may fit facts or be in error	Nursing intervention can assist in maintaining the clients blood pressure within normal limits

framework—for example, Maslow's hierarchy of needs or a self-care framework—and makes descriptive interpretations of the clients condition in relation to that framework. For example, the nurse who uses the needs framework might categorize data and define the clients problem in terms of elimination, nutrition or protection needs.

In a more simplistic example, inductive reasoning is like looking at the pieces a jigsaw puzzle and attempting to describe the whole (without seeing a picture of the completed puzzle). As the puzzle puts more and more pieces together, the whole picture becomes clearer. In deductive reasoning, the puzzler sees the whole picture and puts the puzzle together by organizing the pieces into border pieces, or colors, or some other grouping.

In critical thinking, the nurse also differentiates statements of fact, inference, judgment, and opinion. Table 14.2 shows how these may be applied to a client. Evaluating the credibility of information sources is an important step in critical thinking. Unfortunately, we cannot always believe what we read or are told. The nurse may need to ascertain the accuracy of information by checking other documents or with other informants.

Concepts or ideas or views representing things in the real world and their meanings. Each person has developed their conceptualizations based on experience, input from others, study and other activities. To clearly comprehend a client situation the nurse and the client must agree on the meaning of concept terms. For example, if the client says to the nurse "I think I have a tumor", the nurse needs to clarify what this word means to the client—the medical definition of tumor (a solid mass) or the common lay meaning of cancer—before responding.

Persons also live their lives under certain assumptions. Some people view humans as having a basically generous nature while others believe that the human tendency is to act in their own best interest. The nurse may believe that life should be considered worth living no matter what the condition while the client believes that quality of life is more important than quantity of life. If they recognize that they make choices based on these assumptions, they can still work together toward an acceptable plan of care. Difficulty arises when people do not take the time to consider what assumptions underlie their beliefs and actions.

Attitudes that Foster Critical Thinking

Certain attitudes are crucial to critical thinking. These attitudes are based on the assumption that a rational person is motivated to develop, learn, and grow. A critical thinker works to develop the following attitudes or traits; independence of thought, fair mindedness, insight into egocentricity and sociocentricity, intellectual humility and suspension of judgment, encourage, integrity, perseverance, confidence in reason, interest in exploring both thoughts underlying feelings and feelings underlying thoughts, and curiosity.

- **Independence of thought:** Critical thinking requires that individual think for themselves. People acquire many beliefs as children, not necessarily based on reason but in order to have an explanation they comprehend. As they mature and acquire knowledge and experience, critical thinkers examine their beliefs in the light of new evidence. Critical thinkers consider seriously a wide range of ideas, learn from them, and then make their own judgments about them. Nurses are open minded about considering different methods of performing technical skills—not just the single way they may have been taught in school.
- **Fair-mindedness:** Critical thinkers are fair-minded, assessing all viewpoints with the same standards and not basing their judgments on personal or group bias or prejudice. Fair-mindedness helps one to consider opposing points of view and to try to understand new ideas fully before rejecting or accepting them. Critical thinkers active to be open to the possibility that new evidence could change their minds. The nurse listens to opinions of all the members of a family, young and old.
- **Insight into egocentricity and sociocentricity:** Critical thinkers are open to the possibility that their personal biases or social pressures and customs could unduly affect their thinking. They actively try to examine their own biases and bring them to awareness each time they think or make a decision. For example, a nurse spends extensive time trying to teach a client how to prevent a future recurrence of some problem but is mystified when the client appears uninterested and does not follow the nurse's advice. The nurse's egocentric tendency to assume that all clients are motivated and interested in preventive care (just because the nurse is) resulted in an inaccurate assessment of the

clients desire to learn; both the nurse's and the clients time was wasted. Had the nurse assessed the clients background and beliefs about the problem (that is, had the nurse collected sufficient evidence), the nurse might have identified a problem more relevant to the clients priorities and, thus, developed a better care plan.

- **Intellectual humility and suspension of judgment:** Intellectual humility means having an awareness of the limits of one's own knowledge. Critical thinkers are willing to admit what they do not know; they are willing to seek new information and to rethink their conclusions in light of new knowledge. They never assume that what everybody believes to be right will always be right, because new evidence may emerge. A hospital nurse might be unable to imagine how the elderly wife will care for her husband who has recently had a stroke. However, the nurse also recognizes that it is not possible to really know what the couple can achieve.
- **Intellectual courage:** With an attitude of courage, one is willing to consider and examine fairly one's own ideas or views, especially those to which one may have a strongly negative reaction. This type of courage comes from recognizing that beliefs are sometimes false or misleading. Values and beliefs are not always acquired rationally. Rational beliefs are those that have been examined and found to be supported by solid reasons and data. After such examination, it is inevitable that some beliefs previously held to be true will be found to contain questionable elements and that some truth will emerge from ideas considered dangerous or false. Courage is needed to be true to new thinking in such cases, especially if social penalties for nonconformity are severe. As an example, previously many nurses believed that allowing family members to observe an emergency (such as CPR) would be get in the health care team's way. Others felt that blanket exclusion of family members was unnecessary and extremely stressful for some of them. As a result, nurses initiated research that has demonstrated that family presence can be accomplished without detrimental effects to the nurse, the patient, or the family.
- **Integrity:** Intellectual integrity requires that individuals apply the same rigorous standard of proof to their own knowledge and belief as they apply to the knowledge and beliefs of others. Critical thinkers question their own knowledge and beliefs as quick and thoroughly as they challenge those of another. They are readily able to admit and evaluate inconsistencies within the own beliefs and between their own beliefs and those of another. A nurse might believe that wound care always requires sterile technique. Reading a new article on the use and outcomes of clean technique for some wounds leads the critically thinking nurse to reconsider.
- **Perseverance:** Nurses who are critical thinkers show perseverance in finding effective solutions to client and nursing problems. This determination enables them to clarify concepts and sort out related issues, in spite of difficulties and frustrations. Confusion and frustration are uncomfortable, but critical thinks resist the temptation to find a quick and easy answer. Important questions tend to be complex and confusing and therefore often requires a great deal of thought and research to arrive at an answer. The nurse needs to stick to the issue until it is resolved. For example, the nurses on a unit have tried to establish a policy of selected clients to leave the hospital on a pass rather than have to be discharged and readmitted in the same day. The need for involvement of nursing, medical, administrative, and accounting staff gradually generates solutions to stumbling blocks. The development of the policy moves forward, although very slowly.
- **Confidence in reason:** Critical thinkers believe that well-reasoned thinking will lead to trustworthy conclusions. Therefore, they cultivate an attitude of confidence in the

reasoning process and examine emotion-laden arguments using the standards for evaluating thought, by asking questions such as these: Is that argument fair? Is it based on sufficient evidence? Consider nurses attempting to determine the best way to allocate holiday time off for staff. Should they use seniority, random selection, give preference to those who have children, use "first-come, first-served", or another method?.

The critical thinker develops skill in both inductive reasoning and deductive reasoning. As the nurse gains greater awareness of the thinking process and more experience in improving such thinking, confidence in the process will grow. This nurse will not afraid of disagreement and indeed will be concerned when others agree too quickly. Such a nurse can serve as a role model to colleagues, inspiring and encouraging them to think critically as well.

- **Interest in exploring both thoughts:** A critical thinker knows that emotions can influence thinking and that often feelings underlie thoughts. The rational, critical thinker adopts the attitude that feelings are real and need to be acknowledged. However, feelings needs to be explored to determine whether they are based on reality or interpretations, memories, or fears. Nurses need to identify, examine, and control or modify feelings that are interfering with clear critical thinking. As one example, if a client is injured by a piece of equipment that the nurse reported was malfunctioning but had not yet been repaired, the nurse may feel anger, guilt and frustration. Although the nurse may initially think the client should sue for the injury, to deal with strong negative emotion the nurse can take these steps:
  1. Limit action for a while to avoid hasty conclusions and impulsive decisions
  2. Discuss negative feelings with a confidant
  3. Expend some of the energy generated by the emotion by, for example, walking or exercising
  4. Reflect on the situation and determine whether the emotional response was appropriate.

- **Curiosity:** The internal conversation going on within the mind of a critical thinker is filled with questions: Why do we believe this? What causes that? Does it have to be this way? Could something else work? What would happen if we did it another way? Who says that is so? The curious nurse may value tradition but is not afraid to examine traditions to be sure they are still valid. The nurse may, for example, apply these questions to the issue of moving responsibility for a procedure such as the drawing of arterial blood samples among the nursing, respiratory therapy, or laboratory department staff.
- **Standards and elements of critical thinking:** How can one know whether one's thinking is critical thinking? Paul (1995) proposes that thinkers can use universal standards, shown in Table 14.3. Explicitly stating the standard for critical thinking promotes the reliability and validity of the thinking and thus makes appropriate action more likely. The standards are applied by asking questions to check one's reasoning about the problem. The standards are applied to the elements of thought. These elements may be considered in any order and therefore are presented in a circular scheme.

Applying Critical Thinking to Nursing Practice

Nurses function effectively some part of everyday without thinking critically. Many small decisions are based primarily on habit with minimal thinking involved; examples include selecting what uniform to war, choosing which route to take to work, and deciding what to eat for lunch. Psychomotor skills in nursing often involve minimal thinking, such as

Table 14.3: Universal intellectual standard	
Standard	*Sample question*
Clarity	What is an example of this?
Accuracy	How can I find out if that is true?
Relevance	How does that help me with the issue?
Logicalness	Does that follow from the evidence?
Breadth	Do I need to consider another point of view?
Precision	Can I be more specific?
Significance	Which of these facts is most important?
Completeness	Have I missed any important aspects?
Fairness	Am I considering the thinking of others?
Depth	What makes this a difficult problem?

operating a familiar piece of equipment. But the higher order skills of critical thinking are put into play as soon as a new idea is encountered or a less than routine must be made.

The nursing process is a systematic, rational method of planning and providing individualized nursing care. The phases of the nursing process—assessing, diagnosing, planning, implementing, and evaluating—are discussed in detail in the chapters that follow. The relationship of Paul and Elder's (1995) elements of thought to the phases of the nursing process and application to a clinical example is shown in Table 14.4. In addition to using critical thinking with an individual client, when setting priorities for the day, a nurse employs critical thinking. When analyzing a situation and planning strategies for conflict resolution or change, the nurse manager uses critical-thinking attitudes and skills. The nurse clinician and nurse manager seek to be aware of their thinking while they are thinking, as they apply standards for thinking, and as their thinking progresses.

Problem Solving

In problem solving, the nurse obtains information that clarifies the nature of the problem and suggests possible solutions. The nurse then carefully evaluates the possible solutions and chooses the best one to implement. The situation is carefully monitored over time to ensure its initial and continued effectiveness. The nurse does not discard the other solutions but holds them in reserve in the event that the first solution is not effective. The nurse may also encounter a similar problem in a different client situation where an alternative solution is determined to be the most effective. Therefore, problem solving for one situation contributes to the nurses body of knowledge for problem solving in similar situations.

There are various approaches to problem solving. Commonly used are trial and error, intuition, the research process, and the scientific/modified scientific method.

Problem solving: It is a tool, skill and a process. It is a tool because it can help you solve an immediate problem or to achieve a goal. It is a skill because once you have learnt it you can use it repeatedly, like the ability to ride a bicycle, add numbers or speak a language. It is also a process because it involves taking a number of steps.

You can engage in problem solving if you want to reach a goal and experience obstacles on the way. At the point at which you come up against a barrier you can engage in a

Table 14.4: Relationship of Paul and Elder's elements of thought to the nursing process		
Paul's elements of thought	*Parallels to the nursing process*	*Clinical application*
Information	Assessing	Data: A 45-year-old male Latino complains of severe headache; 20 lb overweight's; blood pressure 180/195 mm Hg. States he has been taking high blood pressure pills only when he has a headache. Is self-employed as a gardener, lives with wife, mother-in-law, and four children. Given these data, a critical thinker is aware that more data must be obtained about the clients cultural health values and reasons for stared behavior. Failure to think critically and to obtain additional data leads to inaccurate goals, diagnosis, and interventions.
Purpose of thinking	Goal setting	Goal: To increase compliance with medication regimen in order to relieve headaches and prevent a cerebrovascular accident (CVA). Thinking critically, a nurse will try to determine the clients goals and to agree to mutual goals
Question at issue	Diagnosing	A critical thinker will defer identifying the clients diagnosis until more data are obtained and the clients priorities are known. This prevents a premature diagnosis based on insufficient data
Points of view	Diagnosing	As a critical thinker, the nurse is aware that the clients point of view may differ from the nurses. Although the nurse may support the Western medical belief system that puts high priority on preventing disease, the critical thinker is also aware that the client may hold diverse views of health and illness, therapy, and preventive measures
Interpretation and inference (conclusions and recom-mendations)	Diagnosing	The critical thinker recognizes that the client erratic use of the prescribed medication may have multiple causes (e.g. troublesome side effects, or belief that illness is due to God's will and is not preventable) and will not infer a diagnosis with etiology until more data are obtained. Failure to think critically can lead to interpretation that are irrelevant, inadequate, and superficial (e.g. an erroneous interpretation that the client problem is lack of sufficient knowledge)
Assumptions (presuppositions)	Diagnosing	The critical thinker makes assumptions in accordance with a broad, unbiased database and mutually set client goals. The critical thinker avoids making unverified assumptions, such as that an increase in knowledge will increase this clients compliance or that this client is motivated to prevent a CVA
Concepts (theories, laws, principles, models)	Diagnosing Planning	The critical thinker uses concepts about motivation, change theory and multicultural nursing to understand the clients behavior and motivation to change. Failure to think critically can lead to exclusive reliance on a simplistic concept, such as "knowledge crates change"
Implications and consequences	Planning Implementing	The critical thinker considers the implication and consequences of selected nursing strategies before implementing plans of care. Plans of care, incusing goals and outcomes, are based on ongoing assessment of the clients cultural values, beliefs, and needs. Failure to think critically may lead to ineffective interventions, such as client teaching that focuses only on resolving a knowledge deficit about the prescribed medication. The critical thinker recognizes that a knowledge deficit may or may not be one of several problems
Interpretation and inference	Evaluating	The critical thinker bases evaluation of client outcomes and the effectiveness of nursing interventions on well-developed, measurable criteria and considers rationally whether outcomes have been validated. Failure to think critically may lead to client noncompliance and an inference that the client did not learn effectively and needs further instruction

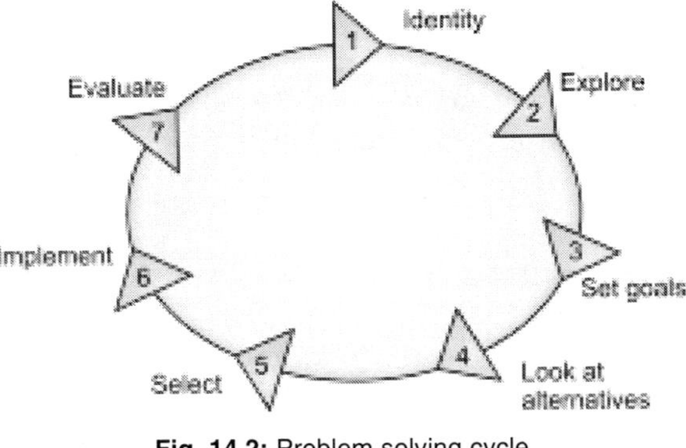

Fig. 14.2: Problem solving cycle

problem solving process to help you achieve your goal. Every time you use a problem solving process, you are increasing your problem solving skills.

1. Seven-step problem solving cycle (Fig. 14.2)
To solve a problem take the steps, one at a time.

Step 1: *Identify the problem*: Identify and name the problem so that you can find an appropriate solution.

Step 2: *Explore the problem*: When you are clear about what the problem is you need to think about it in different ways. Ask yourself.
- How is this problem affecting me others?
- How else experiences this problem?
- What do they do about it?

Seeing the problem in different ways is likely to help you find an effective solution.

Step 3: *Set Goals*: Once you have thought about the problem from different angles you can identify your goals. What is that you want to achieve? Do you want to
- Improve your health
- Increase your time management skills?
- Complete the assignments to the best of your ability?
- Finish the assignments as soon as possible?

Step 4: *Look at alternatives*: After goal decision, you need to look for possible solutions. You can 'brain-storm' for ideas to collect a long list of possibilities. You can seek ideas about possible solutions from others, books or internet.

Step 5: *Select a possible solutions:* From the list of possible solutions, you can sort out which are most relevant to your solution and which are realistic and manageable.

Step 6: *Implement a possible solution:* Once you have selected a possible solution you are ready to put into action. You will need to have energy and motivation to do this because implementing the solution may take some time and effort.

Step 7: *Evaluate:* Just because you have worded your way through the problem solving process, it does not mean that you automatically solve your problem. So you can evaluate effectiveness of your solution by asking yourself (and others):

- How effective was that solution?
- Did it achieve what I wonder?
- What consequences did it have on my situation?

If you feel dissatisfied with the result, then you can begin the steps again and this cycle goes on.

2. Trial and Error

One way to solve problems is through trial and error, in which a number of approaches are tried until a solution is found. However, without considering alternatives systematically, one cannot know why the solutions works. Trial and error methods in nursing care can be dangerous because the client might suffer harm if an approach is inappropriate. However, nurses often use trial and error in the home setting where, due to logistics, equipment and patient lifestyle, hospital procedures cannot work as effectively (e.g. there may be no pole from which to hang an IV bag or no electricity to plug in a device).

3. Intuition

Intuition is the understanding or learning of things without the conscious use of reasoning. It is also known as sixth sense, hunch, instinct, feeing, or suspicion. As a problem-solving approach, intuition is viewed by some people as a form of guessing and, as such, an in appropriate basis of nursing decisions. However, others view intuition as an essential and legitimate aspect of clinical judgment acquired through knowledge and experience. The nurse must first have the knowledge base necessary to practice in the clinical area and then use that knowledge in clinical practice. Clinical experience allows the nurse to recognize cures and patterns and begin to reach correct conclusions.

Experiences is important in improving intuition because the rapidity of the judgment depends on the nurse having seen similar client situation many times before. Sometimes nurses use the words "I had a feelings", to describe the critical thinking element of considering evidence. These nurses are able to judge quickly which evidence is most important and to act on that limited evidence. Nurses in critical care often pay closer attention than usual to a client when they sense that the clients condition could change suddenly.

Although the intuitive method of problem solving is gaining recognition as part of nursing practice, it is not recommended for novices or students, however, because they usually lack the knowledge base and clinical experience on which to make a valid judgment.

4. Research Process and Scientific/Modified Scientific Method

The research process is a formalized, logical, systematic approach to solving problems. The classic scientific method is most useful when the researcher is working in a controlled situation. Health professionals, often working with people in uncontrolled situations, require a modified approach to the scientific method for solving problems. For example, unlike experiments with animals the effects of diet on health care complicated by a person's race, lifestyle, and personal preferences.

Table 14.5 compares the research process or scientific method with the modified scientific method. Critical thinking is important in all problem solving processes as the nurse evaluates all potential solutions to a given problem and makes a decision to select the most appropriate solutions for that situation.

Table 14.5: Comparison between the research process and the modified scientific method

Research Process (Scientific Method)	*Modified scientific method*
State a research question or problem	Define the problem
Define the purpose of or the rationale for the study	
Review related literature	Gather information
Formulate hypothesis and defining variables	Analyze the information
Select a method to test hypotheses	Develop solutions
Select a population, sample and setting	
Conduct a pilot study	Make a decision
Collect the data	Implement the decision
Analyze the data	Evaluate the decision
Communicate conclusions and implication	

Levels of Thinking

There are six levels of thinking/learning within cognitive hierarchy of behaviors.

Level 1: Knowledge: It involves recall of facts, principles and terms in the forms in which they are learned.

Keywords: Who, What, When, omit, where, which, choose, find, how, define, label, show, spell, list, match, name, relate, tell, recall, select.

E.g. When did ——————Happen?
Which one ——————?

Level 2: Comprehension: It represents the lowest form of understanding. The student knows what is being communicated without relating it to other material or seeing it in its fullest meaning. It demonstrates understanding of facts and ideas by organizing, comparing, translating, interpreting, giving descriptions and stating main ideas.

Keywords: Compare, contrast, demonstrate, interpret, explain, extend, illustrate, infer, outline, relate, repharse, translate, summarize, show, classify.

E.g. What facts or ideas show....?
Which is the best answer....?

Level 3: Application: It involves the use of abstractions in concrete situations such as nursing or other specific situations. It is solving problems by applying acquired knowledge, facts, techniques and rules in different way.

Key words: Apply, build, choose, construct, develop, interview, make use of, organize, experiment with plan, select, solve, utilize, model, identify.

E.g. What would result if.....?
Can you make use of the facts to .....?

Level 4: Analysis: It is examining and breaking information into parts by identifying motives or caused; making inferences and finding evidence to support generalizations.

Key words: Analyze, categorize, compare, contrast, discover, dissect, divide, examine, in spite, simplify, survey, take part in, test for, distinguish, list, distinction, theme, relationships, function, motive, inference, assumption, conclusion.

E.g. What are keep parts or features of ....?
What motive is there.....?
What evidence can you find.....?

Level 5: Synthesis: It is compiling information together in a different way by combining elements in a new pattern or proposing alternative solutions.

Keywords: Build, choose, combine, compile, compose , construct, create, design, develop, estimate, formulate, imagine, invent, make up, originate, plan, predict, propose, solve, solution, etc.

E.g. Can you propose an alternative....?
Can you formulate a theory for.....?
What facts can you compile......?

Level 6: Evaluation: It is presenting and defending opinions by making judgments about information, validity of ideas or quality of work based on a set of criteria.

Keywords: Award, choose, conclude, criticize, decide, defend, determine, evaluate, judge, justify, measure, compare, mark, rate, recommend, prioritize, prove, disprove, etc.

E.g. What is your opinion of ....?
Would it be better if......?
How would you rate the....?

Decision Making

Nurses make decisions in the course of solving problems, for example, in each step of the nursing process. Decision making, however, is also used in situations that do not involve problem solving. Nurses make value decisions (e.g. to keep client information confidential); time management decisions (e.g. taking clean linens to the clients room at the same time as the medication in order to save steps); scheduling decisions (e.g. to bathe the client before visiting hours); and priority decisions (e.g. which interventions are most urgent and which can be delegated).

Decision making is a critical-thinking process for choosing the best actions to meet a desired goal. Decisions must be made whenever several mutually exclusive choices are available or when there is an option to act or not. For example, the individual who wishes to become a nurse is the United States has several possible courses of action: a diploma program, an associate degree program, or a baccalaureate program. Therefore, they must evaluate the different types of programs, as well as personal circumstances, to make a decision appropriate to their situations.

Nurses must make decision and assist clients to make decisions. When faced with several client needs at the same time, the nurse must prioritize and decide which client to assist first. The nurse may (a) look at advantages and disadvantages of each option, (b) apply Maslow's hierarchy of needs, (c) consider which tasks can be delegated to others, or (d) use another priority setting framework. When a client is trying to make a decision about what course of treatment to follow, the nurse may need to provide information or resources the client can use in making a decision. Nurses must make decisions in their own personal and professional lives. For example, the nurse must decide whether to work in a hospital or community setting, whether to join a professional association, and whether to carry professional liability insurance.

Here are sequential steps to the decision making process:

1. Identifying the purpose. The nurse identifies why a decision is needed and what needs to be determined.
2. Set the criteria. When the nurse sets the criteria for decision making, three questions must be answered: What is the desired outcome, what needs to be preserved, and what needs to be avoided? For example, for a client with pain, the criteria would be as follows:
   a. What needs to be achieved? Relief of pain
   b. What needs to be preserved? Physical functioning, cognitive functioning, psychologic functioning, client comfort
   c. What needs to be avoided? Central nervous system depression, respiratory depression, nausea.
3. Weight in criteria. In this step, the decision maker sets priorities or ranks activities or services in order of importance from least important to most important as they relate to the specific situation. Because the weighting is specific to the situation, an activity may be ranked as most important in one situation and of less importance in another situation. For example, if a client with the pain has terminal cancer, pain relief may be more important than avoiding the side effects of the pain medication.
4. Seek alternatives. The decision maker identifies all possible ways to meet the criteria. In clinical situations, the alternatives may be selected from a range of nursing interventions or client care strategies. Pain may be treated with oral or injectable medications, as needed (PRN) or on a schedule, or without pharmacologic intervention at all, instead using complementary alternative modalities (CAM).
5. Examine alternatives. The nurse analyzes the alternatives to ensure that there is an objective rationale in relation to the established criteria for choosing one strategy over another. For pain that results from a procedure (such as removal of a foreign object, CAM may not be strong enough relief and oral medication may be effective but act too slowly, so as intravenous narcotic might be the better choice.
6. Project. The nurse applies creative thinking and skepticism to determine what might go wrong's as a result of a decision and develops plans to prevent, minimize, or overcome any problems. If the intravenous narcotic is selected what safety procedures need to be in place, for example, narcotic antidote and supplemental oxygen?
7. Implement. The decision plan is placed into action. The pain treatment is begun.
8. Evaluate the outcome. As with the nursing care, in evaluating the nurse determines the effectiveness of the plan and whether the initial purpose was achieved. How does the client rate the level of pain following the procedure.

Developing Critical Thinking Attitudes and Skills

After gaining an idea of what it means to think critically, solve problems, and make decisions, nurses need to become aware of their own thinking style and abilities. Acquiring critical thinking skills and a critical attitude then becomes a matter of practice. Critical thinking is not an "either-or" phenomenon, people develop and use it more or less effectively along a continuum. Some people make better evaluation than others; some people believe information from nearly any source; and still others seldom believe anything without carefully evaluating the credibility of the information. Critical thinking is not easy. Solving problems and making decisions is risky. Sometimes the outcome is not what was desired. With effort, however, everyone can achieve some level of critical thinking to become an effective problem solver and decision maker.

- **Self-assessment:** The nurse should reflect on some of the attitudes discussed earlier that facilitate critical thinking, attitudes such as curiosity, fair-mindedness, humility, courage, and perseverance. A nurse might benefit from a rigorous personal assessment to determine which attitudes he or she already possessed and which need to be cultivated. This could also be done with a partner or as a group. The nurse first determines which attitudes are held strongly and form a base for thinking and which are held minimally or not at all. The nurse also needs to reflect on situations where he or she made decisions that were later regretted and analyses thinking processes and attitudes or asks a trusted colleagues to assess them. Identifying weak or vulnerable skills and attitudes is also important.
- **Tolerating dissonance and ambiguity:** The nurse needs to take deliberate efforts to cultivate critical thinking attitudes. For example, to develop fair-mindedness, one could deliberately seek out information that is in opposition to one's own views; this provides practice in understanding and learning to be open to other viewpoints. It is a human tendency to seek out information that corresponds to one's previously held beliefs and to ignore evidence that may contradict cherished ideas. This perspective is true for both the nurse and the client. Elders may have great difficulty accepting the pervasiveness of technology or that people don't stay in the hospital as long as they did in the 1970s or that having a diagnosis of cancer does not always mean that one is going to die. On the other hand, elders have a wealth of knowledge and experience and often know better than the health care provider what will work well and be acceptable to them. Nurses should increase their tolerance for ideas that contradict previously held beliefs, and they should practice suspending judgment.

  Suspending judgment means tolerating ambiguity for a time. If an issue is complex, it may not be resolved quickly or neatly, and judgment should be postponed. For a while, the nurse will need to say, "I don't know" and be comfortable with that answer until more is known. Although postponing judgment may not be feasible in emergency situations where fast action is required, it is usually feasible in other situations.
- **Seeking situations where good thinking is practiced:** Nurses will find it valuable to attend conferences in clinical or educational settings that support open examination of all sides of issues and respect for opposing viewpoints. Cultivating a questioning attitude, using either Socratic questioning or another technique, is vital. Nurses need to review the standards for evaluating thinking and apply them to their own thinking. If nurses are aware of their own thinking—while they are doing the thinking—they can detect thinking errors.
- **Creating environments that support critical thinking:** A nurse cannot develop or maintain critical thinking attitudes in a vacuum. Nurses in leadership position must be particularly aware of the climate for thinking that they establish, and they must actively create a stimulating environment that encourages difference of opinion and fair examination of ideas and options. Nurses must embrace exploration of the perspective of persons from different ages, cultures, religions, socioeconomic levels and family structures. As leaders, nurses should encourage colleagues to examine evidence carefully before they come to conclusions, and to avoid "group think", the tendency to defer unthinkingly to the will of the group.

15 CHAPTER
Intelligence, Aptitude and their Measurement

Intelligence

Intelligence is the ability to understand the world, think rationally or logically, and use of resources effectively when faced with challenges or problems. People know more about the measurement of intelligence than about the nature of intelligence. Perhaps we do know quite a lot about the nature of intelligence but there are differences of opinions as to what exactly, should be the scope and the meaning of the term 'intelligence.' Still all of them do use this term very freely and we do understand something definite by this term. An interesting experiment will be to think of a person whom we consider to be very intelligent and then start writing down one after another the various qualities because of which we consider to be very intelligent to be intelligent. Intelligence should not be confused with what we mean by intellect, though it is related to intellect or knowledge. It is quite possible (though it may not often happen) that a man with a high degree of intelligence may be poor intellectually simply for the reason he never attempted to use his intelligence and build up his intellect. Intelligence is some kind of ability which characterizes one's manner of dealing with his environment and his problems. Some people define intelligence as the capacity to meet a novel situation by a properly fitting response. Some others will add speed and success to an intelligent response. Some speak of intelligence as the capacity to deal with abstract intellectual operations connected with arithmetical and verbal reasoning. An intelligent act can be easily differentiated from an unintelligent act. Intelligence is a useful capacity in furthering our welfare.

Intelligence comes from the Latin verb 'intelligence' which means to understand. The word 'intelligence' forms part of our ordinary stock of words which we use everyday. In the field of psychology, too, the word intelligence finds a fairy comprehensive use. As mention below:

- It is general method capability to reason, solve problems. Think abstractly. Learn and understand new material and profit from past experience.
- Intelligence is the global capacity of an individual to act purposefully. To think rationally and to deal effectively with his environment.
- It is an innate mental ability for comprehension and reasoning quickly and correctly.
- It shows the capacity to learn difficult task and the ability to solve increasing difficult problems.
- Intelligence is the ability to adapt to one's surroundings.

- The effective all-round cognitive abilities to comprehend, to grasp relations and reason.
- It is the ability to deal with cognitive complexity.
- It is innate, general, cognitive ability.
- It is an mental activity consisting of grasping the essential in situation and responding appropriately to them.
- Intelligence is what you do when you don't know what to do.
- Intelligence is a ubiquitous individual difference and a hypothetical construct reflected in a variety of behaviors which demonstrate a cognitive capacity for thinking, reasoning, learning, and adapting.
- Intelligence can be defined as the ability to assimilate factual knowledge, to recall either recent or remote events, to reason logically, to manipulate concepts (Either numbers or words), to translate the abstract to the literal, and the literal to abstract, to analyze and synthesize forms, and to deal meaningfully and accurately with problems.

DEFINITION

Intelligence is the capacity for learning and the ability to recall, integrate constructively, and apply what one has learned; the capacity to understand and to think rationally.

It has been defined in a number of ways by the scientists. Some of these definitions are given below:

"Intelligence is an inferred characteristic of an individual, usually defined as the ability to profit from experience, acquire knowledge, think abstractly, or to adapt to changes in the environments."

1. According to Wells, 'intelligence is the property of recombining our behavior pattern so as to act better in a novel situation.' In William Stern's opinion, 'Intelligence is the ability to adjust oneself to a new situation.' So *Intelligence is the ability of adjusting in a new situation.*
   This definition are faulty in the following respects:
   a. They fail to clarify the full scope of intelligence.
   b. Intelligence and adjustability are not the same. Intelligence is innate but adjustability is mostly learnt.
2. Ebbinghaus and Thorndike define intelligence as the ability to make profitable use of past experience. In other words, intelligence is that ability of learning. So *Intelligence is the ability to avail of past experience.*
   The following defects found in this definition:
   a. Learning and intelligence are not identical because learning depends on many factors besides the latter.
   b. This definition too does not describe the full scope of intelligence.
3. According to Garret, one may define "intelligence as including the ability demanded in the solution of problems which require the comprehension and use of symbols." In Terman's opinion "Intelligence is the ability to think abstractly." So *Intelligent is the ability of abstract thinking.*
   This definition suffers from the following defects:
   a. Abstractly thinking is not intelligence, it is only a part of intelligence.
   b. This definition fails to describe the complete scope of intelligence.
4. In Wechsler's opinion "intelligence is the aggregate or global capacity of an individual to act purposefully, to think rationally and to deal effectively with his environment." Computing the different powers of intelligence, Husband has said, "an intelligent person

uses past experience effectively, is able to concentrate and keep his attention focused for longer periods of time, adjusts himself to a new and unaccustomed situation rapidly, with less confusion and with fewer false moves, show variability and versatility of response, is able to see distant relationships, can carry an abstract has a greater capacity of inhibition or delay and is capable of exercising self-criticism." So Intelligence is the conglomeration of any powers.

Actually Husband has given a very good description of an intelligent person but intelligence cannot be accepted to be the sum total of all these qualities. The psychologists however, differ in considering intelligence as a single ability or a collection of many abilities. A description of the different theories concerning the nature of intelligence will help to understand the various interpretations of the form of intelligence.

Type of Intelligence

1. According to *Sternberg's Triarchic* Theory of Human Intelligence (1995), it is of three types.
   i. Analytical Intelligence
   ii. Creative Intelligence
   iii. Practical Intelligence.

- **Analytical Intelligence:** It is academic problem solving skills, 'based on combined operations of execution, performance and knowledge. These three operations will enable us to encode stimuli, hold information in short-term memory, make calculations, perform mental calculations, mentally compare different stimuli retrieve information from long-term memory. And hence, it is helpful to memorize things.
- **Creative Intelligence:** It involves insights, synthesis and the ability to react to noval situations and stimuli. It consists of ability which allows people to think creativity and adjust creatively and effectively to new because they assess an individual's ability to apply existing knowledge to new problems.
- **Practical Intelligence:** It is the intelligence which operates in the real world. People with this type of intelligence can adapt to, or shape their environment. It is not only influenced by mental skills but also attitudes and emotional factors. So, practical intelligence is a combinations of.
  - Adapt to the environment in order to have goals met.
  - Changing the environment in order to have goals met.
  - Do not work, moving to a new environment in which goals can be met.

2. Garden (1999) Proposes eight types of intelligence.
   i. *Linguistic Intelligence:* Involved in reading, writing, listening and talking.
   ii. *Logical-Mathematic Intelligence:* Involved in solving logical puzzles, deriving proofs and performing calculations.
   iii. *Spatial Intelligence:* Involved in moving from one location to another or determining one's orientation in space.
   iv. *Musical Intelligence:* Involved in playing, composing, singing and conducting. Furthermore, Gardner believes that automechanics and cardiologists may have this kind of intelligence in abundance as they make diagnose on the careful listening to patterns of sounds.
   v. *Bodily-kinestetic Intelligence:* Involved in using one's body (or parts of it) to perform skillful and purposeful movements, e.g. Dancers, athletes and surgeons.

vi. *Intrapersonal Intelligence:* Involved in understanding oneself and having insight into one's own thoughts. Actions and emotions, e.g. self-understanding.
vii. *Interpersonal Intelligence:* Involved in understanding of others and one's reactions to others. Being high in social skills, psychologists, teachers and politicians are supposed to be high in this type of intelligence.
viii. *Naturalistic Intelligence:* It involves the ability to understand and work effectively in the natural world, e.g. Biologists and Zoologists.

FACTORS AFFECTING INTELLIGENCE

1. **Biological factors:** Evidence suggests that genetic variation has a significant impact on IQ , accounting for three-fourths in adults. Despite the high heritability of IQ, few genes have been found to have substantial effect on IQ, suggesting that IQ is the product of interaction between multiple genes.

   Other biological factors correlating with IQ include ratio of brain weight to body weight, and the volume and location of gray matter tissue in the brain.

   Because intelligence appears to be at least partly dependent on brain structure and the genes shaping brain development, it has been proposed that genetic engineering could be used to enhance the intelligence of animals. A process sometimes called 'biological uplift' in science fiction.
2. **Environmental factors:**
   Family: Evidence suggests that family environmental factors may have an effect upon childhood IQ. On the other hand, by late adolescence, this correlation disappears, such that adoptive siblings are no more similar in IQ that strangers. Moreover, adoption studies indicate that, by adulthood, adoptive studies are no more similar in IQ than strangers, while twins and full siblings show an IQ correlation.
   - Nature versus nurture: The nature component appears to be much more important that the 'nurture' component in explaining IQ variance in general population.
   - Culture: Cultural factors also play a role in intelligence.
3. **Ethical issues**: Since intelligence is susceptible to modification through the manipulation of environment, the ability to influence intelligence raises ethical issues.
   - Transhumanist Theories: Study the possibilities and consequences of developing and using techniques to enhance human abilities and aptitudes.
   - Eugenics: It is a social philosophy which advocates the improvement of human hereditary traits through various forms of intervention.
   - Neuroethics: Considers the ethical, legal and social implications of neuroscience and deals with issues such as difference between treating a human neurological disease and enhance the human brain. Neuroethical issues.

Theories of Intelligence

I. FACTOR THEORIES

Intelligence is a collection of specific distinguishable abilities. Intelligence is hypothesized to consist of a few major factors. Many have used statistical technique known as factor analysis. The technique is a way of identifying groups of abilities or behaviors or traits that are related to one another. In the area of intelligence testing, the technique is usually applied to several specific subjects.

I. Psychometric (factor analytical) theories: These are based upon analysis of scores of large number of individuals on various intelligence test using a statistical technique called Factors Analysis (FA).

Spearman's two factor theory: Spearman factor analyzed the results of children's performance on various tests and found that many tests were moderately positively correlated. He concluded that every intellectual activity involves both a general factor ('G' or general Intelligence) and a specific factors (s) and differences between individuals are largely attributable to difference in their 'G'. The G accounts for why people who perform well using one mental ability also tend to perform well in others, and is entirely innate.

G-factor theory: Charles Spearman (1927) proposed that a broad general intelligence (G) factor lay beneath the surface of mind. Spearman noted that a number of different cognitive tasks and intellectual measures tend to be correlated with one another, i.e. people who score high on one tend to score high on others as well. Spearmen believed that each individual intellectual task taps both general intelligence or G and some other ability, "S", specific to the particular task.

Burt and Vernon's hierarchical model: Burt (who was a student of Spearman) agreed that there's a G factor common to all tests, but also thought that the two factor model was too simple. He and Vernon elaborated and extended Spearman's model by identifying a series of group factors (major and minor) in between G and S factors. The G is what all tests measure, the major group factors (V: ed and k:m) are what some tests measure (some to a greater extent than others),the minor group factors are what particular test measure whenever they are given, while specific factors are what particular tests measure on specific occasions.

With this model, each child can be ranked on a single scale of (innate) intelligence, giving the dominance of G in the hierarchy.

Hierarchical theory: Some including Vernon (1950) proposed that elements of G-factor theory and the multifactor theories be combined to form a hierarchical theory. In this theory intelligence is punctured as a sort of pyramid. At the top of pyramid is G, general intelligence which shows up in virtually all kinds of intellectual activity. Underneath it are several moderately specific abilities factors like Thurstone primary mental abilities. At the bottom of pyramid are a large number of highly specific abilities, similar to Spearman's S factors.

Thurstone's primary mental abilities: Using 14-year-old and college students as participants, he found that not all mental test correlate equally. Rather they appear to form seven distinct factors or groupings, which he called Primary Mental Abilities (PMAs) namely:

- Spatial (s): The ability to recognize spatial relationships.
- Perceptual speed (P): The quick and accurate detection of visual detail.
- Numerical reasoning (N): Ability to perform arithmetical operations quickly and accurately.
- Verbal meaning (V): Understanding the meaning of words and verbal concepts.
- Word fluency (W): Speed in recognizing single and isolated words.
- Memory (M): The ability to recall a list of words, numbers or other materials.
- Inductive reasoning (I): The ability to generate a rule or relationship that describes a set of observations.

Multifactorial theories: In contrast to Spearman, several theories have concluded that intelligence has multiple components. These theories generally corrected with one another that with other tests.

One of the most influential of the multifactor theories grow out of the work of factor analyst LL Thustone (1938). He identified primary mental abilities, which include verbal comprehension, word fluency, perceptual speed, memory, numerical ability and reasoning. Thurstone developed a number of tests to measure these abilities called Primary Mental Abilities (PMA) Test. Another multifactor theory given by JP Guilford (1967). It is a three dimensional theory. This model indentifies 120 factors of intelligence. Each factor is represented by cell in the cube and is some combination of these three dimensions, i.e. five kinds of contents (5 × 6 × 4 = 120). Guilford concept to intelligence also includes divergent thinking, which is closely related to creative or original problem solving as opposed to convergent thinking, which is involved in solving problems with a single correct answer.

II. Guilford's structure of intellect model: This represents the most extreme alternatives to Spearman's two-factor theory, and totally rejects the notion of a general intelligence factor. Guilford's classified a cognitive task along three major dimensions:

- Content (what must the participation think about?)
- Operations (what kind of thinking is the participant being asked to perform?)
- Products (What kind of answer is required?)

He identified five kinds of content, five kinds of operation and six kinds of product which multiplied together, yields a total of 150 distinct mental abilities. He set out to construct tests to measure each of 150 abilities, and tests have been devised to assess more than 70. However, people's scores are often correlated, suggesting that the number of basic mental abilities is much small than Guilford assumed.

II. PROCESS-ORIENTED THEORIES

The focus of these theories is intellectual processes, i.e. the patterns of thinking that people use when they reason and solve problems. These theories talk about cognition and cognitive processes rather than intelligence.

a. **Jean Piaget's theory of cognitive development Piaget's theory** (1970) is a prominent process theorist. In Piaget's view, involves an interplay of biological maturation and interaction with environment. He viewed intellectual development as an evolution of cognitive process. According to Piaget, cognitive growth occurs in the following steps (Table 15.1).

Jean Piaget (1896-1980) emphasized the ways that children think and acquire knowledge. Piaget described four major stages leading to the capacity for adult thought, these are:

Sensorimotor stage (Birth to 2 years): From the beginning, the child is concerned only with satisfying basic needs and comforts. The self is not differentiated from the external environment. As the sense of differentiation occurs, with increasing mobility and awareness, the mental system is expanded. The external environment and their effects on him or her. Knowledge is gained regarding the ability to manipulate objects and experiences within the environment.

Preoperational (2-6 years): The children use symbols and language more extensively that sensorimotor stage. They learn without the use of reasoning; unable to think logically or

Table 15.1: Piaget's stages of cognitive development		
Years		
First 2	Sensorimotor	Incorporation of reflex patterns. First only to repeat then to maintain and then to produce new changes in the environment increasing understanding of means end relationships. Then object constancy, beginning of true thought and internalized problem solving seen.
2-7	Preoperational	Unsystematic reasoning, internal representations and languages development egocentrism, animism and faulty reasoning about cause-effect relationships. The substage development and symbolic play and Perceptional or Intuitive (4-7 years) stage of reasoning centered on appearances rather than implication. Trial and error method used. Reality and fantasy are confused.
7-12	Concrete operational	Systematic reasoning, logical and reversible but limited.
12 Onwards	Formal operational stage	Logic, reasoning from hypothetical proposition evaluating hypotheses, reality present.

deductively, can name objects but not classes of objects. Language development progresses and reality is often given to inanimate objects. Children can't deal with moral dilemmas, although they have sense of what is good and bad. They are egocentric and also use a type of magically thinking.

Concrete operations (6-12 years): It is so named because children operate and act on concrete, real and perceivable world of objects and events. They show ability to classify objects, egocentric thought is replaced by operational thought. They can regulate themselves, and they begin to develop a moral sense and a code of values.

Formal operations (13-15years): It is so named because young person's thinking operates in a formal, highly logical, systematic and symbolic manner. The individual is able to think and reason in abstract terms can make and test hypotheses using logical and orderly problem solving. A degree of egocentrism returns. Most individuals achieve cognitive maturity, the capability to perform all mental operations needed for adulthood, in middle to late adolescence.

- Hospitalized children who are in the sensorimotor stage have not achieved objects permanence and therefore suffer from separation anxiety. They are vest off if their mothers are allowed to stay with them overnight.
- Children at the preoperational stage, who are unable to deal with concepts and abstractions, benefit more form role playing of medical procedures and situation than by having them verbally described in detail, e.g. a child who is to receive IV therapy is helped by acting out the procedure with a toy IV set and dolls.
- As the children could not understand the cause and effect may interpret physical illness as punishment for bad thoughts or deeds.
- Adolescent's thinking may appear abstract.

Nurse can explain the procedure to an individual of the basis of his intellectually ability. She knows to what extent, she can explain. Otherwise she educated the parents/relatives about necessary details other patient.

During any nursing procedure, the nurse must always understand the particular age and his/her cognitive ability.

b. Bruner's theory: Ferome Bruner (1973) is a process theorist. Babies according to Bruner, have a highly action oriented intelligence. Older children and adolescents know things internally and symbolically, i.e. they are able to internalize symbols or representations, of objects and sections. Reward and punishment are important in its use and development.

c. Information-processing approach: According to Fishbein (1984), the information processing approach as the steps or processes. People go through in solving problems. One person may be more intelligent, because he/she move through the same steps more quickly or efficiently, or is more familiar with the required problem solving steps.

According to it, break intelligence down into various basic skills that people employ to take in information, process it and then use it to reason and solve problems. Robert Sternberg (1984), distinguished between information, process components (Components are the steps one goes through to solve problem whereas metacomponents are the kinds to knowledge one has about how to solve the problem).

Individual Difference in Intelligence

In almost all psychological characteristics, individual differ from one another. In fact, modern psychology deals a great deal with these individual differences. All the psychological tests are meant to measure these difference in intelligence, people differ considerably. Some are very superior and some are idiotic. From the lowest to the highest level we find a whole range of levels of intelligence. And also find that a majority of people will be somewhere around the average. This factor of intelligence and several other psychological factors and biological measurements are said to follow the "Normal Probability Curve". This means that very few will be at the lowest level and similarly, very few will be at the highest level. The number will increase as go up from the lowest point till reach the average. A large number of people will be possessing intelligence around the average point. Then again, the number decreases till we finally come to the highest level. If we draw on a graph paper marking the amount of intelligence along the vertical axis, the graph will take the shape of a bell. It is useful to remember this point since in advanced psychology, frequent use is made of this principle in making psychological measurements and calculations.

- *Mental defectiveness:* The normal people will come within the range covering slightly below and slightly above the average. As we go further down the scale we have what is called mental defectiveness. Below a certain point when the amount of intelligence possessed is not sufficient for the person to lead a normal life, we call him a mental defective. This mental defectiveness is of various grades. Usually, they are brought under the following groups. Nearest to the normal group come those who are called 'morons'. These morons have sufficient intelligence to learn certain simple routine and semiskilled work. The best among the morons can be taught various jobs and they do them very well without any supervision. With proper institutional care and proper methods of teaching, they can be saved from being a burden to society. They may not do very well in regular academic learning. But they can be taught to do very useful work. These morons can sometimes be a danger to society sine they can be easily led into delinquency and other social evils. This is particularly because they do not have enough intelligence to realize the significance of their actions. Mental defectives requires sympathy and understanding and they must be taught and trained by people who are specially trained for this purpose.

Just below the morons comes the group of defectives called the 'imbeciles'. The imbeciles cannot do much useful work. The best of the imbeciles may be taught to do some very simple routine jobs and even that under supervision. But they do learn to protect their lives against simple physical dangers such as water and fire. They can seldom learn to read. They can engage themselves in simple conversation, and most of them can be taught to look after their personal needs such as washing, feeding and clothing. Naturally, these people need more of institutional care than the morons.

The lowest group is called the 'idiots'. They are much worse off than the imbeciles. They cannot take care of their personal needs even. Very seldom, they learn to wash and dress themselves. They can express themselves only in a few monosyllables. Almost like a baby, they cannot avoid physical dangers to life. They can learn practically nothing. Thus they become a very great liability to the family concerned and to the society in general.

- Mental effectiveness may be because of various causes. Sometimes the cause may be physical because of some early disturbances in the central nervous system. Sometimes, it is inherited from the parents. Whatever be the cause very seldom mental defectiveness can be treated satisfactorily. In some cases, where a small amount of defectiveness is caused by some glandular deficiency, medical treatment may produce some improvement. But on the whole the chances of improving mental defectiveness are title. The best that we can do is to study the amount and extent of defectiveness and arrange to give suitable education and training. The parents also must be taught to take a realistic view and face the facts with cheerfulness and courage. They should not develop any tendency of rejecting the child or showing indifference. The resources of an ordinary parent will not be sufficient to meet the demands of the proper training of a defective. So in an enlightened state, there should be sufficient number of schools and institutions meant for such people.

Advantage of Intelligence Quotient

As already explained how the IQ of an individual is obtained. It must be noted however that the IQ of an individual is always constant. If a boy has a mental age of eight at his chronological age of six, his IQ becomes $8/6 \times 100 = 133.3$. Thus would mean that this particular boy is very bright. The IQ of this boy at the age of ten will still be 133.3. This means his mental age when he is ten years old will be 13.3 years. Thus it will be seen that the mental age is increasing every year but not the IQ. This fact is called the "Constancy of IQ". However, some psychologists have questioned this fact seriously and have conducted experiments to see whether the IQ cannot be increased by giving special attention to a particular child and by giving him favorable learning facilities. These experiments have shown that if a child from a poor environment is given special training and education quite early in life, it is possible to increase his IQ by a few points. But these experimental results were not sufficient disturb the hypothesis of the constancy of IQ.

The idea of intelligence quotient or IQ was utilized first of all in 1916 in the Stanford Binet tests. IQ is the ratio between mental age (MA) and chronological age (CA). The chronological age is determined from the date of birth and the mental age by intelligence tests. For example, if the average score of the children of 13 plus in age turns out to be 75 in some tests then any child whose score reveals an average of 75 will be said to have a mental age of 13, whatever be his chronological age. Mental age does not increase with the chronological age. Having understood the mental age properly, it is easy to understand IQ. The equation for the calculation of IQ is as follows:

$$IQ = \frac{MA \times 100}{CA}$$

As is evident from the above equation, to calculate IQ the mental age is divided by the chronological age and then multiplied by 100. To take an example supposes a four years old child has a mental age of three years. His IQ will be calculated with the help of the following equation:

$$IQ = \frac{3 \times 100}{4}$$

The concept of IQ became very popular and was hailed as a great boon to teachers and others. Since the results of ordinary school examinations depend upon a number of factors, the IQ came to be accepted as the true mark of one's intellectual capacity. Thus in the assessment of the abilities and difficulties of school pupils, IQ came to be used very freely. Even admissions to various courses in some countries were based only on one's IQ. Employers measured the IQs of applicants for jobs. It became almost a fashion to speak of one's IQ.

But in recent years, psychologists began to realize that one single score as the IQ does not really give a good picture of the assets and liabilities of an individual either in the school situation or in other situations. The comparative ability in the different aspects of mental functions should be known before we can form an idea of the capacities of a boy. Even for giving training and education, such an analysis is necessary so that necessary emphasis can be given. Thus in recent years the extreme importance that was once given to the IQ has been on the decline though it is still used in all such records. A short pen picture giving his differential capacity for different abilities such as the primary abilities we mentioned earlier, is preferred.

Limitations of the Concept of IQ

Actually the IQ reveals the mental ability of the individual on the basis of which he can be directed about his future. Here, it is essential to keep in sight the limitations of the idea of IQ. Its main limitations are as follows:

1. IQ is not the quantity of a person's intelligence
2. All the tests do not yield the same IQ consequently, none of the IQ as indicated by any one test is completely reliable
3. No person is devoid of intelligence so that IQ does not start from zero
4. IQ changes at least once in every three years
5. Even when a person is examined by the same test a number of times, the IQ shows a change. This difference differs from test to test. For example, in Wechsler Bellevue Test the difference is upto 5 points whereas in the Stanford-Binet tests it is upto 4 points.
6. IQ is the result both of heredity and environment. Thus a change in environment may change the IQ. According to Garret, the good or bad environment may show a difference of 10 points.

In this context, some other important things known from experiments are:

1. There is a possibility of increase in IQ along with a rise in the social and economic status and a possibility of decrease in IQ with a degradation in social and economic status.
2. The IQ generally remains constant from 5 to 14 years of age.
3. The mental level develops gradually.

Classification According to IQ		
IQ	Classification	Percentage
140 or above	Very superior	1-5
120 to 139	Superior	11
110 to 119	Bright	18
90 to 109	Average or normal	48
80 to 89	Dull normal or backward	14
70 to 79	Very dull	5-10
0 to 69	Feebleminded	2-5

IQ and Success in School Work

Researchers have made it clear that there is no invariable relation between IQ and success in school work. But in children with a higher IQ there is a possibility of success in school work.

It has been seen from different experiments that some kind of relation between the fathers occupation and the children IQ is to be observed. The IQ of children of fathers in a particular occupation was found to be higher than that of children whose fathers worked in some others spheres. The following table clarifies this relation:

Fathers occupation	*IQ of offspring*
Rural or urban laborer	96
Semiskilled	99
Ordinary clerk, shopkeeper	104
Clerk, merchant	107
Semiemployee, manager	111
Employee	116

This relation between fathers occupation and the child's IQ can neither be attributed solely to heredity nor to environment. Actually, both these factors determine it. People engaged in different occupations have different levels of intelligence and the environment in their homes is also different which affects the child. In this too, the environmental factor is the more important. Upon getting a superior environment, the son of a laborer may also exhibit an IQ higher than that of the son of a businessman. In fact, the experimental proofs available at present are inadequate to allow the acceptable of any definite relationship between the father's occupation and the child IQ. Though there is undoubtedly some relation between the two.

Feeblemindedness

Feeblemindedness is less than the average deficiency of intelligence. In the words of Woodworth, 'Feebleminded persons are so deficient in intelligence that they cannot manage their own lives without supervision. Thus it is clear that the feebleminded person is a problem for his family as well as for society.

The feebleminded persons are divided in the following three classes according to their intelligence:

1. Idiots—Idiots cannot protect themselves even from common danger. They cannot avoid a vehicle. They will put their hands in the fire and jump in deep water without hesitation. They can neither keep themselves clean nor clothed. They cannot eat themselves nor fulfill other needs. Except some few words they cannot speak any language. They are the least intelligent.
2. Imbeciles—Imbeciles are more intelligent than idiots. They can avoid common dangers. They can speak but cannot write. They cannot do any useful job. Very few imbeciles can learn some useful task and fewer can learn, bathing, cleaning, putting on clothes, though not without supervision.
3. Morons—These are the most numerous among feebleminded persons and also the most intelligent. They can fulfill their daily needs without supervision. They can also learn to do some useful jobs, for example looking after the animals, carpentry, sewing, etc. But to earn a living, they require the supervision of a person who may understand their limitations. Without such a supervision, they will waste money and time and become delinquents.

   Assessment of Intelligence: In the modern civilized society efforts are being made to cure feebleminded persons so that they may lead a normal life. Ordinarily the morons can be taught to earn their living. But the idiots and imbeciles are a constant problem. They can however, be made harmless, by the provision of favorable environment.

Assessment of Intelligence

Assessment: Assessment of intelligence is done by various scales, processes and purposes. Common theses used in psychiatric processes are:

i. Stanford-Binet Intelligence Scale
ii. Wechsler's test
iii. Uzgiris Hunt scale
iv. Bhatia's Battery test

One of the achievement of modern psychology is the development of scientific devices of measuring the general mental ability or intelligence. These are called intelligence test. These are the result of belief that intelligence exits in a certain amount that varies from individual-to-individual.

I. BINET-SIMON TEST/INTELLIGENT QUOTIENT (IQ)

In 1905, Alfred Binet introduced the concept of the Mental Age (MA), which is the average intellectual level of a particular age. The intelligence Quotient (IQ) is the ratio of MA to CA (Chronological Age), multiplied by 100 to eliminate the decimal point.

$$IQ = \frac{MA \times 100}{CA}$$

An IQ of 100, or average, results when chronological and mental ages are equal. Because it is impossible to measure age associated changes in intellectual power after the age of 15 with available intelligence tests, the higher divisor in the IQ formula is 15. One way of expressing a person's relative standing with a group is by percentile. The higher the percentile, the higher the rank within group. An IQ of 100 corresponds to the 50th percentile in intellectual ability for the general population.

IQ is a measure of relative intelligence determined by a standardized test. IQ is a measure of present functioning ability, not necessarily of future potential. Although under ordinary circumstances, is stable throughout life. The IQ itself does not indicate the origins of its reflected capacities—genetic (innate) or environmental. The most used intelligence test must measure a variety of skills and abilities including verbal and performance, early learned and recently learned, timed and untimed, culture free, and culture bound.

Terman classified level of intelligence as follows:

Levels	*IQ*
Idiot	0-25
Imbecile	26-50
Moron	51-70
Borderline	71-80
Low normal	81-90
Normal	91-110
Superior	110-120
Very superior	121-130
Genious/near genious	140 and over

II. WECHSLER ADULT INTELLIGENCE SCALE (WAIS)

The Wechsler Adult Intelligence Scale (WAIS) is the best standardized and most widely used intelligence test in clinical practice today. It was constructed by David Wechsler at New York University Medical Centre and Bellevue Psychiatric Hospital. Designed in 1939, the original WAIS has gone through several revisions. The latest revision, the WAIS-III, is designed for persons 16 to 89 years of age. A scale for children ages 5 through 15 years has been devised (Wechsler Intelligence Scale for Children-III (WISC-III and a scale for children ages 4 to 6½ years (Wechsler Preschool and Primary Scale of Intelligence-Revised (WPPSI-R).

The WAIS comprises 11 subtests made up of six verbal subtests and five performance subtests, which yield verbal IQ, a performance IQ, and a combined full-scale IQ, a performance IQ, and a combined full-scale IQ. Intelligence levels are based on the assumption that intellectual abilities are normally distributed (in a bell-shaped curve) throughout the population.

Importance of Intelligence Tests

In the present day life, intelligence tests play a great part. In many countries, admissions are made to Universities and technical courses only on the basis of intelligence and other psychological tests. For appointments to various aspects posts also, intelligence tests are used to rate the merits of candidates. In many parts of the world, these tests are replacing letters of recommendation. They also replace the results of examination. Without discussing here the details of the merits and demerits of examination results, it may be just mentioned that the examination results are often misleading with regard to the ability of a candidate. Examinations mostly test knowledge. This may or may not be an indication of one's intelligence. But doing well at the examinations is also important, since, to discharge our duties in life a certain amount of intelligence as well as knowledge is necessary. But the popularity of intelligence tests has been due to the fact that examinations are poor tests of one's intelligence. During the last fifty years a large number of psychologists have given their time and attention to the consideration and development of proper intelligence tests. They have been studied from the point of view of psychology and mathematical principles involved in statistics. Modern psychology makes so much use of statistics that one cannot be good student of psychology without learning statistics sooner or later.

During the beginning of this century, the school authorities in France wanted to take some measure to spot out those students who could not do well in their studies because of lack of innate ability or intelligence required for studies. For this purpose, one of their psychologist by name Alfred Binet was commissioned by the French government. Thus he made the first attempt to construct intelligence tests. Since this work was the first of this kind, naturally the tests which he produced where not perfect and later psychologists have greatly improved on them. But even today some revised forms of these tests are in use. But Binet made an important and lasting contribution.

Naturally before constructing tests the question arises, how exactly can intelligence be measure. Some kind of quantitative device must be made before measuring. Binet very brilliantly hit upon the idea of what is called 'the mental age'. A seven-year-old boy may perform intellectual functions that are normal to a seven-year-old boy or he may be better worse. All these three possibilities are there. If he is the same as the average for the normal group then Binet said his mental age can be said to be seven which is the same as his physical age or more commonly called the chronological age. If his intelligence is the same

as the average of the six-year-old boys, then his mental age is only six. Thus the mental age of a boy is expressed in terms of the age group to which his psychological functioning belongs. With this general framework, Binet constructed tests that should be passed or completed by each particular age group. After a good deal of preliminary work, he finalized a test of thirty questions of increasing difficulty.

Types of Intelligence Tests

Intelligence tests are classified as follows according to the activities prescribed in them:
1. Verbal tests
2. Nonverbal tests.

As the name itself suggests, verbal tests make use of language while the nonverbal tests include such activities which do not necessitate the use of language. Both these types are suitable for individual as well as group tests. Consequently. Verbal and nonverbal tests are further subdivided into two classes—individual and group. Thus, finally there are four types of intelligence tests:

i. Verbal individual intelligence tests
ii. Nonverbal individual intelligence tests
iii. Verbal group intelligence tests
iv. Nonverbal group intelligence tests.

i. ***Verbal individual intelligence tests:*** The very name verbal individual intelligence tests suggests that there are intelligence tests given to individuals or in other words they are meant to test the intelligence of individuals. Language finds adequate use in them. Binet-Simon test and the various revisions are all included in this classification.

The State manovigynashala of Uttar Pradesh has made a variety of material, from solid objects to difficult questions. The activities in the beginning are simple like constructing a bridge or a tower of blocks or fitting in irregular wooden blocks in their proper place supplied for them. At the same time at the end of the tests there are difficult question which need considerable thinking. This test is divided into several age groups. The higher groups use language and its use gradually declines with the age group. For example, the two year group includes the following activities:

1. The form panel with three holes
2. Recognition of objects by name
3. Recognizing the organs of the body
4. Making a tower of blocks
5. Naming an objects from its picture
6. Word order.

1. *Opposites.* A number of words are given for which opposite words are to be given in a stipulated time. The list will naturally contain words of varying difficulty.
2. *Verbal comprehension.* Here again another list of words and phrases will be given. Meanings or short explanations have to be given for these words.
3. *Analogies.* Three terms are given, the first two having a particular relationship to each other and a fourth term has to be found out so that the relationship between the third and fourth out so that the relationship between the second. Example:- (i)Dogs: Bark: Donkeys: the correct answer is 'Bray'. (ii)Hill: Mountain: Pond:- The answer of course is 'lake'.
4. *Classification.* In this, usually five terms will be given, four belonging to one and the same category, and one which does not belong to this category has to be detected and underlined or scored off as directed. Example:- (i) Mohammed, Krishnappa, Lakshmi, Sunder, Akbar ali. Of these five terms Lakshmi is the name of a woman, whereas the other four belong to one category, viz. the male sex. So the term 'Lakshmi' has to be underlined; ii)River, pond, tank, well, lake. Here river has flowing water, whereas the other four contain stagnant water. Hence 'river' has to be underlined.

Reasoning test: Some batteries of test contain also some questions for which answers are to be supplied. These are mostly based on one's capacity to reason. Some may even take the form of riddles. Example:- three boys are sitting in a row. Sankar is to the left of Gopal. Chander is to the left of Sankar. Which boy in the middle?

Following directions: A series of connected directions and conditions are given which must be carefully followed to get the correct answer. Example:- (i) If Monday was called Wednesday and Tuesday was called Thursday, what would Thursday be called? (ii)if an elephant is bigger than a horse, put a cross mark within the circle drawn at the end of this question, provided Monday follows Sunday. If not put a dot.

ii. ***Nonverbal tests of intelligence:*** The type of intelligence test discussed till now create two difficulties. (1) they all involve so much of language and vocabulary that it is difficult to administer them to the people of different nationalities. (2) They also assume a certain culture and familiarity with particular types of objects that are used by some people. Hence psychologists began to think of devising intelligence tests that would be free from these defects. During the First World War a need for such new type of tests arose when the American Army wanted to recruit their men on the basis of psychological tests. Many of those men could not read and write properly. Thus nonverbal test began to be developed and we now have a large number of them. These nonverbal tests are also called 'Performance Tests'. This name comes from the fact that in these test one has to perform some kind of motor activities are of various degrees of complication suitable for testing different levels of intelligence. Some are simple tests which are used for a particular purpose. some are complicated and arranged in a series of increasing difficulty.

Some of the well-known nonverbal tests are: Alexander's Pass along Test, Healey's Picture completion Test, Cube Construction Test, Block Design Test, Picture Arrangement Test, Matrices Test, tests with geometrical designs involving the principles of classification, series completion, etc. all these tests are not used simultaneously to test a particular individual. Different psychologist prefer different test from this list. This list itself is not complete. These are several more/some of these tests particularly the Goddard Form Board Test is used with children suspected of mental defectiveness. Some of these a clear idea of the principles involved. Some of these tests would appear to be very simple until we actually attempt to do them. Just seeing the tests will not give us a correct idea of them. The modern tendency in intelligence testing is to have a composite battery of test containing almost equal number of verbal test and nonverbal tests. This is an attempt to make sure that no factor of intelligence is left untested.

One of the best known examples of this type of composite tests is the one devised and arranged by David Wechsler of Bellevue Hospital, New York. The test is known as the Wechsler Bellevue Test. There are two forms of these tests, one for the adults and another for the children. There are also some other well-known composite test consisting purely of performance tests. Two of them are the Pintner-Paterson Test and the Cornell-Coxe Test.

Group tests and individual tests

Intelligence tests can also be classified under the categories of group tests and individual tests. Group tests as the term indicates are given to a group of subjects at a time. Naturally they must all start at one time and finish at the same time, just like an examination. So here the time factor is constant. One's intelligence is measured in terms of the amount of work successfully completed within the given time. Individual tests on the other hand need not necessarily depend on a constant time factor. The individuals ability can be measured in terms of the total time required for completing a job. Here the work will be constant but the time taken will vary. We actually have both these types of tests. It is kind of apparatus to be used, are individual tests. It is not practically possible to have 50 or 60 sets of these materials to test the group at one time. The Wechsler Bellevue test is an individual test. Most of the verbal test need only paper and pencil and so they are usually group tests. Any number of copies of the test can be printed like an ordinary question paper and a large group can be tested together. Of course group tests can also be used as individuals tests.

Construction of the Test for Intelligence

The following subtests are described in the order in which they are presented to the subject.

i. **Verbal skills/Language test:** In these subject makes use of language, for which instructions are given in words-written, oral or both. The test content is loaded with verbal material which may include variety of items as below:
   a. *Information:* This subtest covers general information and knowledge and is subject to cultural variables. Persons from low socioeconomic groups with little schooling do not perform as well as those from high socioeconomic groups with more schooling.

b. *Comprehension:* The ability measure subject's knowledge of social conventions and common sense and examines qualities of a person's reasoning and thinking by posing questions about proverbs and how persons ought to behave under certain circumstances.
c. *Arithmetic:* The ability to do arithmetic and other simple calculations is reflected on this subtest, which is adversely influenced by anxiety, poor attention and concentration.
d. *Similarities:* This subtest is a sensitive indicator of intelligence. It covers the ability to abstract by asking subjects to explain similarity between two things.
e. *Digit span:* Immediate retention is measured in this subtest. Subjects are asked to learn a series of two to nine digits, which are immediately recalled both forward and backward. Anxiety, poor attention span, and brain dysfunction interfere with recall.
f. *Vocabulary:* Subjects are asked to define 35 vocabulary words of increasing difficulty. Intelligence has a high correlation with vocabulary, which is related to level of education.

2. **Performance test:** It is complete nonverbal or nonlanguage tests of intelligence for testing one individual at a time. The contents and responses are in the form of performance and language is not used and includes items which require responses in terms of motor activities.
   a. *Picture completion:* This subtest initiates the performance part of the WAIS and consists of completing a picture in which a part is missing. Visuoperceptive defects become evident when mistakes are made on this test.
   b. *Block design:* This requires subjects to match colored blocks and visual designs. Brain dysfunction involving impairment of left-right dominance interfere with performance.
   c. *Picture arrangement:* Subjects are required to arrange a series of pictures in a sequence that tells a story (e.g. a person committing a crime). In addition to testing performance, this subtest provides data about a subject's cognitive style.
   d. *Object assembly:* Subjects must assemble objects such as the figure of a woman or an animal, in the proper order and organization. Visuoperception, somatoperception, and manual dexterity are tested.
   e. *Digit symbol:* In this final subtest of the WAIS, subjects receive a code that pairs symbols with digits. The test consists of matching a series of digits to their corresponding symbols in as little time as possible.

Examples of Binet's tests of 1905

1. No. 5 Unwrap chocolate from paper
2. No. 9 Name objects pointed out in a picture
3. No. 11 Memory for 3 digits
4. No. 14 Give definition of house, fork and mama
5. No. 15 Memory for sentences of 15 words
6. No. 16 give difference between paper and cardboard, fly and butterfly
7. No. 24 find rhymes
8. No. 25 Complete simple sentences by adding one word
9. No. 30 Differentiate between linking and respecting, between being said and bored.

After such a beginning was made by Binet, later psychologists took up the work and made improvements along various lines. One psychologist soon pointed out that the intelligence of an individual could be measured in terms of what he called the intelligence quotient, commonly known as IQ. The mental age is divided by the chronological age and for convenience sake this fraction is multiplied by 100. Thus the formula becomes

$$IQ = \frac{MA}{CA} \times 100$$ (MA is mental age and CA is chronological or physical age)

And also have different kinds of intelligence tests to suit various purposes, such as to be given to large groups at a time, to be given to people who are illiterate, etc.

A careful study of Binet's tests, examples of which have been already given will show that the questions mostly relate to a knowledge of the immediate environment of the child. The idea behind this is that depending on the intelligence, the child is bound to acquire some knowledge of the various objects that come within its daily activities. Of course, this is a reasonable assumption. An intelligent child will observe and learn more easily than a moron or an idiot. An intelligent child will learn sooner to use all things like a spoon or scissors than a child which is mentally defective. However, two objections were raised against this presupposition of Binet: (1) A child which comes from a better environment in whose home there are a number of playthings and furniture, books and other gadgets will be in a more advantageous position than another child which comes from a comparatively ill-equipped home. (2) The second objection is that children who have a better vocabulary will have an undue advantage since all the tests are verbal. It is in answer to this criticism that soon the nonverbal tests were developed. Of these two, the first criticism initiated a great deal of research work. Naturally, the definition of intelligence and understanding of its nature are connected with this question.

Intelligence must not be confused with knowledge obtained from one's environment, though intelligence certainly is related to the capacity for acquiring knowledge. A proper intelligence test must also test one's capacity to acquire knowledge and also the extent to which one is alert to his environment. This meant that a common test cannot be constructed for large areas of the world which may have different cultures, different languages, different modes of life, etc. Tests can naturally be constructed for smaller units within which there would be more or less common environmental conditions for all the children to be tested. For example, it would be very difficult and unfair to construct one common test for children in a city and for the children in an out of the way village, or say, children of the hill-tribes. Still, this fact has been taken as a challenge by some psychologists who have attempted to construct tests avoiding the influences of cultural factors. Such tests are called 'culture-free tests'. It may be mentioned however, that such attempts have not yielded any appreciable results. But the problem is a very complicated one. The idea that the tests should as far as possible deal with the capacity and the ability to perform certain intellectual functions came to be developed. Intelligence tests came to be constructed more and more on this new principle. This is a distinct departure from the original work of Binet. Spearman whom we have already mentioned is practically responsible for initiating this new line of intelligence-test construction. His tests are meant to measure one's ability to see relationships as mentioned earlier. When dealing with intelligence. It has been agreed upon generally that testing one's ability in verbal manipulation and one's store of vocabulary should also form part of a good intelligence test. Thus modern intelligence test consists of different parts dealing with verbal and nonverbal capacities. When different kinds of tests are put together to form one composite test, it is called a "battery" of tests. Nowadays such batteries are more commonly accepted than a single tests. This is because a battery will be testing different aspects, and we can be confident that we are including as many different aspects as possible.

It is not possible for the beginner to appreciate fully the various steps involved in the construction and standardization of an intelligence test before it is ready for use. Three important processes are involved: (1) Finding out suitable items that will really test the intelligence. This will depend on the definition that we give to the term intelligence. We cannot ask a man what he ate for breakfast in order to determine his intelligence. His answer to that question will not give any idea of intelligence. It will be irrelevant as far as testing intelligence is concerned. This aspect is called the validity of the test. Thus the first task is to select valid items that would really test intelligence. (2) Further the test must be stable and consistent. Other conditions being the same, the test must give the same results should not depend upon chance factors. This aspect is called the reliability of the test. (3) Then there is a process called standardization. After constructing a valid and reliable test on the basis of preliminary testing of large numbers of people we must find out norms for difference groups to which the test may be applied. The norms are usually based on the average achievements of these various groups. If the same test is used for a city population of students and for a rural population the intelligence will have to be different. Within the city group the norms may be higher. If, for example, 50 percent success is the average and hence gets an IQ of 100 in the city population, this average score may be less than 50 percent population. Thus test have to be standardized separately for different groups.

All these processes are very technical, but very interesting. In these processes statistics is used to a large extent and so any student of advanced psychology must have a fairly good knowledge of statistics.

ii. Nonverbal individual intelligence tests: It is quite apparent from the above sample that in verbal tests the child's knowledge of language is more in demand, and therefore the use of these tests is limited to students and literate persons. But these verbal tests cannot be used in the case of literate individuals as these tests involve and extensive use of language which fails as a medium to measure the individual intelligence are tested with the help of nonnature of these tests. These tests involve the least possible use of the linguistic ability and are similarly almost unaffected by knowledge derived from books. An example of these nonverbal test is the Performance Intelligence tests.

It would be in keeping with the context of our discussion to understand in detail the performance intelligence test as an example of the nonverbal individual intelligence tests. The world performance is usually applied to test which requires a minimum use of understanding and language. Thus, these tests make use of items requiring performances and not language and these tests for children is Merrill-Palmer Block Building Test. Besides Seguin form Board it includes block building test as well. In the figure given below a four year-old-girls is making structure by means of blocks as demonstrated by the tester.

Another example of the performance intelligence test is the Porteus Maze test. In it, paper and pencil mazes are used. For his tests, Porteus created mazes for children from 3 to 14 years. It gets difficult, corresponding to the increase in age. The subject is allowed two chance and if he fails in the attempts then the conclusion is that his intelligence is not of that age level. Children of 12 to 14 years are given four opportunities. These tests designed by Porteus not only measure intelligence, but they also reflect the temperature of the individual. It is distinguished from the other test in as much as that it includes some aspects ignored by such tests as the Stanford-Binet test. A comparatively simple example of the performance intelligence test is the form board test. Among them the test Seguin and Goddard deserve special mention. In the from board test, there are numerous blocks and a board in which there are holes corresponding to this block. The subject has to fit the blocks in these corresponding holes in the board, the time taken and mistakes committed being noted from which the score of the test is calculated.

Some difficulties are faced in the both the verbal and nonverbal types of individual intelligence test. They are roughly as follows:

1. *The difficulty of time:* The individual intelligence test takes an hour usually and only one person can be tested at one time. Obviously, at this rate it would be essential to have a very big number of trained examiners and in spite of that it would be difficult to test all the people.
2. *Need for experienced examiners:* The second obstacle in the individual intelligence tests is the need for experienced examiners because the correct result cannot be arrived at if the examiners are inexperienced. At the same time, the availability of such a large number of trained personnel is almost impossible.

Notwithstanding these difficulties, in some circumstances the individual intelligence test become unavoidable. This is because the level of accuracy reached by the individual intelligence tests, in the assessment of a person's intelligence, is beyond the reach of the group intelligence tests.

iii. *Verbal group intelligence tests:* The group intelligence test owe their origin and development to the difficulties from which the individual tests suffer. As the name suggests, these tests are designed to test the intelligence of a group and not of an individual test. All the people in the group are given the same directions and have to perform the same activities. Even the score of the result of group intelligence tests is calculated by machines thus dispensing with the necessity of skilled examiners, resulting in an economy of time.

Army alpha and beta test: An excellent example of group intelligence test is afforded by the Army alpha and beta test, which were evolved during the World War I in order to test the American soldiers. For example, it revealed separately the feebleminded, men capable to becoming skilled specialists, men capable of becoming officers, men needing some training, etc.

Naval and army general classification test: Due to the success which attended these tests, some group tests for classification of naval and Army soldiers were evolved during the World War II. Of these two particular forms deserve mention. These two are: (1) Naval General Classification tests and (2) Army general classification tests.

With the type of calculations made by Cruze, some one billion people were tested by the military general classification tests during the years 1941 to 1946. In these tests there are three subjects viz. those relating to vocabulary problems, relating to mathematics, and relating to problems of counting blocks.

Even after taking all the precautions, some difficulties are discernible in the verbal group intelligence tests which can be eliminated only by reverting to the individual intelligence tests. It is due to these difficulties that the individual intelligence tests are considered more realistic than the group intelligence tests. The difficulties of the verbal group tests are fundamentally as follows:

1. *Difficulties relating to cooperation in tests*—In these tests it is difficult to judge whether the examinee is extending his full cooperation or not.

2. *Difficulty relating to the balance of the subjects*—In these tests it is difficult to determine whether the physical and emotional balance of the examinees is even or disturbed.
3. *Difficulty relating to the ease of the subject*—In the verbal group intelligence tests it is difficult to ascertain if the examinee is feeling at ease and free or restrained.
4. *Possibility of cheating by the subject*—Another difficulty in these tests is that no one can testify whether the person has written the answer himself or copied it from his neighbor. In spite of the difficulties which arise in the verbal group intelligence tests, they have their own advantages due to which they are used comprehensively. As has been said before, the advantages are the same as the difficulties of the individual intelligence tests.

iv. Nonverbal group intelligence tests: As has been mentioned earlier, the verbal intelligence tests are meant only for the literates because of the requirement of linguistic ability. It is for this reason that the nonverbal group intelligence tests have been developed the examinee making a minimum use of language but performing, instead, many activities. One example of the nonverbal intelligence tests is Cattell's Culture free Test and NIIP Test.

In these nonverbal group intelligence tests, the examiners have to explain to the examinees even the simplest directions which are also demonstrated as far as possible. All this is done to make least possible use of language. There are some performance tests in these group intelligence tests, in which the examinee draws some lines according to his abilities, fills in some empty spaces, draws some simple figures, or performs some simple activities. Some psychologists do not give credence to these nonverbal tests in their role of measuring intelligence of the subjects, while on the other hand some psychologists consider them to be better than verbal tests. For example, in Alexander's opinion a complete performance battery will be a better measure than a complete verbal battery.

The truth is that even if nonverbal group intelligence tests are not more important than verbal tests, they are certainly not less important than these tests. Some of their characteristics are as follows:

1. *Comparison of various human group:* The first obstacle in the comparison of human groups of various languages and cultures is the difference in their language. This obstacle can be overcome by the nonverbal group intelligence tests and a comparison between different human groups is rendered possible.
2. *Testing of illiterate soldiers:* The verbal group intelligence tests are manifesly inapplicable to illiterate soldiers for the testing of their intelligence. Consequently, the abilities of illiterate soldiers are assessed by employing the nonverbal group intelligence tests and the possibilities of their learning are known.
3. *Intelligence testing in children:* The linguistic ability is very low in the case of children and consequently the verbal group intelligence tests cannot be given to them. Apparently, intelligence testing of children will have to be done by the nonverbal group intelligence tests.
4. *Advice to some specific classes:* The above exposition on the nonverbal group intelligence tests has made it obvious that these tests have proved most successful with some specific classes of people. Thus, the results of these tests render great assistance in advising people of this group.

Uses of Intelligence Tests

The uses of intelligence tests includes the following:

1. These tests are very useful in the education of children. We can grade them properly and give them the proper quality and quantity of work that would be suitable to them. We can also use the test for finding out whether a boy's failure is because of a lack of real ability or because of a lack of application and work.
2. For all tests of vocational aptitude and vocational selection intelligence test is a basic necessity. Different kinds of jobs require different tests become very useful.
3. For all tests of personality also intelligence testing is necessary. Intelligence is an important component of one's personality. Hence without a knowledge of one's level of intelligence it is not possible to get an accurate picture of the personality structure and functioning.
4. Modern intelligence tests have also helped us to discard old ideas that girls are less intelligent than boys and that a particular race as a whole is inferior to other races in intelligence. Actual testing has shown that in intelligence, taken as a composite characteristic, boys and girls do not show any appreciable difference. In one or two particular factors the average score for the boys may be better or worse than the average score for girls. Similarly, psychologists have also tested various racial groups with appropriate tests. The results have led them to discard the old beliefs of some people that some races as a whole are better than others in intelligence.
5. One more interesting use of the intelligence test may be mentioned. Intelligence tests were first constructed on the basis of the meaning of intelligence that we had. But these test have returned the compliment as it were. When testing became highly developed, these tests and the process of their construction have sharpened and made clearer the very concept of intelligence. It was the existence of intelligence tests that made it possible to develop the theory of factors and the composite nature of intelligence. These intelligence tests have helped us to understand more fully the nature of intelligence itself.
6. *Use in selection:* The results of intelligence tests can be properly used for selection of suitable candidates for educational and professional activities, e.g. admission to a special educational program, identification and offer of scholarship, selection of suitable job.
7. *Use in classification:* It helps to classify individuals according to their mental make-up. In the school, it is possible for the teacher to classify the students according to their class as background, average, bright and gifted and thus arrange in homogenous grouping to provide them with proper educational opportunities according to their individual capabilities.
8. *Use in assessment for promotion:* The results of intelligence tests along with the achievement test can be successfully used for promotion of students to the next higher classes. Besides this, such tests can be used in the promotion of people in their profession and social career.
9. *Use in provision of guidance:* The result of intelligence tests may be successfully used in providing educational, vocational and personal guidance to students by teachers. Personal problems like what courses or special subjects one may study, how one should proceed on one's course of learning, what professions or occupation should be aimed at by a particular individual, etc. may be successfully solved on the basis of the results of intelligence testing.

10. *Use of improving the learning process:* Results of the intelligence testing may prove helpful to teachers to plan the teaching-learning activities. In this connection, Crow and Crow (1973) wrote, results of intelligence tests can help a teacher to discover what the child can learn and how quickly he can learn, as well as the teaching methods that should be applied and the learning content to be utilized to guide the learner to use this mental potentialities to their utmost.
11. *Use in setting level of aspiration:* According to Sawrey and Tilford (1964): One should aim for what he desires. In other words one should be very carefully to set one's level of aspiration neither too high nor too low, if one ventures to be successful. Intelligence tests can serve this purpose.
12. *Use in diagnosis:* The other use of intelligence testing relates with its capacity to diagnose, distinguish and discriminate the difference in the mental functioning of individuals. Like diagnosing the cause of problematic behavior and suggesting possible remedial action, arranging suitable educational program in view of the varied individual differences found in the mental functioning of the learners.
13. *Use in research work:* The results of intelligence tests can be used in carrying out research in the fields of education, psychology and sociology, e.g. to ascertain whether individual differences in mental capacities are the results of heredity or environment or both; how mental capacities grow with age, experiences or training.

Alterations in Intelligence and Learning

The concept of intelligence is difficult to define. It can be considered as the sum of those aspects of mental life which relate to general cognitive abilities necessary for adapting to the environment.

- Learning disability: Abnormal intellectual development may be due to slowness in development (retardation) or distortions in development, or a combination of these. One major functional consequences of intellectual impairment is learning disability. It is rare for intellectual functioning to be impaired to the same degree for all skills. However, the child with significant impairment of such skills, is considered as having disability or mental retardation.
- Gifted children: Those children with high measured intelligence, generally an IQ over 140 or is remarked as having all-round ability. The child faces behavioral and emotional problems, arising because of the child being set a part from others less talented children.

The management of problems related to giftedness is largely educational. Problems arising from factors other than the giftedness can be dealt with as in the nongifted group with family or individual assessment and treatment.

Though the father of the psychological tests for intelligence, in his press interview in June 1978, expressed doubt about the efficiency of the intelligence test for measuring the intelligence of individuals, the use of these tests for last several decades has shown that they can give at least some idea about the grade of the intelligence of a person, provided the test has been modified according to cultural conditions. Thus a knowledge of the intelligence test, as given in this chapter, is certainly immensely valuable for the nurses. They cannot only have some idea about their own grade of intelligence but also predict the behavior of their patients. For example if a person is feebleminded, the Nurse should be quite prepared to hear nonsensical talks from him. Similarly, if a person is very highly intelligent, he is likely to be very sensitive as well and requires a very considerable behavior from the Nurse. Thus a knowledge about the nature of intelligence and its measurement may be useful to the Nurse in understanding herself, her colleagues as well as her patients.

Aptitude

Aptitude is a natural ability or propensity. It is the capacity of a person to achieve along specific ways. It makes the special abilities and achivements in special area.

The people differ from one another and within themselves in their performance in one or the other fields of human activity such as leadership, music, art, mechanical work, teaching, etc.

In everyday life, we usually come across individuals who under similar circumstances surpass other persons to acquire certain knowledge or skills and prove themselves more suitable and efficient in certain specific jobs. Such persons are said to possess certain specific abilities or aptitudes, besides general intellectual abilities or intelligence, which help them in achieving success in some specific occupations or activities.

Nursing personnel requires high degree of aptitude for being a good nurses to take care of their clients in efficient and effective manner.

DEFINITIONS OF APTITUDES

According to Bingham (1937) Aptitude refers to those qualities characterizing a person's way of behavior which serves to indicate how well learn to meet and solve certain specified kinds of problems.

According to Traxler (1957) Aptitude is a condition, a quality or a set of qualities in an individual which is indicative of the probable extent to which he will able to acquire under suitable training, some knowledge, skill or composite of knowledge, understanding and skill.

According to Freeman (1971) An aptitude is a combination of characteristic indicative of an individual's capacity to acquire (with training) some specific knowledge, skill or set of organized responses, such as ability to speak a language, to become a musician, to do mechanical work.

So an aptitude is a condition or a set of characteristics regarded as symptomatic of an individual ability to acquire with training some (usually specified) knowledge, skill or set of responses such as the ability to speak a language, to produce music thus an aptitude is a natural ability to acquire relatively general or special types of knowledge or skill.

NATURE OF APTITUDE

- An aptitude may be considered a special ability or specific capacity besides the general intellectual ability which helps an individual to acquire a required degree of proficiency or achievement in a specific field.
- An aptitude is the interaction of heredity and environment. An individual is born with certain potentialities and begins to learn immediately. Thereafter, everything he learns, enables him to learn still more.
- It embraces any characteristics with the general mental ability of an individual, but aptitude is related to specific abilities. Thus, the knowledge of intelligence of an individual predicts his success in a number of situations involving mental function or activity. Whereas the knowledge of aptitudes acquaints us with those specific abilities and capacity to succeed in a special field or activity. Therefore, to predict an achievement

in some particular job, training courses, we need to know more about one's aptitudes (specific abilities) rather than his intelligence or general ability.

- Usually, interest and aptitude go hand in hand. A person must have an aptitude for activity and an interest in a given activity to get desirable success. But, interest and aptitude both are not one and the same thing. For say, a person may be interested in a particular activity, job or training but may or may not have the aptitude for that. In such cases, the interest in a particular situation/course may be due to some other temptation or persuasion like ambitions of the parents, getting an appointment or job, provision of stipend or financial help, prestige associated with the work.
- It is measured by tests of general mental ability which are used to facilitate prediction of scholastic success.

APTITUDE AND THEIR TESTS

In vocational and educational guidance aptitude tests are very much important because aptitude determines one's success in a particular subject, or vocation. It goes without saying that without mechanical aptitude it is difficult for a person to succeed in vocations involving mechanical jobs. Thus aptitude tests help in the choice of proper vocations for a person as well as in the selection of proper personnel for a particular job. An example of aptitude tests is The Crawford Small Parts Dexterity Tests. In this tests there are holes for pins and screws. The subject takes up the pins one by one with the help of tweezer and puts them in a hole and then a collar on them. After fitting all the pins and collars he does the same with the screws. In the end he fits these screws with the help of screw driver. This test helps to discover mechanical aptitude for jobs involving mechanical functions.

A knowledge of the aptitudes, their measurements and conditions will be helpful to the Nurse to develop a proper aptitude for her profession and to guide those around him in entering professions according to their aptitudes. This will also give her an optimism in her own future success. If she has an aptitude for her profession she is bound to be a successful Nurse whatever impediments she might meet in her path.

MEASUREMENT OF APTITUDES

The terms intelligence, ability and aptitude are often used interchangeably to refer to behavior that is used to predict future learning or performance. However, subtle difference exist between the terms. Like intelligence tests, aptitude tests measure a student's overall performance across a broad range of mental capabilities. But aptitude tests also include items which measure more specialized abilities—such as verbal and numerical skills—that predict scholastic performance in educational programs.

Previously these tests can be divided into the following types according to the specific nature of the aptitude tested by them. These are:

1. Mechanical aptitude tests
2. Musical aptitude tests
3. Art judgment tests
4. Professional aptitude tests to measure the aptitudes for professions like teaching, salesmanship, research work, etc.
5. Scholastic aptitude tests, i.e. test to measure the aptitude for different courses of instruction.

Instead of utilizing specific aptitude test for specific aptitude in very specific field or area, the trend at present, has now changed towards multiple aptitude tests battery to find the suitability of people for different professions requiring different abilities on the basis of scores in the relevant aptitude tests in the battery. These are General Aptitude Test Battery (GATB) and the Differential Aptitude Test (DAT).

1. **General aptitude test:** Battery developed by the Employment Service Bureau of USA, has 12 tests. Eight of which are paper—pencil tests as for name comparison, computation, vocabulary, arithmetic, reasoning, form matching, test matching, three dimensional space, etc. The other four require the use of simple equipments in the shape of moving pegs on boards, assembling and dissembling rivets and washers. From the scores obtained by the subject, the experimenter is able to draw inferences about the nine aptitude factors: intelligence, verbal aptitude, numerical aptitude, spatial aptitude, from perception, clerical perception, motor coordination, finger dexterity and manual dexterity. The GATB has proven to be one of the most successful multiple aptitude barriers particularly for the purposes of job classification.
2. **Differential aptitude test (DAT):** Developed by US psychological corporation. It has proved more successful in predicting academic success and found specially useful for providing educational and vocational guidance to secondary school children. The tests induced in the battery of DAT are the following:
   a. Verbal reasoning: It is a measure of ability to understand concepts framed in words. It is aimed at evaluation of the students ability to abstract or generalize and to think constructively, rather than simple fluency or vocabulary recognition. The words used in these items come from history, geography, literature, science, or any other content area.
   b. Numerical ability: These items are designed to test understanding of numerical relationship and facility in handling numerical concepts. This test is a measure of the student ability to reason with numbers, to manipulate numerical relationships and to deal intelligently with quantitative materials. Educationally, it is important for prediction in such field as mathematics, physics, chemistry, engineering, and other curricula in which quantitative thinking is essential. Various amounts of numerical ability are required in occupations such as laboratory assistant, book-keeper, statician and shipping clerk, carpentry, tool making and other crafts as well as in professional related to the physical sciences.
   c. Abstract reasoning: This test is intended as a verbal measure of the students reasoning ability. It has many picture test yielding ambiguous scores because they require the student to discriminate between lines or areas which differ but slightly in size or shape. This test supplements the general intelligence aspects of the verbal and numerical tests.
   d. Clerical speed and accuracy: This test is intended to measure speed of response in a simple perceptual task.
      - Perceptual ability: Ability to perceive words and numbers with speed and accuracy.
      - Intellectual ability: Ability to grasp the meaning of words and symbols.
      - Motor ability: Ability to use various types of machines and tools like type writer, duplicator, cyclostyle machine, punching machine etc.
   e. Mechanical reasoning: This tries to test 'mechanical aptitude' which is a combination of sensory and motor capacities plus perception of spatial relations, the capacity to

acquire information about mechanical matters and the capacity to comprehend mechanical relationships.

f. Space relations: It is the ability to visualize a constructed object from a picture of a pattern and an ability to imagine how an object would appear if rotated in various ways for measurement of space perception. It means that these test require mental manipulation of objects in three dimensional space.

g. Language usage: This test has two sections.
   - Language usage—I: Spelling
   - Language Usage—II: Grammar

   These tests check a number of words correctly spelled and measure the student's ability to distinguish between good and bad grammar, punctuation and word usage.

Value of Aptitude Testing

- They are excellent predictors of future scholastic achievement.
- They provide ways of comparing a child's performance with that of other children in the same situation.
- They provide a profile of strengths and weaknesses.
- They assess differences among individuals.
- They have uncovered hidden talents in some children, thus improving their educational opportunities.
- They are valuable tools for working with handicapped children.

Uses of Aptitude Tests

1. **Instructional:** Teachers can use aptitude test results to adapt their curricula to match the level of their students, or to design assignments for students who differ orderly. Aptitude test scores can also help teachers from realistic expectations of students. Knowing something about the aptitude level of students in a given class can help a teacher identify which students are not learning as much as could be predicted on the basis of aptitude scores. For instance, if a whole class were performing less well than would be predicted from aptitude test results, then curriculum, objectives, teaching methods, or student characteristics might be investigated.
2. **Administrative:** Aptitude test scores can identify the general aptitude level of a high school. This can be helpful in determining how much emphasis to help identify students to be accelerated or given extra attention, for grouping, and in predicting job training performance.
3. **Guidance:** Guidance counselors use aptitude test to help parents develop realistic expectations for their child's school performance and to help students understand their own strengths and weaknesses. These tests are found to be very useful in helping the youngsters as well as youth in the selection of special courses of instruction, fields of activities and vocations.

16 CHAPTER Psychological Testing

Importance of Psychological Tests

Importance of psychological tests is fairly evident from the preceding exposition of the subject. Before proceeding to a study of the various kinds of tests, it is essential to know the kinds of psychological test that are in use, and the principal elements active in them. Defining psychological tests, Mursell writes, "A psychological test, then, is a pattern of stimuli selected and organized to elicit responses which will reveal certain psychological characteristics in the person who takes them". In this way, psychological tests are an organization of some stimuli. These stimuli are selected with some special, objective in view.

Psychological tests have been proved to possess great utility in many spheres. Briefly, the utility and importance of mental tests can be observed in the following spheres:

1. Guidance—As has been indicated earlier, psychological tests are indispensable in all forms of guidance.
2. Appointments—Psychological tests are nowadays resorted to for the appointment of appropriate individuals to various jobs in private and governments services. It has the doubly beneficial effect of securing proper and desirable jobs for individuals according to their interests, inclinations, intelligence and abilities, as well as ensuring that the highest level of efficiently is achieved by the right man being in the right job. In this way, both the employed as well as the employer are benefited.
3. Selection for training—An individual can benefit from training for some particular job only if he is initially in possession of the requisite intelligence, abilities and qualities, beside the necessary interest in the work involved. It is evident that the individual should be tested in respect of these qualities before any training is imparted to him. Hence, in all advanced nations of the world, all kinds of training institutes make use of psychological tests for selecting the required candidates. Psychological tests are further used for selection of candidates for the National Defense Academy in the country. Such use of psychological tests for the sensation of personnel in training schools is constantly on the increase.

   Some psychological characteristics of the persons being tested. Stimuli present in psychological tests are called test items, and they can be of several kinds—pictures, figures, wooden blocks, word groups, sentences and figures, etc. And the way in which these stimuli uncover psychological characteristics will be evident from a description of each of them.

4. Prediction—The term indicates the forecasting of success in the case of an individual. While guiding the individual, a psychologist can normally make fairly accurate predictions as to the degree of success that one is likely to achieve. The prediction is based upon psychological tests; the greater the capacity of a psychological test to assist in prediction, the greater is its validity and its reliability.
5. Diagnosis—Before giving any guidance, the directing psychologist makes a diagnosis of the problem present before him. He gives suggestions for alleviating a certain condition only after he has decided upon a diagnosis since it is only upon diagnosing some problem that he reaches the root causes, and psychological are test essential for diagnosis; without them a proper diagnosis cannot be achieved.
6. Research—Psychological tests are of use even in the field of psychological research. Intelligence tests, interest inventories, personality tests, tests of mental abilities and personality qualities help in research in these specific directions.

Classification of Psychological Tests

Psychological tests are of various kinds. They have been classified from various different standpoints. Classifications are as follows:

1. Classification according to method of testing — Tests have been divided into two classes; in this case classification is based on the method involved.
   a. Individual tests—These tests are administered to one individual at one time, as indicated by the term denoting them. They include performance tests. In addition to these, they also include tests that require linguistic ability. Some examples of these are Stanford-Binet intelligence test, Wechsler-Bellevue intelligence tests. Kohez's block design test, Rorschach's inkblot test and TAT test, etc. These tests are particularly appropriate for testing of individuals, but they are not financially suitable as they are expensive, in addition to requiring more expert training than in many other cases. Secondly, they are less objective than group test.
   b. Group tests—In this category the tests included are performed upon a large number of people simultaneously. Some examples are the group intelligence tests of the Psychological Burean of Uttar Pradesh, interest lists, vocational lists, etc. They are more objective and less expensive, requiring very little, if any, specialized training they may prove expensive. But in these tests no real rapport between the subject and the examiner is established. Hence they are the individual tests. Nevertheless, they have proved really useful in the case of educational and vocational guidance requirements.
2. Classification According to the Medium of Instruction—In these tests, classification is based upon the medium of teaching of the subjects. The psychological tests, from this viewpoint, are divided into the following two classes:-
   a. Verbal tests—This classification comprehends tests in which questions are orally asked, linguistic and concerned abilities being essentially required. One of the best examples of verbal tests is Dr Sohan Lal's intelligence test utilized at Utter Pradesh Bureau of Psychology. These tests are not intended for and cannot be used in the case of illiterates, only slightly educated persons and small children, since such people lack linguistic ability.
   b. Nonverbal tests—This classification includes that tests do not require the use of language, but substitute figures, pictures, block and other implements for it. Examples

of it are Pidgon's nonverbal tests and Raven's progressive matrices. Their particular felicity lies in the fact that they can be applied to the testing of illiterates, very slightly educated individuals and very young children. This category includes all nonverbal tests.

3. Classification according to the objectives of testing—Division of test on the basis of their individual objective or aim leads them to be put into the following categories:-
   a. Intelligence tests—These help to test the intelligence in the form of both verbal and nonverbal tests. They can be administered both to the individual and to a large group.
   b. Testing of mental abilities—In this are included the various tests of mental abilities such as tests of spatial ability, artistic ability, mechanical ability, etc.
   c. Interest test—These tests help to discover the interest of the individual, some examples of which are strongs vocational interest blank, and colors vocational inventory. Both of them are described in detail at a later stage. Besides these, the vocational interest list devised by the Bureau of Psychology, Uttar Pradesh, is also an effective test.
   d. Aptitude tests—These tests are devised by combining the different tests of mental abilities.
   e. Personality tests—These help to find out the individuals personality traits or characteristics. The main methods of personality testing are Rorschach's Ink Blot Test and TAT.
4. Classification According to Level of the Intelligence—Nowadays, all educationists agree that the success of education depends upon the student being provided education of a kind that accords with his level of intelligence. Hence individual students are classified and stratified according to their level of intelligence, and different curricular and extracurricular programs devised for the three categories of students, the brilliant, the average and the retarded. The classification is based on intelligence tests. It is not only in the field of education but also in various vocations, armed forces and industries that intelligence tests are used to classify individuals so that they can be given the proper kind of work that is within their capacity to perform with reasonable success.

Characteristics of Good Tests

1. Reliability—The higher the degree of reliability that results of a test have the greater is considered the reliability of the test itself. And the reliability of its conclusion means that if the same test is performed upon the same individual more than once, results obtained in each individual list should be the same or commensurate with the first one, if it is modified by changed circumstances.
2. Validity—The validity of a test lies in the fact that it succeeds in testing the particular quality which it is designed to test. For example, intelligence test can be valid only if they, in fact, tests correctly the intelligence level of the individual subject.
3. Objectivity—A test can achieve a high level of objectivity only if the answer to each of its various questions is distinct and precise and if there is no difference of opinion, regarding it among the various examiners. Its efficacy lies in the fact that the conclusion or result is in no way influenced by the examiners individual thoughts or opinions, so that the conclusions or results are obtained no matter what the number of examiners who examine the same subject.
4. Comprehensiveness—Another feature of a good test is its comprehensive nature. This feature involves inclusion of all features or qualities allied to the one in question. It will

provide information on qualities concerned with the one quality actuality being tested. In this manner, in a comprehensive test, questions cover the quality in question as well as allied qualities so that no aspect of the measured or tested ability escapes attention.
5. Discriminating power—This term applies to the ability which helps to distinguish between persons with greater or less ability so that they score more or less points or marks.
6. Utility—This feature concerns the extent to which a particular test can be used with facility. And for this it is essential that the question asked should be simple, the method easy, the time involved less and the expenses negligible.

Of the above mentioned characteristics, the most important are validity and reliability. Hence, both these qualitics will be described in detail here.

These tests provide a relatively standardized objective measurement of certain aspects of the patients such as intelligence, personality, memory, symptom profile, etc.

Aims: The main aims of psychological assessment include:
1. Clarify diagnostic uncertainty
2. Specify the severity of symptoms and other difficulties
3. Assess patient strengths
4. Measure cognitive functioning
5. Inform differential treatment assignment
6. Focus the therapeutic intervention
7. Role include the patient into a therapeutic stance, i.e. interest in his own strengths and areas needing assistance
8. Monitor treatment response.

The psychological assessment depends on collecting information by:
a. Document studies—Case notes which are retrospective, official studies, e.g. census, etc.
b. Mail questionnaires—Cheap and easy but slow response rate, hence it is sample biased.
c. Self-rating questionnaires—Cheap, easy, sensitive to changes but may be answered questionnaires cannot be complex.
d. Observer-rated interview—May be structured, semistructured or informal. Allow great flexibility and accuracy but are expensive, and require training.

The sources of error in psychological assessment includes—
a. Response set—Subject (patient) always tends either to agree or disagree with questions.
b. Bias towards center. Subject tends to choose the middle response and shun extremes (e.g. in a questionnaire with three choices to every 'Nil' 'Occasionally' and 'often' the subject answers 'Occasionally' more often).
c. Social acceptability—Subject chooses the acceptable answer rather than the true one.
d. Halo effect—The answers are chosen to 'fit' with previously chosen answers; response become what is expected by the observer.
e. Hawthorne effect—Researchers alter the situations by their presence.

Areas of assessment: The major areas of psychological assessment include:
a. Cognition
b. Personality traits and disorders
c. Personality psychodynamics (Projective and objective tests)
d. Enabling factors for treatment
e. Symptoms of various psychiatric disorders
f. Environmental demands and social adjustment.

A. COGNITION

i. Stanford-Binet scale: The French psychologist Alfred Binet and Physician Theodre Simon developed this scale in 1905. The 30 items comprising this 1905 scale were arranged in ascending order of difficulty. In 1908 revision, Binet and Simon introduced the concept of Mental age. The intelligence quotient (IQ) was proposed by William Stern in 1912 and incorporated by Lewis Terman (1916). The ratio IQ was measured by formula:

$$IQ = \frac{\text{Mental Age (MA)}}{\text{Chronological Age (CA)}} \times 100$$

Unlike the Wechsler-Bellevue Scales, the same items are not administered to and scored for all subjects; each age level is defined by a series of items which measure various intellectual capacities. The score is expressed in terms of both IQ and mental age attained over all the test items.

ii. Wechsler adult intelligence scale (WAIS): David Wechsler, American Psychologist in 1939. It is one of the most commonly utilized test to measure adult intelligence. It is used in age group from 16 years to adulthood.

Components: It has two major scales (Table 16.1) with subtests, i.e.

Table 16.1: Major scales

Verbal Scale	*Performance Scale*
1. Information (range of general information)	1. Digit symbol (a timed virumotor coding test)
2. Comprehension (Practical Reasoning and interpretation of proverbs)	2. Picture completion (Identification of details missing in line drawings of familiar objects and living things)
3. Similarities (Abstraction and verbalization of the properties common to objects)	3. Picture arrangement (Sequential arrangement of cartoon drawings to depict a theme)
4. Arithmetic (calculations of problems presented orally)	4. Block design (time construction using mosaic blocks of designs conforming to pictures presented on cards)
5. Digit span (Repetition and reversal of numbers given orally by the examiner)	5. Object assembly (Timed construction of puzzles)
6. Vocabulary (definition of words)	

Verbal scale reflects retention of previously acquired (and frequently over learned) factual information and the performance scale reflects visuospatial capacity and virumotor speed on relatively novel problems. Neurologically normal but culturally disadvantaged persons may obtain a relatively low verbal IQ (e.g. because of a limited range of information and vocabulary) whereas it is not unusual for highly educated and widely read persons to have a particularly high verbal IQ. The performance scale is less dependent on formal education but appears to be more sensitive to normal aging. The discrepancy between Verbal IQ and Performance IQ is generally less than 15 points.

Specific impairment on the performance scale occurs in patients with right hemisphere (particularly posterior) lesions.

Exceptions: A physical handicap, neurological deficit, abnormal behavior or cultural differences may necessitate modification of standard testing procedures or substitution of other cognitive tests such a Leiter Scale and Raven's Progressive Matrices (for patients with deafness or auditory agnosias) or Peabody Picture Vocabulary test (for patients unable or unwilling to speak or cooperative with WAIS).

The tests used of neuropsychological assessment in clinical psychiatric settings is best described as the identification of behavior deficits most likely associated with established patterns of organic impairment.

Purposes. The uses of neuropsychological testing include:
1. Learning disabilities in children and adolescents.
2. Neurological disorders (e.g. head injury, dementia, epilepsy, etc.).
3. Emotional and Attentional disorders (Table 16.2).

Inferences		
	Subtest	*Factor Tested*
1	Information and vocabulary	General intelligence, learning ability, alertness to the world around him (Vocabulary score declines least with age)
2	Comprehension	Test of common sense and ability to evaluate past experiences (i.e. reveals about personality and gives clues to the diagnosis of schizophrenia or psychopathic personality)
3	Arithmetical reasoning	Intellectual capacity (influenced by age, education, anxiety and inaction)
4	Memory span for digits	Retentiveness and also defects in attention and concentration (may reflect organic impairment or marked manifest anxiety)
5	Similarities	Capacity of abstraction and reasoning
6	Picture arrangement	General intelligence as applied to social situations
7	Picture completion	Tests lower levels of intelligence and ability to distinguish things
8	Block design	How a person goes about discovering patterns and analyzing form (also indicates organic defect)
9	Digit symbol	Association between symbols (measures, intelligence and is affected by poor schooling as well as by inattention)
10	Object assembly	Intellectual capacity (i.e. creative, mechanical and conceptual abilities)

On the basis of IQ, the population is divided into 7 groups as shown in Table 16.2

Table 16.2: Division of population on the basis of IQ

Group	*IQ*	*Percentile rank*
Very superior	Above 129	98-99
Superior	120-129	91-97
High average (Bright Normal)	110-119	75-90
Average (Normal)	90-109	25-74
Low Average (Dull normal)	80-89	9-24
Borderline	70-79	3-8
Mentally deficient (mental retardation)	Below 70	1-2

N.B. Disproportionate impairment on the verbal scale is primarily associated with left hemisphere damage (in right handed person) when aphasia is present).

Tests

i. **Bender (Visual Motor) Gestalt Test:** The most widely employed graphic tests of constructional apraxia (inability to copy the figures given) appropriate for administration to both children and adults (5 years to adulthood). It was developed in 1938 by Lauretta Bender for assessing maturational levels in children. The tests material consist of nine figures (Items A and 1 to 8).
This test is interpreted from 2 types of errors:
   a. *Closing in phenomenon.* Patient uses pan of the model to be copied in making construction.
   b. *Visual neglect.* Partial or total failure to copy left half of the construction (indicate unilateral spatial inattention or neglect associated with right hemisphere disease).

ii. **Memory Problem.** Failure to repeat of Bender designs after 45-60 seconds indicate memory problem and need further specific test for memory. The other tests used for neuropsychological assessment are given in Table 16.3.

Table 16.3: Instruments used to measure cognitive functioning

Sl. No.	*Instrument*	*Age of patient (years)*	*Type of (Administration)*	*Description*	*Scoring features*
1	Stanford-Binet	2-5 Adult	Objective test (individual)	Performance on problem solving and developmental tasks	Average IQ scores on age appropriate items
2	Wechsler Adult Intelligence Scale (WAIS)	16- Adult	Objective Test (individual)	166 items sampling intellectual skills	Full scale, verbal and performance IQs
3	Wechsler Intelligence Scale of children—Revised (WISC-R)	5-15	Objective Test (individual)	187 items sampling intellectual skills	Full scale, verbal and performance IQs
4	Wechsler Preschool and Primary scale of Intelligence	4-6.5	Objective test (individual)	Taps 6 verbal areas and 5 performance areas	Full scale, verbal and performance IQs
5	Halstead-Reitan	6-Adult	Structural Assessment (individual)	Items sampling intellectual, tactual auditory and kinesthetic functions	7 summary sources for clinical interpretation
6	Luria—Nebraska	6-Adult	Structural assessment (individual)	269 items sampling intellectual, motor sensory and expressive skills	14-T scores for clinical interpretation
7	Otis Quick Scoring Mental Abilities test	5-Adult	Objective (Group)	Performance on verbal and non-verbal dimensions of intellectual functioning	Verbal, performance and full scale IQ

B. ASSESSMENT OF PERSONALITY TRAITS AND DISORDERS

The personality traits need assessment to develop a treatment plan for various reasons, e.g.

a. Traits or disorders may be the focus of intervention.

b. Traits may either help or hinder the development of a therapeutic relationship with the patient.
c. Traits may exacerbate or be related to the incidence of certain symptoms (e.g. depression).

Some of the widely used and psychometrically sound instruments available for assessment of personality are given in Table 16.4

Table 16.4: Instruments available for assessment of Personality

Instrument (Inventory)	*Type*	*Description*	*Scoring*
Eysenck Personality Inventory (EPI)	Self-report	57 Yes/No items, parallel forms	Scores on extroversion and neuroticism
16-Personality Factor Inventory (16-PF)	Self-report	3 equivalent forms of 106-187 items each	Scale scores for person. 16 personality traits
California Personality Inventory	Self-report	468 items	Scores on 18 scales and a special scale
Personality Research Form	Self-report	352 items	Score on 22 personality traits
Million Clinical Multiaxial inventory	Self-report	175 items, true/false format	Base rate scores on 20 clinical scales
Structured analyses of social behavior	Self-report	36-72 statements of interpersonal behavior rated true/false	Internalized attitudes regarding self and significant others

C. ASSESSMENT OF PERSONALITY PSYCHODYNAMICS (PROJECTIVE AND OBJECTIVE TESTS)

The term 'projective test' (based typically on Ego's defense mechanism—Projection) was coined by LK Frank. These tests are used to assess the psychodynamics factors as drives, unconscious wishes, conflicts and defenses. The importance of providing information about personality dynamics and structure that are outside the conscious awareness of the patient is the most important rationale for using these tests. The most widely used tests are—Rorschach Inkblot Test, Thematic Appreciation Test (TAT) and Minnesota Multiphasic Personality Inventory (MMPI).

The other used tests are—children apperception test (CAT), sentence completion tests (SCT), symptom checklist—90 (SC-90), Figure Drawing, etc. Some of the projective and objective tests used for adults are given in Table 16.5.

a. Projective Tests

i. **Thematic Apperception Test (TAT).** This test, developed by Morgan and Murrary, is typical of the group. From ten to twenty of a series of thirty pictures are shown. These are designed to permit identification with persons of both sexes and of different age levels, in some the details are quite indefinite and ambiguous. The subject projects his personality into the situation by building stories about each picture. The interpretation of the test depends upon the figures with which the subject seems to identify, the characteristic mood prevalent in the stories, endings, formal features, topical generalization, and other dynamic clues. More so than many projective devices, the TAT reveals the content of the patients fantasies.

ii. **Rorschach test.** The Rorschach is the best known of the projective techniques. Introduced by the Swiss psychiatrist Hermann Rorschach (1884-1922), it has been

Table 16.5: Instruments for the assessment of personality dynamics and patient enabling factors						
Sl. No	*Instrument*	*Type*	*Description*	*Scoring*	*Merit*	*Demerit*
1	Rorschach Inkblot test (Herman Rorschach 1921)	Unstructured (Projective tests)	10 ambiguous inkblots, Responses scored on multiple criteria	Accuracy of form, location use of color, shading, etc. provide summary scores	Most widely used projective device and certainly the best researched, considerable interpretative data available	In terms of validity, Rorschach remains as enigmatic device, as often as it proves useful, it fails
2	Thematic Apperception Test (TAT) (Henry Murray)	Unstructured (Projective Test)	20 ambiguous cards depicting a number of scores	Affects, outcomes and other qualities	A widely used method that, in the hands of a well-trained person, provides valuable information	Not generally accepted scoring system results in poor consistency in interpretation, time-consuming administration
3	Sentence completion test (sack)	Structured (Projective test)	A number of devices available, all sharing the same format with more similarities than differences	Responses to half completed sentences	Brief administration time; can be useful adjunct to clinical interviews if given before hand	Stimuli are quite obvious as to intent and subject to easy falsification
4	Holtzman inkblot technique (Holtzam)	Unstructured (Projective test)	Two parallel forms of inkblot cards with 45 cards per form	Accuracy of form, location, use of color, etc. provides summary scores	Only one response is allowed per cared, making research easier	Not widely accepted and rarely used, not directly comparable with Rorschach interpretation
5	Minnesota Multiphasic Personality-Inventory (Hathway & Mc Kinley, 1967)	Structured (self-report or objective test)	566 items checklist true/ false format	t-score for 13 criterion scales (numerous subscales)	Provides wide range of data on numerous personality variables	Tends to emphasize major psychopathology. Needs revision under current normative data
6	Symptom checklist - 90	Structured (self-report or objective)	90 items checklist, 5 point intensity scale	T-scores for 9 symptoms clusters	Provides a unitary index of global pathology	Tends to emphasize major psychopathology
7	Million Clinical Multiaxial Inventory	Structured (self-report or objective)	175 items, true/ false format	Base rate scores 20 clinical scales	Brief administration item corresponds with DSM-III-R diagnostic classifications	In need of more validation research. No information on disorders severity

complexly elaborated. The test consists of a standard series of ten inkblots, some in black and white and some colored. These are shown, one at a time, to a subject who is instructed to state what the blot looks like to him or of what it reminds him. Responses are recorded verbatim.

The typical Rorschach scoring symbols and their meaning are given in Table 16.6 Some popular responses for different Rorschach cards are:

1. Any winged animal or topographical detail
2. Two animals
3. Two persons
4. Animal skin
5. Winged animal
6. Animal skin, lamp post
7. Cartoon like figures, ornamental things
8. Two animals, emblum
9. The clownish figures blowing pipes, deer head, head-like structure
10. Call-like structures, various other animals, caterpillar, lungs, trachea, etc.

iii. **Sentence completion test.** Various tests have been devised which require that the patient completes sentences beginning in some such way as 'I become very angry when..... 'or' other people think I....' Although this type of test is more transparent than most projective tests and generally does not utilize uniform scoring instructions, it is a useful supplementary source of data on how the patient wishes to present his attitudes about himself and toward others. Both mood and content are noted in relation to such areas as home, work, sickness, immediate family, etc.

iv. **The draw-a-person test.** This test, originated by good enough and further explored by Machover, is believed to provide data about the patient feelings and perceptions of bodily image. The subject is asked to draw a person and later to draw the opposite sex. Intuitive analysis is carried out concerning structural factors (placement of figure on the page, etc.) and content factors (parts of body used, emphasized, or de-emphasized, etc.)

v. **Word association test.** The word association test popularized by Jung consist of a series of 50 or more words which are presented to the subject one at a time. Mixed in the list are words assumed to be related to conflicts of this patient or words which generally produce emotional reaction. The type of association given to these words, together with signs of emotional disturbance such as delayed to responses, suggests that the key delayed to responses, suggests that the key word is related to a hidden complex.

vi. **Picture-Frustration study (P-F).** This test, developed by Resenzweig, consist of 24 cartoon like pictures, each representing two persons who are involved in a mildly frustrating situation of common occurrence. One figure in each picture is shown saying certain words which either frustrate the other individual or help to describe what is frustrating him. After examining the picture the subject writes in the blank space the first reply that enters his mind. The answers are scored in terms of the directions and type of aggressions (i.e. extrapunitive if directed out upon the environment, intrapunitive if directed upon himself, or impunitive if the aggression is turned of). Similarly the responses are scored in terms of whether the patient is concerned more with the nature of the frustrating situation (obstacle-dominant), with protecting himself (ego-defensive), or with which solution of the problem is most

Table 16.6: Typical rorschach scoring symbols and meanings		
	Scoring	*Meaning*
Location (where it is seen)		
W	Use of whole blot	Approach to problems and to life
Z	Organization toward whole	Usual, popular
D	Usual detail of blot	Ability to organize
Dd	Rare or unusual area	Critical
S	White space	Oppositional
DW and Do	Abnormal responses	Pathological
Content (what is seen)		
H	Living human being	Wealth of associational material
Hd	Detail of human figure	Identifies easily with other people
A	Animal	
Ad	Details of animal	
At	Anatomy (X-rays, surgical specimens, etc.)	
Obj	Objects	Overconcern with illness
N	Nature (landscape, trees, etc.)	Immature identifications
T	Topical (fire, blood, sex, etc.)	Overvalent preoccupation
Form-level (how well it is seen)		
+	Superior form	Stability, good intellectual control
–	Poor form	Distorted, conceptual thinking
Originality (how commonly it is seen by others)		
P	Popular, seen by 1 of 5 persons	Conforming
O+	Good original responses (1 to 100 records)	Superior, original thinking
O–	Poor original response	Bizarre thinking
Determinant (how or why it is seen)		
From		
F	Responses on the basis of contour or from alone	Intellectual control
Movement		
M	Human like action	Creative imagination
FM	Animal like action	Instinctual drives, immature
m	Inanimate movement or force	Inner tensions
Color		
FC	Colored object with form	Good emotional control
CF	Color with indefinite form	Affective lability
C	Color only, form disregarded	Uncontrolled emotions
Shading and surface		
FK	Shading suggesting three dimensions	Self-awareness
K	Shading as diffusion (smoke, clouds, etc.)	Anxiety
Fc	Surface shading (hairy, fur rug, etc.)	Sensitivity
c	Shading as texture (furry shiny, etc.)	Oversensitive, sensuous
C	White or black as a color	Dysphoria, depression

important (need-persistive). Interpretation is in relation to group norms and is suggested as giving some indication of the patients usual behavior when under frustration.

b. Inventories. In addition to tests of intellectual functions and projective tests, various self-administered inventories may be helpful. Not only are such paper-and-pencil tests economical in time but, because of their structure, they are also more reliable sources of personality data with many patients than are projective tests.

two examples will be cited here of the large number of general personality inventories available to the psychologist.

i. **Minnesota Multiphasic Personality Inventory (MMPI).** The patient is asked to consider 566 statements about himself and to answer, if possible, whether each statement seems 'true' or 'false' ('Cannot say' is also available). In the analysis a variety of scales are applied to the items. These include four validity scales; the 1 (lie), the F (failure of normal response), the K (test-taking attitude), and the P (evasiveness) scale. The clinical scales include the Hs (hypochondriacal), D (depression), Hy (hysteria), Pd (psychopath), Ma (mania), Mf (masculinity-femininity), and Sc (schizophrenic), An Si (social introversion) scale is also available. The patients score on all of these composes the MMPI profile. The experienced psychologist makes his diagnoses by scanning the profile and giving weight to the various scoring combination that occur. Overall, the Minnesota Multiphasic Personality Inventory is a useful adjunct to other diagnostic techniques in defining self-attitudes, certain aspects of ego functioning and type of symptomatology is a useful adjunct to other diagnostic techniques in defining self-attitudes, certain aspects of ego functioning, and types of symptomatology.

ii. **Guilford-Martin Temperament Profile.** This is a more recent inventory, not dissimilar to the MMPI and aimed at predicting various types of job and social performances as well as uncovering tendencies towards self-preoccupation, shyness, depression, emotional lability, leadership potential, inferiority feeling, etc.

The tests used for personality assessment for children are given in Table 16.7.

Table 16.7: Some personality tests for children

	Test	*Type*	*Description*	*Scoring*
1.	Child Behavior Checklist	Objective assessment of children 4-16 years	118 items on 3 point scale (never, sometimes, frequently)	Assesses behavioral aspects of personality for different age-groups
2.	Personality Inventory for children	Objective rating for 6-16 years of age group	600 behavioral and personality items	Assesses a member of dimensions including adjustment, ego strength, depression, social skills, delinquency
3.	Children Apperception Test (CAT)	Projective (Unstructured)	10 cards that depict animal figures in a number of settings	Dynamic interpretation and also concerning familial relationships
4.	Draw-a-person (Draw-a-family)	Projective (Unstructured)	Patients drawings on a blank sheet of paper	Assesses personality conflicts, self-image, ego functions, visual-motor coordination, etc.
5.	Rorschach	Projective (Unstructured)	Patients association to10 inkblot drawings	Assesses personality conflicts, ego structure and function, defensive structure, thought process, affective integration
6.	Tasks for Emotional Development	Projective (Unstructured)	Patient makes up stories after viewing stimulus pictures	Assesses personality conflicts

D. ASSESSMENT OF ENABLING FACTORS FOR TREATMENT

In clinical practice, accurate diagnosis is not sufficient for determining optimal, specific treatments. The optimal treatment depends on many other nondiagnostic factors which include characteristics fo the patient that will affect the acceptance, utilization and absorption of the treatment that is recommended.

Unfortunately, this area of assessment has been insufficiently attended to by clinical psychologist. Findings from the traditional tests have been used unsystematically to make inferences that may be of some assistance in treatment planning. These include inferences concerning degree of insight, psychological sophistication, and defensive alignment. Psychological tests can be used for assessing these dimensions as given in the Table 16.8.

Table 16.8: Psychological tests

	Instrument	*Type*	*Description*	*Scoring*
H.	**Cognition**			
i.	Brief Cognitive Rating scale (BCRS) (Reisberg et. al., 1983)	Semistructured interview	5 axes (for concentration, recent and past memory, orientation, and functioning) on 7 point severity	Useful for diagnosis and clinical course of disease
ii.	Global Deterioration Scale (GDS) (Reisberg et. al., 1983)	Unstructured interview	7 point scale	
I.	**Adverse Effect of Drugs**			
i.	Abnormal Involuntary Movement Scale	Observers' Rating	Examination of patient, rated on 5 point of severity (0 to 4)	Assesses adverse effects of drugs
J.	**Eating**			
i.	Eating Attitudes Test (EAT) (Garner and Gardinkel, 1979)	Self-report	40 items rated on six-point frequency scales	Assesses attitude and behaviors associated with
ii.	Bulimic Investigatory	Self-report	33 items 2 subsets (Symptoms Scale and severity scale)	Assesses subjects with bulimia nervosa
K.	**Self-Concept**			
i.	Tennessee Self-concept scale	Self-report	100 items, true/false format, 14 scale	Assesses different aspects of self-assessment
L.	**Rating of long stay patients (Chronic Patients)**			
i.	Standardized Psychiatric Assessment Scale (Krawiecka et. al., 1976)	Observer Rating (Clinical Interview)	8 items, (4 on patients replies, 4 by interviewers observation), each rated on 5 point scale	Assesses chronic patients and changes in their conditions (due to rehabilitation)
ii.	Psychological Impairment Rating Scale (Jablensky et. al., 1980)	Observer Rating (Clinical Interview)	97 items (with 10 sections each item rated on a 3 scale)	Assesses chronic patients and changes in their condition (due to rehabilitation)

E. ASSESSMENT OF SYMPTOMS

The major constellations of symptoms that may require assessment include anxiety, elation and depression, thought disorder, suicidal intensions/behaviors, aggressive behaviors, and substance abuse including abuse of food, alcohol and drugs.

There are number of instruments that have been developed for the assessment of a wide variety of symptoms.

F. ASSESSMENT OF ENVIRONMENT DEMANDS AND SOCIAL ADJUSTMENT

The interaction between the patient and the pressures of the environment has been studied in many disease but the most important are with coronary heart disease (Jenkins Activity Survey), schizophrenia (how expressed emotions affects the course of schizophrenia), marital and social adjustments.

17

CHAPTER

Motivation

Introduction

Motive is a state within the individual that under appropriate circumstance initiates regulates behavior in relation to goal.

The word itself comes from the Latin word, movere, which means, 'to move'. Motivation is what 'moves' people to do the things they do. For example, when a person is relaxing in front of the television and begins to feel hungry, the physical need for food might cause the person to get up, go into the kitchen, and search for something to eat. If the hunger is great enough, the person might even cook something. The physical need of hunger caused the action (getting up), directed it (going to the kitchen), and sustained the search (finding or preparing something to eat). Hunger is only one example, of course. Loneliness may lead to calling a friend or going to a place where there are people. Motivation is the process by which activities are started, directed, and continued so that physical or psychological needs or wants are met.

Motivation is a process of stimulating people to action to accomplish desired goals. It refers to the way in which urges, drives, aspirations, stirrings or needs direct, control or explain the behavior of human being.

Motivation is the force within the individual that influence or directs behavior. Because motivation comes from within the person. Manager cannot directly motivate subordinates. The humanistic manager can, however, create an environment that maximizes the development of human potential. Management support, collegial influence, and the interaction of personalities in the work group can have a synergistic effect on motivation. The Nurse as manager must identify those components and strengthen them in hopes of maximizing motivation at the unit level. All human beings have needs that motivate them. The leader focuses on the needs and wants of individual workers and uses motivational strategies appropriate for each person and situation. Leaders should apply techniques, skills and knowledge of motivational theory to help nurses achieve what they want out of work. At the same time, these individual goals should complement the goals of the organization. The manager bears primary responsibility for meeting organizational goals, such as reaching acceptable levels of productivity and quality.

Motivation is an inferred process within an animal or person that causes that organism to move towards a goal. Motives are inferences from behavior (the things that are said and done). They may be conscious or unconscious. Motives also help in making predictions about behavior. Motivation includes all those internal conditions which begin an activity or sustain it. Motive is different from stimulus because it is there even before the stimulus. In the absence of internal motive there cannot be any response, however intense the external stimulus may be. Motives includes those internal factors which control the activity of the living beings. It does not include mechanical or reflex actions because they depend on the physical structure and the external environment. Such mechanical behavior is observed in less developed animals. Their changing physical and mental conditions control their behavior. Motives depend on the changing physical conditions and past experience. A burnt child dreads the fire because the memory of burning is always present in his mind. Thus it is clear that motivation explains the 'why' of behavior. Why a certain people behave in a particular way can be known by an enquiry into his internal motivating factors. Sometimes this 'why' can be inferred from external behavior also. For example, the influence of the sex motives can be inferred by a particular behavior of a pair of male and female. The cause of a particular behavior towards the child shows tender motive in the mother. There can be one motive behind different actions and different motives behind the same action. A man may throw a rupee towards a beggar due to disgust and also due to pity. A soldier may save a person from drowning due to altruistic motive and also to take him to gallows. So the real motives behind the behavior and experience of the individual in social situations.

Characteristics of Motivated Behavior

The general characteristics of motivated behavior are as follows:

1. *Energy mobilization:* The motivated behavior is energy mobilization. The most peaceful animal becomes frightening in times of emergency. This is due to the mobilization of energy. This process of the mobilization of energy is chemical as well as physical. This process cannot be perceived directly, but when there is some difficulty in the attainment of the object of motive this process is seen in the form of extra energy. The animal tries to attain the object with as much energy as is the impetus of the motive behind it. A hungry dog takes the bread even while beaten. It is often observed that some of the persons brought up in the poor families are very preserving and laborious. Some men perform such inhuman actions due to the sex urge which they would never do in ordinary conditions. When the need is excessive the process of metabolism in the body is also increased in the same proportion and the nervous energy also increases in the same ratio.
2. *Persistence:* Motivated experience or behavior is persistence. The man cannot leave its work without achieving the goal of its motive. A nomad wandering in search of food keeps on roaming so long as he does not get it. The fighting persons keeping on fighting till either of them is down or runs away. Sometimes some motivated actions go on for years. A young man in search of a job goes on laboring for several years till he gets a suitable one. A lover determined to conquer his beloved, does not leave her even in the face of great difficulties. Even in the motivated behavior of cripples and weak persons much patience and persistence is observed.
3. *Variability:* The motivated behavior is variability. A motivated person has a goal, hence he continuously changes his activities with the view of attainment of goal. A person trapped in a house on fire tires new devices to come out of it. Sometimes he tries this way, some times that and this change of behavior goes on till he succeeds in coming out of the house. A man with the goal of earning money tries many ways for it. Sometimes he purchases a lottery ticket while at other times he is busy in some business. In fact the motivated person goes on changing his ways till he arrives at the way successful for the

achievement of the aim. In the beginning his behavior is trial and error, but after he knows the successful way he always follow it.

4. *Restlessness for the attainment of the goal:* The motivated behavior is goal-directed. The restlessness observed in such a behavior persists so long as the goal is not achieved. For example the goal of hunger is food. Till the food is taken, there is persistent restlessness due to hunger. After the food is taken this restlessness disappears. The goal may be conscious or unconscious. Sometimes the man knows the goal of his motive, but at other times it is only after long efforts and trial and error that he knows the real object which will bring his restlessness to an end. The physical and the mental motives have physical and mental goals respectively. It is this goal which distinguishes between mechanical action and the behavior.
5. *Extinction of restlessness after the attainment of the goal:* The motivated behavior is the extinction of restlessness after the achievement of the goal. The restlessness of the motivated behavior exhibits itself in following way of the fulfillment of some internal want or desire and extinguishes as soon as that want or desire is fulfilled. A thirsty man roams in search of water. As he gets water and drinks it the restlessness is gone.

There are only two ways to get rid of the restlessness of the motive. Either the tension should be removed or it should be changed. The tension should be removed by the attainment of the object. Sometimes conflicts are observed due to tensions between more than one motives at the same time. Some tensions may be removed immediately while some take days or years to be extinguished.

Motivation Theory

Traditional management philosophy, which emphasizes paternalism, worker subordination, and bureaucracy as a means to predictable but moderate productivity. In this philosophy, high productivity means greater monetary incentives for the worker, and workers are viewed as being motivated primarily by economic factors. This traditional management philosophy is still in use today. Many factory and assembly line production jobs as well as jobs that use production incentive pay are based on these principles. The shift from traditional management philosophy to a greater focus on the human element and worker satisfaction as factors in productivity began during the human relations era (1930-1970). The best-known human motivation studies in this era were the Hawthorne studies conducted by Elton Mayo (1953).

ABRAHAM MASLOW

Most nurses are familiar with Maslow's *hierarchy of needs* and theory of human motivation. Abraham Maslow (1970) believed that people are motivated to satisfy certain needs, ranging from basic survival to complex psychological needs, and that people seek a higher need only when the lower needs have been predominantly met. Maslow's hierarchy of needs is depicted in Figure 17.1. Although Maslow's work helps to explain personal motivation, his early work, unfortunately, was not applied to motivation in the workplace. His later work, however, offers much insight into motivation and worker dissatisfaction. In the workplace, Maslow's work contributed to the recognition that people are motivated by many needs other than economic security.

Because of Maslow's work, managers began to realize that people are complex beings, not solely economic animals, and that they have many needs motivating them at any one

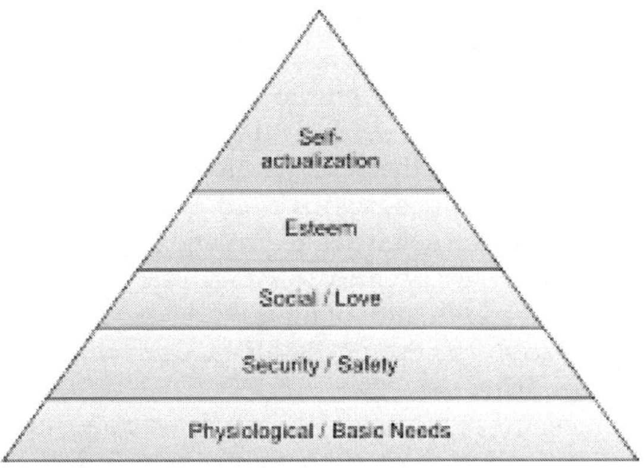

Fig. 17.1: Maslow's hierarchy of needs

time. It also became clear that motivation is internalized and that if productivity is to increase, management must help employees meet lower-level needs. The shifting focus on what motivates employees has tremendously affected how organizations value workers today.

BF Skinner was another theorist in this era who contributed to the understanding of motivation, dissatisfactions, and productivity. Skinner's (1953) research on *operant conditioning and behavior modification* demonstrated that people could be conditioned to behave in a certain way based on a consistent reward or punishment system. Behavior that is rewarded will be repeated, and behavior that is punished or goes unrewarded is extinguished. Skinner's work continues to be reflected today in the way many managers view and use discipline and rewards in the work setting.

Frederick Herzberg (1977) believed that employees can be motivated by the work itself and that there is an internal or personal need to meet organizational goals. He believed that separating personal motivators from job dissatisfies was possible. This distinction between *hygiene* or *maintenance factors and motivator factors* was called the Motivation—Hygiene theory or Two Factor theory. Table 17.1 motivator and hygiene factors influenced by Herzberg.

Herzberg maintained that motivators or job satisfiers are present in work itself; they give people the desire to work and to do not that work well. Hygiene or maintenance factors keep employees from being dissatisfied or demotivated but do not act as real motivators. It is important to remember that the opposite of dissatisfaction may not be satisfaction. When hygiene factors are met, there is a lack of dissatisfaction, not an existence of satisfaction. Likewise, the absence of motivators does not necessarily cause dissatisfaction.

Table 17.1: Herzberg's motivators and hygiene factors

Motivators	*Hygiene factors*
Achievement	Salary
Recognition	Supervision
Work	Job security
Responsibility	Positive working conditions
Advancement	Personal life
Possibility for growth	Interpersonal relationships and peers
	Company policy
	Status

For example, salary is a hygiene factor. Although it does not motivate in itself, when used with other motivators such as recognition or advancement, it can be a powerful motivator. If, however, salary is deficient, employee dissatisfaction can result. Some argue that money can truly be a motivator, as evidenced by people who work insufferable hours at jobs they truly do not enjoy. Some theorists would argue that money in this case might be taking the place of some other unconscious need. Some people in Herzberg's studies, however, did report job satisfaction solely from hygiene or maintenance factors. Herzberg asserts that these people are only temporarily satisfied when hygiene factors are improved, show little interest in the kind and quality of their work, experience little satisfaction from accomplishments, and tend to show chronic dissatisfaction with other hygiene factors such as salary, status, and job security.

Herzberg's work suggests that although the organization must build on hygiene or maintenance factors, the motivating climate must actively include the employee. The worker must be given greater responsibilities, challenges, and recognition for work well done. The reward system must meet both motivation and hygiene needs, and the emphasis given by the manager should vary with the situation and employee involved. Although hygiene factors in themselves do not motivate, they are needed to creat an environment that encourages the worker to move on to higher-level needs. Hygiene factors also combat employee dissatisfaction and are useful in recruiting an adequate personnel pool. Vaughn's (2003) study showed that among the numerous retention factors suggested by Herzberg's Two Factor theory, nurses most desired a sense of recognition and achievement.

Victor Vroom (1964), another motivational theorist in the human relations era, developed an *expectancy model,* which looks at motivation in terms of the person's valence, or preferences based on social values. In contrast to *operant conditioning,* which focuses on observable behaviors, the expectancy model says that a person's expectations about his or her environment or a certain event will influence behavior. In other words, people look at all action as having a cause and effect; the effect may be immediate or delayed, but a reward inherent in the behavior exists to motivate risk taking. In Vroom's expectancy model (Fig. 17.2), people make conscious decisions in anticipation of reward; in operant conditioning, people react in a stimulus-response mode. Managers using the expectancy model must become personally involved with their employees to understand better the employee's values, reward systems, strengths, and willingness to take risks.

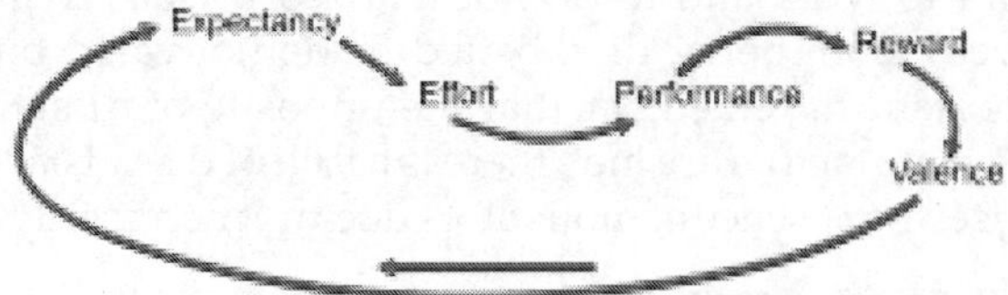

Fig. 17.2: Vroom's expectancy model

David McClelland (1971) examined what motives guide a person to action, stating that people are motivated by three basic needs: achievement, affiliation, and power. Achievement-oriented people actively focus on improving what is: they transform ideas into action, judiciously and wisely, taking risks when necessary. In contrast, affiliation-oriented people focus their energies on families and friends; their overt productivity is less because they view their contribution to society in a different light from those who are achievement oriented. Research shows that women generally have greater affiliation needs than men and that nurses generally have high affiliation needs. Power oriented people are motivated by the power that can be gained as a result of a specific action. They want to command attention, get recognition, and control others. McClelland theories that managers can identify achievement, affiliation or power needs of their employees and develop appropriate motivational strategies to meet those needs.

Saul Gellerman (1968), another humanistic motivational theorist, has identified several methods to motivate people positively. One such method, stretching, involves assigning tasks that are more difficult that what the person is used to doing. Stretching should not, however, be a routine or daily activity but an activity used to help the employee grow. Martin (2005) maintains that the manager's role should be "I'm not out to get you. I'm out to make you better."

Another method, *participation*, entails actively drawing employees into decisions affecting their work. Gellerman strongly believed that motivation problems usually stem for the way the organization manages and not from the staffs unwillingness to work hard. According to Gellerman, most managers "overmanage"—they make the employee's job too narrow and fail to give the employee any decision making power. Indeed, nursing autonomy in decision making was shown to be only moderate in a study of 317 nurses by Mrayyan (2004), who concluded that autonomy could be increased by effective management support.

Douglas McGregor (1960) examined the importance of a manager's assumptions about workers on the intrinsic motivation of the workers. These assumptions, which McGregor labeled *Theory X* and *Theory Y* (depicted in Table 17.3), led to the realization in management science that how the manager views, and thus treats, the worker will have an impact on how well the organization functions.

Table 17.3: McGregor's Theory X and Theory Y

Theory X Employees	*Theory Y Employees*
Avoid work if possible	Like and enjoy work
Dislike work	Are self-directed
Must be directed	Seek responsibility
Have little ambition	Are imaginative and creative
Avoid responsibility	Have underutilized intellectual capacity
Need threats to be motivated	Need only general supervision
Need close supervision Are motivated by rewards and punishment	Are encouraged to participate in problem solving

McGregor did not consider Theory X and Theory Y as opposite points on the spectrum but rather as two points on a continuum extending through all perspectives of people. McGregor believed that people should not be artificially classified as always having Theory X or Theory Y assumptions about others; instead, most people belong on some point on the continuum. Likewise, McGregor did not promote either Theory X or Theory Y as being the ultimate management style, although many managers have interpreted Theory Y as being the ultimate management model. No one style is effective in all situations, at all times, and with all people. McGregor without making value judgments, simply stated that in any situation, the manager's assumptions about people, whether grounded in fact or not, affect motivation and productivity.

The work of all these theorists has added greatly to the understanding of what motivates people in and out of the work setting. Research reveals that motivation is extremely complex and that there is tremendous variation in what motivates different people. Therefore, managers must understand what can be done at the unit level to create a climate that allows the worker to grow, increases motivation and productivity, and eliminates dissatisfies that drain energy and promote frustration.

Classification of Motives

Motivation is a word used to refer to the reason for engaging in a particular behavior. There are different types of motivation. Sometimes people are driven to do something because of an external reward of some sort (or the avoidance of an unpleasant consequence), as when someone goes to work at a job to make money and avoid losing possessions such as a house or a car. When the motivation is external (coming from outside the self), it is called **extrinsic motivation**. In extrinsic motivation, a person performs an action because it leads to an outcome that is separate from the person (Ryan and Deci, 2000). Other examples would be giving a child money for every 'A' on a report card, offering a bonus to an employee for increased performance, or tipping a server in a restaurant for good service. The child, employee, and server are motivated to work for the external or extrinsic rewards.

Motivation involves the action people take to satisfy unmet needs. It is the willingness to put effort into achieving a goal or reward to decrease the tension caused by the need. *Intrinsic motivation* comes from within the person, driving him or her to be productive. To be intrinsically motivated at work, the worker must value job performance and productivity. Parents and peers play major roles in shaping a person's values about what he or she wants to do and be. Parents who set high but attainable expectations for their children, and who constantly encourage them in a nonauthoritative environment, tend to impart strong achievement drives in their children. Cultural background also has an impact on intrinsic motivation; some cultures value career mobility, job success, and recognition, more than others.

Rewards resulting from *extrinsic motivation* (which is motivation that is enhanced by the work environment) occur after the work has been completed. Although all people are intrinsically motivated to some degree, it is unrealistic for the organization to assume that all workers have adequate levels of intrinsic motivation to meet organizational goals. Thus, the organization must provide a climate that stimulates both extrinsic and intrinsic drives. The intrinsic motivation to achieve is directly related to a person's level of aspiration. Extrinsic motivation is motivation enhanced by the job environment or external rewards.

Because people have constant needs and wants, they are always motivated to some extent. In addition, because all human beings are unique and have different needs, they are motivated differently. The difference in motivation can be explained in part by our large and small group cultures. For example, because some culture values material goods and possessions more highly than many other cultures, rewards in this country are frequently tied to those values.

Since motivation is so complex, the leader faces tremendous challenges in accurately identifying individual and collective motivators. Organizations also have cultures and values. Motivators vary among organizations as well as among units in organizations. Even in similar or nearly identical work environments, large variations in individual and group motivation often exist. Much research has been undertaken by behavioral, psychological, and social scientists to develop theories and concepts of motivation. Economists and engineers have focused on extrinsic fiscal rewards to improve performance and productivity, whereas human scientists have stressed intrinsic needs for recognition, self-esteem, and self-actualization. To better understand the current view that both extrinsic and intrinsic rewards the necessary for high productivity and worker satisfaction, one needs to look at how motivational theory has evolved over time.

Different classifications of motives have been affected from different viewpoints, e.g. psychological and physiological, innate and acquired, personal and social. They have been given different names also, e.g. needs, motives, propensities, etc. The theory of instincts is included in this. Two types of classification of the motives are the more popular—innate and acquired. The innate motives include instincts, physiological and psychological needs and personal propensities while the acquired motives account for the social and the learned personal needs.

RS Woodworth has divided into the following three categories:

i. *Organic needs*—Those motives which are aroused by the bodily conditions, e.g. hunger, thirst, etc.
ii. *Emergency motives*—Those motives which are aroused when the environmental conditions demand a strong and quick reaction, e.g. the motive of escape.
iii. *Objective motives*—The object of these motives is behavior towards people and the objects in the environment. This class of motive is comprehensive.

Other psychologists have classified motive under primary and complex needs while some classify them as innate and acquired. The later classification will be the one on the basis of which the following description will be made, because it is the simplest classification.

BIOGENIC MOTIVES

Biogenic motives are also called Biological or Innate motives. Biological or Innate motives are not learned, they are inborn. They are the primary, vital, physiological and biological needs which the person brings with him upon his entry into this world. Their fulfillment is indispensable and of primary importance. They are also necessary for the protection of life. The equilibrium of the body and the mind is disturbed, if they remain frustrated, and it can be restored only when these needs are satisfied. The microscopic cells of the body led the psychologists to a hypothesis of drives, which are internal motor activities. They are found both in men and animals, the only distinguishing features being the modes of their fulfillment. Some of the major ones are:

1. *Homeostasis*—This is a specific organic need, in which the body tries to keep the condition of blood under control because the equilibrium of the body is disturbed if the quantity and proportion of water, salt, oxygen, carbon dioxide, acid, sugar, protein, fat and glandular excretions in the blood is in any way altered. The body has an urge to maintain the normal balance. This balance requires water, oxygen, etc. from the environment. Thus, homeostasis is the origin of many activities in which the nervous system takes part. The individual knows the means of satisfaction of some needs while knowledge of other means is supplied by experience and learning. When a person feels an urge for the first time, he has not thinking of the source from which his satisfaction is to come. But once his urge is satisfied some way or the other, he discovers the means by which he may allay his hunger in the future.

2. *Regulation of temperature*—This is the second specific need of the body. The hypothalamus in the brain is the instrument which regulates the body temperature so that there is never any very substantial difference. Perspiring, trembling, lighting a fire, donning clothes, fanning oneself, installing cooling system, etc. are all perceptible or imperceptible activities caused by the hypothalamus.
3. *Sleep*—This is the third specific need of the organism, the importance of which cannot be denied. The activity of sleeping consumes the individuals maximum share of time. Sleep is the natural reaction of the organism to fatigue and an absence of stimuli. Its center, too, is the hypothalamus which induces sleep, when acted upon chemically. Experiments indicate that a person is not completely inactive in his sleep. Generally, he alters the posture of the body after every twelve minutes. Every person has individual and unique habits of sleep. Sleep is habitual. If a person stays awake indefinitely, his capacity of attention and his interest and energy become lax even though he may complete many of his activities as usual.
4. *Hunger*—The stomach makes contracting and expanding motions when it is empty. These may vary in frequency from 10 to 20 or 25 a minute. Investigations and experiments have shown that there is a close relation between blood chemistry and hunger. The reduction of the sugar in the blood starts hunger sensations, while its excess reduces the hunger. But it cannot be said that blood chemistry is the only factor upon which hunger is dependent because the deficiency of proteins, fats and carbohydrates also result in hunger. Mostly, man demands some particular type of food and not just food, when he is hungry. The choice is regulated by the deficiency in the body. When the feeding was done by the cafeteria method, in which the child may eat anything he likes, in any way which he may prefer and as much of it as he likes, the children soon started to pick out the food by more vision or by smelling. This experiment proves that children develop properly if only they are fed in accordance with their wishes. Generally, there is no difference between the food suggested by doctor and food individually selected. The choice of food is neither by trial and error only nor by the motivation of bodily needs exclusively. The physiological need furnish a motive for the selection of food by trial and error. Human beings eat more if they eat in a collective group. The taste, smell and shape of the food have a marked effect on its selection by human beings. As a general rule, habits are important is eating though these habits may be violated under certain circumstances. There are many harmless things which people do not like to eat. The rejection of a particular food by some individual does not indicate that it is harmful for him. In animals too, the hunger may be due to causes other than the biological needs. In experiments on hen, it was found that she starts eating merely by the sight of a heap of grain. She stops eating but starts again if the grain if first removed and then replaced. She also starts eating if she sees other hens doing so, even when she has no appetite. A similar type of behavior may be seen in human beings.
5. *Thirst*—Thirst, too is a specific organic need, similar to hunger. A person is very restless and active if he is denied water for much length of time, even though every other need is satisfied, and this is an unmistakable sign of some deficiency. The throat and the mouth become parched due to the diminution of water in the salivary glands which is the result of a reduction of water in the blood. Consequently, there is a strong desire to imbibe water or some liquid. Sometimes due to some social reasons, man does not show restlessness even when extremely thirsty. Thirst cannot be definitely or indefinitely quenched by a mere wetting of the mouth and throat. This proves that the cause of

thirst is not the drying up of the mouth and throat but rather the decrease in the normal quantity of water in the blood. In experiments, the dogs drank the water they needed. This ratio seems to be the result of the balance maintained by the pituitary hormones. Besides the specific needs mentioned above, the excretions of the waste products in the form of perspiration, urea, etc. and the need for physical exercises is felt in men as well as in animals. They are both important for the body. The physiological needs mentioned so far are of vital importance for the life of the animal and are consequently vital physiological motives.

6. *Sex*—It is an organic need and it is a means of giving birth and sustaining the species. It is known by the seasonal menstrual changes in the female mammal. Its manifestation has become very complex, in view of the restrictions placed by the society, though its importance cannot be denied. The urge of the sex motive is due to the excretion of a gland. In the male it is caused by the excretion of the sex gland, while in the female due to that of the ovaries. The circulation of the blood carries it to the brain, the resulting behavior being of a type not normally observed. The normal activity due to this motive is an interest in the members of the opposite sex, and a particular type of behavior towards them, the goal being the mating of the male and the female. In the lower species the sex activity is related to the seasons, being the highest in spring when the daylight is of a longer duration. The light has an effect on the brain via the eyes, and it excites the sex instinct. A distinction between sex drive and lust, similar to the one made in the case of hunger and appetite, must be made. While the drive for sex is based upon the sex organs, lust is kindled by either the beauty of femininity of the female or the masculinity and strength of the male which act as stimuli, besides the organs. The proximity of a member of other sex may also create lust. In human society cinema, colorful clothes, make up, etc. are elements which excite lust.
7. *Maternal Behavior*—Maternal behavior exhibits the love and affection a mother has for her child. It is believed that this form of behavior is the consequence of pituitary excretion, the prolactin which affects the brain and causes a specific type of behavior in the mother towards the child. She makes many and varied attempts to protect and look after her children, to get near them when they are separated from her. It is seen sometimes that the behavior of a particular female towards her offspring's is not exemplanary. She deserts them. It cannot be concluded from this that the maternal drive in completely absent but only that there is a more powerful motive at work in the female at the time. Thus a mother fearing disgrace or pursuing some other motive of prudence, may abandon a child without it being essentially assumed that she is indifferent towards the parting.

GENERAL MOTIVES

There are some general motives which are common to most living beings. Woodworth calls them emergency motives, but they are also called general needs. The major ones are as given below:

1. *Escape*—The urge to escape is natural in danger when there is a possibility of physical change. This urge is active in a dangerous situation. We jerk our hand away when it is pricked. A man shrinks his foot if it steps on a thorn. The natural reaction to danger is the preparation for protection against it.

   The signals of approaching danger are importance in the urge to escape. These signals are different living beings and are received by diversified sources. They are innocuous and the danger lies in the comprehension of their meaning. An interesting experiment was carried out to test his. A nonpoisonous snake was given to some people to touch. Children below two years did not show any fear while three to four-years old ones tried to get away from it. Older children ran away from it and college students undoubtedly exhibited fear. In this way, children do not fear many things of which the elders are afraid.

The means of escape to which a person may resort are not the same. To take an example some people daydream in order to escape from danger and they do so through imagination. A man afraid of other persons in society begins to love solitude. Some people become ill when they want to avoid some painful duty. This method of escape is employed by soldiers. Some of them become ill as soon as war begins.

2. *Combat Motive*—This motive is universally available. Its strongest stimulus is resistance. It is a common experience that if you approach a cat, she will bare her teeth and prepare to attack. If you restrain the movements of a child by holding its hands, legs, head, etc. it will go red in the face, start screaming and struggling. Make fun with an irritable person or obstruct the culmination of the motive in a child and the struggle will start. Usually, the struggle is a reaction to the obstruction in the fulfillment of the motive.

   The aim of combat is to remove or overcome the obstacle. An internal, physical and emotional tension persist till the person either gets rid of the obstacle or overcomes it. The pattern of the struggle or combat does not conform to any universal law and therefore differs in different persons. The same rule applies to the instrument used in action. Usually, it is the male who does the fighting. He fights with members of other species and those of his own group of certain things. The characteristic female excretion probably suppresses the urge of combat. Some men threaten before they fight. Some achieve this by showing their teeth, others by screaming, while still others do it by thumping on the chest. Age, intellect, social and cultural factors, etc. alter the methods of combat. The civilized man manifests his combative tendencies by indirect methods of revenge. One form of combat, which is very common in civilized societies, is the fighting of cases in law courts. It is difficult to accept combat as instinct, drive or an internal motive has been hindered. Struggle is the result of anger but sometimes anger is expressed in some others way. An employee, rebuked by his senior cannot retaliate back to him for fear of losing his job, so he gives vent to his anger on his wife or children. Our tendency to combat is sometimes excited by the sight of other while fighting. Playing or watching a game in progress or boxing in films are all outlets for the tension of combat. In the family, the parents restrict many tendencies of the children thus generating a feeling of ill will in them, while the children worry the parents who in their turn, feel disgusted with their children. Brothers and sisters compete with each other for the love of their parents. In the same way, the husband and wife also quarrel on some point or the other. A harmless outlet for these tensions is necessary to preserve serve the peace of the family. Play is adequate for the children. The elder people may be given an opportunity to have their say because it is better to get it off their chests.

3. *Curiosity*—This is a fundamental motive which has no particular bodily basis. When a child is confronted with an unfamiliar object, a desire to know or understand is naturally generated. Every person has a urge to know new things and see new places. A child, given a new things, will turn and twist it to gain some knowledge of it. A child is always ready to ask questions and his questions are endless. You may reprove him because you are tired of his questions but he will never be exhausted on this account. If the

child's curiosity is not repressed, he will continue his search till he has acquainted himself with his surroundings. These are the children who become great inventors, scientists and explorers if they preserve their curiosity upto adult age. This is an important motive from the biological point of view. It makes the animal become familiar with his environment.

4. *Urge to play*—As a general rule, the urge to play is present in almost every animal of higher species. It is an innate tendency which has no specific center in the body though it does depend upon its general condition. A tired or convalescent person does not relish the idea of engaging in a game. The desire to play manifests only when the person has adequately rested and is healthy. A game is played when the person has enough energy and is not forced to spend it one some activity related to his livelihood. Children like to play than the grown-ups because they have practically none of the problems of life to struggle with.

   The pattern of playing varies with the culture or the race and with the individual in the race. Some of the forms which playing takes are jumping, chasing, catching, fighting, sexual behavior, construction and turning and twisting of objects. Often, children are seen copying their elders at play. If is incorrect to interpret this to mean that play is a means of preparation for adult life. Playing definitely assists the activities of adult life by strengthening the tissues and making them efficient to carry out some activities. But it cannot be accepted that play aims at the preparation for the life in future. The fundamental motive is the need for physical exercise and it may be expressed in any form, being directed by the environment in its expression. The mastery motive or the sex drive may be the alternative causes for this urge to play.

5. *Humor or laughter*—The tendency to laugh is nearly universal and it is a special tendency present in human beings only. The activity of laughing does not vary much but the mirth-raising situations do vary with the individual. No rule can be laid down to state the incident capable of raising laughter in a certain person. Some are amused if they see some person slipping on a banana skin or falling in a cycle accident or horse carriage overturning, while others may find nothing funny in these accidents. But leaving aside individual traits there are some occurrences on which people generally do laugh. For example, we laugh at another person's mistakes or we are amused on perceiving another in an embarrassing position. It is not uncommon that boys laugh when they talk of girls who, in their turn, not harboring any charitable feelings for the boys, laugh at the expense of the boys. Grown-up boys and young people are vastly amused by sexual jokes. It is seen sometimes that people laugh more at broad and indecent jokes. Psychoanalysis may think that such type of talk being prohibited and such suppressed by society a tension is created, the slackening of which, on hearing such talk, leads to laughter. This does not lead to the conclusion that every type of humor is a safety valve for the evacuation of suppressed sexual tendency. It is, of course, established that there is a lessening of tension in laughter, and due to this view point, the safety valve theory is the best. Laughter is a tendency similar to play to get rid of tensions. It is natural to feel light and delighted after laughing.

So far we have treated of innate motives which are also called primary motives because they are directly related to the biological needs of the organism. These motives are active almost throughout life though the methods of satisfying them are modified with age and experience. These motives are universal because they are hereditary. A major share of them are directly or indirectly related to the physiological condition of the organism.

Though most of the motives depend upon the physical condition of the organism it is not correct to conclude that all the motives are physical or innate. The innate motives originate within the organism but there are other motives which are related to object outside the organism. Woodworth calls them objective tendencies.

SOCIOGENIC MOTIVES

Sociogenic motives also called acquired motives or secondary motives. Some motives are the result of social situations. Gregariousness is a social motive. A child is unable to fulfill his physiological needs unaided. He learns the ways of the fulfillment from others. Thus, a developed individual fulfills his needs in accordance with the laws of society. This leads to a socialization of his needs, a process in which the individual develops many needs and motives, causes of which are difficult to trace. An example of this is the difficulty in locating physiological causes of the lust for money, search for fame and literary and esthetic tendencies of the modern man. It is apparent that many of the motives and needs of the individuals are learned in society. They may be called secondary or nonvital motives. Some learned motives, which are found in most of the individuals in a greater or lesser degree, will be now described. These being very numerous, only the major ones will be dealt with here.

(a) General Sociogenic Motives

1. *Praise and Blame*—The tendency to win praise and avoid blame motivates human behavior in nearly all societies. Every person wants to be praised by other people even though he may not like to be praised by them directly. Similarly no one likes to be defamed or humiliated by others. Generally, the notion of right and wrong is linked with praise and blame. A person learns to praise worthy behavior and avoids a detestable one. A child fights shy of punishable behavior but gladly behavior which may earn him the love of his mother. Later, this tendency takes the form of praise and blame because praise is fruitful and blame is harmful. Even a person indifferent to the derogation or flattery by others pays attention to the praise or blame accorded to him by his own conscience which is the product of the social convention about right and wrong. The experiments carried out to study the affects of praise or blame establish that they definitely effect the person. The effect of flattery is comparatively more than the effect of derogation.
2. *Mastery Motive*—Alfred Adler has accepted the mastery motive to be the most important motive in human life. According to him man tries to master others in every field of life. Nietzsche believes "Will to Power" to be the major motive in life. According to Darwin there is a struggle for existence at every step in nature and it is the fittest who survives. It follows that every one tries to attain power. Primitive people living in groups have a leader who maintains his masterly position by force. Besides the leader there are other people situated at difference levels. Mastery may be ascertained by age, power or intelligence and these criteria of mastery change with the time and place.

   As a consequence of the mastery motive a competitive tendency and a tendency to rivalry is found in most societies. When competing a person invariably puts in greater efforts, and even more so when the competition is personal rather than in groups.

   But these facts cannot go uncontradicted. The mastery motive, being acquired, is not inevitably found in every society. The tendency of self-assertion is so rare in Arapesh of

New Guinea that it is an abnormality there. This tendency is uncommon among Zuni and Hopi Indians. Among these people the best man is not allowed to participate with the other competitors. In certain studies, it was seen that the Zuni children did not try to get ahead of others in question competition and hesitated in showing results better than others. Why are they so different from other societies in this respect? The elderly people in their society discourage the tendency of self-assertion in infancy whereas this tendency is encouraged right from the start in other societies. In comparison with the Western society, the Indian child is taught to live peacefully, believe in God and depend on luck. Therefore, an Indian is comparatively less active than a member of the Western society.

3. *Aggression*—This is an expression of the mastery motive. There is a great diversity in this tendency, which is the result of the different existing ideals and rules in a society. In India, for example, the Nagas are known as Headhunters while many other Himalayan tribes are very peaceful. In a civilized society murder is considered a wrong and no woman marries but among some Nagas it is that person who doesn't cut heads who finds is difficult to find a bride. The Arapesh tribe of New Guinea discourages the aggressive tendencies, while on the other side, the Mundugumors encourage it from childhood. Therefore, the aggressive tendency, like the mastery motive cannot be accepted to be innate and universal. It is an acquired motive existence depends upon social conditions.
4. *Self-submission*—As opposed to the tendency of self-assertion, some psychologists have accepted the tendency of self-submission as natural. Undoubtedly, the child has many occasions for self-submission, being helpless before his elders. These childhood impressions are important and lasting but it is correct to call the submissive tendency a learned motive because it is usually learnt in the family and society. Being comparatively weaker than men, women have a greater tendency to self-submission but in some South American sea island the women are the leaders and the men follow them in political and economic matters. It varies in degree in different persons, and it may even be completely absent.
5. *Gregariousness*—This tendency makes a person live in a group with the rest of the tribe. It is expressed in the form of herd behavior. But this tendency is neither innate nor universal. While many people live in groups there are some who detest. In fact it is learnt, due to some advantages of the society. A person gets sex, love, company, etc. in a group, and he is enabled to satisfy his many tendencies.
6. *Imitation*—Though imitation is seen very much in the human beings it is not compelling. Even if the existence of any such instinct is given credence its field is very limited. It is common knowledge that a child learns much of his behavior by imitating others, sometimes without a knowledge of what he is doing. As compared to animals, the power of imitation is stronger in human because they can make more minute distinctions. It is not necessary that man may observe all the details or that he may imitate immediately but imitate he does. Imitation is very important in human learning.
7. *Sympathy*—This is an experience of another person's emotional response. Seeing another person is serious trouble, a sympathetic person experiences a similar, though less intense, feeling. Some people cannot keep back their tears when they see another crying. Some people are seen crying for hours upon seeing a tragic story on the cinema screen. Take a look at the ladies coming out of the picture house after seeing a tragedy and you will see marks of crying on many faces. But this reaction is not seen in every one. Some

people laugh, not only to people in pain but even when they are causing grave pain to others. What would you say of such people? They are devoid of sympathy. The news of the death of hundreds of people in Germany makes you curious but even the death of a distinct relative makes you unhappy. Why is it so? Actually, sympathy cannot be said to be innate. A major part of it is conditioned response while the remainder, too, is in some way a learned motive.

(b) Personal Social Motives

In addition to the above same social motives found in each individual, i.e. there are considered as "Personal Motives". In the social environment every individual develops many social motives. The motives that are acquired in the social environment are known as social motives. They have been mentioned earlier, but in addition to the general social motives described there, individuals also develop various kinds of personal motives of a social nature. While the general social motives described there, individuals also develop various kinds of personal motives of a social nature. While the general social motives can be seen in every individual, these personal motives are not universally present. For example, all people do not indulge in the use of intoxicants. Secondly, whereas the social motives of a general sort assume more or less the same form in all individuals, the person social motives have different forms in different individuals. For example, the attitudes and interests, life-goal, level of aspiration, force of habit and unconscious motives, etc. of individuals differ according to their own propensities and inherited qualities. Hence, in the study of the individuals social behavior the personal social motive are also important besides the biogenic and the general social motives. Here, these personal social motives will be elucidated.

1. *Life-goal*—People of all conditions and states, sexes, age levels and cultural levels, have some or the other goals in their lives. It is these goals that direct all the activities and conduct of their lives. It is these goals that provide the incentive whereby the individual is enabled to work industriously. It is these goals that form his personality. Their function is important on the conscious as well as the unconscious level. Usually the life-goal is to a great extent formed and determined in childhood but it is modified as the circumstances of the individual change. It is possible that the child who today wants to enter the medical profession may change his mind tomorrow and may prefer to become an advocate because he observes many features in the medical profession that do not concur with his own conception of life. But though the life-goal of an individual is subject to change, yet some or the other life-goal is invariably in front of the individual to guide him.

   Life-goal is the object at the attainment of which the entire life of the individual is directed. This is to a large extent based upon the philosophy of life. Philosophy of life cannot be said to be the motivating force because it is usually cognitive. The motivating factors are those life-goals which are formed on the basis of the philosophy of life. The goal of life changes if the philosophy of life undergoes any alternation. For example, those people who consider that the goal of life consists in no more than eating, drinking, making a home and amassing physical objects are likely to look upon their business as the goal of their lives. In this way, one wants to become a doctor, another a pleader, another a mill owner, and another a businessman. But there are other people whose philosophy of life does not set such a high store by the physical attainments and material success. For them the study of literature, philosophy, art, science or some other high object is the real and the most valuable goal of life. The object of the lives of these people is to become philosophers, literators, scientists and other intellectual people. There are yet others who consider this life well spent only when it is dedicated to the service of other people. And with this concept as their philosophy of life, they aim at public service, social welfare, etc. Yet another class of human beings takes an entirely different view of life, their philosophy being one of eat, drink and be merry. Their sole aim in life is the amassing of material wealth so that they may enjoy life and get pleasure out of it.

2. *Level of Aspiration*—Just as no person in the world is devoid of a goal and a philosophy of life, similarly every person maintains many aspirations. These are not all alike. While one wants to live in peace, another desires to be the possessor of vast wealth. One person may not desire to have more than can satisfy his needs for four square meals a day and cloth enough to keep him within the bounds of decency while another person may not find it possible to rest satisfied unless he has a beautiful house, a car, and all the accessories that go with symptoms living on grand scale. Levels of aspiration do not differ only on the basis of physical attributes, rather different levels of aspiration may also be seen in other fields. For example, there are many people who profess in other fields. For example, there are many people who profess to be religious, but all religious aspirations are not the same. The majority of these religious functions from time to time, and this satisfies them. But then one does come across people for whom the spread of religion and their own spiritual development becomes the strongest aspiration. Similarly, everyone, the author, philosopher, politician, social worker, leader, actor and men of every other description have their own individual aspirations that are not to be found in the common mass of humanity. Whatever the level of aspiration, or whatever the aspiration animating the heart of man, aspiration does not lose its importance in the life of man. The thoughts and conduct of the individual are formed according to these aspirations. He is perpetually involved in the effort of satisfying them. One man is day and night busy in gathering wealth while another has no compunctions as to the mid-night oil as he is intent upon becoming a famous author. Yet another person is bent upon standing first in the examination and to this end he diverts all his energies. If enthusiasm and motivation are to be maintained intact in the life of man in their function as the mainsprings of action, it is essential that aspirations must inevitably be present, although it is equally necessary that they be balanced by the mind.

Every individual develop aspirations according to his condition and his station in life. A general rule applicable to the economic aspect of this phenomenon is that an individual born in a poor family is likely to have lower aspirations than one born in a richer family. But this is not to be treated as an invariable rule since it often happens that the economic aspirations of a person born in a poor family are very high while on the other hand some people born in a rich family have practically no economic aspirations. In actual fact, the level and form of the individuals aspirations is not conditioned by his circumstances alone. It is not uncommon that within the same family, one member has a religious aspiration while another person has economic aspirations, and even within the field of economic considerations, one has higher aspiration while another has lower. The most important consideration in the formation of aspirations, and the level and form that they take, is the interaction between the individuals inherited qualities and tendencies and the conditions of the environment. Whatever be the dynamics of their formation, the level and form of an individuals aspiration are very important for his life and conduct even though they are susceptible to change as the conditions change.

3. *Interests*—Every individual has many diverse interests. Some interests concur with some people while others coincide with the interests in other people. It is rather difficult for the interests of two individuals to be identical. Interests exert a very important influence upon the individuals behavior. We like the object that concurs with our interest and it awakes in us a desire to possess it. But we neglect the object what does not interest us. This interest also has a close relationship with attention. A person tends to pay maximum attention to the object that coincides with his interests. In other words, his attention is attracted towards it unconsciously. The object that does not interest the individual will not normally attract his attention. We do like objects that are detrimental to our interest, and we desire to stay away from them. Interest are based to a certain extent upon innate behavior or nature and tendencies, but they are also formed to some extent by circumstances. Some interest continue throughout one's life while others change as we grow in mental stature or as our status in life changes. But whatever be their conditions, their importance in life and conduct does not diminish.
4. *Attitudes*—Interests governs an individuals attitude towards various objects. Different people have different attitudes towards the same object because their interests do not coincide. Attitudes are both favorable and unfavorable. In either condition, they exert a very important influence upon the individuals product. If we form an unfavorable attitude towards some object, we try to avoid it and run away from it, while on the other hand we, or any other individual, would like to possess or to be in company with the object towards which a favorable attitude has been formed.
5. *Force of habits*—Another important factor in human life is the force of habit. As long as we do not form the habit of some or the other activity we are free to do it in any way that we please but when that activity becomes habitual we are compelled by force of habit to do it in the customary way. For example, people who habitually use abusive language find it difficult if not impossible to contain themselves and to be decorous but they cannot help themselves. People who have made a habit of arising early in the morning do not have to make any special effort if they want to do so but in the case of person who is a late riser conscious effort is required if her is to arise with the birds. It is within one's means to form habits that one choses, but once the habit has been formed it is very difficult to break it and it requires much affection before it can be removed. Even when he is aware of the failings and condemnable points of his habit, an individual cannot break himself of them. It is evident then that force of habit is an important motive. Concerning this importance James has written, "Habit is the enormous flying-wheel of society, its most precious conservative agent—It alone prevents the hardest and most repulsive walks of life from being deserted by those brought up to tread therein. It keeps the fisherman and the deck hand at sea through winter. It holds the miner in his darkness and nails the countryman to his log cabin and his lonely farm through all the months of snow, it protects us from invasion by the natives of the desert and the frozen zone. Although James has assumed too much correlation between the power of habit and his own American environment, yet it does sufficiently illustrate the force of habit in life. It need not be pointed out that the force of habit is a potent motive in human behavior.
6. *Drug Addiction*—The motivation given by drug addition can be understood in the context of habit as a motive. People who acquire the habit of some or the other drug cannot get rid of that habit. They experience much difficulty and pain if they make any effort at

abandoning that habit of drug. The reason behind this inability is that once the habit of some drug has been formed, that particular narcotic becomes a necessity for that individual and he finds it difficulty to do without it. He is constantly motivated to partake of that drug. The driving force of this drug addiction is so strong that it can drive a man to obtain the drug even if he has to fight and contended against the strongest physical elements such as storm, rain, thunder, etc. He is compelled to search it till he can get his hands on it. The craving does not let him ret till he has satisfied his desire. The strength of the motive of drug addiction can be most poignantly and most effectively seen in the lives of the unfortunate people who are drug addicts. Such people are forced by their inner craving to sacrifice even the most valuable thing in life so long as that craving remains unsatisfied. A person who is himself no drug addict can form only a very hazy picture of the mental state of the people who are cursed with this mental and physical affection. Nowadays, efforts are being made to solve this problem by approaching it psychologically.

UNCONSCIOUS MOTIVES

In addition to the above motives Dr. Sigmund Freud has laid much stress upon the unconscious motives that govern human life and behavior. According to Freud, the unconscious, is a very big part of the human mind, and its activities, though unknown to us, control and guide many of the activities of the conscious mind. Researchers upon the nature and the content of the unconscious mind have revealed that it has a very great importance in human life. It is the unconscious mind that guides, directs and motivates dreams. The unconscious has an important hand even in daydreams. The root causes of mental diseases are traced to the unconscious mind. Causes of forgetting are concealed in the unconscious. It also plays an important role in our imaginings. Even the common forgetfulness that would usually attract no attention is explicable only on the basis of the unconscious. The forgetting of names, the slip of the tongue and of the pen, mistakes in mental or physical activities are all explained by the unconscious. The tendencies originating in the instincts that remain dissatisfied remain within the unconscious from where they are transported to the conscious level only through various forms of normal behavior such as dreams, daydreaming, forgetting, etc. They can be understood only through the analysis of the unconscious, and this understanding can be used to remove many mental aberrations and cure abnormal behavior. Many of the things learnt by us sink to the unconscious mind and are presumed by us to be forgotten only because they do not remain on the conscious level of our existence. It is these that lend insight and help considerably in further learning. It is through these that many people manifest unusual insight into literary and artistic works. Much of the inspiration that artists get for the creation of artistic beauty in drawing, literature, music, dancing, etc. arises in these tendencies of the unconscious mind because they are the medium through which the suppressed tendencies and desires are the satisfied.

The unconscious can be exploited considerably in fashioning human behavior. It usually happens that the conscious and the unconscious tendencies are conflict, leading to various kinds of abnormalities in the behavior or the individual. But if the unconscious can some how be controlled and its cooperation elicited, then our conduct, abilities, qualities, achievements can be reflected in a better light, and a more impressive form. It is expected that psychological research in the future will be able to throw more light upon the working of the unconscious and its consequent importance as a motivating element in human behavior.

IMPORTANCE OF MOTIVES

So far we have explained in details the description of the biogenic and the sociogenic, both the general and personal motives. The next question that concerns us is the choice between them as to the most powerful and influential motive among them. The answer to any such inquiry must be preceded, by some information as to the fundamental need of the human organism among all its various needs, followed by these needs which requires fulfillment after these primary needs. With regard to the question of the importance of the needs, it is a fact of general agreement that the most important are the physiological and biological needs because in the event of their not being satisfied the very existence of the organism is endangered, and once the organism is destroyed, there can be no need for any such consideration. This opinion is undoubtedly reasonable and rational but where the fulfillment of the physiological needs conflict with the social, the intellectual or the spiritual needs, then the situation becomes comparatively complex. It is the view of a particular class of people that when an individual is faced with complete extinction he ipso facto possesses the right to proceed to any length to prevent any such catastrophe, i.e. the needs that insure the continuity of existence are the most important. But on the other hand, another school of thought looks upon the physiological and biological needs as secondary to the social and the intellectual of the spiritual needs. And as to which of these two will predominate in a particular individual depends upon the personality, character and philosophy of life of the individual. Even among the biological or physiological needs, different ones are considered more important by one thinker and other by some other thinker. For example, it has been said that a person afflicted by extreme hunger is capable of doing practically anything to assuage his hunger. But much the same sort of categorical statement can be made with regard to the sexual tendency, and in the opinion of some thinkers it is this tendency which is the most powerful and influential. Freud believed the motivation provided by the sex instinct to be the most powerful in human life and conduct. Others believe the physiological needs to be the relatively more important ones.

Just as some people lay more store by the physical needs of the organism there are some thinkers in whose opinion it is the psychological requirement that is the more important. For example, it is Adler's view that the will to power, the motive of self-assertion are the most important motivating factors in human life. K Horney has believed the safety needs to be the more important. In Goldstein's opinion the more important need is that of self-actualization. Although there is no justification for setting up one particular need as the more important from among the complex of needs that are to be found in all individuals, yet if individual differences are neglected it can be stated definitely that among the most important motivations of human behavior are the biological or physiological motives. And even among them, the motives of sex and hunger are relatively more powerful. Among these two, the motivation of hunger has been appropriately considered as the more powerful since the impulse for sexual intercourse may be aroused only when the stomach is full, not before. In this connection the remarks of Guetzkow and Bowman are enlightening; they write, "It was the rare individual who continued courtship at the end of starvation. Budding romances collapsed, and some men wondered how they could have been so interested in that girl". This example clearly depicts the state of complete inactivity of all other motives that prevails when the individual is hungry.

MOTIVATION AND NURSES

After the biological and the physiological motive, the psychological motives may be considered to be powerful. These include safety needs, need for affection and possession, need for gaining respect and admiration, need for self-assertion, etc. The next motives that can be considered to be powerful are those that have been described in the section under personal social motives. And finally, the important motives to be considered are the general social needs. In this way, in proceeding from the most powerful to the least, motives can be arranged in the following order of their relative importance:

1. Physiological and biological motives
   a. Hunger
   b. Sex
   c. Others.
2. Psychological motives
3. Personal social motives
4. General social motives.

As mentioned above motives and drives are active in the life of patients as well as that of nurses. While the nurse has to keep an eye over the motives of the patients and keep them well under control though not suppressed, she must also keep her own motivation in tact because there is a constant interaction between her own motives and that of the patient. By an insight into the dynamics of motivation she cannot only maintain her mental health and stay gay and cheerful but also use the patients motives for an early cure. Knowledge about physiological needs such as hunger and sleep, etc. will help her in the physical care of the patient whole the knowledge of psychological needs will give her an insight into how to use them favorably for cure. In brief the knowledge of motivation process will help the nurse in her profession as follows:

1. It will help her in maintaining her own mental health
2. It will be useful in her adjustment with the doctors, patients and relatives of the patients
3. It will give her an insight into the etiology of the patients behavior, thus leading to better understanding
4. It will facilitate the process of cure
5. It will help her in diagnosing the disease
6. It will give her job satisfaction
7. It will improve her relations with her colleagues
8. It will help her is solving most of the interpersonal relationships.

Motivation as such affects learning. In the absence of motivation either there will be no learning or very little learning and the learned activity shall be forgotten very soon. On the other hand, sufficient motivation will release energy in the process of learning. The motive gives energy for the continuation of the process of learning. It is due to the motive that a student goes on studying attentively for weeks, months and years. Just look at a boy desirous of learning how to cycle and you can very easily see the role of motivation is this activity. He tries to learn cycling with perfect attention and with all his energy. He fails several times and gets cuts and bruises, but he does not cease to make effort. If he does not succeed one way he adopts another way. So long as he does not learn cycling, a restlessness is seen in him, so much so that he often dreams of cycling. After he learns cycling he seems to be very happy and is seen crying now and then, here and there. This importance of motivation in learning has been widely utilized in education. A good teacher tries to incite motive in the students before beginning some new chapter or before asking them to learn something new. As he succeeds in doing so, half of the work is over, because now he has only to guide the student, for the rest the student learns himself. Learning is a voluntary activity. The more difficult the subject of learning is, the more efforts will be necessary to learn it and consequently the more motivation is required for it.

Motivation is not only required in teaching but also in learning for one self. Hence the intelligent student develops motivation in his studies. By motivation the learning becomes active. In it, the interest and attention are spontaneous. Motivation has the same place in learning as energy in mechanical function.

PSYCHOLOGY OF HAPPINESS IN MOTIVATION

Happiness, a state of well-being and contentment that is much to be desired. The supporters of the **positive psychology movement**, a viewpoint that recommends shifting the focus of psychology away from the negative (abuse, anxiety, depression, all the things that can go wrong) to a more positive focus on strengths, well-being, and the pursuit of happiness (David G Myer 1993). According to Myers and others happiness is the key to many things; the perception of the world as a safer place, healthier and more satisfying lives, and even the ability to make decisions more easily. Happy people are also more likely to help others.

Myers (1993) lists 10 suggestions for becoming happier that are based on his many years of research.

1. **Realize that enduring happiness doesn't come from success:** Money, power, and fame do not guarantee happiness. If people don't have wealth, they may be in miserable, unhappy circumstances but the reverse is not necessarily true: Money really doesn't buy happiness.
2. **Take control of your time:** People who feel in control of their lives by good time management skills are also happier people. Setting goals and breaking those goals down into steps can help a person see progress on a daily basis. Make lists and cross off items as they are finished.
3. **Act happy.** Put on a happy face. When people smile, it releases chemicals that make them feel better, and when they frown, the opposite occurs. Think happy, talk happy, act happy, and you will be happier.
4. **Seek work and leisure activities that engage your skills.** Doing things that are challenging without being overwhelming can result in more happiness in both work and leisure activities. There can be more happiness in tending one's garden than in taking a world tour.
5. **Join the 'movement'.** Exercise, particularly aerobic exercise, will not only help you to feel better and look better physically, but also it relives depression and anxiety. Get moving and get happier.
6. **Give your body the sleep it wants.** Sleep deprivation is bad for the mind, the body, the mood. Sleep-deprived people are crabby, whereas people who have time to sleep and rest adequately are typically happier.
7. **Give priority to close relationships.** A good social support system just can't be beat. Friends offer support and help to get you through the bad times. Take time to nurture friendships and relationships.
8. **Focus beyond the self.** Not only do happy people help other people more readily, but also they are happier for doing so. Helping other makes people feel good.

9. **Keep a gratitude journal.** Writing down the positive things that you have such as a good things that happened today, the friends you saw, and things that you did and enjoyed, also boost a sense of well-being. Stop and smell the roses.
10. **Nurture your spiritual self.** People with a strong sense of faith also tend to be happier. Communities based on shared belief system about faith provide a good support system. These communities can also given a sense of purpose and provide hope during times of stress. People involved in these communities also tend to help others, too.

STRATEGIES FOR CREATING A MOTIVATING CLIMATE IN AN ORGANIZATION

In addition to providing a climate that promotes joy in people's work, the leader-manager can do many other things that create an environment that is motivating. Sometimes, fostering a subordinate's motivation is an simple establishing a supportive and encouraging environment. The cost of this strategy is only the manager's time and energy. The strategies should be used consistently to create a motivating climate as given below:

1. Have clear expectations for workers, and communicate these expectations effectively.
2. Be fair and consistent when dealing with all employees.
3. Be a firm decision maker using an appropriate decision-making style.
4. Develop the concept of teamwork. Develop group goals and projects that will build a team spirit.
5. Integrate the staffs needs and wants with the organizations interests and purpose.
6. Know the uniqueness of each employee. Let each know that you understand his or her uniqueness.
7. Remove traditional blocks between the employee and the work to be done.
8. Provide experiences that challenge or "stretch" the employee and allow opportunities for growth.
9. When appropriate, request participation and input from the subordinates in decision making.
10. Whenever possible, give subordinates recognition and credit.
11. Be certain that employees understand the reason behind decisions and actions.
12. Reward desirable behavior; be consistent in how you handle undesirable behavior.
13. Let employees exercise individual judgment as much as possible.
14. Create a trustful and helping relationship with employees.
15. Let employees exercise as much control as possible over their work environment.
16. Be a role model for employees.

Managers also can create a motivating climate by being a positive and enthusiastic role model in the clinical setting. Managers who frequently project unhappiness to subordinates contribute greatly to low unit morale. A burned-out, tired manager will develop a lethargic and demotivated staff. Therefore, managers must constantly monitor their own motivational level and do whatever is necessary to restore their motivation to be role models to staff. The attitude and energy level of managers directly affect the attitude and productivity of their employees. Managers must be internally motivated before they can motivate others. It is imperative that discouraged managers acknowledge their own feelings and seek assistance accordingly. Managers are responsible to themselves and to subordinates to remain motivated to do the best job possible. McConnell (2005) maintains that there is little difference between workers and their managers when it comes to consideration of what motivates them to work.

Nursing is a stressful profession, and managers must practice health-seeking behaviors and find social supports when confronted with stress or else risk burnout as a result. Weber (2004) states that "good leaders recognize what motivates and drives them not only in their professional but also in their personal lives and have discovered that mastering personal leadership is an essential ingredient in leading others". Burnout and other forms of work-related stress are related to negative organizational outcomes such as illnesses, absenteeism, turnover, performance deterioration, decreased productivity, and job dissatisfaction. These outcomes cost the organization and impede quality of care. Davidhizar and Hart (2006) maintain that there are many ways managers can take responsibility for their own happiness, such as keeping appropriate humor in the workplace, practicing joy building, and keeping the work environment fun and comfortable. These activities can be self-motivating and great antidotes to the burnout and negativism that befall many managers. Perhaps the most important strategy for avoiding burnout and maintaining a high motivation level is self-care. For self-care, the manager should seek time off on a regular basis to meet personal needs, seek recreation, form relationships outside the work setting, and have fun. Friends and colleagues are essential for emotional support, guidance, and renewal. A proper diet and exercise are important to maintain physical health as well as emotional health. Finally, the manager must be able to separate his or her work life and personal life; the manager should remember that there is life outside of work and that time should be relished and protected. Ultimately, the decision to practice self-care rests with each nurse.

Leadership roles and management functions associated with creating a motivating work climate as given below:

Leadership roles

1. Recognize each worker as a unique individual who is motivated by different things.
2. Identifies the individual and collective value system of the unit and implements a reward system that is consistent with those values.
3. Listens attentively to individual and collective work values and attitudes to identify unmet needs that can cause dissatisfaction.
4. Encourage workers to "stretch" themselves in an effort to promote self-growth and self-actualization.
5. Maintains a positive and enthusiastic image as a role model to subordinates in the clinical setting.
6. Encourage mentoring, sponsorship, and coaching with subordinates.
7. Devotes time and energy to create an environment that is supportive and encouraging to the discouraged individual.
8. Develops a unit philosophy that recognizes the unique worth of each employee and promotes reward systems that make each employee feel like a winner.
9. Demonstrate through actions and words a belief in subordinate that they desire to meet organizational goals.
10. Is self-aware regarding own enthusiasm for work and takes steps to remotivate self as necessary.

Management Functions

1. Uses legitimate authority to provide formal reward systems.
2. Uses positive feedback to reward the individual employee.
3. Develops unit goals that integrate organizational and subordinate needs.

4. Maintains a unit environment that eliminate or reduces job dissatisfiers.
5. Promotes a unit environment that focuses on employee motivators.
6. Creates the tension necessary to maintain productivity while encouraging subordinate job satisfaction.
7. Clearly communicates expectation to subordinates.
8. Demonstrates and communicates sincere respect, concern, trust, and a sense of belonging to subordinates.
9. Assigns work duties commensurate with employee abilities and past performance to foster a sense of accomplishment in subordinates.
10. Identifies achievement, affiliation, or power needs of subordinates and develops appropriate motivational strategies to meet those needs.

Nurses also sometimes or many times have to act as leaders or manager in their respective institutions or hospital should always inculcates and use alone strategics for creating a motivating climate.

18 CHAPTER Emotions

Introduction

Emotion is an acute disturbance of the organism, as a whole psychological in origin involving behavior, conscious experience and visceral functioning.

The word 'Emotion' is a derivative of the Latin word 'Emovere' which means 'to move away from', 'to excite', 'to shoulder'. Thus emotion is a state of the individual which deprives him of his equilibrium. In fear, his teeth are clenched together, his body shudders and signs of perspiration may be seen upon his forehead. Emotions shake a man violently. Even when the object of his anger is no longer present, the person's arms twitch uncontrollably. Emotions stimulate the energies of the creature and assist him in dealing with emergencies. In an emotional condition he performs actions which he is incapable of performing in a normal state. But sometimes, though comparatively infrequently, a person is absolutely stupefied and fails to perform even the ordinary activities. These mutually contradictory results bear testimony to the fact that it is difficult to define emotion. Though psychologists have not differentiated between motive, and emotion, everyday experience shows that there is some difference. Similarly, some psychologists do not find any difference between physical activities and emotions. But experiments reveal this difference which is by no means negligible.

Emotion is a complex pattern of bodily and mental changes including physiological arousal, feelings, cognitive processes and behavioral responses to a personality significant situation.The physiological arousal includes neural, hormonal, visceral and muscular changes. The feelings include both a general affective state (good-bad, positive-negative) and a specific tone, such as joy or disgust. The cognitive processes include interpretations, memories and expectations. The over-behavioral responses include expressive reactions (crying, smiling) and action oriented responses (screaming for help).

Emotions can be defined as the 'feeling' aspect of consciousness, characteristics by a certain physical aroused, a certain behavior, that reveals the feelings to the outside world, and an inner awareness of feelings.

Feeling is defined as pleasant or unpleasant experience associated with an idea.

Emotion is a psychophysiological state arising due to a feeling. Emotions consist of three elements. Physiological changes in the body and face. Cognitive interpretations of events, and cultural influences that shape the experience and expression of emotion.

Mood is pleasant or unpleasant experience associated with a real or an imaginary idea, place or a situation. When an emotion persists for a period, it constitutes mood.

Affect is the cross section of mood, when doing mental status examination. Emotion is an affective experience that accompany generalized inner adjustment, mental and physiological stirred-up states in the individual and shows itself in his overt behavior.

Emotion is a mental and physiological state arises spontaneously rather than through conscious effort associated with a wide variety of feelings, thoughts and behavior. Emotions is a complex set of interactions among subjective and objective factors mediated by neural/ hormonal systems, which can:

- Give rise to affective experiences such as feelings of arousal, pleasure/displeasure.
- Generate cognitive processes such as emotionally relevant perceptual affects, appraisals.
- Activate widespread physiological adjustments to the arousing conditions.
- Lead to behavior that is often, but not always expressive, goal directed and adaptive. Emotion are classifies into two form as given below:

Primary emotions: These are those emotions that an individual feels first, as a first response to a situation. These are unthinking and instinctive responses that an individual has for example, if we are threatened, we may feel fear. When we hear of a death, we may feel sadness. Typical primary emotions fear, anger, sadness and happiness.

Secondary emotions: These appear after primary emotions, may be caused directly by them, just like primary and secondary colors. They may come from more complex chains of thinking. For example, news of wartime victory may start feelings of joy, but then get tinged with sadness for the loss of life.

Nature of Emotions

Certain characteristics of emotions forms the nature of emotions:

1. Emotions mostly occur when our safety of our social prestige or any such basic need is thwarted or challenged.
2. Even in such a challenging situation if we meet the situation by reasoning and thinking then the emotion does not surge up. The emotional response is always weakened by the application of our reasoning process. So the two experiences seem to be opposed to each other.
3. Each emotion has certain definite muscular and outward behavior. Ordinarily each emotion is said to have its own expressive behavior. Based on these there are experiments where a subject is asked to identify the emotion by looking at a photograph. Of course here it may not be always possible to be very accurate signs.
4. It has also been found that when we have emotions there are certain internal activities and disturbances going on in what is called the autonomic nervous system, the ductless glands and the visceral organs. We would presently discuss what these are.
5. Unlike the feelings, emotions are very strong in intensity.

Emotional experiences tend to show some characteristics. As given below:

1. Emotions is an affected state of the organism, say joy, sorrow, love, hatred, etc.
2. Emotion is a form of energy mobilization. It helps the individual to overcome the obstacle at the emergency situations like fear or anger.
3. Emotion is very brief. It starts very abruptly and ends soon after the incident is over.

4. Emotion deals with physiological and psychological changes, both subjective and objective aspect.
5. Emotions involve internal changes and disturbance in autonomic nervous system, ductless glands and visceral organs.
6. Emotional experiences also include other activities like perception, learning, consciousness, memory, etc.
7. A strong emotional experience leaves a kind of after—feeling affect, called mood. After the outburst of fear or anger, we remain in a fearful or anguish mood for sometime.
8. Emotion may be innate but it grows to specific patterns with the growth, intelligence, with maturation and learning.

FEELINGS AND EMOTIONS

An emotion is a strong feeling. It is a conscious stirred-up state of an organism. It experienced as certains feelings, pleasant or unpleasant, accompanied by marked physiological changes involving both visceral and peripheral areas.

Good part of life is directed and determined by feelings and emotions. Thinking is often influenced by emotions and how we feel about certain things. Even perception is determined not always by the outside stimulus but by internal feelings, desires and aversions. Thus as motives of behavior, feelings and emotions are very important and should be understood. Sometimes, of course, the feeling or the internal state may not accurately correspond to the external behavior. This happens when we deliberately do some acting, e.g. the actor on the stage need not necessarily feel angry when in a particular scene he fights with sometime. But in practical life the internal feelings and the outside behavior are closely related. For a fuller and clearer understanding of these experiences of ours, it is necessary to distinguish between emotion and feeling. It may not be very easy to do so. Yet for practical purposes it is possible to distinguish between them. This distinction will become clearer as we deal with these two kinds of experiences separately in the following paragraphs.

Both emotion and feeling are closely related to one another. They both depend on the brainstem in the nervous system. Pleasure, pain, fear, anger and love, etc. involve feeling as well as emotions. Consequently, many of the emotions are included in feelings. Feelings may be pleasant and may be painful too. Similarly, emotions may be caused either by happiness or by sorrow.

Significance of Feelings

Feeling is a term which is always used for various kinds of experiences. It is one of those "multi-purpose" terms. When we are not sure of an answer we say 'I feel it is so'. We talk of the feelings of pleasure, familiarity, excitement, happiness, worry, love, disgust and so on. It would be a very good exercise to take a pencil and paper and write down the various kinds of occasions for which we use the term 'feel'. We could also try to classify them under certain definite categories. Feelings like pleasure, happiness, joy, delight, etc. will come under one category characterized by a desirable, pleasant feeling tone. Terms like displeasure, grief, discontent, sadness, etc. will come under one category characterized by a tone of unpleasantness and avoidance. Terms like desire, longing, hopeful, etc. will come under another category characterized by a tone of anticipation and expectancy. Terms like resentment, indignation, fury, etc. will come under the category characterized by a tone of excitement. In this manner we can enumerate many more experiences coming under different categories. Some have noticed that each state of feeling has three distinguishable characteristics.

1. It is pointed out that each feeling whether anger, pleasure, desire or sadness can be said to have a certain pleasant or unpleasant tone.
2. All these feelings are also found to have a certain tone of excitement or numbness, e.g. pleasure has a tone of excitement. Anger also has a tone of excitement. Sadness has a tone of numbness.
3. We also find that most feelings have a tone of tenseness or a tone of relaxation. Some people use the word expectancy for the term tenseness. All feelings connected with our waiting for something to happen will be characterized by the expectancy tone. In the same way when our feelings are referred to something that has already happened there is a tone of release or relief. A feeling of longing will have more of the expectancy tone. A feeling of sadness will have a tone of release since the sad event has already happened.

To make these characteristics clear, we shall try to take three examples and find out what characteristics they have. A feeling of joy, for example, is characterized by a pleasant tone, an excitement tone and a release tone. A feeling of anxiety, for example, is characterized by a tone of unpleasantness, excitement and a tone of tenseness. A feeling of anger will be characterized by a tone of unpleasantness, a tone of excitement and a tone of tenseness. The reader could try in a similar manner to find the characteristics of some more feelings.

A feeling has also got certain other characteristics of its own, distinguishing it from experiences like sensation and emotion. Feeling is an internal experience but it is not felt in any one particular part. We may sometimes say that I feel a pain at the back of my hand. Here we are using the term feeling in a different sense. It is actually directed towards perception of the part where the pain is felt. A pain may be unpleasant. The real unpleasant feeling connected with it has no definite location in any part of the body. In this matter it is different from the sensations. A visual sensation is experienced at the retina of the eye. In other words a sensation is localized but in a feeling of pleasure or grief or anxiety the whole organism is involved. Feelings need not always be strong. Sometimes they are very mild and exist just as dull and background states.

An interesting experiment will be to find out the different kinds of things that give us a feeling and pleasure or a feeling of annoyance. If we actually do this experiment we would find that we differ from one another, except in certain things which will be common to all. We will all be pleased at a sweet taste and sweet odor. Similarly we would all be annoyed if we miss the last bus that would take us to our college or office in time. But if we try to make a list of 20 or 30 things that give us a feeling of annoyance and another list of things that give us pleasure, quite a number of things would be peculiar to each individual. Thus we find that these feelings also depend upon one's past experience, training and learnt habits. Such a study may also help us to understand our weakness, our prejudices and may help us to understand why people like us or dislike us.

In spite of such a close relation between feelings and emotion they are not identical and this difference should not be lost sight of. Feeling is the reaction of pleasure or pain originated by the sense organs, which results from sensation. For example, the observation of a rainbow in the sky results in a feeling of happiness. When a thorn pricks the foot, a feeling of pain is generated. Thus, feeling is sensory and simple, whereas, on the other hand, emotions are more complex. They can be aroused not only by the existing circumstances but also by a recollection of these circumstances. Players are excited by the imagination of derision of their failure in the game. We are filled with hatred when we are reminded of disgusting circumstances. Another difference between emotion and feeling is that while feeling is aroused by sensory emotion, reaction is activated by thoughts and imagination, not by sensations. It follows that there is a difference between emotion and feeling from the mental view point. The difference between their mental qualities is the result of the contributory circumstances from which they originate. Emotion manifests at a more complex level, and new elements are introduced in it. The pleasure which we receive by listening to a good discourse or by reading a good book is not due to the words as such but due to the thoughts expressed by these words. The pleasure which arises out of listening to an oration by a famous leader is due not to the voice of the leader but rather to his opinions.

In the list of feelings given earlier we have also used certain experiences which can properly be called emotions. Anger is an emotion, though we use the term feeling with reference to it. With regard to emotions also we begin by saying 'we feel'. We say we feel angry, we feel afraid and so on. That is why these two are often confused with each other. But technically we use the term emotion for very strong experiences like anger, fear and love. Emotion is defined as "a stirred up—up state of the organism". This definition is so given because in all emotions there is a strong disturbance of the whole organism. There are strong internal changes and definite major external signs such as clenched fists, biting of teeth, shivering of the whole body, loud laughter, etc.

Emotion is a disturbed glandular and muscular activity. Woodworth rightly says that "each emotion is a feeling and each is at the same time a motor set". In this way, emotion is a state of the individual in which the body is externally as well as internally very profoundly upset. This may be clarified by the example the execution of an impulsive activity, or by the failure of such an activity. Therefore, anger is directed upon the interfering object to oneself, though not always because sometimes anger is directed to oneself. When angry, clenching of the fist, grinding of the teeth, elevation of the eyebrows, vociferating, kicking, attacking, trembling, these and other physical activities, or rather disturbances are apparent. The activities in an emotional condition of anger are the opposite of the activities of a person who is struck with fear. In anger many persons become aggressive.

Emotions occupy a very important position in a person's life as they motivate many of his endeavors. The man who gives his life for his country with a smile on his face, who fights in the battlefields, who performs acts of valor and bravery is urged on not by his thoughts and mind but rather by his emotions. A life devoid of emotions is insipid and unattractive. Love, affection, etc. are not the only emotions by which life is made worthy of living. The same can be said of grief, anger, etc. It is commonly experienced that emotion increases energy mobilization in the organism. It is borne out by the fact that when afraid we escape from danger in a way which surprises even us. An angry person performs courageous acts of which he is undeniably incapable of in a more tranquil condition of the mind. A person in love makes sacrifices for the object of his emotion which he would not make in an unemotional state. The love for their offspring spurs the parents on to great sacrifices.

The presence of emotion makes the individual lose control over his brain, the results of which may be beneficial or harmful. When in the grip of anger a man does things which are unfair. A sexually excited person is seen behaving like an animal. An extremely excited person resembles in insane. He fails to distinguish between good or bad and does either with equal enthusiasm. Consequently, he either reaches eminent heights or degenerates to the level of animals.

In practice and experience, it is evident that emotional instability is harmful to the body and mind as many mental and physical aliment result from it. But is equally harmful to suppress them in an effort to control them. Psychoanalysts have made a detailed analysis of the disease arising from such repression. As a matter of fact, in order to control emotions, it is necessary to see that the occasions which excite them are as few as possible. They can also be kept in check by autosuggestions. The emotions become enfeebled through desire if an attempt is made to use them rarely. If the excitement connected with some emotion is conditioned by some other emotion, the painful emotion can be eliminated. Control of emotions can be facilitated if an innocent or useful method can be devised to form an outlet for the animation.

There are many internal and external physiological changes in emotion. Normally emotions cannot be recognized from their external signs, though with practice some of the emotions can be recognized. In practice, we know that our emotions make an impressions on others. Thus we try to conceal our baser emotions, e.g. hate, fear, etc. Culture requires us to conceal our emotions but is the emotion which reveals to us the depth of the experience in other's mind. Though people make an effort to conceal their emotions, at some juncture it becomes necessary to make as complete an exhibition as possible. It is not enough that the lover experiences love for his beloved, exhibition of his love is also necessary. Sometimes another person's behavior necessitates an exhibition of anger. It is correct to put on an appropriate display.

Another substantial difference between emotion and feeling is that the former is more comprehensive than the latter. Feeling is a part of emotion. Emotion includes feeling and it is, therefore, something more than a feeling. This closeness of relation of the two often causes people to forget the difference between them. In emotion some glands inside the body excrete some specific types of juices. But there is no excretion in the case of feeling. In feeling, there is more neural excitement than in emotion. At a certain stage, even a tendency to become active is perceived.

Emotion is vigorous than feeling and it upsets the whole body. The individual loses his stability and his control over the situation. Consequently, the necessary reaction is impeded in its execution and behavior is disturbed. The derangement is present in feeling too, but not as much as in emotion. In a way, a slightly disturbed state indicates feeling and a greater disturbance points to emotion. In an emotional state, the behavior of a person is more excited, vigorous and disturbed than in feeling. In emotion a man sometimes transcends every type of limit, sometimes being completely paralyzed. Feeling never attains such a frenzied state.

Significance of Emotions

It would have been already observed that emotions form a very important part of our behavior. They are responsible for the finest in human achievements and for the worst in history. The most noble in human character and the most despicable in his behavior are all directed by emotions. Sympathy, love, pity, etc. have produced the finest of our conduct and achievements. Anger, hatred, jealousy, etc. have likewise produced the most horrible and meanest things in the human history. We pride ourselves saying that as human beings we are rational animals. But very often we find that our behavior is directed by our emotions very important in one's life a proper understanding of their functions and possibilities becomes a necessity for everyone.

As a child grows to adulthood his emotional life undergoes a good many changes, mostly through learning and training. A child freely gives vent to the muscular and motor expressions of the emotions. If it is angry it kicks about, rolls on the ground, tears the clothes, etc. But a normal adult will not do these. We gradually learn to control some of the overt expressions of our emotions. According to the accepted standards of civilized life such a control is necessary and must be learnt. Further, the child may get upset and give emotional responses even to weak and insignificant stimuli. Not getting a piece of sweet, and being left alone by the mother, may both evoke the same degree of anger and displeasure. But as the child goes it learns to adjust the strength of its emotions to the strength of the stimulus. This also is a characteristic of adult emotional response and it has to be learnt. Further, the stimuli that evoke emotional responses in a child are few and limited to its immediate surroundings and needs. But such a limited scope of emotional response will not be adequate for an adult. If there is a calamity in a far off country a cultured man must feel sympathetic. If a bully troubles a weaker person or a woman or a child, one should take note of it and must help the helpless, though not out of anger, at least of a righteous indignation. Here again, we find the adult to be properly called a man, has to learn to apply his emotional experiences to diverse situations going beyond his own immediate needs. Again the emotions of children are not organized and balanced. The adult has to learn to organize and balance his emotions properly to behave in a steady, dependable and mature manner.

This process of proper emotional development is closely related to one's development of desirable character. Emotional responses give rise to what are called sentiments. In ordinary life we do not always have only one kind of emotion to a particular person or institution. Sometimes one likes his teacher and has pleasurable emotions. At times when the teacher is strict the emotion may be one of hatred or fear. But, in the long run the student forms a permanent composite mental attitude towards the teacher. This attitude is based on past experiences of various emotional responses. Such an attitude or disposition is called a sentiment.

Similarly one may mostly have the emotion of love towards the mother or father. Yet there would be occasions when experiences of fear and anger were also shown. Still on the whole, a disposition of love and affection is developed. That will be the organized sentiment. Similarly we may all feel patriotic about our country and show a kind of affection and love. But occasionally, because of the behavior of the general mass of people or because of the behavior of some leaders we may feel disgust and a kind of hatred to our own country may develop. Here again the sum total of all these emotional experiences will be expressed through a particular sentiment that we build up towards our country. Like this, all of us build up a large number of sentiments towards people, objects, abstract ideas, moral ideas, religious values, institutions, etc.

When all these sentiments are further organized by an individual towards one particular value then he develops a character. Characters is developed by the proper organization of these sentiments around and some deep convictions or purposes in life. Thus to develop good character one must have proper sentiments. To have proper sentiments one must have properly balanced emotions. Thus control and organization of emotions form the foundation for building up a sound character which we all admire. Man is respected as a person only to the extent of his character. It is possible to organize all our emotions just like a child around our own immediate personal needs and gains. All the sentiments would also be organized with this end in view and will be characterized by selfishness. This would naturally produce a very low type of character indeed. But, on the other hand, if one organizes his emotions and sentiments around higher values such as truth, goodness and beauty, the resulting character will also be in the deepest sense, true, good and beautiful.

There are so many reason for emotions are very important in individuals life. A few are as given below.

- **Survival:** Nature developed our emotions over millions of years of evolution. As a result, our emotions have the potential to serve us today as a delicate and sophisticated internal guidance system. Our emotions alert us when natural human need is not being met for example, when we are afraid, our need for safety is unmet. When we feel rejected, it is our need for acceptance which is unmet.
- **Decision making:** Our emotions are a valuable source of information. Our emotions help us make decisions. Studies show that when a person's emotional connections are severed in the brain, he cannot make even simple decisions. Why? Because he does not know how he will feel about his choices.
- **Boundary setting:** When we feel uncomfortable with a person's behavior, our emotions alert us. If we learn to trust our emotions and feel confident expressing ourselves we can let the person know we feel uncomfortable as soon as we are aware of our feeling. This will help us set our boundaries to protect our physical and mental health.
- **Communication:** Our emotions help us communicate with others, e.g. facial expressions convey a wide range of emotions. If we look sad or hurt, we are signaling to others that we need their help.
- **Happiness:** When our needs, especially emotional needs are met, we feel happy. Our emotions and feelings let us know when we are unhappy and when something is missing or needed.
- **Unity:** The emotions of empathy, compassion, cooperation and forgiveness have potential to unite us as a species.

In other words, emotions:

- Determine personal viability of individual
- Prepare us for action individual for action
- Shape our behavior individual behavior
- Regulate social interaction of a person
- Facilitate communication nonverbally
- Facilitate adult-child relationship and thus helps in alround development
- Make life worth living by adding value to experience to human being
- Allow individual to respond flexibly to thier environment (approaching good, avoiding bad)
- Have a central place in moral education and moral life through conscience, empathy and many specific moral emotions such as shame, guilt and remorse.

For each distinct emotion, there are three components:

- **Subjective experience:** It is feeling what an individual believe or existing within his own mind/thought, e.g. happiness, sadness, anger and so on.

- **Physiological changes:** These occur, involving autonomic nervous system (ANS) and the endocrine system, over which we have little, if any, conscious control. However, we may become aware of some of their effects such as gooseflesh, sweating and butterflies in the stomach, etc.
- **Associated behavior:** Such as smiling, crying, frowning, running away, laughing, fighting, etc.

Instincts and Emotions

The study of emotion raises a number of difficulties. It is not even possible to give a simple and definite list of emotions. Some people talk of only three primary emotions, such as anger, fear and love. Others give a much longer list. They associate emotions with various organic needs of the individual commonly called instincts. William McDougall, for example, gives a list of 14 such instincts and 14 emotions associated with them. According to him each instinct arouses an emotion. Some of these fourteen are:

Instincts	*Emotions*
Escape from danger	Fear
Parental instinct	Tender feeling
Mating or sex instinct	Sex emotion
Combat	Anger
Submission	Feeling of humility
Assertion	Feeling of superiority
Laughter	Feeling of amusement
Gregariousness	Feeling of loneliness

This scheme of McDougall may appear to be easy, but as the student advances in his knowledge of psychology he will become aware of a number of controversial problems. Even the term 'instinct' is not commonly used in modern psychology. Some people feel that the term instinct is more appropriate for certain behavior of animals and birds. There we find some rigidity, a definiteness and a certainty of the occurrence of some behavior on particular occasions. When a bird attains a certain age, without having learned it from anybody, it goes and builds a nest almost in a stereotyped manner. This kind of exactness is not found in human behavior. So some people have advocated that the term instinct should be properly applied only to animal behavior. Yet in man also, we do find some basic and innate urges such as the desire to preserve one's self, the sex urge, the desire for company, etc. Since more of training and adaptability are noticed in the case of man as compared to animals, different terms are used to explain such behavior. Some of these terms are, biological needs, urges, drives, unlearned motives, innate propensities, etc.

So any emotional experience even after it has ceased leaves behind a kind of 'after feeling' called mood. We must have all experienced these moods. After we have had an outburst of anger, for a much longer time we would be in an angry mood and when we are in this mood we are liable to become angry again even with a slight provocation. Similarly after an experience of intense fear, we would be in a frightened mood for a much longer time and any unexpected sound or event will make us afraid again.

Views of Emotions

a. **Organic school** (of emotion). It argues that emotions are primarily a matter of biology, of physical events that like a thumping heart, are not voluntarily controlled. It maintains that feeling comes first and thoughts follow or are unrelated to emotion. There are several evidences in support.
   - Emotion seems to appear before cognition does
   - Limbic system (emotional brain) is involved with emotions whereas cognitive processes are controlled by another part of brain
   - Pure sensory input is enough to stimulate an emotional response without interference from higher mental processes
   - Feelings and thinking are often unrelated.

b. **Mental school** (of emotion). Scientists seek psychological explanations of emotion, e.g. in beliefs, judgments and interpretations of events. According to this school:
   - Thoughts come first
   - Simple sensory reactions cannot properly be called emotions
   - Emotions have never been easily assigned to one part of the brain or another
   - The causes and effects of emotion spread rapidly across both brain hemispheres
   - New therapies have had great success treating emotional disorders by changing unrealistic thinking.

Emotions have also raised another interesting but somewhat different problem for some psychologists. We know that all emotions arise when we perceive a particular situation. But if we analyse this further we find that in what we call emotions there are two distinct types of phenomena taking place. (a) A kind of feeling on the mental level such as anger or fear. (b) A mass of bodily changes that take place in the organism. We have already referred to these physiological changes that stir up the whole organism.

The theories of emotion are interesting views of scholarly theorists. Each of these theories explains the order of events that occur when an emotion is present. Each theory is a hypothesis waiting to be tested out. There are four theories of emotions.

Theories of Emotion

There are a number of theories to explain the origin and classification of emotions whereas some theories explain the relationship of bodily states and the emotions. Few important theories are:

I. James Lange theory (proposed in nineteenth century) by American psychologist, William James and the Danish physiologist, Carl Lange. According to this theory (Fig. 18.1).

- We perceive the situation that will produce emotion
- We react to the situation, and then
- We notice our reaction.

This theory believes that emotion results from the perception of one's own bodily reactions. In this view, each emotion is physiologically distinct (Fig. 18.1). But doubts have arisen as to:

a. Whether, especially in the more subtle and less intense emotions, the bodily expressions can be perceived, i.e. in general, one's perception of internal changes is not very acute.

b. Bodily changes are not enough to produce emotion, i.e. by just injecting substances such as epinephrine, we should be able to generate similar emotions but this is not the fact.

c. Emotions occur faster than visceral changes.
d. The same bodily changes occur in many different emotions.

This theory was proposed by American psychologist William James and physiologist Carl Lange. This theory proposes that emotions occur as a result of physiological reactions to events. The emotional feelings result when an individual becomes aware of a physiological response to an emotion provoking stimuli. Thus, separate and distinct physiological activity is required for each emotion.

According to this theory, you see an external stimulus that leads to a physiological reactions. Your emotional reaction is dependent upon how you interpret these physical reactions, e.g. I am trembling, therefore I am afraid.

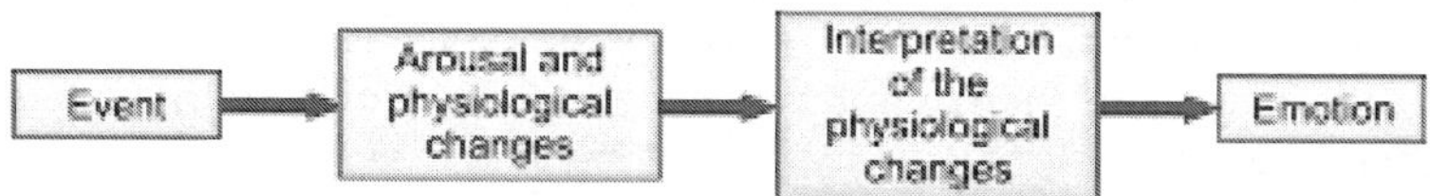

Fig. 18.1: James-Lange theory

II. Cannon-Bard Theory proposed in 1920's by Walter Cannon and Philip Bard. According to this theory, felt emotion and bodily responses are independent of each other and both are triggered simultaneously (c.f. James-Lange Theory). This theory states that emotion originates in the hypothalamus of the brain, which controls both emotional feeling and behavior and in this view, all emotions are physiologically similar (Fig. 18.2). But the scientists are still not sure whether perception of lower brain activity is the basis of felt emotion.

This theory was originally developed by *Walter Cannon* and later upon by physiologist *Philip Bard*. This theory proposes that an emotion-provoking stimulus is transmitted simultaneously to the cortex, providing the feeling of emotion and the sympathetic nervous system causing physiological arousal.

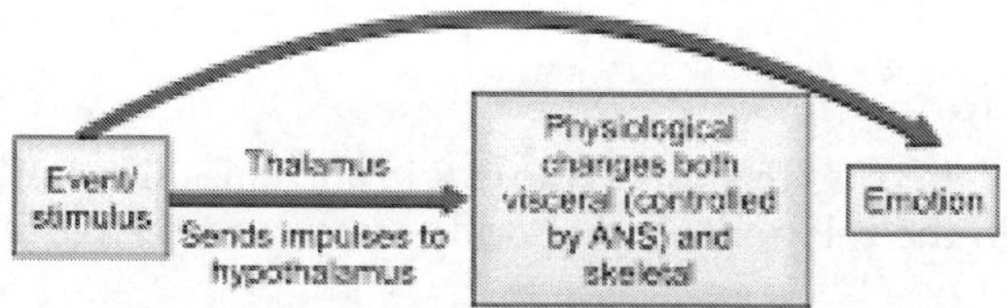

Fig. 18.2: The Cannon-Bard theory of emotion

III. Schachter Singer Theory: This theory is also called two factor theory or cognitive labeling theory. This states that for an emotion to occur there must be physiological arousal and second, there must be an explanation for the arousal.

So, there must be some kind of attention getter and the reason why it got that specific person's attention. It accounts for the subjective interpretation. It does not account for specific physiological states associated with some emotions.

According to this theory, the emotion we feel is due to our interpretation of an arousal or stripped up bodily state. The sequence of events in the production of emotion is:

- Perception of a potential emotion producing situation
- An aroused bodily state which results from this perception and which is ambiguous
- Interpretation and labeling of the bodily state so that it fits the perceived situation (Fig. 18.3). According to this theory arousal and interpretation are two important factors.

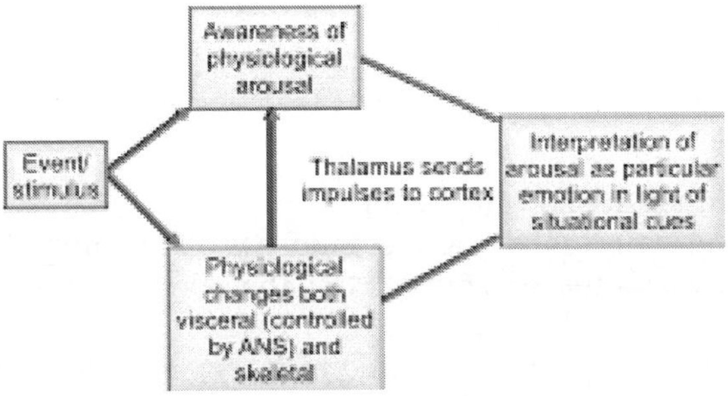

Awareness of physiological arousal

Event/ stimulus

Thalamus sends impulses to cortex

Interpretation of arousal as particular emotion in light of situational cues

Physiological changes both visceral (controlled by ANS) and skeletal

Fig. 18.3: Schachter-Singer Theory of emotion

IV. Cognitive-Appraisal Theory of emotions

a. **The Schachter-Singer theory** described above is often called a cognitive theory because it involves thoughts about the cause of the perceived state of arousal.

b. **Richard Lazarus et al Cognitive theory:** It emphasized the appraisal (evaluation) of information from several sources. This is a cognitive theory because appraisal involves cognition or the processing of information from the environment, the body and memory. The different reactions to the same stimulus occur because of differences in the subjects appraisal of the stimulus.

Lazarus theory of emotion: It most heavily emphasizes the cognitive aspect. This theory that an emotion-evoking stimulus or event triggers a cognitive appraisal, which is followed by the emotion and physiological arousal. Reappraisal of potentially emotion-producing situation is an important component of this cognitive theory. Reappraisal is also a way of coping with stressful situations.

- It has been believe that each theory holds a bit of truth, but to which one is completely right is not possible. They are theories, so can be tested but they can never be proven.

Table 18.1: Three theories of emotions

James Lange Theory	*Cannon-Bard Theory*	*Schachter-Singer Theory*
Perception of an environmental situation which might result in emotion.	Perception of an environmental situation which might result in emotion.	Perception of an environmental situation which might result in emotion.
Reaction to the situation with specific patterns of bodily activity.	Patterns of activity produced in lower brain areas (e.g. the hypothalamus).	A generalized state of bodily arousal which is perceived.
Perception of pattern of bodily activity results in a felt emotion—a different one for each pattern of bodily activity.	1. Patterns of lower brain activity perceived in cerebral cortex as felt emotions. 2. Patterns of bodily activity exopressing the emotion.	Interpretation of the reason for the generalized arousal state. Felt emotion depends upon the reasons given for the generalized arousal stage.

V. Theory of Relationships among Emotions

Robert Plutchik has proposed a descriptive theory that is concerned with what are called primary or basic emotions and the ways they can be mixed together. Plutchik assumes that the relationship among emotions differ in three ways—intensity, similarity to one another and polarity or oppositeness (Table 18.1). He drew a spatial model (Fig. 18.2) representing the relationships among the emotions. Within each primary emotion segment, the strongest varieties of the emotion are at the top of the segment, with progressively weaker varieties toward the bottom, e.g. Grief is stronger than sadness, which in turn is stronger than pensiveness.

VI. Theories about Emotion and Motivation

The difference between some motives and emotions is often minimal, fear, for example, is an emotion but it is also a motive driving behavior because people engage in goal directed behavior when they are afraid. According to proposer of this theory, Leeper, it is the emotional tone which provides the motivation for long sequences of behavior. Motives are important in arousing and sustaining activity, in producing exploratory reactions, in facilitating learning, in governing performance or habit use, in helping produce problem solving learning, in helping govern choice between alternatives in producing willingness to endure penalties to reach some goal or a willingness to forego some reward, and in influencing thought content and sensory perceptions.

Figure 18.2. A diagram of theoretical model portraying the dimensions of human emotions. Each vertical wedge-shaped segment—the one composed of the subsegments grief, sadness, and pensiveness, for example—represents a primary emotion. *Intensity* of the primary emotions is shown from the top down in each segment. Conflicting emotions are placed opposite each other around the figure, while similar emotions are placed near each other around the figure.

Table 18.2: Three theories of emotions

	Robert Plutchik	*Carroll Izard*	*Paul Ekman*	*Silvan, Tomkins*
Primary emotions	Fear Anger Joy Disgust Anticipation Surprise Sadness	Fear Anger Joy Disgust Surprise Contempt Shame Sadness Guilt Acceptance	Fear Anger Happiness Disgust Surprise Sadness	Fear Anger Enjoyment Disgust Interest Surprise Contempt Shame Sadness

Another theory by Tomkins maintains that emotions provide the energy for motives whereas motives or drives simply give information about some need or condition of the body.

FACTORS CONTROLLING EMOTIONS

- Cultures influence the experience and expression of emotions. Display rules are the culture's way of regulating how, when and where a person may express (or must suppress) an emotion. Emotional work is the effort a person makes to display an emotion he or she does not really feel.
- Body language: For example, gesture, posture, bodily movement, touch and mannerism determine the body language and differentiate different cultures.

- Gender: Women and men often express their emotions differently. Women are more likely to reveal fear and loneliness whereas men are more likely to behave aggressively. Women do more emotional work than men. Girls tend to prefer "face to face" friendship, based on shared feelings whereas boys tend to prefer "side by side" friendship based on shared activities.
- Other factors, e.g. age, status, experience, arousal interpretation (appraised), previous learning, facial expression (facial feedback), situations, etc. are important in the origin of motives and expression of emotions.

Measurement of Emotions

Before measuring emotions, one must be able to characterize emotions and distinguish them from other states. Now, emotions are best treated as a multifaceted phenomenon consisting of following components: behavioral reactions, expressive reactions, physiological reaction and subjective feelings.

1. **Nonverbal instruments to measure emotions:** It consists of instruments that measure either the expressive or physiological component of emotion.
   a. **For expressive reactions:** It is the facial, vocal, and postural expression that accompanies the emotion, e.g. anger comes with fixed stare, contracted eyebrows, compressed lips, vigorous movements, raised voice, almost shouting.
      - Facial expression instruments are Facial Expression Analysis Tool (FEAT), Facial Electromyography (EMG) for facial muscle activity.
      - Vocal expression instruments measure the effects of emotion in multiple vocal cues, e.g. average pitch, pitch changes, speaking rate, voice quality and articulation.

   b. **For physiologic reactions:** Emotions show a variety of physiological manifestations that can be measured with a diverse array of techniques. Examples are instruments that measure blood pressure, skin responses, heart rate, adrenaline levels, brain waves, papillary responses, tears and perspiration. Some ANS instruments such as IBM's emotion mouse and variety of wearable sensors can help the computers to gather multiple physiological signals while experiencing an emotion and polygraph—Lie Detector.
2. **Verbal instruments to measure emotions:** These assess the subjective feeling component of emotions, i.e. thoughts which are observed indirectly through:
   - Spoken and written words on rating scales
   - Answers to open ended questions on surveys and during interviews
   - Responses to projective instruments, sentence stems, etc.
   - Self-assessments or perceptions regarding the behavior and intentions of others
   - Other cognitive operations such as rational/logical thinking.

   Verbal instruments used are self-reports, rating scales, pictograms (e.g. self-assessment manikin or Sam) and PREMO (Product emotion).

Some psychologists have tried to find out the relation between these two apparently distinct types of experiences. The physical changes may involve running in the case of fear and hitting or biting the teeth in the case of anger. We normally believe that these physical changes take place because of the corresponding mental feelings. We would say, for example, that we run because we feel afraid, we beat because we are angry. This explanation making the physical changes, the effect of a particular mental state sounds very simple and easy. But this position has been seriously questioned by two people by name William James and Carl Lange. On the basis of observations they claimed that the mental sate or the feeling of anger or fear arises because of the physical changes. According to them the physiological changes are primary and occur first. So they say, we are afraid because we run. We are angry because we beat. This position may appear to be strange. But it is not without truth. If we see a snake and instead of running we try to beat it, then the emotion is not really fear. It is anger tinged with some fear. We would also notice that the more we run, the more the feeling of fear. Experiences like these strengthen this theory. Their explanation is usually referred to as James-Lange theory of emotions.

Other psychologists have however questioned this position and in psychological literature one would find interesting controversy about it. Such confusions arise perhaps because we divide emotion into these distinct and different kinds of phenomena, viz. the physiological and the psychological. Actually the whole emotional experience involves both physiological and psychological phenomena in a composite manner and any emotional experience should be stated as one single phenomenon in the light of the circumstances that have provoked it. We could perhaps take two of the strong fundamental emotions as examples and make some more observations regarding them. This is done to provide a pattern for studying all other emotions as well.

For selecting officers and men for the fighting forces, it would be very necessary to find out the limit to which one can bear such startling stimuli. When the emotion of fear is very strong it may sometimes disorganize our whole behavior system and we may simply shiver and stand still. We may not have the necessary energy or will-power even to run or to take any other steps which will give us safety. The various stages of physiological changes that a strong experience of fear can produce would be an interesting study.

Emotional States of Expression

Emotion is a very complex and intricate psychological process involving different states or expression of emotions.

1. POSITIVE EMOTIONS

a. **Joy:** Joy or happiness has shades of enjoyment, satisfaction and pleasure. There is a sense of well-being, inner peace, love, safety and contentment. There is an existence of both positive thinking and positive activities. Zest and cheerfulness are its secondary emotions.

b. **Love:** Love arises from a feeling of profound oneness. Love can be, romantic, religious or familial. Affection and lust are secondary emotions.

c. **Laughter:** Some of the physical benefits of laughter are:
   - Increases muscular and respiratory activity
   - Stimulates CNS and CVS
   - Increases antibodies
   - Decreases levels of stress hormones
   - Increases pain tolerance
   - Improves your relationship.

d. **Hope:** If your life has hope, purpose, and meaning, then you will be happier and healthier.

2. NEGATIVE EMOTIONS

a. Fear: It is a response to some danger that is about to happen. It is a survival mechanism that is a reaction to some negative stimulus. Nervousness and horror are secondary emotions.

Anger or rage: It would be interesting to find how children make this response. Children, if interfered within their movements, at once show all the signs of anger. They kick about and struggle and show their extreme dislike. Under certain circumstances if the interference, is not beyond a certain point they may only become more restless. But as they are definitely thwarted in their movements, they develop anger. It has been found by experiments that in this matter also there are individual differences from child to child. One could also notice in children under such circumstances a general restlessness as if an unusual amount of energy has been released cases, we might find that even breathing is very much disturbed sometimes resulting in holding the breath for a long interval. We also notice that at such times event the small child seems to be much stronger physically than what it would be ordinarily. In the adult also we find the same pattern of experiences associated with anger.

b. Sadness: It is necessarily related to feeling of loss and disadvantage. If this feeling drowns the person, it may lead to a state of depression. Disappointment and shame are its secondary emotions.

c. Anger: It is evoked due to injustice, conflict, humiliation, negligence or betrayal. If the anger is active, the individual attacks the target, verbally or physically. If the anger is passive, the person silently sulks and feels tension and hostility. Its secondary are rage, irritation and disgust.

Fear: Children show the response of fear usually to two types of situations, such as a sudden loud sound or that of losing their support and balance. A simple and basic pattern of this type of response which we call fear seems to be what is known as "the startle pattern". Though this is more commonly found with children, even the adult behaves in this way suddenly an unexpected loud sound is heard.

Here also there are individual differences. There is an interesting story about Napoleon. He was well known as a man who never showed any signs of fear. When he was taken a prisoner some of the officers wanted to play a practical joke on him. They arranged to have tea around a table with Napoleon. When the tea was sipped, they arranged for powerful cannon to be fired just near the room to see what would happen. When the cannon was fired even though those officers knew about it they all were startled and they split their tea shaking and dropping the cups. It is told that the sound had absolutely no effect on Napoleon. He was continuing to sip his tea calmly as if nothing had happened.

d. Surprise: It means the showing up of an unexpected result. It is accompanied by raising of eyebrows, horizontal lines on forehead, open mouth, wide open eyelids and so on.

Simple and Complex Emotional States

The importance of emotion, in practice and experience, is paralleled by the difficulty of its control. It is more desirable to transform emotions and direct them into productive channels than to suppress these emotions to cast them off. Proper use can thus be made of emotions in life. We have to pass through emotional states which are, in practice, either simple or complex. In the simple emotional state, generally there is only one emotion. In the complex state more than one emotion is involved. For example, aversion is a combination of anger and interest; hatred is a mixture of anger and aversion with a dot of fear; kindness includes love and sympathy. Simple emotion can be observed in children and the complex emotions in grown up persons. Simple emotions are innate. Complex emotions are being constantly developed in social conditions. For example, jealousy is propagated in the child by the arrival of a new child. It is imperative to study a few examples of the simple and complex emotions in order to understand them better. Grief and joy exemplify the simple emotions while love and hate illustrate the complex emotions.

1. *Grief*— This emotion results from damage to an object of one's desire. Grief is felt when a loved person or object is hurt or if one's desires are frustrated. The lengthening of the face, contraction of the chest, tears, catching of the throat, crying, fainting, sobbing, etc. are some of the signs of grief.

2. *Joy*—Joy is the opposite of grief. The expansion of the chest, lighting up of the face, smiling and laughing, glittering eyes, jumping about, clapping, dancing, etc. are all the external signs of joy. This is the result of the gratification of one's desires. Success after struggle brings joy.

Love and hatred are described below as examples of complex emotions:

3. *Love*—It is a complex emotion, a mixture of pity, sympathy, affection, love and prominently sex. Some people believe it to be lust. McDougall believes it to be the emotion aroused by the sexual instinct. It is, sometimes manifested as a permanent emotional tendency as in the case of a mother's love for her child. At this stage it is generally transformed into a sentiment. A child's love for his parents if often a sentiment. Selfishness and selflessness may found in love in different degrees, as both are commonly present in it. In different states either selfishness or unselfishness may dominate the other. Pure selfish love and pure unselfish love are rather the exceptions than the rule. Being a complex emotion, the external changes in love are extensive and they depend on the nature of the person, the intensity of love and the surrounding conditions. Taking on the lap, caressing or fondling, kissing, embracing, sighing, thrilling, etc. are all signs of love.

4. *Hate*—McDougall calls hate a compound emotion. According to his way of thinking, hate includes anger, fear and aversion. Some white people hate the black people. They are angry with everything they do. They want to stay way from the black and they are afraid of them.

Physical Changes in Emotion

Emotion results in physical changes which can be classified as external changes and internal physical changes.

External Physical Changes

Generally emotion is identified with physical change. An emotion is guessed on the basis of external physical changes. If a person grinds his teeth we say that he is angry. When a person trembles it is remarked that he is nervous. In happiness our face lights up, in sorrow our eyes are filled with fears and in surprise our eyes dilate. In this way, a difference in the expression of the eyes, nose, mouth, forehead, etc. is discernible in emotion. A persons voice is altered and he adopts fresh posture. These are the external changes in the manifestation of emotion. These will now be described in detail.

1. *Facial expression*—When under the influence of emotion the facial expression of the person is the first to be altered. It is easiest to read the emotions of pleasure or pain from the

face. No amount of effort can successfully disguise the facial contortions in strong emotion, from an experienced observer. In pleasant emotion, it is said that the face lights up with delight, this lighting up refers to the muscular expansion. Similarly, it is said that the face hangs dawn, the reference is to the contraction of the muscles. Prevalent sayings, such as blushing with shame or averting the eyes, expansion of the eyes in fear, elevation of the eyebrows in anger, are used to describe the changes in facial expressions in emotions. Many psychologists have experimented in order to determine the meaning of a variety of facial expressions. Some experiments seem to indicate that the facial expression by themselves are insufficient to enable a distinction to be made between the emotions, but the data collected from these experiments are faulty because: (1) It is difficult to get the normal emotion in the artificially created situation in the laboratory. (2) In different cultures the mode of expression of the various emotions is not uniform. (3) Even if the normal emotion is produced in the laboratory, it is necessary to photograph it at high speeds. (4) In the recognition of emotions, experiences and instruction are indispensable. In reality it cannot be said with any degree of certainty that it is not possible to recognize emotions from the facial expression. Even after the effects and impressions of the society, there is a degree of similarity. It is easy to recognize the conflicting feelings of pleasure and pain in Leonardo da Vinci's sketches.

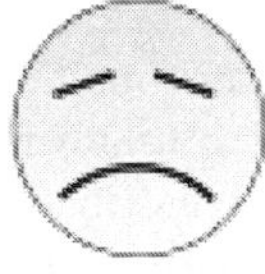

Fig. 18.4: Facial expressions

2. *Vocal expression*—Emotions can be expressed through the medium of voice and through this medium similar emotions can also be aroused in others. In expression of emotions the pitch and loudness of the voice changes. The voice of an angry person is house and loud whereas a happy person's voice is rhythmical and sweet. Some of the stronger emotions can be thus distinguished by hearing the voice. Sometimes even language can successfully excite emotions.
3. *Postural expression*—In an emotion state the posture is affected too. These changes are not similar in all societies and in all the members of any society. When frightened, a person may be seen running or standing will. In love, embracing, kissing, etc. may be observed but these show substantial changes in different societies due to the effect of culture. When angry some people use foul language, others pace about in a frenzy and still others attack somebody. Rubbing hands, clenching fists, standing erect, sitting with a bowed head, hiding, flinging the arms about, etc. all indicate emotion but the identification of emotion depends upon the person and the society to which he belongs and is possible only after adequate information.

Physiology of Emotion

Certain parts of the brain and hormones also play an important part in the activation of emotional experiences. It regulates autonomic nervous system, brain structure and hormonal influences.

Autonomic nervous system (ANS): Autonomic nervous system prepares the body for emotional responses via its two divisions — sympathetic nervous system and para-sympathetic nervous system. The sympathetic nervous system is more active with mild unpleasant stimulation while the parasympathetic division is more active with mild pleasant stimulation. Physiologically strong emotions like fear or anger activate the body's emergency reaction system which prepares the body to deal with danger. Sympathetic nervous system directs the release of hormones from the adrenal gland which further stimulate the internal organs to release blood sugar, raise blood pressure and increase sweating. The parasympathetic nervous system make us calm by inhibiting the release of these hormones.

Brain structures: Among the brain structures, the hypothalamus and the limbic system are the structures which control systems for emotions, patterns of attack, defense and flight. The brain structure most closely associated with fear is 'amygdala'.

Cerebral cortex, the outermost of the brain tissue, is involved in all complex emotions. The cortex provides the associations, memories and meanings that integrate psychological and biological experiences. There are different emotional centers is in the cortex for processing positive and negative emotions. The left hemisphere seems to be involved in positive emotions like happiness while right hemisphere is playing a role in negative emotions like anger. This discovery of hemisphere specialization is known as lateralization of emotions.

Hormones: Hormones play an important role in regulating emotions. During emotional states, there is an increase in the hormonal level in the blood and urine, because hormones are released when one releases emotional stimuli. Androgens and adrenocorticoids are important ones.

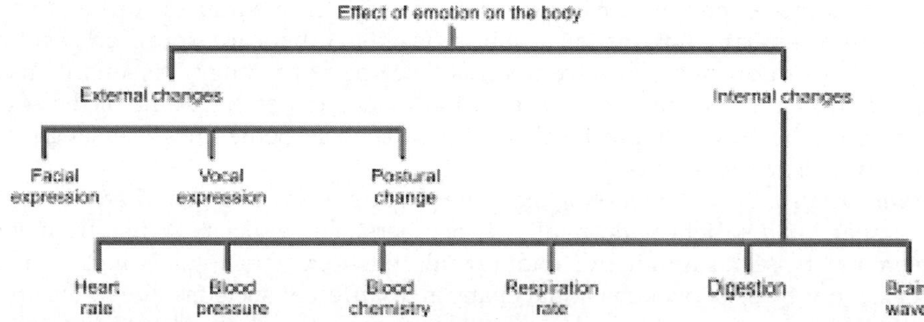

Physiological Changes

We have stated earlier about the physiological changes, but we did not stop to enumerate them. Some of these important changes are:

1. Facial expressions. Various muscles of the face, including the eyes, the lips, the nose and the forehead undergo changes by way of twisting and taking different poses. Facial expressions of emotions is a study by itself. Most of the emotions have their characteristics facial expressions but it may not be easy to spot out significant poses for some of them.
2. Gestures and movements of the hands. Gestures may involve movement of the whole body sometimes.
3. Voice gets affected. When excited the voice becomes loud and high pitched. Under fear the voice takes a sinking and low tone.
4. Breathing and heart beating also get affected. Sometimes they may be retarded and at other times they are accelerated.
5. Blood pressure also affected. We all know the simple advice that patients suffering from blood pressure should not be put to experiences of strong emotions. It was reported

once (though it is difficult to vouchsafe for its truth) that a patient suffering from blood pressure collapsed and died when he go the news of winning a very fat prize amount in a raffle.

6. There are other changes of miscellaneous nature associated with emotions such as "the hair standing on end" stimulation of the sweat glands, the tongue getting dry, etc.
7. One general feature with regard to physiological changes that take place under emotion is the fact that under emotion we have an unusual amount of energy at our disposal. When we are fighting a fire, for example, or when we are running away from danger we are able to run much faster and the energy at our disposal seems to be much more than that available ordinarily for us. (Some of us who may never win a prize at a race may perhaps even beat the champion if we were chased by a cobra). We would have even noticed a comparatively weaker person when under strong anger, overcoming a much stronger man in fight. Thus there is a release of an abnormal amount of energy helping us to meet the dangerous situation and thus preserve our well-being.
8. Perhaps one other important change should be mentioned. When experiencing emotion we undergo a change in our resistance capacity to electrical current. The body or properly speaking the skin normally has a certain resistance to electrical current. But under emotion this resistance is decreased. This can be demonstrated with an apparatus called "Psychogalvanoscope" (of course the experiment is conducted with electrical currents that are weak enough for the ordinary person to stand). This physiological change is important because this change is used for detecting and measuring emotions experimentally.

The Ductless Glands

In our body there are a number of glands which maintain and stimulate the normal process of growth. Physiology deals with all these in detail. In psychology we are concerned with some of them called the ductless glands. They are called ductless glands because these glands have no ducts or pipes through which their secretions are carried to the blood. The secretion is directly delivered into the bloodstream. They are also called endocrine glands. These secretions are called hormones. These hormones have the power to accelerate or retard the activity of the body and its organs. These endocrine glands are: *the thyroid gland, the parathyroids, the adrenal glands, the gonads, the pituitary glands and the pancreas.* Of these, perhaps the first four are more important. We mentioned earlier among the various physiological changes that take place with some emotions, an increase of energy as one. This increase in energy is actually due to the interplay of these hormones.

The thyroid gland which is located at the base of the neck secretes a hormone called thyroxin. Thyroxin is useful in the metabolism or the chemical activity of the body. If this hormone is not adequate the amount of oxygen consumed becomes less and metabolism is affected. When the thyroid is active to an abnormal extent, the individual becomes restless, irritable and unstable. Thus, the thyroid can influence personality and temperamental characteristics.

The adrenal gland which is located near the kidneys produces from its inner area a *hormone,* called *adrenin.* Adrenin is a very potent *hormone* having various effects on our general physiological working. If a small extra quantity is injected into the blood it can produce changes, such as strong and rapid heart-beat, delay in the activity of the stomach and intestines, release of extra sugar from the liver, retarding muscular fatigue, etc. Thus we find that the accelerated activity and increased physical strength and stamina during some emotional experiences are due to an extra discharge of adrenin.

Gonads secrete *hormones* which are particularly connected with the sex functions and the development of the individual. The pituitary gland is sometimes called "the master gland" because by its *hormone* it controls the activity of other endocrine glands.

A more detailed study of the glands is important for understanding the physiological bases of different types of personality. These hormones play a significant part in one's mental health and vigor. In recent years we have been able to understand more and more the significant part played by these glands in the general welfare of the body-mind organism. When all the glands function normally we speak of the condition as a good "endocrine balance". A proper balance of the erections of the different glands is necessary to ensure physical and mental health.

Autonomic Nervous System

Earlier we discussed the structure and functions of the central nervous system. But there is another system called the autonomic nervous system. It is actually a part of the central nervous system is controlled more by the thalamus and the interbrain than by the cerebral cortex. It is also involved more in our emotional life. We said earlier that one of the characteristics of emotion is that, if we bring the cerebral cortex into action and reason out things, the emotion tends to disappear. Thus we see that emotions are related to the interbrain rather than to the cerebrum. The autonomic nervous system has its own important functions to perform. Most of the organic changes mentioned above in connection with emotions and the endocrine glands are all controlled directly by this autonomic nervous system. The autonomic nervous system has its own important functions to perform. Most of the organic changes mentioned above in connection with emotions and the endocrine glands are all controlled directly by this autonomic nervous system. The autonomic nervous system has its own nerves that are connected to the various glands and internal organs, such as heart, lungs, liver, stomach, kidneys, etc. The autonomic nervous system has got two functional divisions called the parasympathetic division and the sympathetic division. The parasympathetic division controls glandular activities that are needed for the health of the organism while not in any dangerous or critical situation. These needs include nutrition, oxidation, promoting growth, sex functions, etc. In the normal state all these biological functions are controlled and promoted by the parasympathetic part of the autonomic nervous system. The sympathetic divisions comes into activity when the individual is in a state of danger or emergency. The extra energy which is needed in a dangerous situation (we have already referred to this) is released and controlled by this sympathetic system through the relevant endocrine glands. The liberation of adrenin in an emergency is largely controlled by this sympathetic division of the autonomic nervous system. When the sympathetic division has taken over, naturally, some of the biological needs controlled by the parasympathetic division will not be attempted to. In other words, when the sympathetic division functions the parasympathetic functions are withheld or suspended. This happens because they perform opposed functions. For example, when there is a danger it is more important to overcome that then to digest one's food or to attend to some other biological need. The threat to the very existence of the organism should be attended to first. If one frequently gives himself up to strong emotions rousing up the sympathetic division and thus obstructing the parasympathetic division, it is possible that the endocrine balance will be upset resulting in some diseases called psychosomatic disorders (such as gastric ulcers and asthma).

Internal Physical Changes

Besides the external changes mentioned above, there are some internal physiological changes too, in an emotion state. When surprised, our breathing almost stops. Our heart beats faster when we are angry. But these internal changes can be known only when they are measured by instruments. Some major changes are detailed below:

1. *Change in heart beat*—Generally, the heart beats faster or slower if the individual is disturbed. This fact is utilized by literary people as they mention this fluctuation of the heart beat to show the presence of emotion. The face is flushed or blood-shot in anger because the alternate contraction and expansion of the blood vessels send an excess of blood to that part of the body. The blood pressure of all those who were present rose when Scott, during his experiments, exhibited some sexually exciting photographs.
2. *Blood pressure changes*—We saw above how the heart beat changes and affects the blood pressure, this change, being very prominent, is very noticeable and is generally considered to be a good indicator of emotion. It is measured with a Plethysmograph. It can be used as a lie-detector, though its validity is restricted to the inexperienced deceiver because only such a person will be disturbed or upset at the prospect. Contradicting all that we have been asserting all along are some experimental results which prove that this change is not inevitable. Examining some soldiers injured in war, it was noticed that their blood pressure was not noticeably altered, in spite of the emotional experience of the war, while the visiting relatives were more severely affected, as was proved by their blood pressure.
3. *Change in the blood chemistry*—This is not all, because in an emotional state some changes in the chemical condition of the blood also take place. Another reaction to emotion is the excretion of adrenaline from the Adrenal gland, which puts more sugar in the blood and gives the person a reserve of energy to rely on and face the situation. The effect of adrenaline is felt in other quarters too. There is more sugar in the urine, blood pressure and heart beat increase and some capillaries in the skin start contracting.
4. *Change in the rate of respiration*—It is a matter of common experience that when excited, one's breath comes in short, quick gasps. When a person is feeling sorry or depressed he breathes slowly. These changes are measured with a Pneumograph. Commonly, emotion causes changes in the rate of respiration.
5. *Change in galvanic skin response*—A psychogalvanometer is an instrument used for measuring the resistance of the skin to an electric current. A skin dampened by perspiration offers more resistance than usual. Previously this state was supposed to be the peculiarity of emotion, but it has now been established that the same state will be the outcome of any physical or mental exercise. But still, the response of the skin is present in emotion and is a definite change in the emotional state.
6. *Metabolic changes*—Another important factor in the internal changes is the effect upon the process of digestion. But it has not been finally proved whether the change differs in different emotions or not. Brunswick's experiments on human beings showed that in fear, sorrow, etc. the process was accelerated and happiness left the digestion indifferent.

7. *Changes in brain waves*—The frequency of brain waves is affected in emotion. This change can be measured by instruments.

These are the major internal and external changes but they do not include every one. There are some other physiological changes which are apparent in emotion, e.g. when a person is extremely frightened he may excrete urine, etc. This is a tendency present in every animal and bird. This comprehency study of internal and external physiological changes must have made it very clear that in emotion there are changes though it is not possible to determine with accuracy the connection of a certain emotion with a certain change.

These changes due to emotion will be clarified further from the following chart:

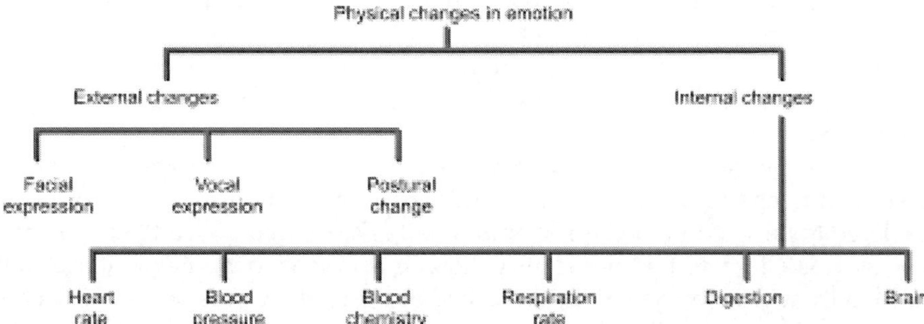

Psychologists do not agree about the importance of physiological changes in an emotional state. The Behaviorists place much emphasis on the physiological changes due to emotion and do not give any credence whatsoever to the mental responses. On the other hand, some psychologists lay an equal emphasis upon the mental changes. Looking at it realistically the physiological changes cannot be assumed to be everything, but then neither can they be neglected and considered insignificant. Similarly, the mental aspect of emotion can neither be neglected nor relied upon exclusively. It is necessary to understand both the aspects to understand emotion completely. As experiments are still being conducted in both these aspects, it is necessary to keep in view the physiological changes as well as the function of the different parts of the brain, while making a comprehensive study of emotions. A fully satisfactory theory of emotions can be evolved in the future only with a balanced viewpoint.

Steps to Control Emotions

1. **Get enough rest:** Most people need to sleep 7-9 hours a night. Less than that may result in intense emotional responses to routine upsets.
2. **Eat well and exercise:** A healthy diet makes you less vulnerable to a host of ills, including out-of-control emotions. Exercise helps you stay heart-healthy and also increases production of endorphins the brain chemicals that keep you calm.
3. **Talk to trusted others:** Have at least two or three people among family and friends that you trust with your most intimate thoughts and feelings.
4. **Learn to solve problems:** Successful problem solving is the key to building confidence you need to meet challenges without giving into hopelessness or helplessness.
5. **Learn to soothe yourself:** Focus on your strengths and your ability to take on difficult situation. Change your responses towards negative judgments about yourself.
6. **Get good information about the stress you face:** Information can defeat fear.

7. **Think! It's possible to have a strong emotion think at the same time:** If your emotions tend to get you into trouble, think through how you want to respond the next time you have feelings like anger, fear, sadness, or disgust.
8. **Take time everyday to do something fun or enjoyable:** Make this time a 'vacation' from your worries and troubles.
9. **Help others in similar circumstances:** It will help you gain new perspective on your own situation.
10. **Consider therapy:** Intense negative emotions that interfere with day-to-day function signal a need for professional help.

Control of Emotions

A child's behavior is more guided by his emotions than by his intellect or reason. His behavior distinctly manifest the influence of emotions such as fear, love, anger, hatred, etc. Some emotions guide him to extremely desirable and likeable forms of conduct but when in the grip of other emotions, his descents to the level of beasts and behaves in the most detestable manner that can only lead to censure from his elders. Experience and behavior show the extent to which emotional imbalance is harmful both to the body and the mind, as it results in all kinds of nervous and mental diseases. But the control of emotions through their repression is no less harmful. Psychoanalysts have made a detailed analysis of the various neuroses that result from such repressions. The best method of controlling emotions, in fact, is to prevent the occasions and opportunities that excite emotions. Auto-suggestion is another means of controlling emotions. If one makes it a practice to avoid using emotion they will weaken through disuse. When the stimulus of one particular emotion is willfully conjoined to another emotion, the undesirable emotion will harmless and innocent channel, then the excitation that accompanies emotions is destroyed, thus facilitation the control of that emotion.

The best method of controlling emotions is their sublimation. It changes the very form of the emotion. A child's conduct can be improved by instilling in him towards good habits, hatred for bad ones, anger for injustice, curiosity towards nature, etc. Once these emotions are conjoined to the right object, his behavior takes a good turn. Sublimation does not destroy the emotion: it only changes the mode of its expression. It achieves the necessary control while avoiding all the damage that is the inevitable corollary of repression. It also avoids the formation of emotional complexes. As psychoanalytic studies have revealed, most of the great poets, authors, scientists, leaders and saints could contribute to human well being only through the sublimation of their emotions. The compositions and creations of both Tulsidas and Kalidas clearly show the results of sublimation of their love for the opposite sex, as a result of which their sexual instinct was sublimated into love of God. Character-development cannot be left to fate. It needs the hardest and unbending effort. And the sublimation of emotions is a very important aspect of it.

Emotions and Health

Emotions play an important role in human life. An uncontrolled emotions plays a vital role in this cousation of many physical disorders.

It is a matter of common knowledge today that emotions, their repressions and expression influence the body and mind of the human being. Again, as the emotions are generally expressed in a social situation, it is bound to effect other persons as well. Thus an emotionally tense situation leads to tension not only within the person but also in his interpersonal relationships. Pointing out to the importance of emotions in health, Dr. Schindler writes in his book *How to live 365 Days a Year,* "Each of us has his own system the greatest known power for good health—the power of good emotions...... By controlling our own emotions we can eliminate half the nagging illnesses that plague our daily lives. Our bodies function well when we are happy. There is an old saying that joy is the best medicine".

Just as emotional maturity and control is useful in maintaining health, lack of emotional maturity and absence of emotional control leads to many physical and mental diseases. For example, persistent emotional disturbances due to anger, fear and worries lead to peptic ulcers, heart disease and epilepsy, tuberculosis, and diabetes. Bronchial asthma, high blood pressure, insomnia, chronic constipation, gastric ulcers and functional colitis are intensified by emotional disturbances. It is clear that most of the diseases require emotional control and emotional health as one of the necessary condition of cure. Good and pleasant emotions contribute to good health. But intense and unpleasant emotions disturb us sometimes to a great extent if they persists. Persist emotional disturbance leads to one of causative factor for psychosomatic disorders.

Emotions and the Nurse

The need of the knowledge about emotions on the part of the nurse. Normally the patients are less self-controlled than the nurses. They are tense, irritable and unbalanced. Therefore, the nurse has to be very patient, mature and balanced in her behavior towards the patients. She has to substitute their negative emotions by positive emotions. She has to replace fear, depression and hatred by hope, courage and love. She should try to eliminate fear, anger, worry, anxiety and resentment from her and from the patients. This requires self-control and healthy interpersonal relationships. Her relationships with the patients and with her colleagues should be friendly, cooperative, frank and sincere. All this requires a knowledge of the what, how and why of the emotions. She should avoid tensions at all cost. She should avoid tensions at all costs. She should cultivate hobbies. She should learn self-control. She should have a thorough knowledge of the dynamics of her own emotions. And last but not the least, she should develop a healthy sense of humor.

Thus, an emotional maturity in the nurse requires a sound philosophy of life, a balanced, healthy and well-adjusted routine, and finally a thorough knowledge of the psychology of emotions, their nature, dynamics and control.

The following suggestions for control of emotions for Nurses:

1. Nurses should learn as much as they can about emotions, their causes, reaction involved and consequences. The more they know about them, the greater is the power they have over them.
2. Try to avoid emergency situations as much as possible. Such situations cause excessive emotional reactions. This can be done if we learn the habit of planning our daily life and our future activities so that we have a few emergencies as possible.
3. Nurses should cultivate hobbies, habits of good reading and wholesome friendships. Get busy in some useful activity. Participate in dramatics, music or games. These activities will direct your attention from the emotion-provoking experiences.
4. A desirable philosophy of life will enable you to avoid mental conflicts and emotional tensions.
5. Try to learn to control unreasonable and excessive external expression of emotions. These external expressions tend to increase the intensity of emotional experiences of the individual. They excite other people and cause further emotionally.

6. A thorough understanding of oneself, one's own limitations and powers helps in controlling one's emotion. Nurses should be able to examine their conflicts and emotions objectively and face facts realistically.
7. A well-developed sense of humor will help nurses forget their petty annoyances and irritations.
8. Try to find humorous elements in situations. Nurses will thus laugh and enjoy life and avoid unpleasant emotional experiences.

The responsibility of a nurse is not only practice her skills and provide physical comfort, it is also reduce the intensity of emotional disturbances as much as it is possible.

When patient comes to the hospital with various problems. Family members, relatives and friends also face discomfort when patient is admitted in the hospital and undergoing treatment.

1. **Help the patient feel comfortable**
   - Give a warm welcome to patient. Let him feel that he is an important guest
   - Do not show judgmental attitude towards patient
   - Orient the client with unit and ward staff to provide feeling of security and assurance of personal safety.
2. **Interact with the patient and relatives**
   - Introduce yourself to the patient
   - Stay with the patient
   - Communicate with him for expression of feelings and release of anxiety.
3. **Alert with basic needs of the patient**
   - Help the patient to determine the unmet needs
   - A nurse should be expert to understand the link of emotions with unmet needs, e.g. need for acceptance when is rejected
   - When physiological needs are met, then comes the next higher needs in hierarchy and meet them.
4. **Understand negatives emotions**
   - Understand the use of defenses by the patient
   - Find out the problem, patient is facing and its cause
   - Clarify the problem that he is facing by comparing the perception of patients' problem with her own perception of that same problem
   - Acknowledge feelings of anger, guilt, helplessness and powerlessness while taking care of.
5. **Promote positive feelings**
   - Deal with the emotions and take more concrete problem solving approach to emotional reactions
   - Encourage exploration of feelings
   - Develop alternative strategies for creating changes that are realistically possible
   - Promote relaxation techniques
   - Promote healthy interpersonal relationships.
6. **Develop empathy**
   - Understand the patients situation, feelings and motives
   - Accept the patient as he is.
7. **Prevent psychosomatic illnesses**
   - Help the patient to relax
   - Arrange for professional help if severe emotional reactions.

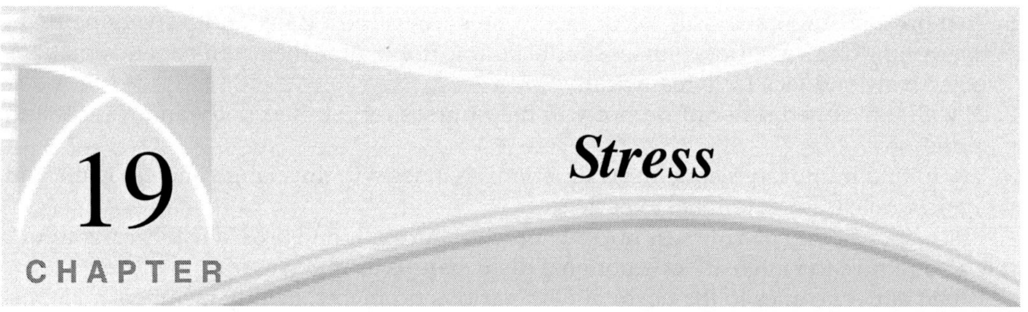

19 CHAPTER Stress

Introduction

Life is stressful and represent a constant, dynamic exchange of energy between people and environment. The organism has innate process to maintain and restore homeostasis under stressful condition. The nature of stress is determined by ones repertoire of resources and coping mechanisms and response to internal and external demands.

Life is really about change. Every day, each person faces some kind of challenge, big or small. Just deciding what to wear to work or school can be challenge for some people, while others find the drive to the workplace or school the most challenging part of the day. There are decisions to be made and changes that will require adapting plans already made. Sometimes there are actual threats to well being—an accident, a fight with the boss, a failed exam, or losing a job, to name a few. All of these challenges, threats, and changes require people to respond in some way.

Stress is a universal phenomena. Everyone in the universe experience it. Parents refers to the stress of raising children, employees talk of the stress of their jobs and students take of their school and colleges. Stress can result from both positive and negative experiences in the life. For example, bride preparing for her wedding. Person to start a new job, and an individual who concerned about taking care of seriously ill persons, etc.

The concept of stress is important because it provides a way of understanding the person as a being who responds in totality (mind, body and spirit) to a variety of changes that takes place in daily life. Stress is an inherent part of everyday living and is encountered throughout the lifespan. Daily interactions with internal and external demands contribute to stress in human beings, who constantly are changing and adapting to their environment.

Meaning

Stress is the term used to describe the physical, emotional, cognitive, and behavioral responses to events that are appraised as threatening or challenging.

Stress can show itself in many ways. Physical problems can include unusual fatigue, sleeping problems, frequent colds, and even chest pains and nausea. People under stress may behave differently; too pacing, eating too much, crying a lot, smoking and drinking more than usual, or physically striking out at others by hitting or throwing things. Emotionally, people under stress experience anxiety, depression, fear, and irritability, as well as anger and frustration. Mental symptoms of stress include problems in concentration, memory, and decision making, and people under stress often lose their sense of humor.

Generally 'stress' refers to a stimulus (stressor) or situation that produces distress. Stress defined as a condition or demand that arises from ineffective coping behaviors that fails to mobilize resources and maintain homeostasis.

Stress as the nonspecific response of the body to any demand made upon it. Although stressors of heat and cold and psychological stressors of failure, success and a new challenge—they elicit essentially the same biological stress response. The absence of stress is death (Hans Selye)

Stress is a physiological or psychological tension that threatens the homeostasis or a individuals psychosocial equilibrium.

Stress is a condition in which the person responds to changes in the normal balanced state. A stressor is any event or stimulus that causes an individual to experience stress. When a person faces stressors, responses are referred to as coping, strategies, coping responses, or coping mechanisms.

STRESSORS AND STRESS

Most people experience some degree of stress on a daily basis, and college students are even more likely to face situations and events that require them to make changes and adapt their behavior: Assigned readings, papers, studying for tests, juggling jobs, car problems, relationships, and dealing with deadlines are all examples of things that can cause a person to experience stress. Some people feel the effects of stress more than others because what is appraised as a threat by one person might be appraised as an opportunity by another. Stress causing events are called stressors, they can come from within a person or from an external source and range from relatively mild to severe.

There are many sources of stress. They can be broadly classified as internal or external stressors, or developmental or situational stressors. Internal stressors originate within a person, for example, cancer or feelings of depression. External stressors originate outside the individual, for example, a move to another city, a death in the family, or pressure from peers. Developmental stressors occur at predictable times throughout an individual's life. Within each developmental stage, certain tasks must be achieved to prevent or reduce stress. Examples of these tasks are shown in Table 19.1. Situational stressors are unpredictable and may occur at any time during life. Situational stress may be positive or negative. Examples of this type of stress include

- Death of a family member
- Marriage or divorce
- Birth of a child
- New job
- Illness.

Events that can become stressors range from being suck behind a person in the 10-times or less lane of the grocery store who has twice that amount to dealing with the rubble left after a tornado or a hurricane destroys one's home. Stressors can range from the deadly serious (hurricanes, fires, crashes, combat) to the merely irritating and annoying (delays, rude people, losing one's car keys). Stressors can even be imaginary, as when a couple puts off doing their income tax return, imagining that they will have to pay a huge tax bill, or when a parent imagines the worst happening to a teenage child who isn't yet home from an evening out.

Table 19.1: Selected stressors associated with developmental stages	
Developmental stage	*Stressors*
Child	Beginning school, establishing peer relationship and adjustments, coping with peer competition
Adolescent	Accepting changing physique, developing relationships involving sexual attraction, achieving independence, choosing a career
Young adult	Getting married, leaving home, managing a home, getting started in an occupation, continuing one's education, rearing children
Middle adult	Accepting physical changes of aging, maintaining social status and standard of living, helping teenage children to become independent, adjusting to aging parents
Older adult	Accepting decreasing physical abilities and health, accepting changes in residence, adjusting to retirement and reduced income, adjusting to death of spouse and friends

Actually, there are two kinds of stressors: those that cause distress, which occurs when people experience unpleasant stressors, and those that cause eustress, which results from positive events that still make demands on a person to adapt or change. Marriage, a job promotion, and having a baby may all be positive events for most people, but they all require a great deal of change in people's habits, duties and even lifestyle, thereby creating stress. Hans Selye (1936) originally coined the term eustress to describe the stress experienced when positive events require the body to adapt.

In an update of Selye's original definition, researchers now define eustress as the optimal amount of stress that people need to promote health and well being.

The degree to which any of these events has positive or negative effects can depend to some extent on an individual's developmental stage. For example, the death of a parent may be more stressful for a 12-year-old than for a 40-year-old.

The Stress Response

When the body is exposed to harm or threat, the result is a cluster of physiological changes that is generally referred to as the stress response—or just stress. All stressors, whether psychological (e.g. dismay at the loss of one's job) or physical (e.g. long-term exposure to cold) produce a similar core pattern of physiological changes; however, it is chronic psychological stress (e.g. in the form of chronic fear) that has been most frequently implicated in ill health.

According to Lazarus, there is a two step process in assessing the degree of threat or harm of a stressor and how one should react to that stressor (Fig. 19.1).

Primary appraisal: The first step in appraising a stressor is called primary appraisal, which involves estimating the severity of the stressor and classifying it as a threat (something that could be harmful in the future), a challenge (something to be met and defeated), or a harm or loss that has already occurred. If the stressor is appraised as a threat, negative emotions may arise that inhibit the person's ability to cope with the threat. For example, a student who has not read the text or taken good notes will certainly appraise an upcoming exam as threatening. If the stressor is seen as a challenge, however, it is possible to plan to meet that challenge, which is a more positive and less stressful approach. For example, the

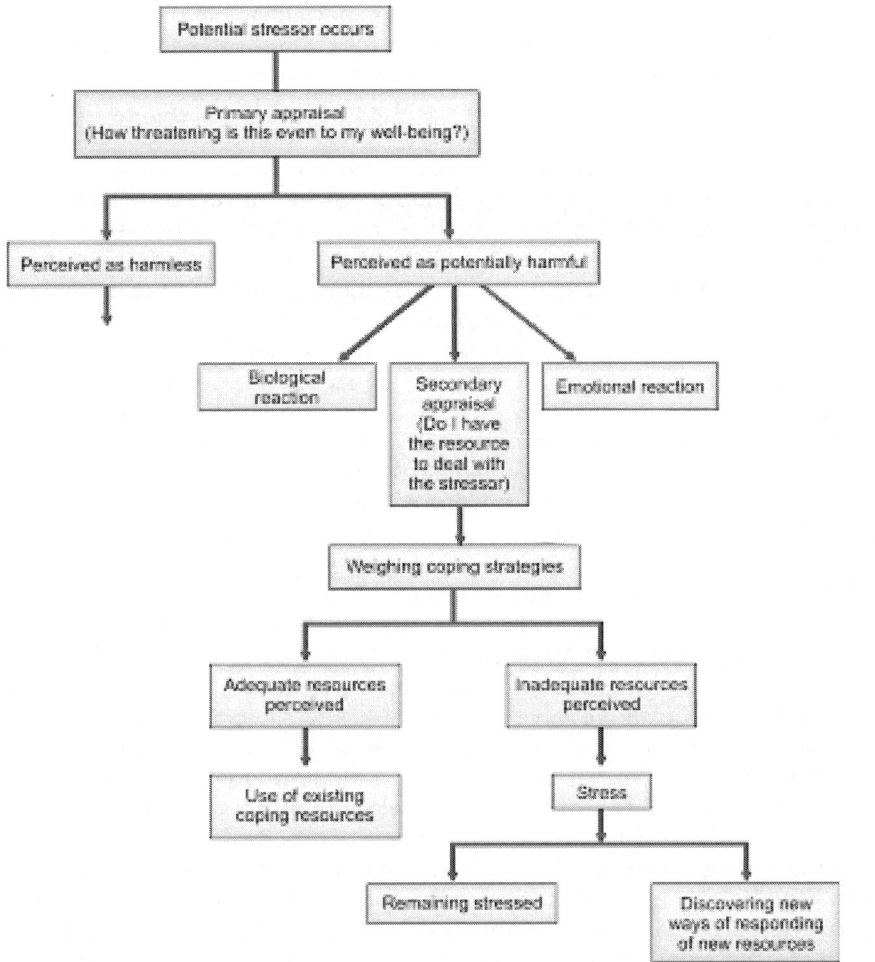

Fig. 19.1: Responses to a stressor. Lazarus's cognitive appraisal approach. According to this approach, there are two steps in cognitively determining the degree of stress created by a potential stressor. Primary appraisal involves determining if the potential stressor is a threat. If it is perceived as a threat, secondary appraisal occurs in addition to the bodily and emotional reactions. Secondary appraisal involves determining the resources one has to deal with the stress, such as time, money, physical ability, and so on. Inadequate resources lead to increased feelings of stress and the possibility of developing new resources to deal with the stress.

student who has studied, read, and feels prepared is much more likely to appraise the upcoming exam as an opportunity to do well.

Perceiving a stressor as a challenge instead of a threat makes coping with the stressor or the harm it may already have caused more likely to be successful, whereas perceiving it as an embarrassment or imagining failure or rejection is more likely to lead to increased stress reactions, negative emotions, and an inability to cope well. Think positive.

Secondary appraisal. In secondary appraisal, people who have identified a threat or harmful effect must estimate the resources that they have available for coping with the stressor. Resources might include social support, money, time, energy, ability or any number of potential resources, depending on the threat. If resources are perceived as adequate or abundant, the degree of stress will be considerably less than if resources are missing or lacking. Using the example of the student and the upcoming exam, a student who feels that she has the time to study and the ability to understand the material in that time that she understood much of the lectures covered on the exam.

With regard to stress there is good news too. Stress is not always bad. In fact, a minimum level of stress is required to lead a productive and creative life. For instance, in case of a student, stress related to poor performance in the examination can gradually lead to better work efficiency and output. But if it surpasses the required and manageable level, the consequences can be highly counter-productive and even fatal. Tolerance level for the degree of stress varies from individual to individual. No absolute standard exists for that. Individual 'A' might not possess the capacity to manage ten stressors at a given point in time, individual 'B' might have the capacity to manage ten stressors only, while individual 'C' might not possess the capacity to handle even one stressor. Some people have the notion that stress indicates some psychological disorder. It is not true. It is not that some of us have it and other's do not. All of us have it. Many of us live days, weeks and even months in a constant state of stress, our body and mind never relaxing and enjoying a moment of peace.

Hans Selye first described the stress response in the 1950s, and he quickly recognized its dual nature. In the short-term, it produces adaptive changes that help the animal respond to the stressor (e.g. mobilization of energy resources, inhibition of inflammation, and resistance to infection); in the long-term, however, it produces changes that are maladaptive (e.g. enlarged adrenal glands). Selye attributed the stress response to the activation of the anterior pituitary adrenal cortex system. He concluded that stressors acting on neural circuits stimulate the release of **adrenocorticotropic hormone(ACTH)** from the anterior pituitary, that the ACTH in turn triggers the release of **glucocorticoids** from the **adrenal cortex**, and that the glucocorticoids produce many of the effects of the stress response. The level of circulating glucocorticoids is the most commonly employed physiological measure of stress. With his emphasis on the role of the anterior-pituitary adrenal-cortex system in stress, Selye largely ignored the contributions of the sympathetic nervous system. Stressors also activate the sympathetic nervous system, thereby increasing the amounts of epinephrine and norepinephrine released from the **adrenal medulla.** Most modern theories of stress acknowledge the major roles of both systems.

The magnitude of the stress response depends not only on the stressor and the individual; it also depends on the strategies the individual adopts to cope with the stress. For example, in a study of women awaiting surgery for possible breast cancer, the levels of stress were lower in those who had convinced themselves to think about their problem in certain ways. Those who had convinced themselves that they could not possibly have cancer, that their prayers were certain to be answered, or that it was counterproductive to worry about it experienced less stress. From the perspective of psychological science, the major contribution of Selye's stress response was that it suggested a mechanism by which psychological factors can influence physical illness. All kinds of common psychological stressors (e.g. losing a job, preparing for an examination, ending a relationship) are associated with high circulating levels of glucocorticoids, epinephrine and norepinephrine; and these in turn have been implicated in many physical disorders. For example, fear or stress prior to surgery has been associated with slower postsurgical recovery, including delays in wound healing.

The relation between chronic fear, stress, and ill health is readily apparent in animals undergoing subordination stress. Virtually all mammals—particularly males—experience threats from conspecifices (members of the same species) at certain points in their lives. When conspecific threat becomes an enduring feature of daily life, the result is **subordination stress**. Subordination stress is most readily studied in social species that form stable dominance hierarchies (pecking orders). What do you think happens to subordinate male rodents who are continually attacked by more dominant males? Several studies have reported that animals exposed to subordination stress are more likely to attack juveniles, to have testes that are reduced in size, to have shorter life spans, and to have lower levels of testosterone and higher levels of corticosterone (a glucocorticoids).

Effects of Stress

Stress can have physical, emotional, intellectual, social and spiritual consequences. Usually the effects are mixed because stress affects the whole person. Physically, stress can threaten a person's physiologic homeostasis. Emotionally, stress can produces negative or nonconstructive feelings about the self. Intellectually, stress can influence a person's perceptual and problem solving abilities. Socially, stress can alter a person's relationships with others. Spiritually, stress can challenge one's beliefs and values. Many illnesses have been linked to stress.

Sources of Stress

Although several specific sources of stress (e.g. marriage, car problems, etc.) have already been mentioned, the reasons why people these events stressful fall into several categories.

Pressure: When there are urgent demands or expectation for a person's behavior coming from an outside source, that person is experiencing pressure. Pressure occurs when people feel that they must work harder, faster, or do more, as in meeting a deadline or studying for final exams.

Time pressure is one of the most common forms of pressure. Although some people claim to "work well under pressure", the truth is that pressure can have a negative impact on a person's ability to be creative. Psychologist Teresa Amabile has gathered research within actual work settings strongly indicating that when time pressure is applied to workers who are trying to come up with creative, innovative ideas, creativity levels decrease dramatically—even though the workers may think they have been quite productive because of the effort they have made.

Uncontrollability: Another factor that increases a person's experience of stress is the degree of control that the person has over a particular event or situation. The less control a person has, the greater the degree of stress. Researchers, in both clinical interviews and experimental studies, have found that lack of control in a situation actually increases post-traumatic stress syndrome symptoms.

The stress increasing effects of lack of control explain the relationship between unpredictability and stress as well. When potentially stressful situations are unpredictable, as in police work, the degree of stress experienced is increased. An unpredictable situation is one that is not controllable, which may at least partially explain the increase in stress. In one study, rats were either given an electric shock after a warning tone or given a shock with no warning. The rats receiving the unpredictable shocks developed severe stomach ulcers.

Frustration: Frustration occurs when people are blocked or prevented from achieving a desired goal or fulfilling a perceived need. As a stressor, frustration can be external, such as when a car breaks down, a desired job offer doesn't come through after all, or experiencing a theft of one's belongings. Losses, rejections, failures and delays are all sources of external frustration.

Obviously, some frustration are minor and others are more serious. The seriousness of a frustration is affected by how important the goal or need actually is. A person who is delayed in traffic while driving to the mall to do some shopping just for fun will be less frustrated than a person who is trying to get to the mall before it closes to get that last minute forgotten and important anniversary gift.

Internal frustrations, also known as personal frustrations, occur when the goal or need cannot be attained because of internal or personal characteristics. For example, someone who wants to be an astronaut might find that severe motion sickness prevents him or her from such a goal. If a man wants to be a professional basketball player but is only 5 feet tall and weighs only 85 pounds, he may find that he cannot achieve that goal because of his physical characteristics. A person wanting to be an engineer but who has no math skills would find it difficult to attain that goal.

There are several typical responses that people make when frustrated. The first is persistence, or the combination of efforts to get around whatever is causing the frustration. Persistence may involve making more intense efforts or changing the style of response. For example, anyone who has ever put coins into a drink machine only to find that the drink does not come out has probably (1) pushed the button again, more forcefully, and (2) pushed several other buttons in an effort to get some kind of response from the machine. If neither of these strategies works, many people may hit or kick the machine itself in an act of aggression.

Aggression or actions meant to harm or destroy, is unfortunately another typical reaction to frustration. Early psychologists in the field of behaviorism proposed a connection between frustration and aggression, calling it the frustrations-aggression hypothesis. Although they believed that some form of frustration nearly always precedes aggression, that does not mean that frustration always leads to aggression. In fact, aggression is a frequent and persistent response to frustration, but it is seldom the first response. In a reformation of the frustration-aggression hypothesis, Berkowitz (1993) stated that frustration creates an internal "readiness to aggress" but that aggression will not follow unless certain external cues are also present. For example, if the human source of a person's frustration is far larger and stronger in appearance than the frustrated person, aggression is an unlikely outcome.

Conflict: Conflict occurs when a person feels pulled toward or drawn to two or more desires or goals but can only achieve or experience one. Lewin (1935) defined three types of conflicts, and his definitions are still used by today's researchers in the area of conflict and conflict resolution.

- Approach-approach conflict. In an approach-approach conflict, a person experiences attraction to two desires or goals, each of which is attractive. Typically, this type of conflict, often called a "win-win situation" is relatively easy to resolve and does not involve a great deal of stress. Because both goals are desirable, the only stress involved is having to choose between them, acquiring one and losing the other. An example of this might be the need to choose between the chocolate cake or key lime pie for dessert or from among several good choices for a date to the prom. "Six on one hand, half a dozen on the other" is a phrase that sums up this conflict nicely.

- Avoidance-avoidance conflict. Avoidance-avoidance conflicts are much more stressful. In this conflict, the choice is between two or more goals or events that are unpleasant. This type of conflict is so common that there are numerous phrases to symbolize it; "Caught between a rock and a hard place", and "lose-lose situation" are some of these phrases. Because neither alternative is pleasant, many people avoid making a choice by delaying decisions. For example, given the choice of risky back surgery or living with the pain, some people would wait, hoping that the pain would go away on its own and relieve them of the need to make a choice. People who are fearful of dental procedures might face the conflict of suffering the pain of a toothache or going to the dentist.
- Approach-avoidance conflict. Approach-avoidance conflicts are a little different in that they only involve one goal or event. That goal or event may have both positive and negative aspects that make the goal appealing and unappealing at the same time. For example, marriage is a big decision to make for anyone and usually has both its attractive features, such as togetherness, sharing good times, and companionship, and also its negative aspects, such as disagreements, money issues, and mortgages. This is perhaps the most stressful of all the types of conflict, causing many people to vacillate or be unable to decide for or against the goal or event. The author experienced a very stressful approach-avoidance conflict when deciding to write this textbook: On the one hand, there would be money, prestige, and the challenge of doing something new. On the other hand, a tremendous amount of effort and time would be required to write the text, which would take time and energy away from other areas of life. Another example is the offer of a promotion that would require a person to move to a city he or she doesn't like—more money and higher status but all the hassles of moving and living in a less than perfect place.
- Multiple approach-avoidance conflicts. When the choice is between two goals that have both positive and negative elements to each goal, it is called a double approach avoidance conflict. For example what if a person had the choice of buying a house out in the country or in the city? The house in the country has its attractions: privacy, fresh air, and quiet. But there would be a long commute to one's job in the city. A house in the city would make getting to work a lot easier, but then there are the negative aspects of pollution, noise, and crowded city streets. Each choice has both good and bad points. This type of conflict also tends to lead to vacillation. Other examples of this type of conflict might be trying to decide which of two people one wants to date or which of two majors one needs to choose.

It is fairly common to face multiple approach-avoidance conflicts in daily life. In a multiple approach-avoidance conflict, one would have more than two goals or options to consider, making the decision even more difficult and stressful. For many college students, deciding on a career is actually this type of conflict.

Models of Stress

Models of stress assist nurses to identify the stressor in a particular situation and to predict the individuals responses. Nurses can use the knowledge of these models to assist clients in strengthening healthy coping responses and in adjusting unhealthy, unproductive responses. Three main models of stress are stimulus-based, response-based, and transaction-based.

A. Stimulus-Based Models

In **stimulus-based stress models,** stress is defined as a stimulus, a life event, or a set of circumstances that arouses physiologic and/or psychologic reactions that may increase the individuals vulnerability to illness. In their classic work, Holmes and Rahe (1967) assigned a numerical value to 43 life changes or events. The scale of stressful life events is used to document a person's relatively recent experiences, such as divorce, pregnancy, and retirement. In this view, both positive and negative events are considered stressful.

Similar scales have been developed, but all scales should be used with caution the degree of stress an event presents is highly individual. For example, a divorce may be highly traumatic to one person and cause relatively little anxiety to another. In addition, many scales have not been tested for age, socioeconomic status, or cultural sensitivity.

B. Response-Based Models

Stress may also be considered as a response. This definition was developed and described by Selye (1976) as 'the nonspecific response of the body to any kind of demand made upon it'. Schafer (2000) defined stress as the 'arousal of mind and body in response to demands made upon them'.

Selye's stress response is characterized by a chain or pattern of physiologic events called the **general adaptation syndrome (GAS)** or stress syndrome. To differentiate the cause of stress from the response to stress, Selye (1976) created the term stressor to denote any factor that produces stress and disturbs the body's equilibrium. Because stress is a state of the body, it can be observed only by the changes it produces in the body. This response of the body, the stress syndrome or GAS, occurs with the release of certain adaptive hormones and subsequent changes in the structure and chemical composition of the body. Body organs affected by stress are the gastrointestinal tract, the adrenal glands, and the lymphatic structures. With prolonged stress, the adrenal glands enlarge considerably; the lymphatic structures such as the thymus, spleen, and lymph nodes, atrophy (shrink); and deep ulcers appear in the lining of the stomach.

In addition to adapting globally, the body can also react locally, that is, one organ or a part of the body reacts alone. This is referred to as the **local adaptation syndrome (LAS)**. One example of the LAS is inflammation. Selye (1976) proposed that both the GAS and the LAS have three stages: alarm reaction, resistance, and exhaustion (See Figure 19.2).

i. Alarm reaction: The initial reaction of the body is the **alarm reaction,** which alerts the body's defenses. Selye (1976) divided this stage into two parts: the shock phase and the countershock phase. During the **shock phase,** the stressor may be perceived consciously or unconsciously by the person. In any case, the autonomic nervous system reacts, and large amounts of epinephrine (adrenaline) and cortisone are released into the body. The person is then ready for 'fight or flight'. This primary response is short-lived, lasting from 1 minute to 24 hours. The second part of the alarm reaction is called the **countershock phase**. During this time, the changes produced in the body during the shock phase are reversed. Thus, a person is best mobilized to react during the shock phase of the alarm reaction.

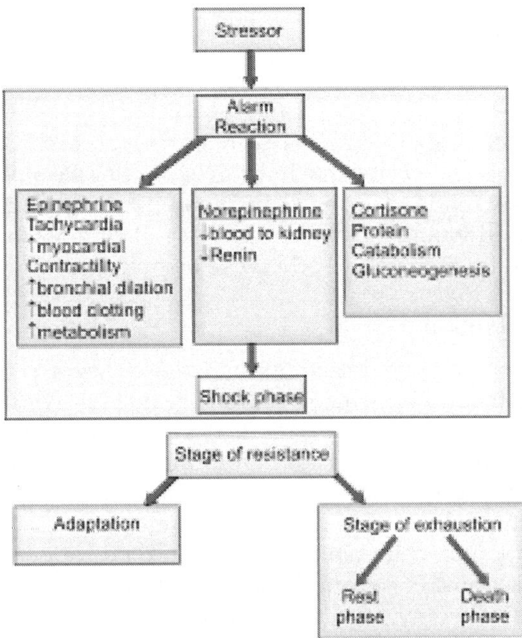

Fig. 19.2: The three stages of adaptation to stress the alarm reaction, the stage of resistance, and the stage of exhaustion

ii. Stage of resistance. The second stage in the GAS and LAS syndromes, the **stage of resistance**, is when the body's adaptation takes place. In other words, the body attempts to cope with the stressor and to limit the stressor to the smallest area of the body that can deal with it.

iii. Stage of exhaustion. During the third stage, the **stage of exhaustion**, the adaptation that the body made during the second stage cannot be maintained. This means that the ways used to cope with the stressor have been exhausted. If adaptation has not overcome the stressor, the stress effects may spread to the entire body. At the end of this stage, the body may either rest and return to normal, or death may be the ultimate consequence. The end of this stage depends largely on the adaptive energy resources of the individual, the severity of the stressor, and the external adaptive resources that are provided, such as oxygen.

Seyle's (1976) general adaptation syndrome encompasses a range of physiologic responses to stressors in the body as a whole (See Figure 19.2). Stressors stimulate the sympathetic nervous system, which in turn stimulates the hypothalamus. The hypothalamus releases corticotrophin releasing hormone (CRH), which stimulates the anterior pituitary gland to release adrenocorticotropin (ACTH). During times of stress, the adrenal medulla secretes epinephrine and norepinephrine in response to sympathetic stimulation. Significant body response to epinephrine include the following:

1. Increased myocardial contractility, which increases cardiac output and blood flow to active muscles
2. Bronchial dilation, which allows increased oxygen intake

3. Increased blood clotting
4. Increased cellular metabolism
5. Increased fat mobilization to make energy available and to synthesize other compounds needed by the body.

The principal effect of norepinephrine is decreased blood to the kidneys and increased secretion of renin. Renin is an enzyme that hydrolyzes one of the blood proteins to produce angiotensin. Angiotensin tends to increase the blood pressure by constructing arterioles. The sum of all of these adrenal hormonal effects permits the person to perform far more strenuous physical activity than would otherwise be possible.

C. Transaction-Based Models

Transactional theories of stress are based on the work of Lazarus (1966), who states that the stimulus theory and the response theory do not consider individual differences. Neither theory explains which factors lead some people and not others to responds effectively nor interprets why some people are able to adapt for longer periods than are others.

Although Lazarus recognizes that certain environmental demands and pressures produce stress in substantial numbers of people, he emphasizes that people and groups differ in their sensitivity and vulnerability to certain types of events, as well as in their interpretations and reactions. For example, in terms of illness, one person may respond with denial, another with anxiety, and still another with depression. To explain variations among individuals under comparable conditions, the Lazarus model takes into account cognitive processes that intervene between the encounter and the reaction, and the factors that affect the nature of this process. In contrast to Selye, who focuses on physiologic responses, Lazarus includes mental and psychologic components or responses as part of his concept of stress.

The Lazarus **transactional stress theory** encompasses a set of cognitive, affective, and adaptive (coping) responses that arise out of person-environment transactions. The person and the environment are inseparable, each affects and is affected by the other. Stress 'refers' to any event in which environmental demands, internal demands, or both tax or exceed the adaptive resources of an individual, social system, or tissue system'. The individual responds to perceived environmental changes by adaptive or coping responses.

Indicators of Stress

What is stress? When your physical, emotional and spiritual abilities are experienced to be less that the environmental pressures and demands, they trigger a stress response. Those that the environmental pressures can be real, imagined or anticipated. Fundamentally you tend to enter into a flight mode rather than a fighter mode. This response occurs both with physiological as well as psychological manifestations. Physiological manifestations include symptoms like palpitations, headaches/ bodyaches, digestion problems, giddiness, lips turning blue or pale, drying of throat, butterflies in the stomach, shivering, stammering, dilation of pupils listless, nausea and other such symptoms. Psychological manifestations include withdrawal, disinterest, irritability, addiction, lack of self-esteem, psychosomatic symptoms, anticipatory anxiety, lack of performance at work place/family/ social groups, dysfunctional marital/ sexual relation and many similar indications.

Indicators of an individual's stress may be physiologic, psychologic, or cognitive.

Physiologic indicators. Responses to stress vary depending on the individual's perception of events. The physiologic signs and symptoms of stress result from activation of the sympathetic and neuroendocrine systems of the body. The lists physiologic indicators of stress as given below:

- Pupils dilate to increase visual perception when serious threats to the body arise.
- Sweat production (diaphoresis) increases to control elevated body heat due to increased metabolism.
- The heart rate and cardiac output increase to transport nutrients and by-products of metabolism more efficiently.
- Skin is pallid because of constriction of peripheral blood vessels, an effect of norepinephrine.
- Sodium and water retention increase due to release of mineralocorticoids, which results in increased blood volume.
- The rate and depth of respirations increase because of dilation of the bronchioles, promoting hyperventilation.
- Urinary output decreases.
- The mouth may be dry.
- Peristalsis of the intestines decreases, resulting in possible constipation and flatus.
- For serious threats, mental alertness improves.
- Muscle tension increases to prepare for rapid motor activity or defense.
- Blood sugar increase because of release of glucocorticoids and gluconeogenesis.

Psychologic indicators. Psychologic manifestations of stress include anxiety, fear, anger, depression, and unconscious ego defense mechanisms. Some of these coping are helpful; others are a hindrance, depending on the situation and the length of time they are used or experienced.

i. Anxiety. A common reaction to stress is anxiety, a state of mental uneasiness, apprehension, dread, or foreboding or a feeling of helplessness related to an impending or anticipated unidentified threat to self or significant relationships. Anxiety can be experienced at the conscious, subconscious, or unconscious level. It differs from fear in four ways:

- The source of anxiety may not be identifiable; the source of fear is identifiable.
- Anxiety is related to the future, that is, to an anticipated event. Fear is related to the present.
- Anxiety is vague, whereas fear is definite.
- Anxiety is the result of psychologic or emotional conflict; fear is the result of a discrete physical or psychological entity.

Anxiety may be manifested on four levels (Table 19.2):

1. Mild anxiety produces a slight arousal state that enhances perception, learning and productive abilities. Most healthy people experience mild anxiety, perhaps as a feeling of mild restlessness that prompts a person to seek information and ask questions.
2. Moderate anxiety increases the arousal state to a point where the person expresses feelings of tension, nervousness and concern. Perceptual abilities are narrowed. Attention is focused more on a particular aspect of a situation than on peripheral activities.
3. Severe anxiety consumes most of the person's energies and requires intervention. Perception is further decreased. The person, unable to focus on what is really happening, focuses on only one specific detail of the situation generating the anxiety.

4. Panic is an overpowering, frightening level of anxiety causing the person to lose control. It is less frequently experienced than other levels of anxiety. The perception of a panicked person can be affected to the degree that the person distorts events.

Table 19.2: Indicators of anxiety levels

Category		*Level of anxiety*		
	Mild	*Moderate*	*Severe*	*Panic*
Verbalization changes	Increased questioning	Voice tremors and pitch changes	Communication difficult to understand	Communication may not be understandable
Motor activity changes	Mild restlessness Sleeplessness	Tremors, facial twitches, and shakiness Increased muscle tension	Increased motor activity, inability to relax Fearful facial expression	Increased motor activity, agitation. Unpredictable responses
Perception and attention changes	Feelings of increased arousal and alertness Uses learning to adapt	Narrowed focus of attention Able to focus but selectively inattentive Learning slightly impaired	Inability to focus or concentrate Easily distracted Learning severely impaired	Trembling, poor motor coordination Perception distorted or exaggerated Unable to learn or function
Respiratory and circulatory changes	None	Slightly increased respiratory and heart rates	Tachycardia, hyperventilation	Dyspnea, palpitations, choking, chest pain, or pressure
Other changes	None	Mild gastric symptoms (e.g. 'butterflies in the stomach')	Headache, dizziness, nausea	Feeling of impending doom Paresthesia, sweating

ii. Fear. Fear is an emotion or feeling of apprehension aroused by impending or seeming danger, pain, or other perceived threat. The fear may be in response to something that has already occurred, in response to an immediate or current threat, or in response to something the person believes will happen. The object of fear may or not be based in reality. For example, the beginning nursing student may be fearful in anticipation of the first experience in a client care setting. The student may fear that the client will not want to be cared for by the student or that the student might inadvertently harm the client.

iii. Anger. Anger is an emotional state consisting of a subjective feeling of animosity or strong displeasure. People may feel guilty when they feel anger because they have been taught that to feel angry is wrong. However, anger can be expressed in a nonalienating verbal manner; it is then considered a positive emotion and a sign of emotional maturity because growth and beneficial interactions result from it.

A verbal expression of anger can be considered a signal to others of one's internal psychologic discomfort and a call for assistance to deal with perceived stress. In contrast, hostility is usually marked by overt antagonism and harmful or destructive behavior, aggression is an unprovoked attack or a hostile, injurious, or destructive action or outlook; and violence is the exertion of physical force to injure or abuse. Verbally expressed anger differs from hostility, aggression and violence, but it can lead to destructiveness and violence if the anger persists unabated.

A clearly expressed verbal communication of anger, when the angry person tells the other person about the anger and carefully identifies the source, is constructive. This clarity of communication gets the anger out into the open so that the other person can deal with it and help to alleviate it. The angry person 'gets it off the chest' and prevents an emotional buildup.

iv. Depression. Depression is a common reaction to events that seen overwhelming or negative. Depression, an extreme feeling of sadness, despair, dejection, lack of worth, or emptiness, affects millions of Americans a year. The signs and symptoms of depression and the severity of the problem vary with the client and the significance of the precipitating event. Emotional symptoms can include feelings of tiredness, sadness, emptiness or numbness. Behavioral signs of depression include irritability, inability to concentrate, difficulty making decisions, loss of sexual desire, crying, sleep disturbances, and social withdrawal. Physical signs of depression may include loss of appetite, weight loss, constipation, headache, and dizziness. Many people experience short periods of depression in response to overwhelming stressful events, such as the death of a loved one or loss of a job; prolonged depression, however, is a cause for concern and may require treatment.

Unconscious Ego Defense Mechanisms

Unconscious **ego defense mechanisms** are psychologic adaptive mechanisms or, in the words of Sigmund Freud (1946), mental mechanisms that develop as the personality attempts to defend itself, establish compromises among conflicting impulses, and allay inner tensions. Defense mechanisms are the unconscious mind working to protect the person from anxiety. They can be considered precursors to conscious cognitive coping mechanisms that will ultimately solve the problem. Like some verbal and motor responses, defense mechanisms release tension. Table 19.4 describes these mechanisms and lists examples of their adaptive and maladaptive use.

Cognitive Indicators

Cognitive indicators of stress are thinking responses that include problem solving, structuring, self-control or self-discipline, suppression and fantasy. Problem solving

Table 19.3: Examples of the effects of stress on basic human needs

Needs	*Example*
Physiologic	Altered elimination pattern Change in appetite Altered sleep pattern
Safety and security	Expresses nervousness and feelings of being threatened Focuses on stressors, inattention to safety measures
Love and belonging	Isolated and withdrawn Becomes overly dependent Blames others for own problems
Self-esteem	Fails to socialize with others Becomes a workaholic Draws attention to self
Self-actualization	Preoccupied with own problems Shows lack of control Unable to accept reality

Table 19.4: The psychological defense mechanisms	
Defense mechanism and definition	*Example*
Denial refusal to recognize or acknowledge a threatening situation	Keerthi is an alcoholic who denies being an alcoholic
Repression "pushing" threatening or conflicting events or situations out of conscious memory	Kusuma, who was sexually abused as a child, cannot remember the abuse at all
Rationalization making up acceptable excuses for unacceptable behavior	"If I don't have breakfast, I can have that piece of cake later on without hurting my diet"
Projection placing one's own unacceptable thoughts onto others, as if the thoughts belonged to them and not to oneself	Kamala is attracted to her sister's husband but denies this and believes the husband is attracted to her
Reaction formation forming an emotional reaction or attitude that is the opposite of one's threatening or unacceptable actual thoughts	Maruthi is unconsciously attracted to Raju but outwardly voices an extreme hatred of homosexuals
Displacement expressing feelings that would be threatening if directed at the real target onto a less threatening substitute target	Anitha gets reprimanded by her boss and goes home to angrily to pick a fight with her husband
Regression falling back on child-like patterns as a way of coping with stressful situation	Four year old Arun starts wetting his bed after his parents bring home a new baby
Identification trying to become like someone else to deal with one's anxiety	Bharathi really admires Dorothy, the most popular girl in school, and tries to copy her behavior and dress
Compensation (substitution) when a person tries to make up for areas in which a lack is perceived by becoming superior in some other area	Mahesh is not good at athletics, so he puts all of his energies into becoming an academic scholar.
Sublimation turning socially unacceptable urges into socially acceptable behavior	Ajay, who is very aggressive, becomes a professional hockey player

involves thinking through the threatening situation, using specific steps to arrive at a solution. The person assesses the situation or problem, analyzes or defines it, chooses alternatives, carries out the selected alternative, and evaluates whether the solution was successful.

Structuring is the arrangement or manipulation of a situation so that threatening events do not occur. For example, a nurse can structure or control an interview with a client by asking only direct, closed questions. Structuring can be productive in certain situations. A person who schedules a dental examination semiannually to prevent severe dental disease is using productive structuring.

Self-control (discipline) in assuming a manner and facial expression that convey a sense of being in control or in charge. When self-control prevents panic and harmful or nonproductive actions in a threatening situation, it is a helpful response that conveys strength. Self-control carried to an extreme however, can delay problem solving and prevent a person from receiving the support of others, who may perceive the person as handling the situation well, as cold, or as unconcerned.

Suppression is consciously and willfully putting a thought or feeling out of mind: "I won't with today. I'll do it tomorrow". This response relives stress temporarily but does not solve the problem. A man who keeps ignoring a toothache, pushing it out of his mind because he fears the pain of having a filling, will not obtain relief of his symptoms.

Fantasy or daydreaming is likened to make-believe. Unfulfilled wishes and desires are imagined as fulfilled, or a threatening experience is reworked or replayed so that it ends differently from reality. Experiences can be relieved, everyday problems solved and plans for the future made. The outcome of current problems may also be fantasized. For example, a client who is awaiting the results of a breast biopsy may fantasize the surgeon as saying, "You do not have cancer". Fantasy response can be helpful if they lead to problem solving. For example, the client awaiting breast biopsy results might say to herself, "Even if the doctor says, 'You have cancer', as long as he also says it can be treated, I can accept that". Fantasies can be destructive and nonproductive if a person uses them to excess and retreats from reality.

Coping with Stress

Coping may be described as dealing with problems and situations, or contending with them successfully. A coping strategy (coping mechanism) is an innate or acquired way of responding to a changing environment or specific problem or situation. According to Folkman and Lazarus (1991), coping is "the cognitive and behavioral effort to manage specific external and/or internal demands that are appraised as taxing or exceeding the resources of the person".

Two types of coping strategies have been described; problem-focused and emotion-focused coping. Problem-focused coping refers to efforts to improve a situation by making changes or taking some action. Emotion-focused coping includes thoughts and actions that relieve emotional distress. Emotion-focused coping does not improve the situation, but the person often feels better.

Coping strategies are also viewed as long-term or short-term. Long-term coping strategies can be constructive and realistic. For example, in certain situations talking with others about the problem and trying to find out more about the situation are long-term strategies.

Other long-term strategies include those that involve a change in lifestyle patterns such as eating a healthy diet, exercising regularly, balancing leisure time with working, or using problem solving in decision making instead of anger or other nonconstructive responses.

Short-term coping strategies can reduce stress to a tolerable limit temporarily but are in the end ineffective ways to deal with reality. They may even have a destructive or detrimental effect on the person. Examples of short-term strategies are using alcoholic beverages or drugs, daydreaming and fantasizing, relying on the belief that everything will work out, and giving into others to avoid anger.

Coping strategies vary among individuals and are often related to the individuals perception of the stressful event. Three approaches to coping with stress are to alter the stressor, adapt to the stressor, or avoid the stressor. A person's coping strategies often change with a reappraisal of a situation. There is never only one way to cope. Some people choose avoidance; others confront a situation as a means of coping. Still others seek information or rely on religious beliefs as a means of coping.

Coping can be adaptive or maladaptive. Adaptive coping helps the person to deal effectively with stressful events and minimizes distress associated with them. Maladaptive coping can result in unnecessary distress for the person and others associated with the person or stressful event. In nursing literature, effective and ineffective coping are often differentiated. Effective coping results in adaptation, ineffective coping results in maladaptation. Although the coping behavior may not always seem appropriate, the nurse needs to remember that coping is always purposeful.

The effectiveness of an individuals coping is influenced by a number of factors, including:

- The number, duration, and intensity of the stressors.
- Past experiences of the individual.
- Support system available to the individual.
- Personal qualities of the person.

If the duration of the stressors is extended beyond the coping powers of the individual, that person becomes exhausted and may develop increased susceptibility to health problems. Reaction to long-term stress is seen in family members who undertake the care of a person in the home for a long period. This stress is called **caregiver burden** and produces responses such as chronic fatigue, sleeping difficulties, and high blood pressure. Prolonged stress can also result in mental illness. As coping strategies or defense mechanisms (Table 19.4) become ineffective, the individual may have interpersonal problems, work difficulties, and a significant decrease in abilities to meet basic human needs (Table 19.3).

Coping strategies are actions that people can take to master, tolerate, reduce, or minimize the effects of stressors, and they can include both behavioral strategies and psychological strategies.

Problem-focused coping: One type of coping strategy is to work on eliminating or changing the stressor itself. When people try to eliminate the source of a stress or reduce its impact through their own actions, it is called problem-focused coping. For example, a student might have a problem understanding a particular professor. The professor is knowledgeable but has trouble explaining the concepts of the course in a way that this student can understand. Problem-focused coping might include talking to the professor after class, asking fellow students to clarify the concepts, getting a tutor, or forming a study group with other students who are also having difficulty to pool the groups resources.

Emotion-focused coping: Problem-focused coping can work quite well but is not the only method people can use. Most people use both problem-focused coping and emotion-focused coping to successfully deal with controllable stressful events. Emotion-focused coping is a strategy that involves changing the way a person feels or emotionally reacts to a stressor. This reduces the emotional impact of the stressor who is faced with a professor who isn't easy to understand might share his concerns with a friend, talking it through until calm enough to tackle the problem in a more direct manner. Emotion-focused coping also works for stressors that are uncontrollable and for which problem-focused coping is not possible. Someone using emotion-focused coping may decide to view the stressor as a challenge rather than a threat, decide that the problem is a minor one, write down concerns in a journal, or even ignore the problem altogether.

Ignoring a problem is not a good strategy when there is something a person can actively do about solving the problem. But when it is not possible to change or eliminate the stressor, or when worrying about the stressor can be a problem itself, ignoring the problem is not a bad idea. Researchers working with people who had suffered heart attacks found that those people who worried about a future attack were more likely to suffer from symptoms of posttraumatic stress, such as nightmares and poor sleep (both factors that increase the risk of a future heart attack), than were the people who tried to ignore their worries.

Using humor can also be a form of emotion-focused coping, as the old saying "laughter is the best medicine" suggest. A recent study on the effects of laughter found that laughter actually boosted the action of the immune system by increasing the work of natural killer cells (cells that attack viruses in the body). In this study, participants were shown a humor video for one hour. Blood samples were taken 10 minutes before the viewing, 30 minutes into the viewing, 30 minutes after viewing and 12 hours after viewing the humor video. There were significant increase in natural killer cell activity and nearly half and dozen other immune system cells and systems, with some effects lasting the full 12 hours after the video.

Emotion-focused coping is highly related to several forms of psychological defenses first proposed by Sigmund Freud, as the next section discusses.

Psychological defense mechanisms: In Freud's writings on psychoanalysis, he stated that when people experience anxiety (stress) from conflicts between the demands of the body's needs and desires and society's rules for proper behavior, there are certain unconscious distortions of thought that can protect their self from that anxiety. These unconscious distortions of the perception of reality are called psychological defense mechanisms and were further explained by Freud's daughter. Although Freudian theory has fallen in and out of favor over the last century, the concept of these defense mechanisms has remained quite useful in clinical psychology as a way of describing people's defensive behavior and irrational thinking.

Table 19.4 lists, defines, and gives examples of some of the more common defense mechanisms.

It may have become obvious that nearly all of these techniques are forms of emotion-focused coping strategies, although their misuse can easily lead to more problems, as many of Freud's patients discovered.

Unlike much of the rest of Freud's psychoanalytic theory, research in cognitive psychology has uncovered some scientific support for the concept of unconscious coping mechanisms at work when people experience stress. Implicit memory, also called procedural memory, is a form of long-term memory in which habits, skills, conditioned responses, emotional associations, and other well-learned procedures are stored. These memories affect conscious behavior, as in being able to balance on a bicycle, but are not stored in conscious awareness and cannot easily be brought into conscious awareness.

Meditation as a Coping Mechanism

Meditation is a mental series of exercises meant to refocus attention and achieve a trance-like state of consciousness. Meditation can produce a state of relaxation that can aid in coping with the physiological reactions to a stressful situation.

Concentrative Meditation. Have you ever found yourself staring out into space, or at some little spot on the wall or table, only to realize that your mind has been a complete blank for the last several minutes?

The state just described is really nothing more than concentrative meditation, the form of meditation best known to the general public. In concentrative meditation, the goal is to focus the mind on some repetitive or unchanging stimulus (such as a spot or the sound of one's own heart beating) so that the mind can forget daily hassles and problems and the body can relax. In fact, Benson found that meditation produces a state of relaxation in which blood pressure is lowered, alpha waves (brain waves associated with relaxation) are increased, and the amounts of melatonin secreted at night (the hormone that helps induce sleep) are increased.

Some people say that if you meditate for only twenty minutes a day, you don't have to sleep at night. The would be nice—think how much more could be accomplished with those extra hours. Unfortunately, although certain meditation groups to make some rather wild claims for meditation, research has shown none of them to be true. What research does show is that concentrative meditation is a good way to relax and lower blood pressure in adolescents and adults, men and women. It isn't the only way, as reading a good book or taking a warm bath also produces relaxation. Even simply resting for the same amount of time as one might meditate can be just as relaxing. The advantage of meditation is that people can do it almost anywhere, even in the classroom just before a big test. (It would be a little difficult to take a warm bath then).

Receptive meditation. The other kind of meditation is less well known and not as easily achieved. It is called receptive meditation and involves trying to expand consciousness outward. The best description of what this is like to think about a time when you were overawed by nature. Perhaps you were standing at the ocean's edge on a starry night and became suddenly aware of how vast the universe really is. Or perhaps you were walking in the woods and listening to all the little sounds of the birds and animals surrounding you. Your attention was focused outward rather than inward, and this is similar to the state that this type of meditation tries to achieve.

The effects of meditation: Regardless of which form of meditation people choose to try, the effects are similar. Meditation for only 20 minutes can produce lowered blood pressure in people with hypertension (high blood pressure). It can calm anxiety help people get to sleep, and help people deal with stress.

Mental health professionals should make an effort to include an assessment of a person's cultural background as well as immediate circumstances when dealing with adjustment problems due to stress.

Religion Beliefs as a Source of Coping

A belief in a higher power can also be a source of great comfort in times of stress. There are several ways that religious beliefs can affect the degree of stress people experience and the ability to cope with that stress.

First, most people who hold strong religious beliefs belong to a religious organization and attend regular religious functions, such as services at a synagogue, mosque, temple or church. This membership can be a vital part of a person's social support system. People do not feel alone in their struggle, both literally because of the people who surround them in their religious community and spiritually because of the intangible presence of their deity.

Another way that religion helps people cope involves the rituals and rites that help people feel better about personal weaknesses, failures, or feelings of inadequacy. These include rituals such as confession of sins or prayer services during times of stress. Finally religious beliefs can give meaning to things that otherwise seem to have no meaning or purpose, such as viewing death as a pathway to a paradise, or the destruction of one's home in a natural disaster as a reminder to place less attachment on material things.

Many religions also encourage healthy behavior and eating habits through their prohibitions on such activities as overeating, drinking alcohol, smoking, drug use, and sexual activity outside marriage. Some research even suggests that people with religious commitments live longer than those who have no such beliefs, although this is correlational research and should not be interpreted as concluding that religious belief causes longer life expectancies.

When stress there is tremendous pressure. The person becomes totally dysfunctional. All of us have to be well-versed with the coping mechanisms of managing stress, both preventive as well as intervention measures as per our need, aptitude and capacity. They have to be made part of our life style, otherwise nonstop can act as a killer in terms of stress, so the milliondollar questions are: how to change thinking and attitudes and how to shape behaviors? This editorial addresses these two questions. The approach are not absolute in nature. Their application varies from individual to individual. Considering one's idiosyncracies, each person may choose those mechanisms which are compatible to his or her personality profile.

Coping Mechanisms for Cognitive Approach

The coping mechanisms for cognitive approach suggested are:

Accept death as basic existential condition: Fear of inevitable. Treat it as an opportunity for growth. Though physical death finished us but the idea of death can serve as a driving force to act and add meaning to living. We can choose to be creative and usefull to our society during span of being in this world.

Carve out a meaning of life: We are born in a meaningless world. You are the one to attach a meaning to your life. Decide on yours aims and ambitions. Decide on ideals of your life within a given cultural setting and even beyond depending on your strength. Think divergently. Living without meaning will lead you to a futility syndrome. Life is like a flowing stream. Its flow will stop if you don't contribute in your own way to it. No absolute meaning can be attached to life. Meaning is relative and subjective. You explore your inner core, decide on your ideals and work towards seeing them gratified.

Realize that stress is in-build in life: Stress cannot be eliminated from life. Take preventive measures. All of us have got to learn to manage stress. Be prepared to face at least ten stressors everyday. View death as an eventuality. Take it as a positive indicator leading to growth and creativity. Live for every moment. Life is a paradox. We have to plan for future and yet live in here and now.

Practice stress incolution: It is a psychological and behavioral analogue to immunization on biological level. It includes three phases: Educational Phases: Understand the ways in which you respond to stressful situations. Rehearsal Phases: Acquire and rehearse new set of thoughts. Application Phase: Get into relaxation, self rewards, discussion and problem solving.

Indulge in cognitive restructuring: What you say to yourself directly influences the things you do. Self statements effect a person's behavior as much as statements made by others. Become aware of your self talk and your inner speech. Modify your negative self talk to positive self talk. If you say to yourself that you are dull, you will start behaving in a dull fashion and if you say to yourself that you are intelligent, you will behave intelligently. Self-statements work like self-hypnosis.

Dispute irrational beliefs: Situations, people and events are not a source of stress. Perceptions and irrational beliefs lead to stress. So confronting/disputing the irrational beliefs and substituting them by positive and rational beliefs reduce stress. Others will not change. You have to change your reactions. Empower yourself. Take control of everything in your life. Do not let loose your ownership. Believe, you can change the whole world. "Stand up, be strong, take the whole responsibility on your shoulders, and know that you are the creator of your own destiny."

Use positive imagery: Healthy imagery and daydreaming help in reducing stress. So, use positive imagery as a stress relieving mechanism. Engage in it to the extent that it does not make you dysfunctional. You can imagine yourself doing challenging task with positive results. It makes you feel good and can help in operationalizing the things which appear beyond your control or impossible.

Listen to your feelings: Feeling is the core of existence. Pay attention to your inner feelings and needs. Do not ignore them. Never suppress them. Make efforts to gratify them. In case you are not able to actualize them, work on them, sublimate them. If you do not, then the result will be frustration and irritability. Suppressing feelings means snowballing them. Regular introspection can be helpful weeping to an extent in private can be therapeutic. Sharing can be good if the other person demonstrates empathy and ensure confidentiality.

Accept responsibility for yourself: All of us must take a responsible stance in work situation as well as personal life. Do not get into the trap of passing on the buck to others. Pat unfortunate events/experiences of life and situations should not be carried along one must shun learned helplessness. Focus on here and now. Make choices and be ready for consequences. People with habitual routine of shirking responsibility have learnt to select a life style in which others can be maneuvered to take responsibility. Such people tend to blame others for their failures."

Accept that you are not in control of the world: Events and people will not follow the course of action you want. Events are beyond your control. Attempts to change people and events is self-defeating. Accept what you cannot change, rather change yourself. Follow " I am okay, you are okay" approach; rather than "your are okay, I am okay" approach. Delete "the other must do", "the other should not be unfair to me", "why me" type of internal dialogues from your personal dictionary of beliefs and values. Unfair things will happen in life. What worst could have happened to the mythological legends like Ram and Sita in Ramayana.

Stop perfectionist attitude: Do not accept mediocrity in your life. Make success as your goal and not perfection. Perfection is like a bachelor's wife. Achieve as per your ability and situational constraints. Accept that you may not be the best. There can be better performers than you. Give them credit. Realize the fact that one cannot get everything in life.

Coping Mechanisms for Behavior Approach

Plan and organization your life and work: Set your goals/objectives and make decisions: define your personalized goals in terms of being: meaningful, measurable, realistic, deciding on 5Wh's; who, why, when , where, what and how well? Develop steps to reach the defined goal—primary, secondary and check steps. Learn to make decisions about how to use time, energy and other resources required in actualization of your goals and objectives. Learn to take risks and manage them.

Management of time: Set priorities. Complete one assignment at a time. Limit telephone calls. Regulate visitors. Stop unnecessary repetitive activities. Limit meetings. Organize and reorganize your work and home environment. Avoid procrastinations. Make weekly and monthly time management schedules. Hang it in front of a place where you can see it conveniently. Get out of your routine one day a week. Good time management enhances performance and reduces stress. Reverse is also true. It is well known that the most busy person has time at his disposal because he knows managing time.

Be assertive: Learn to say NO. Assertion is a form of appropriate behavior—direct, hones and concrete expression of emotions, beliefs, needs and feelings. Learn the difference between assertions, aggression and passiveness. Accept and identify your personal rights and rights of other person. Reduce obstacles to acting assertively like irrational thinking, excessive anxiety or guilt or negative self talk. Develop assertive skills through active practice methods. Avoid bipolar approaches—passiveness and aggression.

Act as a problem solver: Look to say problem objectively. Own responsibility. Make choices. Prepare in advance for expected consequences of your choice. The solution may not be the best, choose the second best or the third best as per the personal, situational, time and other constraints. Do act with mental coolness. Critically and systematically locate the problem, define the problem and cause and effect relationship, find and examine alternate solutions to the problem, choose and implement one or more of these solutions, organize an action plan into a sequence of specific action steps, establish a definite time limit and dates for completing each step, announce publicly your commitment to the action plan among the "significant others", development check points to measure the progress, reinforce/reward yourself for making progress, act here and now and evaluate the results of the chosen solution.

Music/Lyrics therapy: Listening to music may depends on the aptitude and receptivity of an individual. Those with such personality types can get benefited both by the rhythm and harmony of classical/semiclassical music as well as by the lyrics which contain deeper meaning of life and also many times, the answers to various questions of life. Meaningful lyrics directly penetrate into the mind and heart leading to positive mental programming. The act of singing goes many steps further. It is a physical exercise in terms of respiratory involvement and a mental exercise as well. It can also be quite useful in terms of acting as a pranayama, a breathing exercise and also as a medicine for emotional ailments. Music relaxes and calms you. It elevates you to the state of happiness. Music works as an effective therapy. Total indulgence in it generates a feeling of oneness with the Divine: a state of peace and bliss. Cultivate the habit of listening to good lyrics and music. Learn it seek training from an expert.

Laughter therapy: Laughter therapy and humor create relaxation and reduce stress. Laughter and humor act as cathartic medicine to cope with and cure emotional and psychological set-backs. Laughter works as an effective muscle exercise. It is known as internal jogging. Laughter takes you to a higher level of consciousness leaving no scope for stress. Once your mind is free, it enhances creativity.

Take time off your leisure/sublimate energies: Engage regularly in leisure/physical exercises. Sublimate your energies. Get out of your office and home at reasonable breaks. Raise your activity level. Develop and groom your hobbies and interest. Take time off for yourself and your family from your phone routine monotonous work and domestic life. Uses your time management skills for fixing up the slots for such activities. Schedule it in your time management 'to do list'. Visit your close friends, relatives and significant others at some convenient time.

Take nutritious diet and develop proper sleep habits: Develop proper food and sleep habits. They promote physical psychological well being. Quality of diet and proper sleep improve health they enhance physical and mental energy. Choose and take your food thoughtfully. Concentrate on the details of the act. Enjoy your food. Gradually eliminate "Rajasic" and "Tamasic" food habits. Cultivate the food habits, which enhance. "Sathwic" Temperament.

Develop interpersonal communication skills: Interpersonal skills enhance self-esteem. These skills make you a good communicator, helping to have a better self-image. They enrich your social, professional, personal life. Interpersonal skill deficits cause inferiority complex. These reinforce social avoidance and withdrawal. It has a negative impact on professional venture/assignments and personal life. Grooming one's interpersonal skills is absolutely essential for performance in all walks of life. Practice and perfect your interpersonal skills.

Dress up neatly and smartly: Physical appearance reinforce confidence. You feel important and strong. It strengthens your interpersonal skills. Observing hygiene, dressing up pleasantly and smartly is essential for upholding one's sense of well being. Identify the most striking aspects of your physical personality. Take it as your strength. Develop it further. Seek feedback. Focus on it. Nurture it.

Cultivate and mobilize group support: Individuals are basically alone in this world. Yet they have opportunity to relate to other people. People are concerned about preserving their identity, but at the same time strive for connectedness with others. One of the most important elements in managing stress is utilization of a good support system. Supportive relationships are those marked by warmth, empathy and care. Support systems help us to manage stress at least in distinct ways. They give us emotional support. Simply knowing that others understand our situations, care for us and respect our problems provides us a lot of strength. It provides a platform for consensual validation.

Build on spiritual strength/ intelligence: Individuals have an option available to begin the process of developing a spiritual temperament or health, which can be adopted to neutralize the stress. The objective here is to evolve certain spiritual practices from the rich spiritual heritage for our growth and psychological well being. One has to make the choice! It is only the spiritual knowledge, says, Swami Vivekananda, that eternally destroys the miseries of life. Any other knowledge leads to temporary satisfaction of wants. Danah (2002) considers "Spiritual Intelligence", thus assumes a lot of significance. It develop confidence, control, clarity and meaning in every action. Sinha (2004) has identified some indicator of spiritual intelligence like flexibility, self-awareness, an ability to use and face suffering, a tendency to **Music and Lyrics elevates you to a state of Bliss** probe and as fundamental questions, the ability to be inspired by a vision, ability to work against convention, ability to see connection between diverse things, thinks holistically, a desire and capacity to cause as little harm as passive. Spiritual intelligence is reported to enhance creativity. Gradual and rigorous cultivation of values of working with detachment and training self in the control of ego is considered fundamental in Indian spiritual thought. *"Without attachment perform ever the work to be done, doing work without attachment, man indeed attains to the higher. He who abandoning all desires lives and moves without any longings, free from the sense of I or mine, attains to peace."* Bhagavad Gita. We have been taught in our spiritual culture that ego struggles and attachments are the roots of stress. It is not a child's play to eliminate them, because they are inbuilt in human system. However their limits can be consciously kept under check and reduced with gradual efforts. Attempts can be certainly made in this direction by changing our beliefs and following certain practices. To begin with, we need to restructure our cognitions by changing our views about creation, existence and internalize our role in it. Combined with these is the role of **faith** in the Divine and **prayer** which is therapeutic in nature. These heal us eternally. Stress can be a **Motivator** in terms of performance. Individuals have to make a choice.

20

CHAPTER

Attitude, Will and Character

Introduction

Attitudes are derived primarily from social influences. From birth, the human being is enmeshed in social influences. From birth, the human being is enmeshed in social institutions which constitute his environment in the same sense as the physical world. The home, being the primary social unit, has a great influence on the formation of one's attitudes. This is why later experiences cannot easily alter these attitudes. This is also the reason why attitudes gives a consistency to our responses to persons, groups, and other social objects.

The main aim of education is to modify the behavior of the child according to the needs and expectancy of the society. Behavior is composed of so many attributes. One of these important attributes is attitude toward the things idea, person, or object, in this environment. The entire personality and development of the child is influenced by habits, interests and other psychophysical disposition are all affected by his attitudes. Therefore it is important for a teacher to understand the meaning and nature of attitudes, the factors responsible for their formation and development and techniques of their measurement. In the foregoing pages we will try to understand the above aspects.

Attitude is a bent mind, predisposition of certain actions. It is a process by which the individuals learn as a result of experience to orient themselves towards objectives and goals. Attitude is associated with physical neural state, verbal opinion, ideologies and above all integrated philosophy of life. Attitude is the detailed direction of human behavior. Attitude is a stage of sensitiveness and proneness to act. Attitudes can be defined as readiness to acts; mental posture, guide for conduct; feelings, desires, fears, convictions; a state of readiness; a set of organism as a whole; a cumulative perception; predisposition to form certain opinions; thinking one develops a kind of mental set; a tendency process of individual consciousness; a precondition of behavior; precondition of behavior in various degrees of readiness; frame of references that influence behavior.

There are four phases of totality of human behavior: (1) Overt symbolic (speaking, writing, etc.), (2) Overt nonsymbolic (direct muscular act like closing a door, running, etc.), (3) Covert symbolic (thought), (4) Covert nonsymbolic (feeling and emotions). It is only the overt stage (symbolic or nonsymbolic) that can be analyzed. As regards the covert phases of behavior, what any person is actually feeling and thinking cannot be measured and is still anybody' s guess. It is in the light of this distinction that so much controversy as to the nature and measurability of genuine behavior tendencies (attitudes) has risen. For example in the quotation of Shakespeare "One might smile and smile and yet be a villan" it is not simply a case of double thinking but a case of double living as well. Even within the sphere of covert behavior (as in the case of opinion response to verbalized social situations) is not identical with overt nonsymbolic behavior (the actual behavior in an actual life situation).

The concept of attitudes is a hypothetical postulate which implies a broad-based behavior tendency in individuals towards a psychosocial object which precedes on and over behavior. Attitudes have to analyzed in the light of the broad-based pattern of real life situations to which they are related. Attitude cannot be directly observed, but only through inference, as real and substantial ingredients in human nature, it becomes impossible to account satisfactorily either for the consistency of an individuals' behavior or for the stability of any society.

Attitude can be measured through schedules and questionnaires termed as quantitative method. There are three principle sources of data which help in attitude research. These are: (1) Background information such as biographies, case histories, letters, etc. (2)Interviews, (3) Questionnaires, etc. Attitudes are formed through experience which means that they are learnt. Once a person has developed a particular attitude, it may be difficult for him to determine considerations or strong emotional bias has little bearing on the effect or the attitudes on the particular attitude, it may be difficult for him to determine how he acquired it. Once an attitude is formed whether based on rational considerations or strong emotional bias has little bearing on the effect or the attitudes on the person's thinking or behavior.

Definition and Nature of Attitude

Attitudes is a specific mental state of the individual towards something according to which his behavior towards it is moulded. For example, due to difference in the respective attitudes of the Muslims and the Hindus towards cow-slaughter, their behavior towards the cow differs. The nature of attitude will be further clarified by the following definitions:

1. GW Allport (1935) defined an attitude as a "Mental and neural state of readiness, organized through experience, exerting a directive or dynamic influence upon the individual's response to all objects and situations with which it is related". He looked upon attitude primarily as asset to respond in a particular way. He observes, "There is a common thread running through these diverse definitions. Reflexes, unlike attitudes, are more specific, habits are more specific but invariably automatic, instincts are innate and universal as against attitudes, which are acquired and personal. Sentiments are more permanent and hierarchical organized through experience exerting a dynamic influence upon the individuals' response to all situations and objects with which it is related."
He defines common attitudes as " Those attitudes which are uniform owing to the operation of similar environmental and cultural conditions upon similarly constituted beings. Physical environment and culture provide cooperation in the production of common attitudes."

"Social attitudes are individual attitudes directed towards social object and individual attitudes strongly interconditioned by collective or groups contacts" (Bernard).

"An attitude is a mental and neural set of readiness, exerting a directive dynamic influence upon the individual's response to all objects and situations with which it is related". This definition reveals the following facts concerning attitude—

a. Attitude is the mental or neural state of readiness
b. Attitude influences the reactions of the individual
c. Attitude changes the reactions of the individuals.

An attitude is an enduring system that includes a cognitive component, a feeling component and an action tendency. Attitudes involve an emotional component. This is why when an attitude is formed it becomes resistant to change; it does not generally respond to the facts. An attitude involves beliefs as well as evaluations. The upper caste man has an unfavorable attitude towards lower caste. The Indian has an unfavorable attitude toward the Pakistanis. These attitudes involve some knowledge about the other groups (the cognitive component), some feeling of dislike (the affective, evolutional component) and a predisposition to avoid, attack, etc. (the action component).

2. Travers defined "An attitude is a readiness to respond in such a way that behavior is given a certain direction".

Accordingly attitude is responsible for behaving in a particular and definite way. If one keeps a positive and favorable attitude toward an object, he will be attracted towards it, he will admire it and try to achieve it. On the other hand if one has a negative or unfavorable attitude one will try to avoid it and even feel hostile to it. For example, a person having positive attitude towards democracy will respond positively to democratic practices and institutions and negatively to authoritarian procedures. His behavior will speak out of his attitude.

3 Mckeachie and Dayle: Defined "an attitude as an organization of concepts, beliefs, habits and motives associated with a particular object".

This definition takes into account all of the concepts, beliefs, habits and motives associated with the object. The concepts and beliefs associated with an attitude are often referred to as the cognitive component of the attitude, the habit as the action component, and the motives as the effective component. In this way all what one thinks, feels and how does he react expresses one's attitude towards an object. For example, if we take attitude toward a political party, the formation of favorable or unfavorable attitude will be the result of his thinking and feeling towards that party and it will be exhibited overtly through some act tendencies like heated discussion with associates or strangers, casting a vote in favor of the party candidate or doing active party work during the election campaign.

4. Sorenson: Defined "An attitude is a particular feeling about something. It therefore involves a tendency to behave in a certain way in situation which involve something, whether person, idea or subject. It is partially rational and partially emotional and is acquired, not inherent, in an individual.

The definition explains why an individual behaves in a certain way when he is needed to respond to a particular object for which he has developed a positive or negative attitude. He has some what a definite set of feelings, likes or dislikes for that object which partly stands on rational and partly on emotional footings. But in all cases, they are acquired and learned through varying experiences. One's attitude towards one's religion is an acquired tendency or disposition. He is not born with enthusiasm or apathy for this particular religion. He has developed a sort of attachment or favorable feeling towards his religion due to his own experiences from his early childhood. His feeling is partly rational and partly emotional. He may be able to give very good reasons for advocating and appreciating his religion but their basis is partly beneath conscious reasoning.

5. Whittaker: Defined "An attitude is a predisposition or readiness to respond in a predetermined manner to relevant stimuli".

This definition accepts attitude as a predisposition or tendency to behave in a particular and definite way to a particular situation. One's attitude decides one's response to a particular stimulus. For example in responding to all stimuli related with the congress party one has a predisposition or tendency to act in a certain way if one has developed an attitude towards that party.

In this way attitudes are, to a great extent, responsible for the particular behavior of a person about an object, idea or person. But by this conclusion it should not be taken that one's behavior is an absolute function of one's attitude. Behavior by all means is a function of both characteristics of the behaving person and the situations in which he behaves. Hence a person may hold strong attitude and yet, under certain circumstances may behave in quite contradictory to those attitudes. In this way one's behavior towards object related to a particular attitude cannot be safely predicted through that attitude but it can be safely said that it makes the individual respond in a particular way to the particular stimuli.

Therefore, we may understand attitude as a determining acquired tendency which prepares a person to behave in a certain way toward a specific object or class of object subjects to the conditions prevailing in the environment.

6. Kimball Young (1951) defined "An attitude may be defined as a learned and more or less generalized and affective tendency or predisposition to respond in a rather persistent and characteristic manner, usually positively or negatively (for or against) in reference to some situation, idea, value, material object or class of such objects or person or group of persons." The definition of attitude improves upon the definition by Allport in this respect that it introduces the following two elements omitted by Allport:

a. Attitude is generally negative or positive
b. Attitude is a learned or acquired affective tendency.

7. Krech and Crutchfield defined "An attitude, as an enduring organization of motivational, emotional, perceptual and cognitive processes with respect to some aspect of the individuals world." This definition is a specific attempt at the analysis and an exposure of the various elements present in it. In this way, Newcomb has written, "An expression of preference is not an attitude but a motive pattern". Hence in an attitude the processes of motivation, emotion, perception and thought are present. Newcomb writes, "Attitudes are defined in terms of susceptibility to the arousal of motives and not to the carrying out of a particular motive pattern. An individual's attitude towards something is his predisposition to perform, perceive, think and feel in relation to it. From this definitions, it is evident that attitude is a mental or neural set of readiness, system or disposition in which the motivational, affective, perceptual and thought processes are included and due to which the individual's positive or negative activity is directed to the objects, individuals and groups surrounding him.

Characteristics of Attitudes

Attitudes are predisposition of determining tendency to respond in a specified manner. Now the questions arise, should all the predispositions like habits, interests, traits and physiological motives be classified as attitudes? The answer is no. For a more clear distinction an attitude should meet the following criteria:

1. **Attitudes have a subject-object relationship:** Attitudes always involve the relation of the individual to specific objects, persons, groups, institutions and values or norms related to his environment.
2. **Attitudes are learned:** Attitudes as pointed out earlier are learned and acquired dispositions. They are not innate and inherent in an individual. Consequently they may be differentiated from physiological motives. Hunger for example, is an unlearned physiological motive, while preference for a particular food, an acquired tendency, is classified as an attitude. Again, while almost, any suitable member of the opposite sex may satisfy a man's sexual need, when the need becomes attached to a particular person, the attachment (acquired).
3. **Attitudes are relatively enduring states of readiness:** Attitudes represent the states of readiness to respond to a certain stimulus. Physiological motives also do the same. But in their case like hunger and sexual tension the states of readiness disappear for a period when they are gratified. Attitudes, on the other hand, are relatively enduring states of readiness. Consequently, a wife may hold affective attraction to her husband even after the sexual tension has been resolved.
4. **Attitudes have motivational-affective characteristics:** Attitudes have definite motivational characteristics. Other dispositions like habit of writing with right hand do not have any motivational or affective quality; but attitudes toward one's family, nation, religion or other sacred and hallowed institutions have definite motivational affective characteristics.
5. **Attitudes are numerous and varied as the stimuli to which they refer:** We may have a number of attitudes depending upon the number of stimuli to which we respond. Attitude is an implicit response, therefore it stands to be varied with the number and variety of the responses which the individual makes. The changes in environment and the situations further brings variety in the expression of these attitudes. Therefore it is correct to say that attitudes are as numerous as the objects towards which they are directed and the situations in which they are expressed.
6. **Attitudes range from strongly positive to strongly negative:** Attitudes involve direction as well as magnitude. When a person shows some tendency to approach an object he is said to have positive attitude towards it but he when shows tendency to avoid the object, his attitude is described as negative. These positive or negative attitudes may involve intense feelings and vary from the large negative values to the increasingly positive.

The major characteristics of attitude are the following:

1. *Attitude are related with images, thoughts and external objects:* Attitudes are related with images, thoughts and external objects. For example, upon hearing of the Chinese attack on Indian territory, every Indian national developed a negative attitude towards the Chinese aggressors. In this attitude is involved the thought that in attacking India the Chinese have made a most unjustified and immoral move. In this attitude, some imaginary concepts concerning the Chinese aggressors are present in the mind of the individual and these are based upon this knowledge of the Chinese attack. The mental attitude is further influenced by some external objects. Because of this attitude, the individuals is persuaded to contribute his entire wealth to the national defence fund in order to help to expel the aggressor from the country. The relation of the attitude to thoughts, images and external objects is evident from this example.

2. *Attitude are directive for specific direction:* Attitudes guides the behavior of the individual in one particular direction. In the foregoing example which illustrated the nature of attitude, it was seen that due to there being a negative attitude towards the Chinese aggressors the individual was prepared to do his best to help the Indian soldiers who were fighting them. In this way, the behavior of an individual can be predicted if there is knowledge of his attitude towards the Chinese attack. Since attitudes direct the activities of the individual, his reaction can be predicted, by knowing his attitudes.
3. *Affective experience attitude with attitudes:* Various kinds of affective experiences are also attached to attitudes. In the foregoing example may be seen attached emotions of anger, displeasure and sometimes hatred to the attitude of the Indian individuals towards the Chinese attack.
4. *Importance of the unconscious in the creation of attitude:* The unconscious motive is an important factor in the creation of attitudes. Sometimes even the individual himself is unaware of the motives for his attitude towards a particular person or object because in fact the motive is in his unconscious.
5. *Relation between the individual's needs and problems:* Attitudes are related to the person's needs and problems. When China attacked India (1962), every Indian was faced with economic, political and other problems which thereby became all the more glaring. This led to a very direct interference in the fulfillment of his day to day needs since it is only natural for the populace to suffer many hardships. In this way, being related to needs and problems a negative attitude towards the Chinese is developed in the minds of the Indian people.

ANATOMY OF ATTITUDE

All attitudes are not alike in their structure. They differ from one another in a number of characteristics. Attitudes develop in the process of need satisfaction. Individual develops favorable attitudes towards object and belief that satisfy his wants. The individual will develop unfavorable attitude towards objects and person that block the achievement of his goal. The attitudes of the individual are not only developed by satisfaction of wants but also shared by information to which the individual is exposed. The information is frequently used to form attitudes which are in consonant with pre-existing relation attitudes. Many attitudes held by people lack validity, simply because they are not sufficiently will informed. No individual can help to collect all the first hand information and the essential affects about most of the objects. He has to necessarily depend on the opinion of the experts. For a child, experts are his parents; for a student, the teachers; for the writers, the books; for the religious persons, the pundit or priests; for scientists, the findings of the other scientist in their field, etc. Individual is living in a complex world and is at the mercy of various experts and authorities for much of his cognitive content and his attitudes. Thus authorities of experts are sometimes unreliable. At times, the individual himself is unschooled in extracting substance or because of his perception he picks up a fact by himself and runs the risk of being fooled. Finally when he does not find facts either from authorities and experts or from his first hand information he may invent facts by himself and develop an irregular attitude.

PHYSIOLOGY OF ATTITUDES

People have attitudes towards social objects because they (a) help them to organize, simplify and understand the world around them, (b) protect their self-esteem, by avoiding unpleasant truths about themselves, and (c) allow them to express their fundamental values (Triandis, 1971). To these three functions must be added a fourth one, that they help them to conform to the group and thus maximize rewards from the group. Thus attitudes help us to adjust our environment. Once a social object has been categorized, it is possible to react to it in the manner typical of the group to which we belong. This saves us from a fresh decision and all its difficulties and problems. It helps to behave in a smooth manner.

Smith et al (1956) have pointed out that one of the functions of attitudes is to provide "externalization" to some inner problems. The man with unresolved inner conflicts and frustrations can direct his hatred towards the out groups. This is one reason why "agitational" approach to social and political problems is more in vogue in India today than the "constitutional" approach. Even the members of the legislature and the parliament take recourse to agitations whether in favor of prohibition or against cow slaughter. Language problems, border problems, river-water sharing problems and so on have been providing endless opportunities to the political leaders to start agitations to overthrow the duly constituted governments.

Katz (1960) discussed four functions that attitudes perform for the personality: (a) the adjustment function helps to maximize the rewards and minimize the penalties, by agreeing with the majority attitude; (b) ego-defensive functions are served by enabling the individual from acknowledging uncomplimentary basic truths about himself; when a person does not get selected for a job he will say that only people with "influence" get jobs these days, though he may himself have asked some legislator or minister to ring up somebody in the selection committee; (c) value-expressive functions are involved when the expression of the attitudes gives pleasure to the person since they reveal the values he cherishes as, for example, vegetarianism or prohibition; and (d) knowledge functions based on the individuals need to give structure to his universe, to understand it.

Two Major Dimensions of Attitudes

These are two major dimensions (Fig. 20.1) underlie behavior toward any kind of attitude object: (a) positive *vs.* negative affect and (b) seeking *vs.* avoiding contact (Triandis).

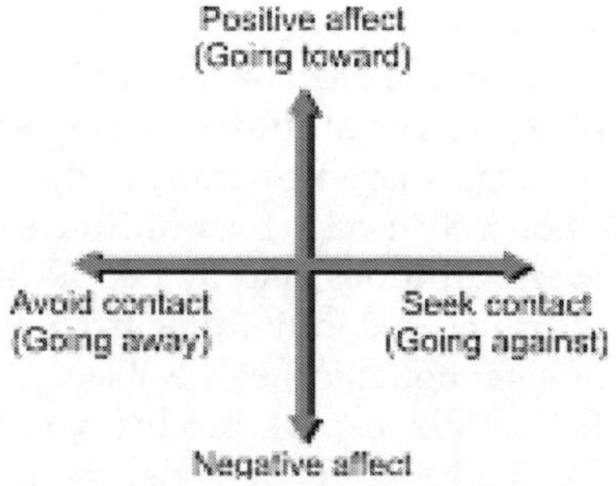

Fig. 20.1: Dimension of attitude

A positive attitude will make a person sacrifice himself to the loved object as in patriotism, for example. A negative attitude may make a person to destroy the government property like the bus or tram or post office. There is seeking contact towards an object with positive affect as in embracing the beloved; there is also seeking contact towards an object with negative affect like in stabbing a person. Thus, when there is seeking contact with positive affect it is "going toward" and when there is seeking contact with negative affect it is "going against". When there is avoiding contact with negative affect there is the behavior of "going away". As an illustration of avoiding contact toward an object with positive affect may be given the behavior of a person towards one whom he reveres; for example, the youth who is fired by zeal with respect to the "Sarvodaya" movement may develop a great reverence to the Sarvodaya leader, Vinoba Bhave; he has a positive affect towards him, but he would not like to go near him; he may stand at a distance and look at him. However, most of our behavior will be along the three types, namely, going toward, going against and going away; the fourth type of avoiding contact with an object with positive affect is rare.

Role of Attitude in Behavior

Individual behavior is a function of internal force such as personality, attitudes and motivation. The attitude of the individual is changed or modified by the information to which he is exposed. Many of the attitudes of individuals lack validity because of their being ill informed and having inadequate information so as to represent the essential facts. Attitude is a complex thing consisting of several components such as intellectual, cognitive, feeling of emotional components, etc.

Attitude is a predisposition directed toward some object or individuals or group of people or the organization. All attitudes are not alike in their structure and they differ in number of characteristics. Changing the attitudes of the people is neither easy nor necessarily rewarding because everyone seeks consistency. We want our beliefs and actions to be concurrent with each other and we feel uncomfortable if they are not. Attitudes have intellectual, emotional and action tendencies and people strive for consistency among them. Attitudes tend to be stable and an integral part of individuals which make it difficult to change. For successful attitude change it is necessary to ensure all three components to change.

Attitudes cannot be changed by mere advising. They cannot be changed by training either. Attitude can be changed or modified by education. This is a long range process that takes into account the whole man, goals, fears habits, history and concepts of individuals about himself. This type of education can be termed as counseling. Change of attitude is man-centered rather than work-centered. It aims at the source rather than result of performance. In an industry very few people make good counselors or educators. A good manager should use every opportunity to counsel, to integrate his subordinates, to develop insight. Counseling cannot be restricted to any special time or place it is a long range and educational process.

Behavior sciences gives us an idea about productivity, positive attitude, positive outlook toward life. In fact, the success or failures in any area is caused by mental attitudes than by mental capacities. The core of positive outlook is to regard life as worth living. The individuals who regard life as meaningless are not only unfortunate but disqualified and unfit in life. The positive living is to change negative attitude to positive one and also confusion to clear thinking, defeat to victory, failure to achievement, frustrations to gratification, hesitation to decision, loneliness to friendship, pessimism to optimism, suppression to fulfillment.

Positive attitude can make an individual stronger and negative attitude weaker. Transactional analysis reveals that people can change. The will to change requires lot of patience and efforts in order to achieve the change. Positive thinking is a continuous process of maturity learning. Maturity means ability to learn and read the life situations. A matured man is never a shirker, never a parasite but cooperative and sincere in the attainment of objectives.

Attitudes have motivational origins. Studies have shown that employees with favorable attitudes are more productive than employees with less favorable attitudes. Studies at brought out information that there seems to be a consistent pattern of relationship between attitudes and opinion on one hand and actual job performance on the other hand.

Attitudes are the motivating forces behind man's social behavior. It is because of attitudes that the individual's behavior exhibits consistency and system. In the absence of a permanent organization the individual would be a new person in every situation. His behavior will be organized only by the immediate pattern of stimuli and his economic needs. But because the individual possessed some or the other attitude towards every person and object his behavior is marked by a continuity. For example, if an individual has a negative attitude towards communism he will always be seen opposing the communist party. But while having beliefs opposed to the communist thought the individual may not indulge in any antagonistic activity. In the same way, when it is felt that the people have a positive attitude towards the governments plan it may be expected that they will do their best in the way of cooperating with the government. Having formed an attitude the individual may come to an instantaneous decision in any matter and he need not contemplate every time.

Social attitudes play an important part in directing man's social behavior. Man's behavior is influenced by his beliefs, assumptions and decisions. And these are affected by the individual's attitude towards different persons and objects. They are the motivating forces. Hence it is only natural for the individual's social behavior to be influenced by these attitudes.

Attitude and belief are fairly intimately related. To put it in the words of Kerch and Crutchfield, "A belief is an enduring organization of percepts and cognitions about some aspect of individual's world. A person's beliefs are not always scientific because beliefs are formulated on opinions even without knowledge although knowledge is helpful in the formulation of beliefs. Beliefs can be real as well as imagined or unreal. Sometimes even faith is the basis of belief, in cases where the individual believes even when any favorable evidence is not forthcoming. When any attitude is based on belief. In the individuals social behavior the greater influence is caused by attitudes because they are the actual motives of behavior. There is no question of a belief being in favor of or against an individual or object. Only attitudes are in favor or against. For example, in India one comes across many people who harbor a favorable opinion for communist philosophy while many others are antagonistic to it. On the other hand, knowing and accepting that the earth is round is a matter of belief and there may be no question of a favorable or unfavorable opinion.

The child develops in a social environment. In this social environment he gains the experience of different objects, individuals, institutions and associations, etc. With differing experiences he formulates different types of attitudes towards them. In this development of attitudes there is some contribution of beliefs, decision and assumptions. In this manner, by the time he attains adulthood, his attitudes become quite firm and these also direct his social behavior. In this way, it is evident that social attitudes play an important role in social behavior. Hence, the social behavior of the individual is better understood if prefaced by an understanding of these social attitudes. But there is also a limit to the accurate prediction of the social behavior of the individual on the basis of the knowledge of his social attitudes because, for one, it is difficult to know an attitude in it's entirely and secondly, attitudes also keep on changing.

Attitudes also influence the individual's abnormal behavior. For example, some people believe in the existence of ghost, witches, etc. and consequently they develop specific and peculiar attitudes towards certain objects and animals such as the temple or the snake. And because of these attitudes they indulge in many kinds of religious rituals. It is difficult to change these attitudes because it is difficult to adduce evidence to the contrary. An individual not only formulates attitudes towards external objects but possesses attitudes even about himself. These attitudes have much importance for his social adjustment. His behavior may become abnormal if he forms a wrong attitude towards himself. For the individual's behavior to be desirable, his attitude towards himself and external objects should be favorable.

It is well known that there was an identity between the social norm expressed as an attitude and the actual behavior towards the ex-untouchables in India. In spite of the campaign carried on by Gandhiji and in spite of Art 17 abolishing untouchability in 1950, even now negative attitude as well as avoidance behavior is to be found in the villages of India where 80 percent of the people live (Kuppuswamy, 1972).

On the other hand, one of the great problems India has been facing is in the area of national integration. As far as the expressed attitudes are concerned Indians are highly nationalistic, they will shout "Jai Hind". They stand in reverence when the national anthem is sung. But in actual behavior casteism, communalism and linguism prevail. Here behavior is at variance with the attitude expressed verbally.

It must be recognized that attitudes are neither necessary nor sufficient causes of behavior. They are only "facilitative causes". Behavior is a function of (a) attitudes, (b) social norms, (c) habits and (d) expectations about reinforcement. When there is consistency between all these four factors, there is consistency between attitudes and behavior. Sugar (1967) tested this formulation. He asked college students (a) whether they liked to smoke (affect toward smoking), (b) whether their friends approve of smoking (norm), (c) whether they usually smoked (habit). Later on he casually offered them cigarettes. It was found that when all the three predictors were consistent, the behavior followed; but when the three predictor variables were not consistent the accuracy of prediction dropped.

Thus, the actual behavior is dependent not on attitude alone but on the other factors like the social norm, habit, etc.

Formation of Attitude

Attitudes are universal, they are either positive or negative attitude of person are the permanent way of ones behaving these are acquired characteristics of a person, which are reflected in his work and behavior.

Many of the attitudes of the individual have their source and support in groups with which the individual comes in alliance. His attitudes tend to reflect the beliefs, values and the norms of his group and to maintain his attitude the individual must have the support of like minded person. The group helps in the formation of attitudes. The son of an unskilled worker, aspiring for middle class status will tend to accept the middle class values and attitudes. His middle class outlook will embrace such diverse objects as sexual practice and political issues. The attitudes of the individual reflect personality.

Attitudes are learned or acquired dispositions. Based on the opinion of Allport, Stagner has suggested that attitudes are formed under one of the following four conditions:

1. *The integration of experiences.* The accumulation and integration of a number of related experiences about an object gives birth to an attitude towards that object. Attitude of Hindus towards Muslims or *vice versa* has been formed in this way.
2. *The differentiation of experiences.* When the new experiences are acquired, they are differentiated or segregated from the already acquired experiences. This segregation or differentiation may tend to make certain attitudes more specific.

3. *Trauma or dramatic experience.* Attitudes are formed with greater speed and intensity on account of the suddenly unusual, shocking and painful experiences. A shopkeeper whose shop has been burnt by the striking students may develop intensely negative attitudes towards all students.
4. *The adoptions of the available attitudes.* A large number of attitudes are acquired in a ready made fashion by simply following suggestions or examples of friends, parents or adopting the mores and traditions of the community and society.

The majority of attitudes held by a person are acquired from the members of the family and from the peer group in early childhood and later. Thus, other people are generally the sources for the formation of attitudes. Most of our attitudes develop within the group to which we belong. Another source is personal experience; they, however, formed by association with other people. The most intense, but rare, are the attitudes formed by a "traumatic experience", like, for example, the shock of being suddenly attacked physically by a member of another communal group. The *cognitive* component of attitudes are influenced by the general tendency to categorization. Such categorizations simplify the situation but they are highly inaccurate because of the simplification. We shall learn more about this when we discuss the problem of "stereotypes".

The *affective* component of attitudes is characterized by the presence of positive or negative emotion. The effective component is influenced greatly by reinforcement and repetition. The positive attitude towards festivals is due to food, the lights, etc. which give rise to pleasure. Similarly the negative attitudes are due to unpleasure associated with individuals, groups or social events.

The *behavioral* component of attitudes are greatly influenced by social norms which are ideas held by a group regarding what is correct behavior and what is not. In the course of socialization children are told by parents about what they should do and what they should not do. The general basis for negative attitude toward Harijans is the fact that parents prevent children from associating with sweepers, cobblers, etc. who are poor, illiterate and dirty. Why do such norms for behavior toward outgroups develop? Triandis and Triandis (1960) have argued that economic conditions place one group in a position of advantage over another group. In order to maintain this position of advantage negative attitudes are developed towards the group with economic disadvantages so that it can continue to be backward. The norms will continue to operate even when economic considerations are not relevant. The upper caste man, for instance, continues to look upon a person as "untouchable" though he may have superior education, wealth, etc. This is how he tries to maintain his self-esteem.

Among the personality variables which determine the formation of attitudes, the most important is child-training which leads to formation of "authoritarian" personality. Adorno et al (1950) showed that people who had stern and punitive fathers and grew up in families organized along hierarchical lines with a powerful father figure, developed the authoritarian personality. Such people accept in group authority figures without questioning them, desire powerful leaders, show obedience and respect for authority, approve severe punishment for deviants and admire military men, athletes and financiers. By contrast those low in authoritarianism prefer equalitarian leaders, show warmth and love in interpersonal relations, are tolerant of deviants, admire scientists, artist and social reformers. Thus, those high in authoritarian scale are highly prejudiced in their outlook while those low in it are tolerant.

Another significant personality variable is "conscience" or inner control. There is a good deal of evidence to show that when the mother is the chief socialize using techniques of discipline like withdrawal of love, the child develops internal controls. But, when the father is the chief socialize using techniques of discipline like physical punishment, the child has weak internal controls; the child does not learn to control himself. People who learn to use internal controls are more likely to act according to their own standards, while those who are under the influence of external controls are more likely to act according to the norms of their in-group.

Thus, the kind of child training to which different individuals are exposed results in different conceptualizations regarding interpersonal relationships. The more positive conceptualization leads to an outlook that people are good, strong and humanistic, they advocate negotiation, etc. to settle disputes. But those who had experience of highly punitive child-training practices are likely to develop negative views of human relations looking upon people as bad and weak and favor settling disputes by violence.

Insecurity is another important personality variable. Sense of insecurity makes a person to be intolerant of ambiguity; so he may opt for "right dictatorship" (fascism) or "left dictatorship" (communism). Insecurity may be caused not only by child training, where the parents punish inconsistently and without explanation, but also by loss of status in adult life.

Among the societal variables determining attitudes are membership of groups. A person is not only a member of some groups, he also aspires to belong to other groups, called "reference groups". A person's attitudes are anchored in his membership and to the reference group.

Thus, attitude formation begins primarily as a learning process during childhood and adolescence. Once the attitudes are formed, the influence of the principle of cognitive consistency becomes increasingly important. The individual is no longer primarily passive. He begins to process the new information in terms of what he has already learned. He tends to reject inconsistent information and accept more readily information consistent with his attitude. Thus, well-established attitudes tend to be extremely resistant to change, but others may be more amenable to change.

Factors Influencing the Formation of Attitudes

Attitudes are unquestionably an acquired disposition and therefore conditioned by learning or acquisition of experiences. Heredity factor does not play any role in the formation of development of attitudes. Environmental forces help an individual to form and develop various attitudes. An attitude at any stage is essentially a product of the interaction of one's self with one's environment. Therefore the factors influencing the formation and development of attitudes can be divided into two parts as follows:

A. Factors within the individual himself

B. Factors within the individual environment.

A. Factors within the individual himself: All individuals do not respond similarity in same situations. The effect of environmental stimuli in acquiring some predispositions is very much conditioned by the growth and development pattern of an individual child. Let us try to emphasize these developmental factors.

- *Physical growth and development:* In the development of attitude physical growth and development plays a significant role. Poor physical health, low vitality and undeveloped somatic structure is responsible for poor emotional and social adjustment and poor social adjustment inevitably an important effect on the formation of attitudes in many different directions. A crippled and undersized girl of fifteen years is unlikely to form the same attitudes as those formed by another girl of fifteen who is tall, well-proportioned and charming for her age. Even the color of the skin, weight of the body or biochemical changes in the body tissues and fluids, for example sex hormones have a vital effect on the development of attitudes through its connection with social adjustment.

- *Intellectual development:* Development of attitudes is conditioned by the growth of intelligence. The components of intelligence like memory, understanding, thinking and reasoning play a significant part in attitude formation as they help in gaining perceptual experience. Due to his limited intellectual capacities a young child is incapable of forming attitudes about remote or complex abstract things. His attitudes are always of a particular kind that are related to his own immediate problems and experiences. With the growth of intellectual capacities an intelligent adult is capable of having more abstract and generalized attitudes.
- *Emotional development:* Emotional development also affects the formation of attitudes. Emotions play a dominant role in overt or covert behavior manifestation and behavior is related to attitudes. As the child develops with age and growth the capacity for varied emotional experiences and attitudes is gradually developed. Emotional maturity helps in social adjustment and seeking social approval. In turn it makes an individual to develop numerous attitudes through his direct or indirect experiences.
- *Social development:* Attitudes are rarely individual affairs. Social interaction and group processes are the key of attitude formation at any stage of human development. Children having poor social adjustment are much more likely to have antisocial attitudes and are less subject to group influences in the formation of other attitudes. Children with healthy social adjustment easily pick up social attitudes from their respective groups.
- *Ethical and moral development:* Each individual develops certain ideals, values and a concept of self in which he has pride. For enhancing his feelings of self-esteem one tries to develop those attitudes that suit his values and ideals. A student who values historical events or objects will have a favorable attitude towards the subject of history. A man who thinks that God is one will not have unfavorable attitude towards the persons belonging to the religions other than his own.

B. Factors within the individuals environment: Leaving aside the individual variations shown through their various personality characteristics on account of the pattern of their growth and development, attitudes are largely borrowed from the groups within one's environment to which one owes one's stronger allegiance. It has now been firmly established that the environmental forces, in the shape of the social groups, institutions and community cast a strong influence shaping the beliefs and attitudes of an individual. Let us try to understand a few important environment factors.

- *Home and family:* In attitude formation and family environment plays a leading role. The child by identifying himself with his parents and other members of the family picks up their attitudes. The family more or less defines for the child the expected roles which he must play in various situations and thus initiates the formation of specific attitudes. The healthy family environment and positive attitudes of the parents and family members brings desirable impact on children in picking up desirable attitudes while parental negative attitude for example of hostility and rejection lead them to imbibe ascendant and aggressive attitudes. In the similar way many antisocial attitudes are said to be product of the faulty upbringing and uncongenial environment of the home and family.

- *Social environment:* Where the family and home environment plays its role in the formation of early attitude, the contact with the people in neighborhood, school, community and society and mores and traditions of the community to which one belongs cast strong influence in reshaping early attitudes and acquisitions of many more new attitudes. As the child grows older and has wider social contacts he is influenced by so many social institutions and groups and as a result he is tries to pick up attitudes of those groups for which he has stronger allegiance or that suits much to his own nature and motives.

In school, the factors like teachers and their behavior, classmates or schoolmates, and their behavior, the teaching methods, curriculum general tone and discipline of the institution all contribute towards attitude formation.

The religious groups, social clubs or constitution where one learns or earns has a definite set of emotional and intellectual environment with the result that the members of the group tend to pick up the characteristic attitudes of the group and in this way social groups play a leading role in attitude formation.

Mass media in the form of newspapers, in radio, and television moving pictures, propaganda literature and advertisement also play a key role in shaping and reshaping the attitudes. Individuals tend to identify them with the views expressed through these agencies. Thereby heroes and heroines of the screen and radio programmers, attractive figures shown in the advertisements and slogans of a popular leader prove a potent source for the formation of attitudes.

No doubt that the attitudes of people tend to be relatively stable but can always be modified at least to some extent. Certain difference in employee's attitudes is inevitable and that is responsible for effectiveness of individuals within an organization. There are certain ways by which it is possible for supervisor and manager to get some inkling of attitudes of individuals such as interpreting the chance remarks of individuals, the behavior of individuals in the work groups, etc. A sensitive supervisor can always get a feeling with respect to the general reaction of his work group even though he cannot pinpoint such reactions specifically. The other way to find attitude change is the analysis of certain factors such as turnover rate, absenteeism and production level. Various methods have been developed for doing this, some of these consisting of questionnaires which are filled out by the employees.

Measurement of Attitude

Measurement of attitude is a highly technical process. So an attempt is made to give a general indication of the various procedures used to measure attitudes.

1. ***Self-report measures:*** Typically attitudes are assessed on the basis of a series of carefully constructed, standardized, statements each with an index. The subject is asked to specify whether he "agrees" or "disagrees" with the statement. Usually each statement is assigned a scale value so that a quantitative index of the attitude may be obtained. When a scale constructed by the Thurstone (929) method is used, the subject simply selects those items with which he agrees. For example, in the Thurstone scale to measure attitudes toward war, the statement "War is glorious" has a scale value of 11.0. "I never think about war and it does not interest me" has a scale value of 5.5. "War is a futile struggle resulting in

self destruction", has a scale value of 1.4. The attitude score is the median of the scale values of the items with which he agrees.

Another procedure which yields similar result is that developed by Likert (1932). In this method the subject has to indicate his response to a statement on a five-point scale—strongly agree, agree, undecided, disagree and strongly disagree; weights of 1, 2, 3, 4, and 5 are given to these responses. The final attitude score is obtained by summing the scores for each statement.

Another technique is the Bogardus (1925) social distance scale where seven statements of varying social intimacy from "would marry" a member of the group to "would not like him to enter my country" are given and the subject is asked up to which degree of intimacy he would like to admit the given social group.

Yet another technique is the "semantic differential technique" developed by Osgood (1957) in which the subject has to indicate on a seven-point scale the quality of the item.

All the various techniques correlate highly with each other; if a person is rated as a highly prejudiced person by one technique, he will be rated in the same way by the other techniques also.

2. ***Observation of overt behavior:*** It has been seen above how La Piere (1934) made a trip around US with a Chinese couple to study the attitude of hoteliers towards Oriental people, on the basis of actual behavior.

Webb et al (1966) have criticized the heavy dependence of social psychologists on self-reports to measure attitudes. They have suggested a series of measured based on actual behavior or on records indicating behavior. For example, the sales records will show the attitude toward food items, or towards the various "soft drinks" like Coca-Cola, Fanta, Limca, etc. Similarly a measure of change in attitude toward "ready-made dresses" could be obtained by analyzing the sales records of ready-made dresses and also analyzing the number of orders given to tailors to make various types of clothing.

3. ***Interpretation of partially structured stimuli:*** The subject may be shown a photo or a picture and asked to describe the scene. This is a "projective" technique. On the basis of the description or story, the subject's attitude toward that social object could be studied.

Methods of Measurement

Attitudes defined as implicit responses or predispositions to objects, persons, ideas, values or situations in the social surroundings. Thereby they are essentially covert tendencies. If we want to measure them, they must by some means, be drawn out into or manifest themselves in the form of overt behaviors. This can be done in the following two ways:

1. **Direct method:** Measuring the verbal report of the attitude
2. **Indirect method:** Interpretation of the attitude from the unsaturated or indirect responses. Let us discuss these methods.

1. Direct method for measurement of attitudes. In this method opinion of an individual about a particular subject in the form of a verbal report is collected and on this basis his attitude about the subject is estimated. Generally the following devices are used for this purpose.

i. Asking the individual directly how he feels about a subject. (questioning and interview techniques)
ii. Asking to check in a list of statements with which he is in agreement. (Check list, etc.)

iii. To indicate his degree of agreement or disagreement with a series of statements dealing with the same subject (attitude scales).

The last mentioned devices are known as attitude scales. These scales are most widely used for the measurement of attitudes. Generally the following two types of scales are popular:

1. Attitude scale: To develop an attitude scale the first step is to write but a large number of statements, as may as hundred or more, each of which expresses a view point of some kind towards the company. Each of these statements is typed on a separate slip of paper and the judge is asked to place each statement in one of several piles (usually 7, 9, or 11), ranging from statement judged to express the least favorable viewpoints to statements judged to express the most favorable viewpoints (7, 9 or 11). Statements judged to express varying degrees of favorableness in between these extremes are placed in the piles that are judged are used in the process, sometimes as many as 100 or more. These judges are assisting the construction of the scale. They are not having their own attitudes measure. The allocation of statements to the several piles is a part of the process of constructing the scale.

The purpose of the allocation is to determine the scale values of the various statements. If all judges tend to place a statement in piles towards the favorable then we can conclude that the statement expresses a favorable towards the company. If the statement is placed by the judges in piles towards the unfavorable end of the series, then we may conclude that an unfavorable attitude end of the series, then we may conclude that an unfavorable attitude is expressed by that particular statement. So we can determine the average location of the statement by the judge. Statements that are scattered by the judge over several categories are eliminated.

The use of different statements in scales measuring the same attitude helps in checking results by a repeat test in order to be sure of conclusion reached and to measure the effectiveness of systematic company effort to improve employee morale.

2. Likert scale: Likert's method is simpler than Thurstone method and does not require the use of judges in scaling the statements. While a number of different procedures were tried and compared but the simplest method described by Likert was found to give results that correlated very highly with more complex methods. Each statement has five degrees of approval and asking the person taking the scale to check one of the five degrees.

- Strongly approved
- Approved
- Undecided
- Disapproved
- Strongly disapproved
- Validity and reliability.

The problem of reliability and validity of attitude scale has two aspects, one relating to the nature of the relationship between real attitudes in day-to-day life and the other relating to the consistency and significance of the measured attitudes themselves.

A scale is constructed in terms of certain conceptual frames of reference and in the final stage the results of a research conducted with reference to this scale are projected back to the very frames of reference where from they originated. Measurement of the behavior provides us with index of the attitude which is thereby defined in terms of behavior. It is in this sense that it seems that attitudes can be measured.

There are three principal methods of establishing the validity of a measuring device: (1) Comparing the results obtained from it with those of another device. The validity of which has been established. (2) Judgment of experts and (3) Internal consistency. The validity of the Likert scale established by a comparison of the same with an already established scale of Thurstone is an example of judgment technique adopted. The usual criterion of validity adopted, therefore, is the evidence of internal consistency among the various statements in a battery.

A. Thurstone's attitude scales: These are also known as equal appearing intervals scales. In constructing such scales a large number of statements representing a variety of opinions on a subject are collected. These statements are then given to a number of judges who are asked to sort the statements in two categories say from "very favorable" to "very unfavorable". Whenever the judges disagree significantly over an item it is rejected. The finished scale, then consists of remaining statements or items that represent clearly defined opinions on the subject. Each of these final statement is then assigned a scale value based on the median scale position given by the judges. If half the judges, for example, had assigned a particular statement to position 4 or lower and half had assigned it to position 5 or higher, the scale value assigned to the statement could be 4:5. Some of the statements from the Thurston's scale for measuring attitude toward the church with the scale values of each statement are shown below:

Items	Scale Value
I believe the church is the greatest institution in America to day	0.2
I believe church membership is almost essential to living life at its best	1.5
I believe in what the church teachers, but with mental reservations	4.5
I believe in religion but I seldom go to church	5.4
I do not receive any benefit from attending church service but I think it helps some people	5.7
I think the church is a parasite on society	11.0

In administering the scale, individuals are asked to check all the statements with which they agree. For each individual, then a scale position is computed as the average of the scale values of all the items he has checked.

B. Likert attitude scale: This scale is more popular than Thurstone's scale. It employs a larger number of items than Thurston's scale and discards the methods of scaling of several judges. In constructing such scale a number of statements or items concerning particular subject are collected. These items each of which clearly represents either a favorable or unfavorable attitude, are then tested for internal consistency, i.e. to see all the statements or are actually concerned with the same subject. The tested items constitute attitude scale. The individual is asked to indicate the degree of his agreement or disagreement with each item on a five point scale. Thus for assessing attitude toward internationalism, the sample items such as follows, are presented.

Encircle one of the symbols preceding each of the following statements. A stands for "Agree", SA stands for "Strongly agree", D for "Disagree", and U for "Undecided". And SD stands for "strongly disagree."

Response	**Items**
SA, A, U, D, SD	We should be willing be fight for our country whether it is in the right or in the wrong.
SA, A, U, D, SD	Our country should never declare war again under any circumstances.

For scoring the items a value of 5 may be given to the responses indicating strong agreement, 4 for simple agreement, 3 for undecided, 2 for simple disagreement and 1 for strong disagreement. Thus, each individual can be assigned a single quantitative score for the measurement of his attitude.

2. Indirect Method for Measurement of Attitude: The process of offering attitude directly from the verbal report or expressed opinion as many limitations. One may conceal one's real attitudes and may to really know what one feels and unable to know one's attitude about situation in the abstract. Even overt behavior is not always a true indication of one's attitude. When politicians kiss babies their behavior may not be a true expression of their attitude towards children.

To avoid this problem, it has been tried to make use of the measurement methods that are indirect or disguised in nature. These methods are also known as interpretive methods. In these methods the subjects are given opportunities to structure their own responses without letting them know the real purpose of the task. The projective techniques used for the assessment of personality are the good examples of these indirect methods. These techniques have been discussed in detail in the chapter 'Personality'. The essence of these techniques is that the subject expresses his covert tendencies while responding to the unstructured stimulus. An intelligent interpretation of his responses may show his attitude towards a particular object or issue.

Now the question arises which of these two techniques – direct or indirect should be used for measuring attitudes. Both of these are the best instruments and have their own values and limitations. Perhaps in my opinion the best method or the procedure adopted for the measurement of attitudes is that one which combines the verbal report and the interpretive techniques. It will surely help us in getting an extensive and intensive measurement of attitudes covering their covert tendency and overt manifestation.

- **Opinion surveys:** Attitude scales help to measure the attitudes of individuals by summarizing data for all employees within a group; such scale can be used to quality as 'morale' of employee groups.

Attitude scales can be useful in indicating the relative level of morale of employees group, they do not enable a management to identify specific factors that may be sources of employee unrest or dissatisfaction. This information can be obtained by the use of questionnaire that provides for giving opinions about specific matters such as working conditions, company policies, facilities, etc. The questionnaire can be distributed by mail to the employee's homes after the employee had been informed about the survey.

The usual practice in opinion questionnaire is that of obtaining a single response to each question in either 'yes' or 'no'. In particular, the employees may be asked to check each item in one of the three boxes; satisfied, neutral or dissatisfied and also check each item as being of great importance.

It is possible to develop questionnaire that can serve both the purposes of obtaining opinions of employees and measuring their attitudes. One method for doing this is described by Harris. He identified 48 questions that would seem to indicate overall morale. Ten judges were asked to check the response to each question that most strongly represents a favorable attitude towards the company. Any question on which checks to the 10 judges did not show at least 80 percent agreement was discarded at this point. Forty-six questions met the criterion and it is interesting to note that there was unanimous agreement on 42 questions.

The questionnaire returned by the employees were then divided into two random halves. After the halves had been satisfied on the basis of several characteristics, such as sex, marital status and length of service and the reliability of this scale was determined by correlating odd vs. even, it was analyzed that items had correlation.

- **Interviews:** Still another method of obtaining information about personnel reactions is the use of interview. In some cases interviews are carried out to find out personnel reactions and are used with present employees either all employees or a sample. The employees are given assurance that the information furnished will not be used for any administrative purpose. To provide such assurance the interviews usually are conducted by representatives of some outside organization such as a consulting firm or university.

In a guided interview, the interviewer asks a series of questions so that each of which may be answered by a simple 'yes' or 'no' or by some other words or phrases. In the unguided interview the interviewer asks more general questions to encourage the employee to express himself.

Difficulties in Measuring Attitudes

From the description of the nature and characteristics of attitude it can be deduced that it contains many elements which it is very difficult to measure. To take but one, the emotions and feelings involved in attitudes cannot be measured and hence attitudes can be measured only indirectly or by approximately guessing about them. Attitudes are internal systems. In this form, they do not possibly admit of any measurement, but the individuals external behavior is generated by inner tendencies. Hence, attitudes can be measured from external behavior. For the measurement of attitudes it is necessary that the immediate circumstances be controlled. The greater the amount or extent of control upon these immediate circumstances the greater will be their success and their reliability. Hence control of the conditions is necessary in the measurement of attitudes. But there are certain conditions which defy any attempts at controlling them. For example, it would be difficult to generate communal attitudes in the laboratory, or artificially anywhereelse. In a situation of this kind the experimenter should keep in mind all the details of the actual circumstances in conducting the experiment upon the attitude. It is therefore evident that the degree of reality which can be obtained in the measurement of attitudes, which in addition, do not offer the same degree of reliability at all can be expected in the measurement of attitudes. The accuracy of the measurement of attitude can be tested by its capacity of prediction. The extent to which any measurement can forecast and predict the future conduct of any individual, it is accurate to that extent:

The following conclusions are to be drawn from the preceding discussion of the measurement of attitudes:

1. Attitudes can be measured only indirectly
2. The greatest possible degree and extent of control should be levied upon the immediate circumstances in the measurement of attitudes
3. In studying attitudes the uncontrolled circumstances should be carefully studied
4. The measurement of attitudes cannot be as reliable or accurate and the measurement of external behavior
5. The accuracy of the measurement of attitude can be judged from the accuracy of prediction of the individuals subsequent behavior.

Attitudes and Nursing

It is clear from the foregoing discussion about the attitudes that success in Nursing profession requires correct attitude. If the nurse develops a correct attitude towards her profession, doctors, colleagues and patients, her adjustment becomes easier and she very easily masters her job. This attitude is not necessarily inborn. It has to be cultivated. Thus a nurse should know as to what are the correct attitudes required in her profession. A list of correct attitudes for a successful and efficient nurse, given by Kempf and Averill will be useful for her:

i. Ambition to do her task well
ii. Conformity with the rules and regulations of the profession for which she is preparing
iii. Willingness to work and to work with effectiveness
iv. Cheerfulness and optimism
v. Interest in the problems and difficulties of other people
vi. Cooperativeness, industriousness, respect for the opinion and judgment of others
vii. Interest in increasing the fund of knowledge underlying effective nursing care
viii. Determination to grow professionally
ix. Maintenance of poise and self-control in all professional situations
x. Maintaining a consistent pride in their profession
xi. Arising to the unexpected without undue panic
xii. Determination to make the patient comfortable by giving attention to small details that mean so much to the patients well being.

In order to get success in her profession the Nurse should develop the above attitudes and change her former attitudes accordingly. This change of attitude will require change in perceptions by new experiences and fresh knowledge; it will also require a control over emotions and drives, which may be hampering her job. Finally, she will have to tap the various formative agencies.

- **Employee attitude and action:** Employee aspirations are like layers and to provide an outlet for each of these ascending desires requires simultaneous emphasis upon company objectives. The interests of both employee and company must be served at same time. The beginning of all efforts to permit the employee to do his best is the assurance of personal security. In addition, the executive has the responsibility that the job itself shall remain secure as a result of constantly lowering departmental costs and improving quality and service. Next to security, the employee hopes for a job that provides a good place to work. Particularly the human contacts and interaction make the work pleasant or burden some.

With job security and working conditions taken care of, the workman's interest moves on to opportunity for advancement in such matters as overall experience, personal standing, responsibility, income and the like. In return he will give his zeal. To operate a department with such opportunities are present, the manager must so competently conduct its affairs in the company interest that departmental progress is recognized. If the employee is to be simulated to do his best, he requires in addition to security, working condition and opportunity, a truly worthy objective which he and his associates are convinced is entitled to their highest efforts. The awaken the devotion of a group of employees is the highest accomplishment to which any executive can aspire. A good manager can earn the willing response, the loyalty, the zeal, the devotion of their employees by so strengthening and advancing the effectiveness of departmental operation that each employees is given opportunity to develop his abilities and to enlarge his opportunities, and to provide a reasonable degree of security, job satisfaction, personal opportunity and an ideal to work.

We have many basic similarities but our backgrounds are different. Our experience have been different. Our hopes and ambitions are different. We are individuals and expect and want to treated as such. Each one of us is born with extraordinary capacities and some have special talents which are most unusual. Manager should try to know what unusual abilities may be concealed behind the routines of his workmen; the manager's attitude is that every single person hopes for an ever-better future for himself. The employee's individual differences, their long ancestry, their high economic value, their extraordinary talents and their inborn ambition if fully appreciated and accepted, provide us with a sound basis for a truly progressive attitude towards the manager responsibility.

In all our activities we can do better if we put our minds to it. Our research and development have/revealed a capacity for increased creativeness that has been far greater than anyone could have dreamed. In fact, there is no end to growth and improvement because of new situations and these in turn invite new suggestions. We have a kind of native wisdom which as years pass enables to form common sense of judgments in the absence of all formalized rules or logic. In fact every persons contains the promise of growth better with time.

The psychology of attitudes: A knowledge of attitudes greatly contributes to an understanding of the reactions of people. Each kind of work acquires a social level or status. Sometimes the mere location of the work becomes a distinguishing feature, even if the work is the same. Other factors influencing the social status of the job are types of work, wages vacations with or without pay, the kind of table or work space and any other feature which tended to go with one kind of work and with another. Social meaning became attached to these distinguishing features, their meetings being derived from attitudes toward social status.

Disagreements, over the nature of a given set of facts are possible because attitudes influence the way the facts are experienced. The degree to which meanings are determined by attitudes varies; but it is important to realize that the meanings and importance of things are influenced by attitudes. Prejudice is individual's unfavorable attitude. The problem is not to judge but to improve attitudes.

Words, thoughts and feelings also derive meanings from the way they are organized. Bread has different meaning and different feeling when grouped with milk than when grouped with water.

Interpretations or groupings of facts tend to be such that they support the attitude existing before the specific interpretation is made. An unbiased person should be able to group facts in a variety of ways and determine which interpretation best match with reality.

Attitudes usually are associated with likes and dislikes and consequently have an emotional content. Thus any conditions which influence emotion is likely to influence certain attitudes. Mood of an individual are temporary predispositions toward having certain emotional reactions. As a consequence, it is to be expected that one's mood will influence the attitudes. Once emotions are stimulated the prevalent attitudes become important factors in determining, whether or not a specific emotional reaction will be applied to an individual or to a group of individuals. Unfavorable reactions to groups are most common during periods of tension, partly because mood tend to be unfriendly at such times and relatively dormant attitudes are revived.

Personality difference and attitudes: Personality difference are highly important in determining the type of attitudes. Some individuals are inclined towards extreme, other toward conservatism and still others avoid extremes. These tendencies seem to be so general that they are sometimes regarded as personality differences. Also, differences in social dependability, decisiveness, and emotionally may influence attitudes on specific topics. Other facts, such as sex and intelligence, have also been shown to have rather specific effects on opinion. Differences in personality make up and intelligence must account for the individual difference which occur when experiences or environments are comparable. To what extent personality differences are inborn and to what extent they are acquired is not known, but undoubtedly some of the differences must be attributed to heredity.

The role of experience in attitude formations is our primary concern here, since this factor is most readily altered. The extent to which attitudes are influenced by experience largely determines the degrees to which they can be controlled and account for group trends among individuals with similar backgrounds. By means of attitude measurement, it has been found that a single situation in a motive can sometimes alter attitudes on racial, social, and economic values. Findings have shown that (i) unemployment disturbs former religious and economic values; (ii) radical students are more inclined to be highly intelligent than nonradical ones, despite the fact that children of professional classes tend to be conservative; (iii) a speech given in person is more effective in influencing attitudes than reading the same speech; (iv) judgments made by individuals in two-person groups are more strongly influenced by the other member when the later is stranger than when a friend more acquaintance; (v) support for civil liberties is significantly associated with increased years of higher education; (vi) beliefs can be changed as a result of suggestion and may shift the attitude from negative to positive attitudes are more difficult to modify than conservative attitudes (vii) radical attitudes are more difficult to modify than conservative attitudes. Most of the attitudes that give us concern can be classified as emotionally unfavorable; and are perhaps the most difficult to change.

Changing of Attitudes

Attitudes are not challenged by telling, advising or showing. *They are not changed by the process called 'training'. They are changed only by education. This is a long range process that takes into account the whole man, his home life, goals, fears, hopes, history and concept of himself.* This type of education is sometimes called 'counseling'. It is man-centered rather than work-centered. It aims at the source rather than the result of performance. In a counseling or educational relationship, however, the manager acts as guide. He does this through perceptive questioning and commencing. The subordinate talks about and expires his own feelings. The subordinate provides almost all the conversations. Only he knows or can find out what is behind his own actions.

Attitudes can be changed in a variety of ways. One of the sources of change is by obtaining new information which may come from other people or through the mass media. Such new information may produce changes in the cognitive component of a person's attitude. There is a tendency for consistency in the component of any attitude. So when there are changes in the cognitive component there may be changes in the effective and behavioral components also. Attitudes may change through direct experience.

However, it must be same age that there is a great difference in situation; in the laboratory and in the college campus significant changes in attitudes may be possible; but as politicians and other propagandists like the advertisers know, the campaigns conducted through mass media are not so successful in producing changes in attitudes among the masses. There must be a "communicator" who holds a particular position on some issue and is trying to convince others to hold the same position. In order to do this, he produces a "communication" designed to persuade people to change their views. This communication is presented in a given "situation". These three constitutes the essential features—the source, the communication and the situation and surroundings. But the communication may not reach the target intact. Probably the communication may not reach the target at all because the lines of communication do not exist.

There is considerable evidence with regard to what is now identified as the "two-step flow of information". Most people do not read newspapers and do not hear the radio. Only a small fraction in the society read newspapers carefully and hear the significant programs on the radio. These people tend to be the most influential members of their community or group. They are called the "opinion leaders", because they have considerable impact on the attitudes of their associates. They pass on the information to their friends. By means of this two-step flow of communication, some of the persuasive material does reach the people. Thus, one of the critical points in propaganda and attitude change is to reach these opinion leaders.

For example, applying these principles to the Indian situation. In 1920 when Gandhi launched his noncooperation program he was able to get practically the whole nation to support him. Thousands of responsible citizens gave up their professions and joined the movement. Tens of thousands of students gave up their studies. This phenomenal situation arose because Gandhi, the source of communication, had already demonstrated in 1917 his capacity as a leader and his fearlessness by the four successful campaigns, namely: (1) Champaran Satyagraha in indigo plantation in north-western corner of Bihar; (2) Ahmedabad Satyagraha and fast to settle the textile mill laborers problems; (3) the Kaira Satyagraha in Gujarat to suspend the land revenue code due to famine; and (4) the abolition of indentured labor system. His communication was the attainment of self-government through "ahimsa" the abandonment of all kinds of violence and through non-cooperation, "a voluntary withdrawal' of all support to the government. He wanted all those who "are holding offices of honor or emoluments" to give them up, and also those who belong to the menial services under the government. Then what about the situation? The movement was launched after the Jallianwala Bagh massacre and Khilafat agitation and the failure of the British Government to satisfy the demands for "Home Rule" by accepting the recommendation of Montague-Chelmsford reforms which only envisaged the transfer of a few subjects in the states to elected ministers. Thus the whole country was seething with discontent. What about the target? Gandhi started for the first time a mass movement. So the people were ready to join a movement which gave promise of the overthrow of the alien rulers. The masses are ignorant; they were mobilized through the "two-step" flow of information. The leaders, who resigned their offices, communicated the message. Thus, not only the 1920 movement, but the other movements launched by Gandhi in 1930 and 1942 were all of the same pattern. He had insight into the needs of the people and could make them sacrifice their all for the attainment of independence.

By contrast, such forces are not in operation either with respect to the Five-year plans or community development program or other national programs. It is only the Bank Nationalization program that had some of these features which could change the attitudes of the people.

As stated earlier attitudes are by no means fixes and unchanging predispositions. They can and do change. The task of attitudes change is very much related to their formation. As discussed earlier attitudes are formed through experiences—direct or indirect. Consequently they may be changed through acquisition of new experiences as Bonner remarks, "Such factors as social, expectancies, propaganda, education and personal experience with different attitudes do make for modifications and shifts in people's predispositions toward objects, persons, ideas and situations in their environment".

Let us try to utilize the knowledge of attitude formation and change in our classroom teaching. The simple question is that can our school or classroom teaching be so equipped as to develop desirable social attitude among the pupils or what should be done to bring changes in the otherwise negative or understandable attitudes of the people? Let us try to think about this problem.

Whether individuals have to develop an attitude or to modify it they have to think about the different factors contributing towards its acquisition. In brief we have to proceed in the following way:

1. Attitude formation is conditioned by the growth and development of an individual in all the dimensions like physical, intellectual, emotional social, and ethical. Therefore, efforts should be made to bring an all round harmonious development in the personality of the child.
2. Home and family establishes the formation of early attitudes. Parents and members of the family should be educated and given proper guidance for helping their children to pick up positive and socially desirable attitudes and family environment.
3. Attitudes toward things are very largely conditioned by one's desire to preserve or to enhance one's feelings of self-esteem. Therefore the self-respect of the students should always be given due consideration while adopting any program at the development of attitudes. They should never be let down and feel that by adopting such opinions or attitudes their status or self-esteem will be lowered.
4. It should be kept in mind that it is easier to develop attitudes positively than negatively. It is, for example, probably more effective to develop a liking for honesty or democracy than to attempt to develop a dislike for dishonesty or autocracy.
5. The attitudes are never taught, they are caught through direct or indirect experiences. Therefore, teacher should not try to teach attitudes directly as facts may be taught. He should make use of indirect suggestions or provide experiences that will naturally tend to result in the desired attitude formation.
6. Social environment as we have seen plays a dominant role in attitude formation. Therefore, attempts should be made to control and modify environmental influences in such a way that desirable attitudes may be developed.
7. Attitudes are rarely individual affairs. Group interaction plays a key role in attitude formation. Therefore, it should be utilized for the development of desirable attitudes. The teacher should utilize his class as a well-organized group for the attitude development. He should try to develop group support for, and expression of, particular attitudes. Group discussions, seminars, skit, drama, and other social or group activities, may be chosen for developing and organizing group attitudes. The important thing is to develop the attitude of a group, the attitude of the members will naturally follow because the individual tends to accept whatever his group accepts and to reject whatever his group rejects.

8. The teacher should not go too far from the opinions and attitudes of his students. Otherwise it will naturally segregate him from the group and he will cease to be a leader. Wise and successful political leaders know this fact and therefore they always carry with them the mass of the voters. Teachers also should take note that they should direct their efforts toward the attainment of reasonable goals.
9. The teacher should bring desirable and essential changes in their method of instructions for developing favorable attitude towards their subjects. They should also learn how to change their own behavior according to the needs of the situations. They should try to produce their own examples for the development of desirable attitude.
10. The audiovisual aids and mass-media may be utilized for developing desirable attitudes among the pupils. The textbooks should be so written that they do not encourage negative or unfavorable attitudes for example disliking for a particular religion, caste, creed, color of a country, liking or temptation for dishonesty, corruption, war, and quarreling, etc. Similarly radio, television, films, newspapers and magazines, etc. should be properly controlled for developing desirable attitudes.

In this way development of desirable attitudes or reshaping of undesirable attitudes is a gigantic task. It needs cooperation of all the forces of environment. Parents, members of the society, teachers, schools and government authorities all need to join hands in this task of desirable attitude formation among the young generation. First of all they should feel the necessity of right attitude formation and then try to bring changes in their own attitudes before planning to bring similar changes in the young generation. In brief, the overall environment, the cultural pattern of the community and outlook of the whole group need modifications and change before bringing the similar change in the attitude of an individual child or adult.

Reason and Will and Character

Both reason and will have important contributions to make to the life of man. But many of the thinkers have unnecessarily stressed the role of the one or the other and have given primary importance to one and secondary importance to the other.

Thinkers supporting the rationalist option lay extreme stress upon the importance of knowledge and reason to human behavior. It is their contention that only reason can guide man along the right path. Only reason can be the determinant or judge in the conflict for supremacy that occurs between different desires. Only reason can determine the propriety of one desire as compared to another conflicting desire. Rationalist thinkers like Kant went so far as to advocate the complete extinction or annihilation of feelings because they almost inevitably instigate the individual and because of passions even the good action of the individual are not balanced.

On the other hand, some thinkers have laid prime importance on passions, tendencies, and drives. It is contended by them that these elements are the real motivating causes in human beings. Ribot has written that there is nothing other than instincts, motivating forces, desires, feelings and emotions at the root of human conduct. In the words of Hume the British empiricist, "Reason is and ought to be the slave of passions and can never pretend to any other office than to serve and obey". In this way, then, thinkers opposing the rationalistic viewpoint have awarded secondary place to reason in life and behavior.

In fact, both the above points of view are partial. If the matter is carefully attended, to, it will be seen and will have to be admitted that both reason and passion have a place in the life of human beings. Hume's view is open to certain damaging objections. To start with, it is not a fact that reason is the slave of passions. It cannot be denied that often people do not attend to reason in the satisfaction of their desires and passions and indulge in completely irrational activity into which they are guided by their passions. But then, on the other hand, reason is given to man in order that he may be possessed of some faculty that can decide when there is a conflict between two or more desires. Even if it is taken for granted that reason is the slave of passions it is not logical or proper to conclude therefrom that it should remain so. On the other hand, the rationalist view is equally one-sided. In the absence of tendencies, passions, desires, etc. what is there for the reason to direct or guide, what is it going to work on? If passions are eliminated from human behavior the very basis for the functioning of reason is also destroyed. Hence, both passions and reasons are of importance to human life.

Impulse, Desire and Will: The presence of some motives at the root of human behavior has been recognized by practically every psychologist. These motives have been given different names such as needs, motives, instincts, etc. by the psychologists. Every desired activity of the individual has its origin in some or the other impulse. And this impulse has its origin in some physical or psychological deficiency in the organism. These impulses or tendencies, either innate or acquired, are the actual motives of conduct. Impulse gives rise to desire. When man feels hunger the devours bread or desires to do so. The impulse of hunger gives rise to the desire for food. But mere desire is not sufficient to instigate the individual to obtain the object; for this, it must be converted into will. Will is the name given to that desire which has been decided to be converted into action. In this way, decision is part of will. When the individual selects one out of many conflicting desires and decides to give it active implementation it becomes will. Desired activity takes place only after it has been willed.

Impulse and Will: In this way, there is an intimate relationship between impulse and will. As Ginsberg has written, "In truth, however, it is mistaken to separate impulse from will as it is to separate sharply sense from thought". There can be no willing without an experience. Thus, the contention of the Rationalists that impulse, reaction, will, etc. are independent in the field of activity and of influence. The actual situation is that the human personality cannot be dissected into different parts in this manner. The personality is a complete whole and functions as a whole. In this unit the impulses, reason, will, etc., influence each other. All these are activated by the self of the individual. In specific circumstances any one of them can be dominant or primary while the rest assume secondary importance. But the importance of none of the others is thereby lessened.

Reason is Social and Individual Life: Defining reason Ginsberg has written, "Its function is that of harmonizing the impulses by subordinating them to broad and coherent ends. It has thus the important function of directing and organizing". It is evident that reason is needed all the more in social life. It is by means of reason that the individual decides upon what he should do. In the struggle that is life the individual is faced by different alternatives in various circumstances. He finds it difficult to choose one of then from among the many that are contending for his attention. It is in just this kind of situation that reason comes to the rescue of the person. It is only too correct that Bertrand Russell has accorded greater importance and greater potentiality to the power of reason over and above the other power.

Conduct based on reason is more balanced and adjusted. It is reason that determines the various functions that the different institutions in society seek to perform. Reason illuminates and clarifies the ideals in the various aspects of behavior. It has two forms, theoretical reason organizes and directs thoughts while its practical aspect guides conduct.

But in the absence of will, the practical reason is incapable of doing anything because its utility is apparent only when its direction or guidance is given practical shape. Elucidating the nature of will, Ginsberg has written: "Will is not a mere idea with no Conative energy, but the whole utility or synthesis of our Conative nature. It is essentially a principle of integration, an effort towards harmony, working within and through complex system of Conative effective interests, and its energy of our whole personality. "In this way, just as reason manifests the cognitive aspect of our personality, will is representative of the affective aspect. All activities in social life originate in will. The will is the determinant in human conduct. In actual fact if the reasoning is proper, the conduct is willed. In the words of Bertrand Russell, "The power of thought in the long run is greater than any other human power". The right kind of thought is rate and difficult but not impotent".

Synthesis of Reason and Will: As a matter of fact, both reason and will have important function to perform in human life. When there are many conflicting desires or many alternative stating the individual in the face, he employs his reason to pick out the best desire or the best alternative, and he then acts on this choice. Following this choice the selected desire or alternative gets the sanction of the will and is then turned into practical application. When reason is absent, the individual generally indulges in incorrect and improper actions. In the absence of will, the individual is like that straw in the turbulent ocean which is tossed form side to side by the strong waves which take it where they will, when they will, how they will. The fundamental motivation of human conduct comes from needs. But it is only by the help of reason and will that the passion, upon his reason and will being equally healthy. The personality of the individual loses its organization when his reason and will find reason to conflict with each other.

Will and Character: Character is the system or organization of sentiments. And in this system one master sentiment rules over all the other sentiments. As long as the individuals sentiments are scattered and lack system, he has no character. Thus any individual who exhibits signs of being led by one sentiment at one time and by another at another time is called characteristics if the term is interpreted in the psychological sense. It is in this sense that it has been remarked that women have no character. In the character formation, the individuals sentiment of self-regard directs his emotions of love, friendship, hatred, etc. From the moral viewpoint a character is high if the master sentiment is high and valuable, but if it is not so, the character is said to be low. In this way, it is one thing for a character to be organized and stable, and another to be high or low. One is a psychological concept while the other is a moral concept.

Here, it is essential to keep it in mind fundamentally, character does not imply moral character. It was the German philosopher Immanuel Kant who chose to interpret the term character in the sense of moral character. In ancient Greece, the term character referred to the moulds used for making coins. In order to prevent the minting of false coins, each mould was so formed as to be difficult of imitation. The same sense continued even into modern English. It is for this reason that some people qualify the term and use the expression ethical character if they want to distinguish between good and bad character. In the words of Skinner, One's character, defined by the history of the word, is all that makes him or her unique, different from everyone else. In this manner, character includes all those special features of an individuals personality that serve to make him distinctive and individual. Yet character is more commonly interpreted to be a system or organization of sentiments.

The intimate relation between character and sentiment is further evinced by the evolution of different kinds of character in different cultures. Sentiment is closely to culture, since in every culture attempts are made to develop certain definite sentiments in an individual of sentiment in society, William McDougall has written, "The growth of sentiments is of utmost importance for the character and conduct of individuals and of societies, it is the organization of the affective and Conative life. In the absence of sentiments our emotional life would be a mere chaos without order, consistency or continuity of any kind, and all our social relations and conduct, being based on the emotions and their impulses, would be correspondingly chaotic, unpredictable and unstable. An individuals social conduct is guided by some values, values that are related to his sentiments. Hence, sentiments have a special significance for the individuals character. For example, individuals who attach much value to sacrifice, service or benevolence usually possess sentiments of patriotism, linguistic attachment or philanthropy. It need hardly be pointed out that in the absence of these sentiments no such values and could possibly survive.

• **Sentiment of self-regard in character-formation:** Much importance is attached to the sentiment of self-regard in connection with formation of character. Mcdougall has gone to far as to consider the sentiment of self-regard as character itself. As has been pointed out earlier, emotions of love, friendship, hatred and parental regard are integrated in self-regard. Importance of the sentiment of self-regard becomes evident once the value of emotions for human character is realized. Love is a complex emotional state, a mixture of pity, sympathy, maternal love, parental regard and most of all sexual instinct. The importance of love for the development of the child's character can hardly be over-estimated. If excessive love spoils the children, the absence of love is equally dementing and injurious as it hinders their mental development. According to modern psychologists, love is more important for child's education than punishment. Man is susceptible to love at all stages of life, the effects of lack of love, sufficient love and excessive love being evident even when he attains adulthood. Hatred is a complex emotion consisting of anger, fear and distaste. Hatred lowers the level of character. But, sometimes, it also helps to support certain other higher qualities of character. For example, the patriots harbor strong feelings of hatred for all who would betray their motherland. Parental affection and friendship both help in developing social qualities in the individual. Parental affection is a composite emotion that includes such emotion as pity, sympathy and love for beings younger than oneself. McDougall believes that the emotion of parental affection is conjoined to the parental instinct. Man is normally found to love his offspring, which he considers a part of his own ego. The feeling of friendship has much social significance. It results in an individual becoming aware of and considering the interests of others for which he is sometimes even induced to forego his own benefit. It is evident, in this way, that a developed sentiment of self-regard is an essential prerequisite for the creation of very high and desirable traits in a character. But the intensity of self-regard varies in degree from culture to culture, although this cannot form a just criterion for considering individuals as having a low character or no character at all.

• **Process of character-formation:** The process of character-formation originates in childhood, to which the child's life in the home and school, and social and cultural life in his surroundings contribute. Character is formed of the organization of sentiments. Sentiments are formed of the organization of emotions. Some emotions are innate while others are acquired. Both the acquired as well as the innate emotions contribute in the formation of sentiments. In social situations different emotions become bound up with different objects due to the simple and natural process of mental association. For example, a child delights in his mother's approach and he manifests the emotion of love towards her. If he comes to harm through the agency of some animal or situation, he learns to fear it. When fear is strengthened by indifference and anger, hatred is generated. Gradually, these various sentiments combine into a complex that is called character. An individuals character is known through the ruling or prominent sentiment which directs all the other sentiments. In the character of a patriot, for example, the sentiment of love of country becomes the sentiment of self-regard, and all other sentiments are directed by it.

Character and habits – Habits are an important element in the individuals behavior. Much of his day-to-day conduct is determined by his habits. Thus, character is expressed in habits, though it cannot be said that character is the sum total of habits.

Character and volition – Volition is a very important element in character. It is will power that develops the character. People of strong wills stick to their principles without flinching, while the weak willed people show a lack of this spirit and are easily diverted from their paths by the least obstruction. Hence, the intelligent teacher tries to develop volition in his students. For this it is essential that every student should be given the maximum possible opportunity for performing some task on his own initiative. This helps to maintain their active tendency, and their volition also improves. The child should be encouraged to complete the day-to-day tasks that are set to him, and when he successfully completes his work, he should be praised. Failure to do this discourages the child, and he develops the sense of lack of confidence. It should also be kept in mind that the student should not be loaded with so many tasks that it becomes impossible for him to perform any, since this too reduces his ability to determine the course for himself.

- **Will and Character in Nursing:** Character, as has been already pointed out, is a fashioned will. In the beginning one has to voluntarily perform certain functions, ultimately they become a part of his character. In the words of Alexander Shand, "Character is the mental and moral equipment acquired for education and environment and is revealed in the conduct of the individual and his relations with people". This definition clarifies the role of character in Nursing profession. The peculiar character of a Nurse, as exhibited by a Florence Nightingale, is due to her education and environment as a Nurse and she is known by that character. We can predict her conduct as soon as we know that she is a successful nurse because she must be having that particular character. That is why as soon as she enters the room of a patient she is greeted with a smile and a hope. A knowledge of the psychology of women character helps the nurse to develop such a character. It is an arduous task but certainly it is that which brings her respect and applause from the community around her.

21 CHAPTER Personality

Introduction

Personality is the unique way in which each individual thinks, and feels throughout life. Personality should not be confused with **character,** which refers to value judgments made about a person's morals or ethical behavior, nor should it be confused with **temperament,** the enduring characteristics with which each person is born, such as irritability or adaptability. Both character and temperament are vital parts of personality. Generally personality is taken as the external appearance of the individual. In philosophy the meaning personality has been the personality the external appearance nor is it the self, but it includes both and much more. The word *persona* was used for the cover, utilized by the actors, to change their appearance, but in the Roman times it was taken as the particular character itself. The second meaning has been taken in the word 'personality'. Thus personality is not a fixed state, but a dynamic totality which is continuously changing due to interaction with the environment. Personality is known by the conduct, behaviors, activities, movements and everything else concerning the individuals. The way in which an individual adjusts with the external environment is personality.

Definitions

Personality is defined as a distinctive and relatively stable pattern of behavior, thoughts, motives and emotions that characterize an individual.

In the words of Munn, 'Personality may be defined as the most of characteristics integration of an individuals structure, modes of behaviors, interests, attitudes, capacities, abilities and aptitudes'. Behaviors require integration. This integration of various traits is found differently in different persons. As a general rule every normal individual has some sort of integration. The personality traits. Thus personality which makes distinction in one man and another.

In the words of Gordon Allport, 'Personality is the dynamic organization within the individual of those psychophysical systems that determine his unique adjustment to his environment.' The personality is the organization of the internal and external activities. It includes the external appearance, abilities, aptitudes and capacities, etc. it is not a collection of the traits, but individuals through his personality. Thus personality manifests in his various activities. Capacities, aptitudes and behavior patterns, which are manifested in the individuals' relation with the environment.

According to Gordon Allport only the relatively stable aspects of behavior should be recognized as personality traits. Allport writes, 'From the evidence now in hand, four important conclusions may be drawn; (1) Personality, defined as the distinctive mode of formed at birth but it may be said to have begun at birth. (2) The earliest distructive adjustments in respects to which infants can be said to differ are in the intensity and frequency of their spontaneous both these factors are primarily products of inheritance. (3) Promaturation to form distinctive habits of adjustment of rudimentary traits; but by the second half of the first year, adaptive responses to the physical environment and to people show so marked distinctiveness. (4) Distinctive qualities noticed early in life tend to persist; the child seems predisposed to learn certain modes of adjustment and reject others. Even before these adaptive forms are clearly defined an observe can often, by the method of 'Porphecy' predict later traits. Irrespective of the methods used in the study of the consistency of early development, the evidence is positive in virtually every case. Thus heredity influences the biological features of personality. As a matter of fact, the heredity does not determine personality completely, nor is it ineffective in it.

Personality can be defined as a dynamic and organized set of characteristics possessed by a person that uniquely influences his or her cognitions, motivations and behaviors in various situations (Ryckman 2004).

Nature of Personality

The term 'personality' is also freely used. But if ask people as to what they mean by the term 'personality' they may get many different by explanations. Often, it will not be a definition but it will only be a description. Many emphasize the physical appearance of an individual as constituting a strong or weak personality. Being tall and well built with a powerful voice may be described as characteristics of a commanding or impressive personality. Some may give emphasis to dress. Some others may give emphasis to the manner in which one talks or generally behaves. Some may even give emphasis to the intellectual strength of a person while describing his personality. Some may equally well-emphasize the moral qualities of a person. Such as person may only be a half-naked fakir to someone else. But to them the moral and spiritual strength of the individual constitutes his great personality, admirable enough to be called the 'Mahatma'. The definitions of the term personality from different people person will get a very interesting assortment of descriptions and explanations. Psychologists have tried to understand the nature of human personality along three definite lines.

1. Individual personality depends to a large extent on how he acts and reacts in a social group. Naturally, how he behaves with people, how the influences people, how he is influenced, all these go to make up what we would understand by 'personality'. To understand human personality purely in terms of the social environment and social stimuli. Many of our characteristics are developed purely to maintain our position in society and to obtain social approval and recognition. the social environment mean here not merely the individuals who compose the society but also the large number of stimuli that comes from the culture of a group. The traditions, customs and manners and philosophy of life practiced by a particular community or race have their effect on the individual within that group. Hence personality may be studied from the point of view of cultural environment. Here of course mean that personality is the sum total of responses to social stimuli but we also include the possibility of the individual dynamically acting on the social environment. The individual is not only a 'response' but is also a stimulus.

2. Personality has been studied from the point of view of the uniqueness of an individual, emphasizing this uniqueness as the chief connotation of the term 'personality'. These people emphasize certain particular qualities such as one's intelligence, one's temperament, one's dynamic nature, etc. intelligence has been agreed by all people as a necessary component of one's personality structure. One's personality will to a large extent depend on the amount of his intelligence. So also temperament is accepted by everyone as an important characteristic in the make-up of one's personality. One's temperament depends upon the manner in which his psychic energy gets organized and expressed. If one frequently experiences strong emotions of anger, joy or fear he develops a particular temperament. One's temperament also depends on how strongly his biological urges are experienced and satisfied. Thus temperament depends on how one controls, deals with, and uses his psychic energy. The dynamic nature will to some extent depend on one's physical health and also on the goals one sets for himself. Though all these factors are generally accepted by everyone, some people try to understand personality by emphasizing these characteristics and by emphasizing the manner in which these characteristics are combined in a particular individual resulting in his peculiar individuality. That, according to them will be one's personality.
3. All the characteristics of human being are generally acceptable as important components of personality some have been tried to take a comprehensive and all-inclusive view and understand by personality the sum total of a persons nature and behavior. These people tried to make a very exhaustive analysis of the human being in order to understand personality. Most of the modern studies are along this line.

Theories of Personality

Personality is an area of the still relatively young field of psychology in which there are several ways in which the characteristic behavior of human beings can be explained. One reason that there is not yet one single explanation of personality that all can agree on is that personality is still difficult to measure precisely and scientifically. At present, there are four main perspectives, or viewpoints, in personality theory:

- *The psychoanalytic perspective* had its beginnings in the work of Sigmund Freud and still exists today. It focuses on the role of the unconscious mind in the development of personality. This perspective is also heavily focused on biological causes of personality differences.
- *The behaviorist perspective* is based on the theories of learning (Chapter 11). This approach focuses on the effect of the environment on behavior.
- *The humanistic perspective* first arose as a reaction against the psychoanalytic and behaviorist perspectives and focuses on the role of each person's conscious life experiences and choices in personality development.
- *The trait perspective* differs from the other three in its basic goals: The psychoanalytic, behaviorist, and humanistic perspectives all seek to explain the process that causes personality to form into its unique characteristics, whereas trait theorists are more concerned with the end result—the characteristics themselves. Although some trait theorists assume that traits are biologically determined, others make no such assumption.

The various *theories,* which explain the development and function of personality, are:

Psychoanalytic Theories

a. Freud's psychoanalysis: Sigmund Freud's (1856-1939) psychoanalysis is a theory of personality and also a method of psychotherapy. Psychoanalytic theory is an approach to psychology that emphasized unconscious motives and conflicts.

i. Structural theory: According to Freud, the personality consists of three major systems. As given below:

- *Id*: The part of personality containing inherited psychological energy, particularly sexual and aggressive instincts; operates according to the *pleasure principle* (i.e. the principle guiding the operation of the id; seeks to reduce tension, avoid pain and enhance pleasure). Id is unconcerned with objective reality and is unaffected by the environment. Id is mainly unconscious part of mind and has two basic instincts—the life or sexual instinct (i.e. libido, which in psychoanalysis is the psychic energy that fuels the life or sexual instincts of id) and the *death or aggressive instincts.* Id may discharge its tension in the form of reflex actions, displacement, physical symptoms or "wishful" thinking (i.e. uncensored mental images and unbidden thoughts).
- *Ego*: The part of personality that represents reason, good sense and rational self-control operates according to *reality principle* (i.e. the principal guiding the operation of the ego; seeks to find socially acceptable outlets for instinctual energies. To overcome the wishes of the id" which conflict with social reality, ego has certain defense mechanisms (i.e. methods used by the ego to prevent unconscious anxiety from reaching consciousness). These deny or distort by the reality and they operate unconsciously. They are often unhealthy patterns that cause emotional problems and self-defeating behavior. Some defense mechanisms are *repression* (i.e., a threatening idea, memory or emotion is blocked from becoming conscious and sent back to the id); *projection* (i.e. one's own unacceptable feelings are attributed to someone else); *reaction formation* (the feeling that produces unconscious anxiety is transformed into its opposite in consciousness); *regression* (i.e. In traumatic situations, going back to previous stage of development showing childish habits or immature behavior), *denial* (i.e. refusal to admit that something unpleasant is happening), etc. These defense mechanisms protect the ego and allow the person to cope with reality. They act like immune system of the mind to protect it from 'anxiety'. Ego operates both at conscious and unconscious level.
- *Superego*: The part of personality that represents conscience, morality and social standards. It has two parts—the ego ideal (moral and social standards in unconscious) and conscience (conscious part of superego). According to Freud, the healthy personality must keep all three forces (id, ego and superego) in balance.

ii. Freud's psychodynamic or functional theory: Dynamics is a term from physics that refers to the motion and balance of systems under the action of outside or inside forces. The term 'Psychodynamic' refers to psychological theories that explain behavior in terms of forces located in the individual, such as drives, motives or in psychoanalysis, instinctual energy. It consists of three components.

- *Unconscious:* Mental processes, such as motives, desired and memories not available to awareness, or conscious introspection. Many ego's defense mechanisms operate at this level. It constitutes about 9/10th part of mind.
- *Preconscious:* The memories or thoughts that can be easily recalled and available to awareness on efforts.
- *Conscious:* Awareness about thoughts or certain things around us.

In dreams, narcoanalysis or hypnosis, one can reach the unconscious. Personality differences in tastes, habits, attitudes and behavior patterns stem from the way people displace their energy from early instinctual preferences (displacement is the shifting of instinctional energy from its original object or activity to a different one). When displacement serves a higher cultural or socially useful purpose as in the creation of art or inventions, it is called sublimation.

iii. Psychosexual development of personality: Freud called these stages. Psychological development depends on the changing expression of sexual energy in different parts of the body as the child matures. The 5 stages are:

- *Oral stage (age-year):* It marks the first year of life and has two stages—the sucking and the biting stages. Oral "fixation" in adulthood may foster excessive oral behavior as in smoking, thumb sucking, nail biting, talkativeness, etc.
- *Anal stage (ages 1-3):* The major issue at this stage is control of bodily wastes, i.e. toilet training. It also has the excretory or expulsive stage and the holding or retentive stage. Fixation at this stage results in compulsiveness, excessive self-control and overconformity.
- *Phallic or Oedipal Stage (age 3-5):* The child wishes to possess the parent of the opposite sex and get rid of the parent of the same sex (called Oedipus complex, i.e. attachment of a boy to his mother or Electra complex, i.e. attachment of girl towards her father). It is resolved in the later stage by identification (i.e. a process by which the child adopts an adult's standards of morality, beliefs, and values as his or her own. In psychoanalysis, identification with the same sex parent occurs at resolution of the Oedipal conflict). It indicates the emergence of Superego. According to Freud, a healthy female resolves 'penis envy' by having children whereas a neurotic female resolves it by trying to be like men (in dresses or career). According to Freud, women do not develop the strong moral superegos that men do and feel inferior or dislike other women and develop unhealthy personality traits of passivity, vanity, jealously and masochism.
- *Latency Period* (6 through puberty). This was not considered very important in the development of personality. As the child learns more about the world, sexuality is largely repressed and the ego expands.
- *Genital stage* (adolescence and beyond): It is the stage when mature heterosexual interests appear. Three major sources of sexual arousal during this stage are memories and sensations from earlier childhood periods, physical manipulation of genitals and other erogenous zones and hormonal secretions. Not everyone reaches the mature stage. The defense mechanisms of the ego and the displacement of instinctual energy may prevent people from reaching mature genital sexuality and keep them fixated on immature forms of sexual behavior.

b. Jung's analytic psychology: Carl Jung (1875-1961) differed with Freud on the nature of the unconscious. In addition to the individuals personal unconscious, there is a collective unconscious, containing the universal memories and history of human kind. Jung also postulated archetypes, i.e. universal, symbolic images that appear in myths, art, dreams and other expression of the collective unconscious. Some of the common archetypes involve god, rebirth, devil, wise old person, mother, trickster or magician, hero, animus (a male archetype present in females) and anima (a female archetype present in males). Jung defined complex as a network of ideas bound together by a common emotion or set of feelings.

Jung also proposed the concepts of introversion (turning inward toward contemplation) and extraversion (turning outward toward others). Jung's ideas, often mystical and complex, have been difficult to test experimentally.

c. **Adler's individual psychology:** Alfred Adler (1870-1937) gave the concept of inferiority complex (i.e. in ability to accept natural limitations, occurs when the need for self-improvement is blocked or inhibited).

According to Adler, people have a desire of superiority, which is not the desire to dominate others but the desire for self-improvement. Adler emphasized the individuals need for others. A key concept is *social interest* (i.e. the ability to feel empathy, cooperate and be connected to others), empathy and concern for others. Social interest reflects the ability to be unselfish, to be sympathetic, to cooperate and to feel connected to other people and to the world. Adler maintained that the real essence of human personality is the *creative self* (i.e. each person actively creates his or her own personality from the raw material of heredity and experience).

The style of life is a result of biological factors, the individuals conscious and unconscious motives, past history and life goals. Some differences between Adler's and Freud's theories are:

- To Freud, human beings were the passive victims of unconscious forces. To Adler, they were the masterful directors of their fate.
- To Freud, creativity was a side effect of sublimation: To Adler, creativity was a basic capacity of the species.
- To Freud, social cooperation was a grudging sacrifice of the id. To Adler, it was the essence of human life.

d. **Horney's psychoanalytic interpersonal theory:** Karen Horney's (1885-1952) key concept was that of basic anxiety, the feeling being "isolated and helpless in a potentially hostile world". Because people are dependent on each other, she believed they often end up in a state of anxious conflict when others don't treat them well. People relate to each other in one of three ways: move toward others; move against others or balances and move away from others. She asserted that it is not women who have 'Penis-envy" but men have "womb envy" but later Bruno Bettelheim argued that both sexes envy the reproductive abilities of the others. Horney also gave concept of basic hostility (i.e. grows out of resentment of parental behavior that led to anxiety).

Psychoanalysis has been criticized due to the following problems:

- *Untestable hypotheses:* Many of the ideas of psychoanalysis are descriptive observations, more poetic scientific and also untestable.
- *Incorrect or time limited ideas:* Freud's ideas that our instincts fill an internal reservoir, fixed amount of aggressive energy and sexual conflicts behind most personality problems, have proven to be incorrect.
- *Patients-represent-everyone fallacy:* Findings on patients cannot be generalized to all human beings.
- *The looking backward fallacy:* It is assumed that if A come before B, then A caused B. Psychoanalysis often made this error.
- An overemphasis on unconscious processes rather than real experiences.
- Psychosexual theory of development is not strictly applicable to all cultures.

Learning and Behavioral Theories

These theories of personality emerged from experiments in classical conditioning, instrumental conditioning and cognitive learning. These theories focus on observable events and behavior.

a. Early social learning theory: According to Dollard and Miller's this theory, one may act indecisive and neurotic when one is torn between approaching and avoiding a certain course of action. At the start of action tendency to approach wins over the avoidance tendency but as the goal is nearer, the avoidance tendency wins over the tendency to approach and the individual retreats from the goal.

Social learning or observational learning occurs when an individual learns something by observing another person doing it, in other words it is learning by modeling. According to social learning theory, behavior is seen as a two way interaction between an individual and his environment, that is, 'Both people and their environments are reciprocal determinants of each other' (Bandura, 1977). Exponents of this theory view the behavioristic approach to learning as one that limits the idea of the potential of an individual and his influence over his own behavior. According to social learning theory, an individual possesses no inherent behavior patterns at birth other than reflexes, so must learn everything else. Such learning occurs as a result of observing the behavior of other people, which allows complex patterns to be acquired in a more efficient way than trial and error. Indeed, some behaviors such as language can only be learned, according to Bandura, by observation of human models, as it is highly unlikely that mere reinforcement of random vocalization would lead to the complex use of speech that forms the everyday language of an individual. Learning, then, is envisaged as behavior that is acquired by observation of modeling stimuli, providing the learner with a symbolic image of such behavior, which may serve as a guide.
Bandura identifies four processes involved in the observation learning situation.

- *Attentional processes:* These processes are concerned with the characteristics of the model and of the observer. In the former, some of the factors which influence learning are variables such as interpersonal attraction between the model and the observer, the usefulness of the observed behavior and the distinctiveness, complexity and frequency of contact with the modeled stimuli. Observer characteristics comprise the level of arousal, capacity to process information, the perceptual set and amount of previous reinforcement.
- *Retention processes:* It is obviously important to remember the modeled behavior if one is to learn from it, so the role of such strategies as rehearsal is crucial. Jeffrey (1974) found that the highest level of learning was achieved when the modeled behavior was first organized and symbolically rehearsed before actually performing the behavior.
- *Motor reproduction processes:* The learner must be capable of actually carrying out the observed behavior and of evaluating it in terms of accuracy.
- *Motivational process:* Modelled stimuli are more likely to be learned if the observer sees some value in them, but the role of reinforcement in social learning theory is one of facilitation rather than necessity. It may take the form of external reward such money, or self-reinforcement, where the learner rewards herself with something when a predetermined behavior has been achieved. For example, she may set herself a number of objectives to achieve for a course and having attained them may reward herself by going out to dinner. The likelihood of the modeled behavior being learned is increased when the observer sees the model being reinforced for performing that behavior. This is termed vicarious reinforcement.

Information can be transmitted by the model in a variety of ways, such as an actual physical demonstrations, by pictures, words and the mass media. Abstract modeling is the term used for process whereby the observer elicits the principles of behavior from a variety of modelled stimuli and applies them to a situation that is similar to the ones which are observed. For example, observation of various models performing a surgical dressing would allow the observer to learn the rules of the procedure and these could then be applied to similar situations. How does social learning theory explain the development of novel or creative responses? Bandura sees the novel response as a utilization of the qualities of many models, to produce anew creative behavior. These are a number of characteristics of both the model and the observer that make learning more likely. Experiments indicate that persons who possess status, prestige, power are more effective models for those kind of behaviors. Individuals who are lacking in self-esteem and confidence and those who are dependent tend to be more easily influence by the behaviors of models who are obviously successful. However, one need to interpret such results with caution, as many confident people readily adopt behavior of those actions are seen to be of value.

b. Radical behaviorism: BF Skinner's approach is exclusively instrumental or operant, i.e. it deals only with the processes by which reinforcement (reward) and punishment influence the likelihood of behavior. Personality is nothing but a collection of reinforced responses. The person behave in certain ways because of the reinforcement responses. We behave in certain ways because of the reinforcement contingencies we experience. Personality composes of behavior based on theories of learning.

The social learning approach to personality includes:
I. Aspects of the individual
II. Aspects of the environment
III. The interaction between them.

According to social learning theorists the identified qualities of the person that they believe influence behavior across many situations are:
- Inherited temperaments
- Skills and talents such as singing, writing, etc.
- Perceptions
- Expectations
- Plans of actions.

Humanist Theories

There is no single theory that represents the humanistic approach, but all theories share a common view that this approach involves the study of man as a human being, with his thoughts, feelings and experiences. This is in direct contrast to the stimulus-response theorists, who study man from the point of view of his overt behavior, disregarding his inner feelings and experiences. Humanistic differs from cognitive theory also, in that the latter is concerned with the thinking aspects of man's behavior, with little emphasis on the affective components. Exponents of humanistic theory claim that the other two theories omit some of the most significant aspects of man's behavior, with little emphasis on the affective components. Exponents of humanistic theory claim that the other two theories omit some of the most significant aspects of human existence, namely feelings, attitudes and values. Humanistic theory is closely related to the philosophical approach called phenomenology, which asserts that reality lies in a person's perception of an event and not in the event itself. The humanistic viewpoint is summarized by Hamachek (1977) as follows:

It is a psychological stance that focused not so much on person's biological drives, but on their goals; not so much on stimuli impinging on them, but on their desires to be or to do something; not so much on their past experiences, but on their current circumstances; not so much on life conditions *per se*, but on the subjective qualities of human experience, the personal meaning of an experience to persons, rather on their objectives, observable response.

Humanistic theory, then is concerned with human growth, individual fulfillment and self-actualization and it is claimed that this approach is 'intuitively right' as it agrees with the ideas most people have about what is uniquely human. However, the behaviorist approach is not considered to be wrong, but humanistic theory prefers to emphasize the affective aspects of man as being of equal importance to the cognitive and psychomotor elements.

There are two main principles that apply to the humanistic approach to learning and teaching, namely teacher-student relationships and the classroom climate. The former stresses the importance of the interpersonal between learner and teacher as a major variable affecting learning and this in turn affects the climate of the classroom. The presence or absence of conflict and tension will depend largely on the quality of relationships within the classroom setting.

Phenomenology is the study of events and situations as individuals experience them, in personality, the study of an individual's qualities from the persons own point of view. Humanists believe the personality is defined by human abilities that separate us from other animals; freedom of choice, free will and self-direction. Humanist approach rejected the psychoanalytic emphasis on hostility, biological instincts and conflict. It also rejects the fragmented approach of the behavioral schools, with their emphasis on describing pieces of the person.

I. Maslow's theory: Human nature consists of some good things, such as joy, rapture, laughter, love, simple daily happiness and are moments of ecstasy. The inner nature of human beings is essentially good, or at least neutral.

Abraham H Maslow (1908-70) was a major exponent of the humanistic approach to psychology, and has also made a significant contribution to motivation theory with his theory of a hierarchy of needs. He coined the term 'third force' psychology because he considered the first force to be Freudian psychotheraphy and the second to be the stimulus-response school. The latter school, he felt, had little relevance to the human personality: 'these extensive books on the psychology of learning are of no consequence, at least to the human center, to the human soul, to the human essence' (Maslow 1971). One of the key concepts he defined was that of 'self-actualization' and he studied the behavior of people who he classified as self-actualizers. Maslow stated eight ways in which an individual self-actualizes, and these include 'experiencing ways in which an individual self-actualizes, and these include 'experiencing fully, vividly, selflessly, with full concentration and total absorption'. He mentions the 'peak experience', which is an ecstatic moment that can be brought on by such experiences as classical music and religious experiences.

For the humanist, the goal of education is to assist the individual to achieve self-actualization, or, as Maslow puts it, 'to help the person to become the best that he is able to become'. This intrinsic approach is in contract to the extrinsic educational ethic, in which the transmission of factual knowledge is seen to be more important than the development of an individual. The ideal college, according to Maslow, would be one in which the main objectives would by the discovery of one's identity and the destiny or vocation for each person.

II. Rollo May's: Major role in the humanist movement emphasizes some of the fundamentally difficult or even tragic aspects of the human condition, including loneliness, anxiety, and alienation. This doctrine holds that human beings have absolute freedom of choice but this freedom carries a price in anxiety and even despair.

III. Carl Roger's client oriented theories: To Carl Rogers, Congruence is the harmony between the conscious self and the totality of the person's unconscious feelings and life experiences. To become fully functioning, congruent people need *unconditional positive regard* (i.e. love or support given to another person with no conditions attached), love and support for the people. Conditional positive regard sometimes may result in incongruence. The suppression of feeling and parts of oneself produces low self-regard, inaccurate perceptions of reality, defensiveness and unhappiness.

The major criticism of the humanistic approach is that many of its assumptions cannot be tested because the terms that humanist use are vague. Critics also say that humanistic psychology is closer to philosophy than science, because it rests on a subjective view of human nature.

Carl R Rogers made his reputation as a psychotherapist, developing a new approach that he called client-centered therapy (Rogers, 1951). This involves the therapist in a non-directive role in which the client is encouraged to develop a deeper understanding of himself. The role of the therapist is to provide a noncritical atmosphere, in which there is no attempt to interpret for the client, but simply a reflecting back of his statements in order to assist him in developing self-awareness.

This concept of client-centered therapy led Rogers to formulate his student-centered approach to learning, which is contained in his most important work on the subject (Rogers, 1969). In this work, he states a number of principles of learning:

1. Human beings have a natural potentially for learning.
2. Significant learning takes place when the subject matter is perceived by the student as having relevance for his own purposes.
3. Those elements of learning which are threating to the self are more easily perceived and assimilated when external treats are at a minimum.
4. Learning which involves a change in self-organization is threatening and tends to be resisted.
5. When treat to the self is low, experience can be perceived in differentiated fashion, and learning can proceed.
6. Much significant learning is acquired through doing.
7. Learning is facilitated when the student participates responsibly in the learning process.
8. Self-initiated learning, which involves the whole person of the learner feeling as well as intellect, is the most lasting and pervasive.
9. Independence, creativity and self-reliance are all facilitated when self-criticism and self-evaluation are basic and evaluation by others is secondary importance.

10. The most socially useful learning in the modern world is the learning of the process of learning, a continuing openness to experience and incorporation into oneself of the process of change.

These ten principles illustrate Rogers' approach to learning and his emphasis on relevance, student participation and involvement, self-evaluation and the absence of threat in the classroom.

Rogers sees the teacher as a facilitator of learning; a provider of resources for learning, and someone who shares his feeling as well as his knowledge with the students. Thus the prerequisites of an effective facilitator of learning are awareness of self, being oneself in the classroom, acceptance and trust of the students and understanding and empathy.

He sees learning as being a continuum, with much meaningless material at one end and significant or experimental learning at the other. The former could describe many curricula, which are seen as virtually meaningless by the student for whom they are intended. Experiential learning, on the other hand, has a number of qualities such as personal involvement, self-initiation, pervasiveness, self-evaluation and meaningfulness. He contracts the kind of learning that is concerned solely with cognitive functioning with that involving the whole person. Teaching, according to Rogers, is a highly overrated activity, in contrast to the notion of facilitation. Teaching by giving knowledge does not meet the requirements of today's changing world; what is required is the facilitation of learning and change and this calls for a different set of qualities in the facilitator. The most important factor is the relationship that exists between facilitator and learner and Rogers suggests a number of qualities that are required for this:

1. Genuineness, i.e. the facilitator comes across as a real rather than as some kind of ideal model. Hence it is important that he shows normal reactions to the students so that they accept him as a real person.
2. Trust and acceptance, i.e. acceptance of the students as a person in her own right as a person who is worthy of respect and care.
3. Empathic understanding, i.e. putting oneself in the student's shoes in order to see and understand things from her perspective.

Rogers suggests that it is possible for the teacher to build into a program the freedom to learn, which students require. This can be done by using student's won experiences and problems so that relevance is obvious and by providing resources for the students in the form of both material and human resources. He also recommends the use of learning contracts that help to make the students have autonomy over their own learning. The goal of education is that of the student becoming a fully functioning person.

TRAITS AND TYPES THEORIES

Trait is a descriptive characteristics of an individual, assumed to be stable across situations, e.g. shy, brave, reliable, friendly, hostile, serious, confident, etc.

A type is a clump of traits thought to describe a certain kind of individual. An "executive type" has the traits of leadership, dominance, high self-confidence and consideration for others.

"Type theories" are used to describe personality, e.g. Hippocraes theory of 4 humors (blood, phlegm, yellow bile and black bile), *Gall's system* of phrenology, and William Sheldon's classification according to ectomorphic, mesomorphic and endomorphic.

I. Trait theories are based on Gordon Allport's theory of common traits, i.e. 3 types of traits—*Cardinal traits* (overwhelming importance to an individual and influence practically everything that person does, e.g. Gandhi and Luther King have common trait of non-violence); *central traits* (that reflect a characteristics way of behaving, dealing with others and reacting to new situation, e.g. warm, neat, humble, shy, etc.) and *secondary traits* (aspects subject to change, e.g. preferences for food, colors, movies, etc.).

II. Cattell's theory of factor analysis: Raymond B Cattell's theory is based on the study of personality traits by using a statistical method called factor analysis. A personality has surface traits (traits visible in a person's words or deeds) and source traits (the underlying causes of surface qualities).

III. Hans Eysenck's theory of extraversion introversion neuroticism (i.e. extent to which a person is anxious, depressed, obsessive and hostile and has trouble coping).
Locus of control: It is general expectation about whether the results of one's actions are under one's control (external locus).

Self-esteem: How people feel about themselves privately (experienced self-esteem) or behave with others (presented self-esteem).

Trait and type theories have been criticized because of circular thinking, "label" a personality receives and may become victimized by it "piece meal" approach to personality and problems of consistency and predictability (i.e. consistency paradox).

Personality is believed to be formed in first few years of life and do not change later on. The basic traits of personality which are stable throughout life are:

- Shyness versus sociability
- Neuroticism
- Aggressiveness
- Consistency.

Biases in the study of personality are:

- Pleasure of pattern
- Perceptual bias
- Cultural bias.

For abnormal personality traits and disorders, see chapter on "Personality Disorders". Read authors text on psychiatric/Mental health Nursing.

Factors Affecting Personality

BIOLOGICAL FACTORS

For sometime there was a discussion among the psychologists about the relation of heredity and environment in the development of personality. In this discussion arguments were given from both sides and data were gathered on the basis of observation and experimentation. It was found by these data that the development of personality depends upon both heredity and environment in the factor influencing personality.

The factors affecting personality can be divided into two classes—(1) Biological, and (2) Social. The biological factors affecting the development of personality are there: (i) Ductless glands, (ii) Physique and (iii) Nervous system.

I. Ductless glands: Ductless glands send their secretions directly to the blood without ducts. Their secretion are called hormones. These hormones are responsible for many changes in the personality. Each gland secretes one or more types of hormones. A description of the effect of some of the ductless glands will show the extent to which personality is influenced by them.

- *Pancreas:* Pancreas sends insulin to the blood. The amount of sugar in the blood depends upon the amount of insulin in it. When the deficiency of insulin, i.e. sugar, is in the body the mental capacities are weakened and the personality of the individual seems less balanced. His mood is changed, temperament becomes irritated and fear increases.
- *Thyroid:* Thyroid gland has a very important function in the development of physical structures as well as mental development. If it is absent since the very birth body and mind of the child do not develop. Cretins, imbeciles, etc. are the result of the absence of thyroid gland. Its destruction causes a disease known as myxedema. This disease creates laziness in man. The activities of the mind as well as those of muscles are slackened. The memory becomes weak, concentration and thinking becomes difficult. In the period of development the excess of the activity of thyroid gland results in rapid physical growth, specially the development of height. An excessive activity of this gland results in tension, irritation, worry and instability in man. Thus with the increase or deficiency in the activity of thyroid gland, the activity of the body as well as of the mind also increases and decreases.
- *Adrenal:* Adrenal gland secretes adrenaline. Adrenaline has an important influence upon personality. Its excess creates hypersexual traits in men or women. Its deficiency in woman is responsible for the absence of the rounded contours and feminine voice. If mobilizes the capacities in the time of emergency. The excess of adrenaline causes rapid heart-beat, high blood pressure dual having less adrenaline feels relaxation in the muscles, more sweat and the pupils of the eye are extended. An entire absence of adrenaline results in the disease known as Addison's disease. In this disease one feels weakness and lethargy in the body, the power of resisting disease is lessened, the increased in sex activity disappears and metabolism becomes slow, the skin becomes black, the power of resisting heat and cold is lessened and behavior becomes irritable.
- *Gonads:* The secretion of the gonads, i.e. sex hormone is an important factor influencing personality. In adolescence there is a special increment in sex hormones. Hence changes are observed in the individuals according to their sex. In the boy one finds the appearance of masculine characteristics such as beard, moustaches, high pitch in voice, etc. while in the girl there is development of mammary glands and appearance of other womanly traits. The process concerning pregnancy, e.g. menses, pregnancy, the bearing of the child and maternal behavior is very much influenced by the hormones.
- *Pituitary:* The hormones secreted by the pituitary glands control other glands. The hormones secreted by the front part of the pituitary gland increase the activity of other glands as well. The hormones secreted by the back part of the pituitary glands control the blood pressure and the metabolism of water in the body. These hormones also effect physical growth. In the time of physical growth the bones and muscles of the individual grow speedily due to the activity of these glands. In its excess, the height can go even 7 to 9 feet. But because after excessive activity this gland becomes very much inactive, these very tall persons die at an early age. If the activity of the pituitary gland is very much deficient during the period of development, the individual remains a midget, though his intellect is normal and the physical structure is not unattractive. If the activity of this gland is normal during the developmental period and becomes excessive afterwards, the hands, feet, nose and lower jaw, etc. become broad. This state is known as acromegaly.

The effect of the hormones is influenced by the hereditary as well as the environmental factors. But still the excess or deficiency in their activity creates some changes quite apparent in the personality of the individual. It is not necessary that the excess of the secretion of any one of the particular glands should always show some special influence in the body, e.g. the excess of sex tendency should not always be supposed as due to excess of the secretion of the sex gland, since different glands also interact upon each other due to which activity of some is increased while that of others is decreased. The sex behavior, for example, is very much influenced by social norms, customs, circumstances, habits and many other things. Hence, in spite of the deficiency of the sex hormones, the individual may appear to be very much interested in sex activities. On the other hand, in spite of the excess of the sex hormones, the individual may not appear to be interested in sexual activities.

ii. Physique: It is sometimes observed in daily life that the fat men are easy going and social, while the thin persons are self-controlled, irritated and unsocial. Thus the physical structure has some relation with the temperament. But even the instances contrary to this rule are not lacking. Hence the relation of physical structure and the temperament has not been definitely established. More studies are required in their direction. The studies conducted so far have been mostly on college students. Before one arrives at some definite conclusion, studies must be conducted on adult persons as well. But even after that, the problem of the basis of correlation remains unanswered. Similarly, by correlation between the temperament and physique the former cannot be taken to be the result of the latter. It should also be remembered in this context that the physical structure makes a difference in other's behavior towards a particular person. It is observed that our behavior towards different individuals is modified, to some extent, according to their physical structure. This difference in our behavior makes a change in their personality. Hence, a particular difference should not be supposed to be due to physical structure alone but also due so other's behavior towards the particular person, though the former may be more important.

iii. Body chemistry: In ancient times, the differences of temperament were supposed to be due to differences of chemical elements in different men. Thus the nervous personality was taken as the result of excess of nervous fluid. It was supposed that the sanguine persons have an excess of blood, the choleric persons an excess of bile, phlegmatic persons an excess of phlegm and the melancholic persons, an excess of spleen. This principle is not accepted in modern psychology, but still no psychologist denies the relation of personality with the proportion of chemical elements in the body. These chemical elements are of two types. Some reach the body from outside while some are created in the body itself. Thus the drugs have sufficient effect on personality. The behavior of the drunkard is an example of such effect. Different types of intoxicating drugs have a clear influence vitamins also causes some changes in the personality. With the increase or decrease of the quantity of sugar in the body, the physical and mental state of the man is very much changed. In convalescence one finds a difference in the individuals personality. Difference is also noticed after a long illness.

Besides the above-mentioned biological factors many other factors influence personality, e.g. sex, intelligence, and nervous system, etc. The difference in the sex of male and female creates a difference in their personality, though it has been established that much of this difference is caused by social and cultural environment. Galton and Goddard believe that intellect is absolutely hereditary. The modern psychologists do not agree with this view though the influence of heredity is not denied. The environment affects intellect, but the development of intellect is ultimately limited. The influence of specific abilities, as that of music, mathematics, etc. on human personality is very well known. Like the intelligence, the abilities are also generally hereditary. According to Kempf, the author of *The Automatic Function and Personality,* the nervous system is one of the important determinants of personality.

SOCIAL FACTORS

The environments of different individuals are very much different from one another and so also their effects, but the influence of environment of personality can be roughly classified in that of home, school and society. All these three play an important part in the development of personality.

The environment of the home has a comprehensive influence on the development of personality. This influence as a general rule, is according to the patterns found in a particular culture. In the family the relation of child with the parents is the most intimate. The cultural development of the child is very much influenced by the behavior of the parents, e.g. a child brought up in Indian family will be very much different in his behavior than another brought up in a Western home. But even in the same culture much difference can be observed in the parent-child relationship in different families, e.g. generally, the child has a respectable place in Indian family, but all Indian parents do not sufficiently love and sympathize with the child. In such circumstances much repression is observed in child's behavior. He becomes an introvert and often enjoys in his dreams, daydreams and imagination things which are denied to him by his parents. The influence of the presence of the parental love is again not the same in the case of all children. A child may become aggressive while another may become submissive in the same circumstances. On the other hand, if the parents show excessive affection towards the child, the child may become an extremist and excessively dependent upon the parents. A child excessively ignored shows different types of conflicts in his personality. Children brought in the psychological clinics for the cure of defects of personality showed that an important cause of their defects was the behavior of their parents toward them. According to Sigmund Freud, the tendency to depend upon the parents in the childhood is manifested in the tendency to depend upon the leader in the adult age. If the child is allowed freedom in the matters concerning his belongings, food, clothes, books, etc. he will develop a habit of freewill; if all these are decided by his parents, he will not get an opportunity to utilize his judgment and so become over-dependent or submissive.

Parents are more powerful and efficient than the child. Hence they are ideals before him. The child wants to become like his parents. Thus he establishes his identification with either of the parents and tries to follow his manners, ways and behavior. The child also fulfills his frustrated desires through this identification. It has been observed that the little boy wears the big shirt of the father and walks proudly like him with a stick in his hand. This identification with the parents in the childhood is later on converted into the identification of the individual with the leader. By the identification with the leader's achievements and sorry in his failures.

In the absence of affection and sympathy, the child often turns criminal. While discussing the causes of criminal tendencies, Healy and Bronner have emphasized three factors, viz. the effort to get rid of the painful circumstances, the tendency to revenge for the mis-behavior of the father, the efforts to satisfy the frustrating desires. Often the child has the curiosity as to where from the younger brother or sister has come. The answer to this question by the parents has an important effect on his personality. The child has a natural curiosity towards the sex tendency. Often the parents try to suppress his curiosity towards sex or they just rebuke when he aks such questions. But the child is not silenced by this. He tries to enquire from the servants or friends in the house. But this leads to guilt conscience. The reactions in the parents about the everyday matters in the family and the relations of the mother and father among themselves also affect the personality of the child. In short, the behavior of parents and the circumstances in family affect the personality of the child.

Development of Personality

It has been observed that the behavior of the oldest and the youngest, the elder or the younger is not the same in the family. Similarly, it has been found that the parent's behavior towards them is not the same. This has led the psychologist Alfred Adler to emphasize the importance of birth order in the development of personality. The birth order of the child fixes his status in the family which decides his roles which effect his personality. The youngest child is treated with affection by everyone, hence he becomes over-dependent. The eldest child becomes self-sufficient and tyrant, because being the only child for some time he does not share his rights and things with others. The birth of another child in the family has an important influence on the first child, since it takes away his monopoly in affection and sometimes he is neglected altogether. Hence he feels jealous with the younger child and tries to regain his rights. On the other hand, the new child is anxious to make his place in his family. The above description of the child's problems based upon the conception of birth order has not been conclusively proved. The researchers have found similar conflicts in different birth orders. Adler has truly said that the individual develops his style of life from the pattern of his early life in the family, but there are no grounds to suppose that this style of life remains unchanged in future. It cannot be denied that the environment in the childhood is one of the most important factors determining personality, but it is difficult to believe with Freud and Adler that the personality of an individual is completely determined in childhood.

The personality of an individual is gradually developed from the days of infancy. In this process of development the environment plays an important part. It has been agreed by all that the family or the home influences the child more than anything else in the proper development of personality. Most of the traits which the child develops are formed in the early days from the patterns of relationships that are established with the members of the family, particularly parents and siblings (brothers and sisters). Even the psychological disorders of later life are the results mostly of wrong pattern of relationships that are obtained in the early days within the home.

Personality may be viewed from the point of view of what it is and how it is composed. This would mean a study of the various traits and how they are organized and personality may be studied from the way it expresses itself on the outer environment stressing the behavior aspect. It is studied more from the point of view of not what it is but what it does. Here, how a person adjusts himself to the society in which he lives, how he meets his daily problems, how he reacts to difficulties, etc. will all be emphasizes. For any proper understanding of personality both these view points are necessary. A modern tendency in psychology is to take such a composite view. This would also mean that in understanding personality we are not carried away mainly by what other people think of an individual from his behavior but what he actually is. This would also emphasize the view that a man's personality depends on how he perceives himself and how he organizes his own desires, fears, experiences, etc. The different stages of infancy, adolescence, youth and old age are very clearly depicted in the physiological development of human beings. The speed and direction of physiological development differs from one stage to another. In the different stages of the physiological development, different changes are visible in the personality of the individual. In some stages these changes are faster and more comprehensive while in other stages the change is comparatively less. This shows a change in the personality too.

1. *The first-six years:* Freud and many other psychologists give much importance to infancy in an individuals life. Some psychologists have claimed the development of personality to start during pregnancy. In Rank's view the development of personality starts in the mother's womb. He further maintains that the very activity of its conception affects the child's personality, the presence or absence of difficulties in it making a difference in the personality. But it has been possible to prove this theory by experimentation. In Freud's opinion, whatever incidents take place in the first three years of child's life permanently mould his character the rest being a mere development of these peculiarities. Suckling, weaning, loving, fondling, scolding, beating, toilet training, etc. all affect the child's personality. The love and affection of the parents have a very significant effect upon the child. Excessive love and affection make a child stubborn and inconsistent. Lack of affection stunts the development of his emotions while proper love gives him emotional stability.

Besides love and affection, suckling also impresses the personality of the child. Experiments indicate that even when the child is not hungry, he does not want to release the breasts. Actually suckling is not merely a mode of satisfying hunger but also a symbol of the mother's love for the child and consequently weaning also affects the child's personality because it sometimes expresses the indifference of the mother towards the child. If the child is suckled for a long time he becomes over-dependent. Early weaning may lead to pessimism and morbidity. An interesting experiment was carried out on college students in this context. They asked their mothers about the ages at which weaning had been carried out, and they were subsequently tested for their sense of security or insecurity. The result indicated an important correlation between weaning and the sense of security and insecurity. Those who had been weaned at an age of 6 to 9 months scored less points in security than those suckled for over 9 months, showed no sense of insecurity whatsoever. This strange result was seen in the light of the fact that in the cultural group from among which these students had been chose, the cause of weaning was not the desire but the inability to continue suckling. This study indicates that the weaning does not have as great an effect as indifference on the part of the mother's indifference. In the first six years, the child learns the adjustment of his needs with the environment. His relations with his mother during this adjustment leave a permanent mark on the development of his personality. The development of a sense of insecurity at this age leads to mental conflict making a child frightened and depressive and aggressive and naughty. Even toilet training affects the child. If, in the teaching of cleanliness, of which parents and other members partake, excessive strictness and resolution are applied, the child may develop compulsive traits. The birth order too has an effect on the child. The relation of the parents among themselves, the social and financial of the family, both leave an indelible mark on his personality. The outlook and reaction of the family members towards the sexual tendencies also tend to affect the child's personality. Unnecessary fear develops a criminal tendency in the child. The intelligent satisfaction of his curiosity has a good effect on his development.

Important characteristics of personality become apparent at a very early age of the child. The differences of will power, friendliness, determination and impressing others, etc. appear at the ages of two or three. By the time a child is five he starts expressing competitiveness. It has been seen from experiments that traits like self-dependence, love for the family, humor, emotional adjustment and reaction to resistance, etc. of the personality appear at the age of one and stay permanent even after adolescence. But some traits show some change. Actually, there is a lot of truth in the fact that the foundation, of the characteristic traits in the personality of individual are laid in childhood.

2. *Prepubertal childhood:* The second stage in the development of human personality continues till the on coming of puberty and it is accordingly entitled the prepubertal childhood. At this stage, the conditions of the school start affecting the development of his personality because commonly, by now, he has started attending school and playing with other children. The child is given a particular place in the family, whereas he has to acquire for himself a position among his colleagues. He thus learns the lesson of equality and justice. His mother does not afford him security in the school, whereby he learns the traits of independence and self-dependence. The child enters his own age group and acquires a role according to his personality, and by living in a group learns the patterns of his future grown-up life. It is at this stage that he learns the lesson of leadership, friendship, sympathy and social adaptation. His success or failure in the group develops many good and bad traits in the child. A child extremely dependent on some one member of the family has difficulty in adjusting in the group, a state which generally results in the origination of a feeling of inferiority. The practices which a child adopts are the ones which have brought him success in his attempts at the adjustment within his group. If obstinacy and self-assertion or aggression are more advantageous he will develop them and if escape is more successful the child will become an escapist.

3. *Puberty and adolescence:* The next stage in the development of human personality is the stage of puberty and adolescence. Puberty is a physiological condition, in which the maturation of sexual organs takes place. It is the link between childhood and adulthood. Adolescence as a psychological state is generally characterized by extensive disturbances.

- Puberty does effect personality. After puberty, the interest in sexual activities becomes specific and developed. Many studies have made it known that the social behavior of girls and boys registers a maturation after puberty. This may be caused by an awareness of the physiological condition in puberty leading to a feeling of adulthood. In this stage the boys and girls identify themselves with adults, their interests becoming adult. Immediately before puberty, there is extensive physiological development and immediately after it the boys and girls start exhibiting the respective physical signs of their sexes. The girls start having menstrual cycles and their organs acquire rounded contours. Boys grow beards and moustaches and their voices become heavy. In this stage the speed of mental development, too, is maximum. Puberty takes place two years earlier in girls than the boys, this being the reason for their earlier exhibition of pubertal changes.
- The psychological state of adolescence affects personality in no small measure. The girls and boys start taking an interest in the persons of the opposite sex. They also experience an increase in the sense of independence. The adjustment of adolescence is a problem which differs with culture. The disturbance of an adolescent in civilized societies is not found in the people of Samoa. In their society unlike the civilized societies,

there are no restrictions on sexual behavior and the individual becomes self-dependent at an early age. The disturbance of the adolescent stage is due to those mental conflicts through which a civilized person has to pass. These conflicts arise from many social problems like sexual adjustment, self-dependence, choice of profession, etc. In this age, if the parents still look on the youth as a child, he will either make a revolt against it or admit to it, the latter course leading to a retrogression in the development of his personality. The indifference to sex education makes these adolescent problems even more intricate. In India, there is more sex education and less sex restrictions in primitive tribes than there is in the Hindu society. Thus the transition from adolescence to adulthood is easier for the tribal youths than the Hindu youths. Absence of the means of satisfying sexual curiosities and a social sense of evil related to them increase the guilt conscience and anxiety of the adolescent, and this does not allow the proper development of his personality. It is a baseless idea that the person becomes entirely new during adolescence or that there is a complete reorganization of his entire personality. Adolescence is a stage in the development of personality and development is a continuous process in which infancy affects adolescence and adolescence affects adulthood.

4. *Adulthood and after:* The fourth stage, following adolescence in the development of personality is adulthood. Many studies or researchers have revealed that equilibrium is at a low ebb in the beginning of adulthood and just before old age, between them there being comparatively better adjustment. Upon entering adulthood a person adopts some permanent occupation, gets married and a lot of change is brought in the personality. After this, till old age, not much change is needed. This outline of the development of personality is not essentially same in all. Actually, it depends on the adjustments of the adult age, one of the problems being economic adjustment. Getting a lower post than anticipated, long periods of unemployment, getting an uninteresting occupation, freedom from dependence on employment, all have profound effect upon the individual. Many serious problems arise in the adjustment with the marriage partner in adulthood. Similarly, incidents like absence of children, death of the offspring, too many children and, in India, too many daughters, tend to keep a man in worry and misery till old age. In brief, as we have said above, occupation, marriage and offspring are essential for an adult. If their condition is satisfactory the person's personality remains balanced but if there is any disturbance it becomes difficult for the person to retain his balance.

5. *Old age and before it:* After adult life, in old age and just before it, many troubles surround the person, major ones concerning the diminution in his physical energies, economic power and social prestige. In old age people who find themselves dependent on others do not retain their mental balance. People who retire with a meagre pension or a provident fund of some thousands are not in a very satisfactory state unless they have developed some occupation from their adult life. A problem of adjustment arises for the mother who has nothing to do after her children have been married off. If now she does not take to some work, religious or social activity the only thing left for her is to criticize the neighboring daughters-in-law or to create unnecessary troubles and obstacles in the lives of the younger generation. It must have become obvious, from this rough outline of the stages in the development of personality, that it means the adjustment with new needs, conflicts and frustrations. New problems of adjustment keep on arising in the different stages in the physiological and psychological development of personality. It is often seen that the

deficiencies of one stage in the development are fulfilled in the next stage. But besides this, in every stage new problems arise whose solution is essential. The development of personality is a continuous process passing through these stages.

Integration of Personality

Personality is the dynamic organization of the psychological traits, exhibited in man's adjustment with the environment. If the organization of psychophysical qualities in personality is not orderly, difficulties will arise in the adjustment with the environment. Such a personality will be called disintegrated.

The integration of personality is necessary in order to effect adjustment with the environment. Adjustment will be natural and easy if this integration is strong. The integration of personality is the integration of all the psychophysical traits of personality. There is an absence of conflicts in it. In it, all mental activities work in an organized way. An integrated personality is flexible, strong and organized, as well as balanced. McDougall has called personality is found in everyone in a lesser or greater degree. If the integration is less than is essential, then problems of adjustment with the environment arise.

The weakness of the Ego is fundamental in the personality problems. Either the persons Ego cannot control the Id's desires and impulses or it cannot adjust with the Superego. For the integration of personality, it is necessary that the person maintains a balanced and realistic outlook. Some failures and frustrations come in everyone's life, and the persons should pursue his life task without being too much disturbed by happiness or sorrow. An integrated approach is the golden path of life. It is only the balance of emotions, needs, imagination and thinking, etc. which can keep the personality integrated.

The definition of the integration of personality must have made it clear that it essentially needs socialization without which the person finds it difficult to adjust with the environment. The social environment is not the total environment of the person and neither is sociability by itself the only adequate trait for adaptation in society, and yet it is an essential trait in the personality. Sociability, as the name suggests, is that tendency by which a person harmoniously mixes with other people of the society and lives with them. An unsocial person is introvert and likes to live alone. He experiences difficulty in meeting other people and having relations with them. In daily life, the problems which arise in his meeting with other people assume alarming proportions while the social man deals with them with ease. For example, the unsocial person feels lonely when he is alone, and bored and restless upon the advent of new people.

Deficiency of integration is seen in the problems of maladjustment with the environment. The reason is that in the absence of integration the personality is unbalanced, there being no proper blending of psychophysical traits. It is not essential that deficiency of integration may render him incapable of work. Many of the famous persons suffered from grave deficiencies in the integration of their personalities, but though this did not hinder or restrict their greatness, their personalities were one-sided. With people of average capacities such deficiency will affect even their skills. It can be said that in case of deficiency in integration of personality, the person can neither be skilled in his behavior nor does he get success in his life's tasks. He not only makes his own life disturbed but also disturbs the peace of others. Thus psychologists help people in the integration of their personalities by giving suggestions.

Types of Personality

Personality is an organismic unity of both physiological and psychological elements. Psychological maladjustments can lead to serious disturbances in the cognitive and emotional life of the person and also psychological upsets can disturb physiological functioning. For example, over activity of the thyroid gland results in nervousness, irritability, in addition to the usual physical symptoms. Under activity of the thyroid will bring about sluggishness, apparent mental deficiency, indifference to emotional stimuli.

The concept of personality types assumes (i) that personalities characteristics are mutually exclusive groups, and (ii) that in each types there are certain mutually dependent and interrelated traits pattern of response that can be inferred from each other. This theory has an obvious appeal because of its simplicity. Even as abstractions types have very limited usefulness and often contribute more to prejudice and to hasty decisions than to sober judgment of real knowledge. The various personality types can be classified as:

1. Humoral types
2. Physical types
3. Psychological types.

HUMORAL TYPE

For humoral types personality we go to back to Galen with his four humors—blood, phlegm, choler (yellow bile) and melancholy (black bile) from which stem the four temperaments. The Russian Physiologists Pavlov brought out the concept of humoral types of personalities. (i) Choleric, (ii) Sanguine and (iii) Phlegmatic.

i. **The choleric:** The choleric temperament, according to Pavlov, is the result of a strong but unbalanced nervous system in which excitation preponderates over inhibition. Characterized by persistence and constancy of purpose, the choleric individuals emotions are very easily aroused. Such individuals are vehement in speech and action and they carry out very swiftly. Choleric individual is bold and ambitious but tends to be incautious.

   Choleric type individual should seek work in which getting excited will be an asset rather than a liability. One would hardly recommend the choleric person to become an advance. But as an actor he would probably do very well. The choleric women excel in jobs which involve selling and public speaking.

ii. **The sanguine:** The sanguine individual is slightly less excitable than the choleric, and does not display the same degree of persistence and consistency. His temperament is the result of a nervous system which functions strongly in a balanced but mobile fashion. He is stable, yet active, courageous, hopeful and cheerful. He is nevertheless somewhat inconsistent. He is courteous, lively, alert and demonstrative.

   Sanguine temperament type succeed in public relations work and various forms of social service while the women make good nurses and teachers. Sanguine men should routine clerical work and women should avoid repetitive factory jobs. Phlegmatic type individuals fit best into jobs which are routine but responsible, e.g. accountancy. Phlegmatic women should do well as secretaries, librarians or filing clerks. They should avoid jobs like fashion model and air hostess.

iii. **The phlegmatic:** Characterized by the inability to be easily aroused to feel or act, the phlegmatic temperament corresponds to balanced but inert nervous system. The phlegmatic individual is stable and calm. He may, in fact tend to cool sluggish or apathetic. Normally quiet and reserved and does not easily become friendly or antagonistic.

iv. **The melancholic:** The melancholic temperament is characterized by slowness of thought and a tendency to be depressed. It corresponds to a feeble type of organization of the nervous system. Consistency and determination are other traits of the melancholic.

The melancholic temperament is best fitted to work where snap decisions and rapid action are not demanded. Melancholic men are likely to do in well occupations where steady application is essential. Such individuals are suitable for jobs which do not involve real sense of initiative and spontaneity.

PHYSICAL TYPE / PHYSIOLOGICAL TYPE

A second theory of personality types depend upon the conformation of the human body. The notion of the body types can be correlated with different types of personality. This was found by Terrus in early Greek medieval concepts. In the 12th century L Rostam distinguished digestive, muscular and cerebral types. Then Ernst Kretschmer at the same time was led by his work with mental patients to develop a three fold physical classification: 1. Pyknic, 2. Asthenic and 3. Athletic.

The Pyknic characterized by a broad trunk, relatively short limbs, round face and tend to gain weight in middle age. The Asthenic has a narrow trunk, long limbs, longer arrow face and rare lean. The athletic has broad shoulders and trunk, narrower hips, well-proportioned limbs and good muscular development.

In psychology, people have been classified on the basis of physiological and mental traits and temperaments.

Physical Types

Physical types in personality are exemplified in the classification of personalities by E Kretschmer in his book *Physique and Character*. Kretschmer has classified people into two classes according to their physical structure.

1. *Cycloid:* These people are fat. Their temperament is extrovert, sociable and happy.
2. *Schizoid:* These people are thin and tall. They are temperamentally self-centered, emotional, reticent, peaceful and lovers of solitude.

Besides these two types, Kretschmer has mentioned many subclasses on the basis of physical structure, some of the main ones being:

1. *Asthenic:* People of this group are short and thin. They are of a self-centered, emotional, dreamy, intellectual, peaceful and solitude loving temperament.
2. *Athletic:* As the name suggests, their built is strong having broad shoulders and slim waists. In behavior they are social, prudent and active.
3. *Pyknic:* The people are fat. Their stomachs protrude and they have round faces. They are naturally happy and sociable.

Types Based on Temperament

Classification of personality has been made on the basis of temperaments, besides the physical structure. One example of such classification can be found in WH Sheldon's book *The Varieties of Temperament*. Before this, the bases of classification were the anthropological measurements, by which the shape and structure of the body people were classified.

On the basis of shape and size. Sheldon classified people into the following groups:
1. *Endomorphic:* Their stomach is big and the large intestines are developed.
2. *Mesomorphic:* In this type the bones and muscles are developed.
3. *Ectomorphic:* Their bones are long and soft while the physical structure is weak.

On the basis, temperament too is classified into the following three classes:
1. *Viscerotonic:* In this type activities of eating predominate. They love comfort and food and seek the love of others. They also sleep deeply. They like others to help them when in trouble. People with endomorphic physical structure fall into this category.
2. *Somatotonic:* The mesomorphic people constitute this group. They are of a brittle, clear and competitive nature, and are generally powerful, daring, authoritative and loud talkers. In troubles they are more active.
3. *Cerebrotonic:* This class includes the ectomorphic types of people. They are controlled, withdrawing and sensing. They are habituated to suppressing their emotions. They love solitude and instead of seeking assistance in trouble, they like to stay within their own limits. They speak slowly and their sleep is disturbed.

Morgan and Gilliland have mentioned four types of personality on the basis of temperament:
1. *Elated:* They are optimistic, elated and happy
2. *Depressed:* These people are pessimistic, depressed and emotional
3. *Irritable:* They are the interfering, irritable and of hot-tempered type
4. *Unstable:* Their mood is unbalanced, unstable and emotional.

Kretschmer found a predominance of the emotional temperament among pyknic.

Asthenic were introverted, shy and serious ranging in temperament from hypersensitive to phlegmatic and duel. The athletic physique was found to be intermediate in temperament.

3. PSYCHOLOGICAL TYPE

The most important classification of personality is done by Jung. On the basis of sociability he has accepted two types of people—extroverts and introverts.
1. *Extroverts:* Those people take more interest in others and like to mix with people of similar temperaments. They are realistic and face the problems of life objectively. They take part freely in any social give and take. They are dominated by emotions, whereby they take decisions quickly and act on them without delay. They are skilled in etiquette. The extrovert group is made up of traders, players, actors, social and political leaders, etc.
2. *Introverts:* As the name suggests, the mental tendencies of these people are directed not outward to peoples around them, but rather inwards to themselves. They are thus self-centered and lovers of solitude. With them, thinking and contemplation predominates. They are busy in their own thoughts and they try to impress others only by their thoughts. They are idealists and think much about future. Usually they take more interest in the natural environment than they do in their social environment. Neither they come to any decision in haste nor do they act on its promptly. They are not worldly wise. They pay more attention to thought than work. Scientists, philosophers and poets come within this group.
3. *Ambiverts:* In the real world these two types are rarely found pure. Mostly some peculiarities of both the extroverts and the introverts are found in people. These intermediate people are called 'ambiverts'. Later still, Jung divided these people into sensing, thinking, feeling and instinctive types.

The above theories of classifying personalities are not accepted in modern psychology. On this subject the following criticisms are important:

1. Experience and observation show that most people cannot be fitted into any one type.
2. The 'type' raises doubts on the subject of cause and effect. It would be incorrect to assert that a certain person is solitude loving because he is an introvert.
3. Types cannot be established by measurement. Only the different traits of personality can be measured. Again, it is not essential that these traits will remain the same in a person.

Thus, the attempt of dividing people into groups is not only without advantage and impractical but also useless.

It was in psychiatry and philosophy that the third chief doctrine of personnel types first emerged. The various scientists like CG Jung and E Soranger may be cited as representatives of 20th century. Jung coined the terms 'Introversion' and 'Extroversion' to describe what he considered to be contrasting types. Introversion was characterized as directing attention and interest inward, with a tendency of excessive daydreaming and careful balancing of considerations before reaching a decision. Extroversion was characterized by outgoingness in attention and interest, responsiveness to external stimuli, dominated by thinking which relates to people and object. The introverted thinker's on the other hand, are prompted by his own inner convictions and may have little to do with reality.

The extrovert thinker would make a good public relations man, barrister, teacher, lecturer, staff supervisor, departmental head, politician, etc. because extrovert performance is best when under observation. The introvert thinker, however, prefers to stay in the background and work unobserved and is consequently 'behind-the-scenes' man. He should not be put in a position where spontaneity of feeling is required because he has to be guided in his feelings by what he thinks a situation demands.

These type of individuals are concerned with feelings and emotions and evaluates the world in terms of pleasant and unpleasant. The extrovert type should choose work in selling, social welfare entertainment, while the introvert types will function best in the world of arts, religion, meditation, etc. and are creative but inclined to be inhibited and withdrawn.

Whichever general attitude one adopts to this concept of personality, actual investigations and methods adopted to understand the composition of personality have been undertaken along two lines. Each line of approach has made vast contributions to our total picture of personality. One method, though it first started only as a factual observation, consists, in trying to understand personality by studying the differences between individuals. Take two of your friends of example. One is always very sociable, freely talks with people, easily makes friends, mostly seems to be jolly and does not seem to take things very seriously. Another is rather quiet, reserved, does not freely discuss about himself, often likes to be left alone undisturbed, etc. We will observe several people falling under one category and several others falling under the other. The question naturally arises whether we cannot understand personality along the line of two types on the basis of the qualities that distinguish mentioned above one psychologists tried to understand and differentiate people on the basis of characteristics which he called *extroversion* and *introversion*.

The extrovert is one who is always sociable, taking interest in others, freely discussing about himself, seldom fond of being alone, etc. The introvert is the opposite of these. Even in the matter of interest the introvert will be characterized by activities which can be done by himself alone. While the extrovert will like to spend his time chatting with a group of people in a club the introvert will like to go out for a long walk alone or to sit down in a corner and read a book or to play a game of chess. This classification of people into extroverts and introverts was first made by a psychologist by name CG Jung of Switzerland. In fact he is one of the greatest of psychologists living today. He is one of the three founders of modern psychology, particularly abnormal psychology, the two others being Freud and Adler. Ever since Jung made this observation the whole the psychological literature has been using these terms, the extrovert and the introvert, in various contexts to understand the nature and behavior of man. But there is a difficulty in making a division of people into these two types. In fact, though we do meet quite a number of people who are extreme introverts, or extreme extroverts a large majority of people fall between these two extremes having the characteristic of both types. Hence there is real difficulty in classifying people into types. However, such an approach is useful in understanding certain components that make up one's personality.

It has been recognized that extreme introversion or extreme extroversion is not very conducive to mental health. It is also known that these characteristics can be modified within certain limits by discipline and training. Hence it is worthwhile for the student to understand whether he is developing habits which characterize any one of these extremes. If so, it is better to attempt by patient discipline and by learning new habits, at a balance of these two tendencies.

Other attempts have also been made to differentiate people into different types based on different categories of qualities. Some people have been found to be very much interested in politics, some are more interested in business matters, some are interested in intellectual pursuit of philosophical and reflective nature, some are in general interested in pursuing esthetic enjoyment. Based on these observations it has been attempted to classify people into the political type, the theoretical type, the economic type, the esthetic type, the social type. There have been many other similar attempts also. But most of these did not gain very much acceptance from the general student of psychology because of the difficulty involved in such a procedure. We very seldom find people who would belong purely to one type. Most of us are of a composite or mixed type. So on the whole 'the doctrine of typology' in psychology has not been very well-received. Still from the works of people like Jung, who followed these principles of differentiation, we have learned a good deal.

The other method has been to study the individual himself, to analyze his make-up as it were. On the basis of a general theoretical idea we try to find out various qualities that are in an individual. Such qualities which make up one's personality are usually referred to as 'traits of personality'. A vast amount of study has been made on this principle of analyzing and differentiating personality traits. Different people have suggested different lists of traits. Sometimes the list becomes very large and one does not know where to stop. Qualities such as sociability, gratefulness, radicalism, conventionality, curiosity, etc. have been mentioned as traits. Enumeration of traits has a serious difficulty. This refers to the very definition and nature of a trait. A question has been asked whether these traits are really independent of each other. It has been noticed that one trait is often linked with another. Also one trait leads to another. They are so interdependent that some people find it difficult to take any single trait seriously. If you take honesty as a trait it will certainly involve some other traits such as sociability, courage, moral character, etc. This kind of groupings will almost become impossible for a neat classification of personality traits. Still, a study of personality traits as undertaken by several psychologists has, like other lines of approach, yielded vast amount of valuable data in understanding human nature.

One other theoretical consideration that has arisen in connection with the study of traits is whether the traits are continuous and permanent in any individual. Studies show that on the whole these traits are developed fairly early in life and they continue to exist right through life. In cases where there in any severe crisis in later life, these traits may undergo a change. A severe disappointment or frustration in life, loss of job, resulting in serious economic insecurity and other critical experiences like this can change a man's basic personality traits. He may give up some particular trait as a result of this shocking experience and develop new traits. Otherwise on the whole these traits are more or less permanent and continuous.

Broad Classifications of Personality

The broad classification of personality are:
1. Sick personality
2. Healthy personality.

Sick personality: The sick personality can also be labeled as "disturbed" or "peculiar" or "crazy". Personality sickness can occur at any stage, the most vulnerable tones are when there are marked physical changes. The causes of personality sickness fall into physical and psychological categories.

Physical conditions may account, for the way a person reacts in different situations and for the kind of adjustment he makes to life in general. The psychological cause of personality sickness is anxiety which stems from self-dissatisfaction. The person is unhappy about himself and dislikes himself to the point where he becomes self-rejectant. The self-rejection includes chronic attitudes of self-disapproval and self-disagreement, self-distrust, feeling of unworthy. In one of its most cruel forms self-rejection included severe guilt. A person becomes self-rejectant when he is unable to gratify his needs and desires because of personal limitations or environment.

Predictable factors in personality sickness are influenced by age, sex, socioeconomic status, family size, popularity, etc. Personality sickness is a matter of grave concern. Personality sickness becomes worse unless diagnosed and treated by a competent and professionally trained person through the diagnoses of its causes. Personality sickness requires an immediate attack involving diagnosing the cause of sickness, reporting the findings to the person, alert him about the cause and nature of the trouble and prescribing the measures. Each of these stages is very difficult. There is no wonder drug for psychological sickness as there are for physical sickness and person himself must assume a greater responsibility for following the prescribed pattern of treatment than is necessary in physical sickness.

Healthy personality: Healthy personality is an image of the 'Self' that the invidiual can accept and live, or without feeling anxious or hostile or without being self-defeated or destructive to others, people with healthy personalities are judged to be well-adjusted. This is because they can gratify expectations. Good physical health contributes to a favorable concept of self. Following are the essential characteristics which should be provided for an individuals healthy personality.

a. Foundation for healthy self-concept should be the early experience
b. Encourage and help the individual to acquire good health and love within his physical limitations

c. Ensure the important needs especially for the achievement, acceptance and affection
d. Provide an environment rich in opportunities for learning how to live successfully with other people
e. Guide in the development of stable self-concept by reducting the gap between his real and ideal self-concept
f. Set an example of good social and personal adjustments
g. Help to increase the self-understanding by better application of one's strengths and weaknesses
h. Help to develop stress tolerance to avoid the self-dislike that leads to self-rejection
i. Help in developing success factors as persistence, accuracy, curiosity, originality, leadership, pride in achievement and creativity in thinking
j. Control the stray behavior and to provide the guidance, help and encouragement which are essential.

The personality pattern of an individual is unique in the sense that it is different from the personality patterns of others in complexity, fluidity, accessibility, resistance to change and centralization. *But a mature personality, is tolerant, responsible, hardworking, self-motivated, modest, independent, with ability to understand criticism and exercise will power.*

Normal and Abnormal Personalities

People have been considering mostly what might be called the normal personality. But they come across people who exhibit very abnormal behavior, suffering from all kinds of psychological disorders from the simple hysteria to the serious disorder which call madness or lunacy. Some of these patients manifest very strange and abnormal patterns of behavior. Individual may be tempted to think that they are completely different from human beings. With some, at any rate, they may not be able to see any connection between their behavior and that of the normal people. Psychology deals with such cases also. In fact there is a branch of psychology called abnormal psychology dealing with such phenomena. People now know that these abnormal behaviors are not really different in kind from the characteristics are merely an exaggerated and distorted form of characteristics which are found in normal men. Thus the difference is only a matter of degree and not of kind. They are not a different kind of people, they are essentially similar to us. Only, some of the characteristics that are in us are exaggerated in them. Personality is expressed in the method one employs in the adjustment with the environment. Every person lives in a specific environment, but this environment continuously changes. The person has to adjust themselves to this dynamic environment, his adjustment depending upon his capabilities, qualities, tendencies, interests and abilities. If the person adjusts himself to the environment and conducts his behavior according to the social norms, his personality is supposed to be normal. A person is called abnormal when he either does not fit into the environment or does not behave in accordance with the current norms of behavior in society. The popular criteria of normality and abnormality differ from society to society and group to group. But the normality or abnormality is determined in a society on its own criterion. Thus, the personality of a Naga may appear abnormal in the Hindu society. It is obvious here that from the scientific view point this changing criterion is totally inadequate, and due to the psychologists have attempted to evolve a universal criterion of normality and abnormality, to distinguish between the two. It can generally be said that a person incapable of affecting adjustment in a civilized society will be called abnormal.

Disintegration of Personality

In Woodworth's opinion, an integrated personality is one in which the several traits, interests and desires and are combined in an effective harmonious unity. The main cause of disintegration is the absence of this very unity. The continual conflict between the different interests or desires of a person and the continuous absence of any harmony are the causes of disintegration. The absence of harmony may be attributed to a number of causes, like personality abnormalities, prolonged conflicts, multiple personality, hysteria or other mental diseases, phobias, weakness of will, the unnatural and abnormal expression of lusts and instincts, insanity, excessive daydreaming and many deficiencies in character, deficient sociability, irritable, energetic or quarrelling temperament, etc. The formation of mutually contradictory habits leads to the dissolution of the organization in personality. The persistent conflict between the desires does not allow the personality to remain organized. Idiots, imbeciles and the like cannot create any harmony between their different interests, desires and tendencies and consequently their personality is disintegrated. Sometimes personality may be disintegrated by being inflicted for a long time with some mental disease or some incurable physical ailment. Even a difficult, pathetic and painful life may lead to disintegration and a similar result may come about if desires are either excessively repressed or left dissatisfied to a great extent. According to Freud the most comprehensive cause of disintegration of personality is the excessive repression of the sex impulse. Another possible cause of personality disintegration is the extreme expression of the tendency of self-assertion. In brief, the main causes of the disintegration of personality are excessive repression of natural tendencies, unhealthy environment, defects of temperament or character, mental ailments and abnormalities and grave deficiencies of the will power and intellect.

- **Conflict:** One of the most important causes of disintegration of personality is conflict. Most of man's activities result from motives. Often, more than one motives arise in the person simultaneously, which originate a doubt in his mind and cause tension. He finds it difficult to decide on the mode of action, this state being psychologically designated 'conflict'. There are two main causes of conflict—1. *Environmental Obstructions*—Many hindrances in the environment create conflicts inside the person. 2. *Personal Deficiencies*—The deficiencies of the character, temperament and personality of the person himself create conflicts between the motives. In reality, the existence of conflict in life is indispensable, without which development is not possible but when these conflicts assume abnormal proportions they become harmful.

The major types of conflicts are as follows:

1. *Approach – Approach conflicts*—In this type, the motives, engaged in the conflict are such that the individual accepts them both and would like to fulfill both, the conflict arising from the fact that both cannot be fulfilled at the same time. A person, for example, wants both a pantaloon and a blanket but has money enough only for one.
2. *Avoidance – Avoidance conflicts*—In this case both the motives are of such a nature that the individual would avoid them if he could. For example, neither does a person want to work nor would he appreciate being called a malingerer.
3. *Approach – Avoidance conflicts*—In this type the motives which conflict with each other are such that one of them the individuals wants to fulfill while the other he wants to avoid. For example, a player would like to participate in a game but would also like to avoid injury.

4. *Double approach – Avoidance conflicts*—In this class of conflicts although the person has come to a decision in one direction he still feels an inclination towards the other allurements, although he cannot alter his decision.

Excessive conflicts indicate a weakness of determination. Strong will power is needed to avoid it or to get rid of it.

Multiple personality: Multiple personality is an example of disintegration in personality. One of the disorders of personality arises because of a phenomenon technically called 'dissociation'. When dissociation works in an extreme form we get what is called 'the multiple personality'. At a particular stage of the development of the individual, a splitting of the personality takes place and two apparently complete personalities develop manifesting themselves alternately. An understanding of the cases of dual or multiple personalities requires a good deal of psychological knowledge, which a beginner cannot hope to have. Even in such an extreme case it can be shown that the phenomenon is only an exaggeration of a characteristic that is seen in normal people. In other words, mild dissociation can be very commonly noticed even in normal people. We all would have behaved at times completely different from our usual manner. We might be perfectly honest people for all practical purposes. But there may be some occasion or a particular area of life where without any diffidence we might tell a lie. We would then be behaving almost like a completely different individual. These two diametrically opposed beliefs or attitudes are never compromised. In fact they are never brought together in the mind of the individual. So, no sense of inconsistency is felt. We are also familiar with various kind of double standards of morality. All these are examples of a very mild form of dissociation. It is this very same dissociation in its most severe form which produces such a strange fact as multiple personality. In between these two extreme forms of dissociation, there are various other stages producing different degrees of psychological abnormality. Hysteria is one such psychological disorder caused by dissociation. Different forms of somnambulism are also produced by this dissociation or splitting of consciousness.

This phenomena of dissociation gives us some suggestions regarding the nature of normality. Let us take a normal person A as an example. A is a student in the nursing class. He has a name and he has a concept of himself. Whatever he does is done with the awareness of himself as a constant entity. It is he who attends the class, it is he who does a good thing and it is he who does some mischief. Whether in the classroom or in the playground, or on the road, or at the home, it is he who does and experiences all these things. All the activities and behavior are integrated around one single point, viz., an idea of himself or his ego. It is because there is such an integration around one point that he is normal for all practical purposes. But in some cases a modified form of integration takes place around two focal points. This gives rise to the development of two selves or two personalities side by side. When the dissociation is complete we have a neat example of dual personality.

One of the aims of psychotherapy as developed in modern times and based on the principles of psychology is to analyze the causes of disintegration and to re-establish an integration around one focal point. The more we draw ourselves together around one strong conflicts in the mind, if left uncompromised and unadjusted, will tend to produce dissociation.

The above example illustrates the signs of multiple personality—the first being that in multiple personality, the personality is subdivided into two or more contradictory personalities. In this, one personality is a happy one while the other is irritable, one is peaceful but the other is restless. Often the present personality does not remember the other personality and even if it does remember it, it thinks of this as another person. The personality which remains for a long time is called the primary state and the personality which persists for a comparatively shorter time is called the secondary state. Commonly things related to the primary state are remembered in the secondary state but things of the secondary state are not recalled in the primary.

A famous example of multiple personality is that of a young woman named Anitha, upon whom so many troubles converged that she developed an extremely religious, ethical and sacrificing character. But at the same time along with this she sometimes showed another personality in which she became very naughty. In order to cure her of this dual personality Anitha was given psychiatric treatment, but in this period personality developed in her. This personality was selfish and aggressive. She thus had three personalities, the first being the primary and the other two the secondary ones. Naturally, in her first condition she had no memory of the other two states and in the other two conditions she remembered the other two as strange personalities.

Cures of Personality Disintegration

To effect cure for personality disintegration, the first thing a psychologist does is to collect the case history of the patient and find out the causes of personality disintegration. The cure of these cause is the cure of personality disintegration, and thus each case of personality disintegration is to be cured by a specific method. It is obvious that there can be no general method which will cure every type of personality disintegration, but in spite of this some methods can be mentioned which will cure different cases of personality disintegration. These are as follows:

1. *Suggestion:* Suggestion is an important method in psychotherapy, one essential of which is that the patient should have complete faith in the psychologist and in his approach. The need for a psychologist who can create respect and faith in the patient is obvious, the possibility of success of the suggestions depending on the extent of the respect and faith. Many mental and neurological ailments are relived on the basis of just his faith. Sometimes autosuggestion also helps the cure, in which the patient gives suggestions to himself. Sometimes even counter-suggestions prove efficacious, being especially effective in cases in which direct suggestions have proved ineffective. In common and simple matters, it becomes necessary for the psychologist to explain the reasons for his cure in order to create faith in the patient. This is called rational suggestion. In brief, the first thing the psychologist does is to create faith in the patient for him and then proceeds to cure the disease by suggestion after profound mutual relations have been established.
2. *Hypnosis:* In a hypnotized state the suggestions are comparatively more effective because the person accepts the suggestions of the psychologist without any objection, being as he is in an inactive or passive condition having completely surrendered himself to the psychologist. Accordingly, when the patient is in a hypnotized state, directions relating to the elimination of mental disease, bad habits and physical defects can be given. These suggestions have succeeded in removing many very dangerous mental diseases during hypnosis. Though it cannot remove all the mental diseases it still retains its importance in curing many defects of personality.
3. *Psychoanalysis:* Psychoanalysis is the best among the different methods employed in the curing of personality disintegration. In psychoanalysis the method of free association is

used to discover the causes of the ailment. The individual lies or sits relaxed and expresses his thoughts and feelings in their natural form. Consequently, this reveals the fundamental cause of his difficulties which are generally the result of repressed tendencies. After these tendencies have come to light harmless modes of their expression are explained to the patient or, instead, they are sublimated, organized and substituted.

4. *Faith cure:* The Christian science of healing is based on faith. Even where there were no scientific explanations astonishing results were observed. The importance of faith in cure has been emphasized in the Indian sacred books. In this method the patient believes that he is getting better day to day and his troubles are being reduced.

At the end, it is essential for the cure of personality disintegration that the person learns to face the situations, that he has self-confidence, that his will power be strengthened, that he understands the situation and that he may learn to sublimate or substitute his tendencies instead of repressing them. And for all this it is necessary that the person should lead as normal a life as possible. Sometimes a change in the environment also proves advantageous. Sometimes physical cure also becomes necessary.

Psychologists have now definitely established that the repression of natural desires creates the dangers of destruction of personality equilibrium and creation of mental diseases and abnormalitics. On the other hand, all desires and tendencies cannot be expressed. For example, the society does not allow the fulfillment of many desires motivated by the sex impulse and there is danger for mental health in their repression. Therefore psychologists have suggested the sublimation of such tendencies by which these are afforded the opportunity of harmless and healthy expression. For example, the sexual tendencies are satisfied by taking part in the fine arts and by being engaged in literature. In the same way, sport sublimates the aggressive tendencies. Sublimation directs human energies along profitable channels and saves them from wastage.

Personality and the Nurse

Personality is something that enables a person to standout as distinct from others. It is the quality of an individual behavior. The nurse needs to know the basics of personality for providing effective care for the patients inhospitals and clients in the community. The nurse interacts with different persons everyday so evaluation of character and personality is essential for planning the nursing care. The nurse interacts with patients, doctors, coworkers and others which needs certain behavior pattern, so the nurse shured develop and practice well-adjustable personality.

The nature determinance of personality must have made it clear that personality is something which is not only inborn but which is mostly to be cultivated in social environment. Now, in order to understand the bearing of personality on Nursing profession one should know the personality traits required in a Nurse. Among the most important personality traits of a successful Nurse are: Mental alertness, self-confidence and credibility, integrity and dignity, sympathetic understanding, gracious manners, friendliness of spirit, kindliness, adaptability and cheerful disposition. These personality traits have to be developed by constant practice for a sufficiently long time. In this process the environment of her profession has a very important role to play and undoubtedly well known hospitals are the best places for developing a sound personality for the Nurse but if she is not so fortunate as to get an ideal environment, she should make the best of whatever is available. Much will depend on her strong will and capacity of adjustment and her skill in making the best of the given opportunities. If she finds the environment absolutely uncongenial, she may try to get her transferred to a better place or leave her job and join elsewhere. In any case she should make all efforts to develop the above mentioned personality traits. This will not only help her in her profession but also bring her cheerfulness and job satisfaction, sure signs of a successful profession.

Tests of Personality

At this point it may be interesting to introduce some of the methods used to determine the various types and the various traits. Two of the common methods are called the questionnaire method and the rating scales. The questionnaire method as used to determine whether a person is an introvert or an extrovert usually takes the form of set of 40 to 50 questions or statements with some suitable directions.

The following are a few statements taken from "The Neymann - Kohlstedt Diagnostic Test for Introversion-Extroversion. The direction to the subject is given as follows:

This test is composed of 50 statements each being followed by the words Yes or No. There is no implication of right or wrong in any of the statements and you are asked to consider them from the viewpoint of personal like or dislike. Read the first statement and if you like the idea it expresses, draw a line under 'Yes'. If you dislike it, draw a line under 'No'. Proceed in the same way with the rest of the statements.

1. Be by yourself a great deal — Yes No
2. Work with many people around you — Yes No
3. Think a great deal before deciding anything — Yes No
4. Dislike having people watch you — Yes No
5. Work better when people praise you — Yes No
6. Often mediate and think about yourself — Yes No
7. Think a great deal — Yes No
8. Pay little attention to details — Yes No
9. Study others rather than yourself — Yes No
10. Change your opinions easily even when formed — Yes No

Here the experimenter already knows which answer indicates extroversion and which answer indicates introversion. The total answers are tabulated and from the ratio of extroversion score to the introversion score the particular individual's extroversion—introversion index is calculated. Whether the actual score will indicate over introversion or over extroversion will also depend on the expected average score for a large group to which the individual belongs. This is so because these personality characteristics will have to be finally judged in relation to the standards obtained in the group to which the individual belongs. An individual who is 5′-10" tall will be called a short man in a society where most people reach the height 6". But he will be considered a giant in another society where the average height is only 5". This same principle has to be applied in all psychological measurements also.

The questionnaire method when used for studying personality traits or general characteristics of personality will usually take the following form:

Questions like the following sometimes even more than a hundred covering all aspects of life may be given to the subject asking him to underline Yes, No or Doubtful.

1. Do you get on well with your brothers and sisters? Yes No Doubtful
2. Did your father try to plan your life? Yes No Doubtful
3. Do you daydream frequently? Yes No Doubtful
4. Do people think you are selfish? Yes No Doubtful
5. Have you strong likes and dislikes with regard to food? Yes No Doubtful
6. Do you usually control your temper? Yes No Doubtful
7. Do ideas often run through your head so that you cannot sleep? Yes No Doubtful
8. Does it make you uneasy to cross a bridge over a river? Yes No Doubtful
9. Is your mother's nature usually cheerful? Yes No Doubtful
10. Do your feelings alternate between happiness and sadness without apparent reason? Yes No Doubtful
11. Were your parents happily married? Yes No Doubtful
12. Do you have recurring and disturbing dreams? Yes No Doubtful
13. Have you ever been afraid of going insane? Yes No Doubtful
14. Are you troubled by shyness? Yes No Doubtful
15. Is your sleep generally sound? Yes No Doubtful
16. Are you troubled by the ideas that people are watching you on the street? Yes No Doubtful
17. Do you suffer from night-mares? Yes No Doubtful
18. Does it make you uneasy to sit in a small room with the doors shut? Yes No Doubtful
19. Do you get discouraged easily? Yes No Doubtful

The rating scale is a little more technical and difficult in its construction. The rating may be self-rating or it may be the rating of a particular trait in others. Sometimes the rating may also be done by a team of expert judges. The rating method attempts to find out the opinion of the subject with regard to the degree to which one particular trait is present or absent in himself or in another. Usually we arbitrarily fix up three degrees or five degrees. This is usually referred to as 'three-point scale' or 'five-point scale'. An example will make this clear.

Do you think it is justifiable to tell a lie?

(A) Always (B) Sometimes (C) Never

The subject has to mark one of these. Here his trait of honesty is measured on a three-point scale (of course, in actual measurement, judgment will not be made on the basis of one question alone). A five-point scale for this will be—Always, often, sometimes, rarely, never. The question may take this form also. My sense of punctuality is: high, average, low. The degrees in a five-point scale will be: very high, high, average, low and very low. In an actual rating scale there will be a number of questions on the various characteristics that we want to study.

The difficulty with regard to these questionnaire and rating scale methods are that we can never be sure of getting frank and scientifically accurate judgments. When we are judging ourselves we may be tempted (even without a conscious desire to tell a lie) to err in our favor. When we are judging others we may tend to be over strict. Also when judging an individual or a group which we like we may tend to be over generous. In actual tests some steps are usually taken to minimize these errors.

Projective Tests of Personality

In recent years some other tests of personality have been developed and have acquired great importance.

They are called the projective tests of personality. There are quite a number of them in use at present, but we will mention two of the most important.

Suppose people are sitting on the beach, a patch of cloud in the sky with an irregular shape. If we look at it and allow our imagination to work on it we may see a number of things supposedly represented by the shape and structure of that cloud. Actually we do not perceive these things there. For perception the proper stimuli must be there. We perceive some irregular shapes and then imagine a host of things because of the associative process. The actual perception is influenced a great deal by our associations. Which association will be roused depends upon our moods and mental states at that moment. If we are happy we may see pleasant and nice things. If we are unhappy we would see unpleasant and frightening things. In fact there is a conflict between the perceptual process and the associative process both working at the same time. In this conflict or struggle between the claims of the actual stimulus and the memories from the associative process good deal of our inner nature and personality make-up would be expressed. It has been found in actual practice that what we see in such a cloud gives a clue to the various changes that go to make-up our personality. In other words we project ourselves on the cloud. The projective tests of personality are based on this sample principle.

If we are shown an accurate picture of a lion and ten of us are asked to say what it is, all the ten of us will say that it is a lion. Since the picture accurately depicts a lion the perceptual process suffers no difficulty. It is controlled and directed exactly in the same manner in all the ten of us and we all say that it is a lion. Suppose now the picture was not very accurate but was very vague and the outline was left in an indistinct manner. If this was shown to all of us might respond in ten different ways, no two persons seeing the same thing in that picture. This difference arises because we are not actually guided by the perceptual process alone. The picture being indistinct starts different associative lines in different people. In doing so we are giving expression to our own inner perceptual and associative organization. In other word, we reveal our inner make-up. As a result of actual experimental observations such tests have come to be accepted as the best indicators of one's personality. The individual reveals himself very frankly because he does not know that he is revealing himself.

A well-known test of this type is the one devised by a Swiss Psychiatrist, Hermann Rorschach by name. He found that irregular inkblots can be used to bring out the personality characteristics of different individuals. He standardized after a good deal of experimentation, ten cards each containing an inkblot which is symmetrical but irregular in outline. The shading is not uniform within the inkblot. Five of these include color also, the other five being only shades of black and grey. The subject who is tested is shown these cards one after another and asked to say all that he sees in them. Though this 'Rorschach test' has gained great importance particularly in the testing program of any psychological clinic, it is not something to be played with easily. The interpretation of the responses given by an individual to a Rorschach inkblot is very complicated and requires a great deal of specialized technical training and experience. An advanced knowledge of clinical psychology and of the psychology of personality is also necessary as a background before one could specialize in the use of the Rorschach test.

Next to the Rorschach test, in importance, is the projective tests called the 'Thematic Apperception Test' (TAT). This test was developed by an American Psychologist by name HA Murray. This test is some what different from the Rorschach test which contains only irregular inkblots. In the TAT we have some pictures mostly of actual human beings depicting particular situation. In one picture, for example, a boy sits with his hands on his chin and a violin in front of him looking as if he is imagining something. It may be that he is worried about something also. The subject to be tested is asked to make up a story based on this picture. Like the inkblots, here also, there is no full story presented in the picture. From the one scene presented, he has to make up an introduction and a conclusion. This means he creates the story from out of his own mind. It has been found on the basis of actual experiments that in creating the story the individual projects himself and reveals unknowingly his own fears, hopes, difficulties, etc. In other words, he projects his own personality into the story.

Another picture contains an old man by the side of a young man. Though the human figures are distinctive it is not clear as to what exactly is happening. The old man may represent the father scolding his son, or advising his son, or taking leave of the son, etc. All such ideas can be seen in the picture depending upon the actual life-history of the subject who is tested. In the actual TAT there are 20 cards like this, 19 containing pictures and one just a blank cared. For this blank card the subject has first to make up a picture of his choice and then write a story on that. Some cards are meant to be given only to boys. Some are meant only for girls. Some are meant for boys and men. Some others are meant for girls and grown up women and some are common to all. The TAT is also quite popular and is extensively used in psychological clinics and laboratories.

When both the Rorschach and TAT are used we may get a fuller picture because the one supplements the other. The Rorschach will easily reveal to us that an individual has an emotional shock or difficulty. But the TAT can give us additional material as to the nature of that shock and the area of life in which that difficulty lies. It may be in his relationship to the parents, it may be his difficulties with his job, it may be his difficulties in his marriage or sex life. All this descriptive material can be obtained more easily from the TAT stories. The difficulty which we mentioned regarding the use of the Rorschach holds good with the TAT which also requires very intense technical training before one can use it.

Based on this principle of projection there are so many other tests also with varying psychological importance and usefulness. Different tests have been devised for testing small children, and no personality testing is supposed to be complete without the use of some kind of projective tests. For children mostly the tests use play materials such as color and brush, drawing materials, toys and dolls, etc. When plenty of choice is given to child by way of these materials, observe how and with what particular things the child plays. From the way it creates a theme with the available play materials, almost similar to the lines of the TAT an understanding of the child's difficulties and problems is attempted.

22 CHAPTER

Development of Human Behavior

Introduction Growth and Development

The terms growth and development represent independant, interrelated and dynamic processes. **Growth** is physical change and increase in size. It can be measured quantitatively. Indicators of growth include height, weight, bone size, and dentition. The pattern of physiologic growth is similar for all people. However, growth rates vary during different stages of growth and development. The growth rate is rapid during the prenatal, neonatal, infancy and adolescent stages and slows during childhood. Physical growth is minimal during adulthood. Mostly these two terms are used interchangeably and taken as synonymous terms. Both relate to the measurement of changes occurred in the individual after conception in the womb of the mother. Change is the law of nature. An individual starting from a fertilized egg, turns into a full-fledged human adult. In this turn-over process he undergoes a cycle of changes brought about by the process of growth and development in various dimensions—physical, mental, social, emotional, etc. Therefore in the wider sense, both the terms growth and development can be used for any change brought about by maturation and learning and essentially is the product of both heredity and environment.

In practical sense both terms are used to denote the changes in the organism's physical as well as functional behavior. These changes which cover physical, emotional intellectual and social aspects of a human life are roughly divided into four major classes namely changes in size, changes in proportion, disappearance of old features and acquisition of new features.

All these types of changes have qualitative as well as quantitative aspects and hence generally, growth and development go hand in hand. And the two terms are to be used collectively. Both, taken together, explain the total changes—functional as well as constitutional changes—in the body and behavior of the individual with the lapse of time after the conception.

Terminology—these two terms have different meanings that can be put in the way given below Table 22.1.

Principles of Growth and Development

As stated earlier growth and development are independent, interrelated processes. For example, and infant's muscles, bones, and nervous system must grow to a certain point before the infant can sit up or walk. Growth generally takes places during the first 20 years of life; development continues after that.

Table 22.1: Different meanings of growth and development	
Growth	*Development*
1. The terms growth is used in purely physical sense. It generally refers to an increase in size, length, height and weight. Change in the quantitative aspects come into the domain of growth.	1. Development implies over-all changes in shape, form or structure resulting in improved working or functioning. It indicates the changes in the quality or character rather than in quantitative aspects.
2. Growth is one of the part of developmental process. In strict sense development in its quantitative aspects is termed as growth.	2. Development is a wider and comprehensive terms. It refers to over-all changes in the individual. Growth is one of its parts.
3. Growth may be referred to describe the changes which take place in particular aspects of the body and behavior of an organism.	3. Development describes the changes in the organism as a whole and does not list the changes in parts.
4. Growth does not continue throughout life. It stops when maturity has been attained.	4. Development is a continuous process. It goes from womb to tomb. It does not end with the attainment of maturity. The changes, however small they may be, continue throughout the life span of an individual.
5. The changes produced by growth are the subject of measurement. They may be quantified and are observable in nature.	5. Development, as said earlier, implies improvement in functioning and behavior and hence brings qualitative changes which are difficult to be measured directly. They are assessed through keen observation in behavioral situations.
6. Growth may or may not bring development. A child may grow (in terms of weight) by becoming fat but this growth may not bring any functional improvement (qualitative change) or development.	6. Development is also possible without growth as we see in the cases of some children that they do not gain in terms of height, weight or size but they do experience functional improvement or development in physical, social, emotional or intellectual aspects.

Development is an increase in the complexity of function and skill progression. It is the capacity and skill of a person to adapt to the environment. Development is the behavioral aspect of growth (e.g. person develops the ability to walk, to talk, and to run).

The change brought about in the individual by the process of growth and development; tend to follow some well-defined principles. These are known as principles of growth and development. These principles are being described below.

1. *Principles of continuity:* Development follows continuity. It goes from womb to tomb and never ceases. An individual starting his life from a tiny cell develops his body, mind and other aspects of his personality through a continuous stream of development in these various dimensions. Growth and development are continuous, orderly, sequential processes influenced by maturational, environmental, and genetic factors.
2. *Rate of growth and development is not uniform:* Although development follows continuity, yet the rate of growth and development is not steady and uniform at all times. It proceeds more rapidly in the early years of life but slows down into later years of infancy. Again at the dawn of puberty there is a sudden rise in the adolescence.
3. *Principle of individual differences:* According to this principle there exist wide individual differences among children with respect to the growth and development in various dimensions. Each child grows at his own unique rate.

4. *Uniformity of pattern:* Although development does not proceed at a uniform rate and show marked individual differences, yet it follows a definite sequence or pattern and somewhat uniform in the offspring's of a species. For example all offspring's of human beings begin to grow from head downwards. Similarly the motor development and language development in all children seems to follow a definite sequence. All humans follow the same pattern of growth.
5. *Development proceeds from general to specific responses:* In all phases of child's development, general activity precedes specific activity. His responses are of a general sort before they become specific. For example the boy waves his arms in general, random movements before he is capable of so specific a response as reaching. Similarly when a newborn infant cries, the whole of the body is involved. With growth the crying is limited to the vocal cords, eyes, etc. In language development, the child learns general words before specific. He uses the word daddy in greeting many men and it is only afterwards that he uses if for his father. Development proceeds from simple to complex, or from a cup, for example, the child must first learn a series of single acts: eye-hand coordination, grasping, hand-mouth coordination, controlled tipping of the cup, and then mouth, lip, and tongue movements to drink and swallow.
6. *Principle of integration:* Where it is true that development proceeds from general to specific or from whole to parts, it is also seen that specific responses or part movements are combined in the later process of learning or development. "Development", as observed, "thus involves a movement from the whole to the parts and from the parts to the whole." It is the integration of whole and its parts as well as of the specific and general responses that make a child developed satisfactorily in the various dimensions of his growth and development.

7. *Principle of interrelation:* The growth and development in various dimensions like physical, mental, social, etc. are interrelated and interdependent. Growth and development in any one dimension affects the growth and development of the child in other dimensions. For example children with above average intelligence, are generally found to possess above average physical, and social development. The asset of growth in one dimension diminished the bright possibility in other dimensions. For example, the children having poor physical development tend to regress in emotional, social and intellectual development.
8. *Development is predictable:* With the help of the rate of growth and development of a child it is possible for us to predict the range within which his mature development is going to fall. For example X-rays of the bones of the wrist of a child will tell approximately what his ultimate size will be. Similarly the knowledge of the present mental ability of a child will help in predicting his ultimate mental development. The sequence of each stage is predictable, although the time of onset, the length of the stage, and effects of each stage vary with the person.
9. *Principle of development direction:* There are two specific facts concerning the direction of the development that development is 'cephalocaudal as well as proximodistal'.
   - Growth and development occur in a cephalocaudal direction, that is, starting at the head and moving to the trunk, the legs, and the feet.This pattern is particularly obvious at birth, when the head of the infant is disproportionately large.

     By cephalocaudal development he means that development proceeds in the direction of the longitudinal axis (Head to foot). First, the child gains control over his hand and arms and then on his legs so that he can stand.

According to the proximodistal tendency of the development, it proceeds from the center to the periphery. In the beginning child exhibits his control over the large fundamental muscles but afterwards due to growth and development of smaller muscles he can exhibit more refined movements. For example a control over finger comes after the control over the arm and the hand.

10. *Development is spiral and not linear*: The child does not proceed straightly on the path of development with a constant or steady pace. Actually he makes advancement during a particular period but takes rest in the next following period, to consolidate his development. In advancing further therefore, he turns back and then moves forward again like a spiral.
11. *Growth and development as a joint product of both heredity and environment:* Child at any stage of his growth and development is a joint product of both heredity and environment. His growth and development is any dimension at all times is directly or indirectly influenced by the forces of heredity and environment. Learning can either help or hinder the maturational process, depending on what is learned. Each development stage has its own characteristics. For example, Piaget suggests that in the sensorimotor stage (birth to 2 years) children learn to coordinate simple motor tasks. Development becomes increasingly differentiated. Differentiated development begins with a generalized response and progresses to a skilled specific response. For example, and infant's initial response to a stimulus involves the total body; a 5-year-old child can respond more specifically with laughter or fear.
    - Certain stages of growth and development are more critical than others. It is known, for example, that the first 10 to 12 weeks after conception are critical. The incidence of congenital anomalies as a result of exposure to certain viruses, chemicals, or drugs is greater during this stage than others.
    - The pace of growth and development is uneven. It is known that growth is greater during infancy than during childhood. Asynchronous development is demonstrated by rapid growth of the head during infancy and the extremities at puberty.

Factors Influencing Growth and Development

The factors that influence growth and development are genetic and environmental. The genetic individual is established at conception. It remains unchanged throughout life and determines such characteristics as gender, physical characteristics (e.g. eye color, potential height), and temperament (e.g. response to stimuli in the environment). Environmental factors include family, religion, climate, culture, school, community, and nutrition. For example, poorly nourished children are more likely to have infections than are well-fed children and may not attain their full height potential.

Stages of Growth and Development

For human organism life starts from a fertilized ovum in the womb of the mother. Not only before birth, but also after birth to many years the child is a helpless organism until or unless he is helped by the continuous process of growth and development and attains maturity. When one attains maturity, one is ceased to be called an adolescent and labeled as an adult member of the society. He is supposed to play a responsible role in the society. Before being called as adolescent, he is named as child or infant, etc. All of these names—infant, child, adolescent and adult, etc. are linked with various stages of growth and development through which the child passes from birth to death.

There are certain common developmental or practical characteristics belonging to each stage. The human organism shows peculiar quantitative and qualitative changes in his body and behavior with the help of which at what particular age an individual belongs to which definite stage of his life.

If include the prenatal period, the life span of a human organism can be divided, conveniently, into the following stages:

Sl. No	*Nature of the stage*	*Period and approximate age*
1	Prenatal stage	From conception to birth
2	Stage of infancy	From birth to two years
3	Childhood stage	From 3rd to 12 years or in strict sense up to the on set of puberty
4	Adolescent stage	From the onset of puberty to the age of maturity (Generally from 13 to 19 years)
5	Adulthood	From 20 year and beyond or in strict sense from the age of attaining maturity till death

There is no absolute rigidity in the above classification in terms of either the division of life span into above mentioned stages or the duration of period mentioned against them. There are certainly great individual differences and so we should not imagine that every child will necessarily have each stage according to the period indicated above.

When using the term growth and development synonymously, the major aspects or areas, in which a human child goes ahead for his complete development, can be mentioned below:

a. *Physical development:* The physical development of the individual includes the development of his internal as well as external organs.
b. *Intellectual or mental development:* It includes the development of intellectual powers like the powers of reasoning and thinking, imagination, concentration, creativity, sensation, perception, memory, association, discrimination and generalization, etc.
c. *Emotional development:* Under this aspect, starting with the basic instinct, the evolution of various emotions takes place and also the emotional behavior is developed to the point of emotional maturity.
d. *Moral or character development:* Moral or character development includes the evolution of moral sense and development of character. The individual develops his ethical and moral codes.
e. *Social development:* Initially the child is selfish and antisocial. Gradually he is developed into a social being by learning to behave according to the rules and norms of his society and makes adjustment to it.

Stages of growth and development: The rate of a person's growth and development is highly individual; however, the sequence of growth and development is predictable. Stages of growth usually correspond to certain developmental changes (Table 22.2).

Table 22.2: Stages of growth and development

Stages	*Age*	*Significant characteristics*	*Nursing implications*
Neonatal	Birth to 28 days	Behavior is largely reflexive and develops to more purposeful behavior.	Assist parents to identify and meet unmet needs.
Infancy	1 month to 1 year	Physical growth is rapid.	Control the infant's environment so that physical and psychologic needs are met.
Toddlerhood	1 to 3 years	Motor development permits increased physical autonomy. Psychosocial skills increase.	Safety and risk-taking strategies must be balanced to permit growth.
Preschool	3 to 6 years	The preschooler's world is expanding. New experiences and the preschooler's social role are tried during play. Physical growth is slower.	Provide opportunities for play and social activity.
School age	6 to 12 years	Stage includes the preadolescent period (10 to 12 years). Peer group increasingly influence behavior. Physical, cognitive, and social development increases, and communication skills improve.	Allow time and energy for the school age child to pursue hobbies and school activities. Recognize and support child's achievement.
Adolescence	12 to 20 years	Self-concept changes with biologic development. Values are tested. Physical growth accelerates. Stress increases, especially in face of conflicts.	Assist adolescents to develop coping behaviors. Help adolescents develop strategies for resolving conflicts.
Young adulthood	20 to 40 years	A personal lifestyle develops. Person establishes a relationship with a significant other and a commitment to something.	Accept adult's chosen lifestyle and assist with necessary adjustments relating to health. Recognized the person's commitments. Support changes a necessary for health.
Middle adulthood	40 to 65 years	Lifestyle change due other changes; for example, children leave home, occupational goals change.	Assist clients to plan for anticipated changes in life, to recognize the risk factors related to health, and to focus on strengths rather than weaknesses.
Older adulthood			
Young-old	65 to 74 years	Adaptation to retirement and changes; for example, children leave home, occupational goals change.	Assist clients to keep physically and socially active and to maintain peer group interactions.
Middle-old	75 to 84 years	Adaptation to decline in speed of movement, reaction time, and increasing dependence on others may be necessary.	Assist clients to cope with loss (e.g. hearing, sensory abilities and eyesight death of loved one). Provide necessary safety measures.
Old-old	85 and over	Increasing physical problems may develop.	Assist clients with self-care as required and with maintaining as much independence as possible.

Theories of Growth and Development

Growth and development are commonly thought of as having five major components: physiologic, psychosocial, cognitive, moral, and spiritual. A discussion of some the major theory relating to these components follows.

Researchers have advanced several theories about the various stages and aspects of growth and development, particularly with regard to infant and child development.

i. Development Task Theory (Havighurst, 1900-1991)

Robert Havighurst believed that learning is basic to life and that people continue to learn throughout life. He described growth and development as occurring during six stages, each associated with 6 to 10 tasks to be learned (Table 22.3).

ii. Freud Theory

Sigmund Freud (1856-1939) introduced a number of concepts about development that are still used today. The concepts of the unconscious mind, defense mechanisms, and the id, ego, and superego are due to Freud's. The Unconscious mind is the part of a person's mental life that the person is unaware of. The concepts of the unconscious is one of Freud's major contributions to the field of psychiatry. The id resides in the unconscious and, operating on the pleasure principles, seeks immediate pleasure and gratification. The ego, operating on the reality principle, balances the gratification demands of the id with the limitations of social and physical circumstances. The methods the ego uses to fulfill the needs of the id in a socially acceptable manner are called defense mechanisms or adaptive mechanisms. Defense mechanisms, or adaptive mechanisms as they are more commonly called today, are the result of conflicts between the id's impulses and the anxiety that attends these conflicts due to environmental restrictions. The third aspect of the personality, according to Freud, is the superego. The superego contains the conscience and the ego idea. The conscience consists of society's "don'ts" usually as a result of parental and cultural expectation. The ego ideal individual strives. Freud proposes that the underlying motivation to human development is a dynamic, psychic energy, which he calls **libido**.

According to Freud's theory of psychosexual development, the personality develops in five overlapping stages from birth to adulthood. The libido changes its location of emphasis within the body from one stage to another. Therefore, a particular body area has special significance to a client at a particular stage. The first three stages (oral, anal, and phallic) are called prudential stages. The culmination stage is the genital stage. Table 22.4 indicates characteristics for each stage.

If the individual does not achieve a satisfactory progression at each stage, the personality becomes fixated at that stage. Fixation is immobilization or the inability of the personality to proceed to the next stage because of anxiety. For example, nurses can assist an infant's development by making toilet training a positive experience, thereby enhancing the child's feeling of self-control. Freud also emphasizes the importance of infant-parent interaction. Therefore, the nurse as a caregiver should provide a warm, caring atmosphere for an infant and assist parents to do so when the infant returns to their care.

Ideally, an individual progress through the tasks of each stage and balance is achieved between the id, ego, and superego. Conflict or stress, however, can delay or prolong progression though a stage or cause a person to regress to a previous stage.

Table 22.3: Havighurst age periods and development tasks

Infancy and Early Childhood

1. Learning to walk.
2. Learning to take solid foods.
3. Learning to talk.
4. Learning to control the elimination of body wastes.
5. Learning sex differences and sexual modesty.
6. Achieving psychologic stability.
7. Forming simple concepts of social and physical reality.
8. Learning to relate emotionally to parents, siblings, and other people.
9. Learning to distinguish right from wrong and developing a conscience.

Middle Childhood

1. Learning physical skills necessary for ordinary games.
2. Building wholesome attitudes toward oneself as a growing organism.
3. Learning to get along with age-mates.
4. Learning an appropriate masculine or feminine social role.
5. Developing fundamental skills in reading, writing, and calculating.
6. Developing concepts necessary for everyday living.
7. Developing conscience, morality, and a scale of values.
8. Achieving personal independence.
9. Developing attitudes toward social groups and institutions.

Adolescence

1. Achieving new and more mature relations with age-mates of both sexes.
2. Achieving a masculine or feminine social role.
3. Accepting one's physique and using the body effectively.
4. Achieving emotional independence from parents and other adults.
5. Achieving assurance of economic independence.
6. Selecting and preparing for an occupation.
7. Preparing for marriage and family life.
8. Developing intellectual skills and concepts necessary for civic competence.
9. Desiring and achieving socially responsible behavior.
10. Acquiring a set of values and an ethical system as a guide to behavior.

Early Adulthood

1. Selecting a mate.
2. Learning to live with a partner.
3. Starting a family.
4. Rearing children.
5. Managing a home.
6. Getting started in an occupation.
7. Taking on civic responsibility.
8. Finding a congenial social group.

Middle Age

1. Achieving adult civic and social responsibility.
2. Establishing and maintaining an economic standard of living.
3. Assisting teenage children to become responsible and happy adults.
4. Developing adult leisure-time activities.
5. Relating oneself to one's spouse as a person.
6. Accepting and adjusting to the physiologic changes of middle age.
7. Adjusting to aging parents.

Later Maturity

1. Adjusting to decreasing physical strength and health.
2. Adjusting to retirement and reduced income.
3. Adjusting to death of a spouse.
4. Establishing an explicit affiliation with one's age group.
5. Meeting social and civil obligations.
6. Establishing satisfactory physical living arrangements.

Self-esteem, self-concept, behavior, ability to interact with others, and ability to adapt to life changes.

Many theorists attempt to account for psychosocial development in humans. Many of these theories explain the development of a person's personality and the causes of behavior.

TABLE 22.4: Freud's five stages of development			
Stage	*Age*	*Characteristics*	*Implication*
Oral	Birth to 1½ year	Mouth is the center of pleasure (major source of gratification and exploration).	Feeding produces pleasure and sense of comfort and safety. Feeding should be pleasurable and provided when required.
Anal	1 ½ to 3 years	Anus and bladder are the sources of pleasure (sensual satisfaction, self-control). Major conflict: toilet training.	Controlling and expelling feces provide pleasure and sense of control. Toilet training should be a pleasurable experience.
Phallic	4 to 6 years	The child's genitals are the center of pleasure. Masturbation offers pleasure. Other activities can include fantasy, experimentation with peers and questioning of adults about sexual topics. Major conflict: the Oedipus or Electra complex, which resolves when the child identifies with parent of same sex. (The Oedipus complex refers to the male child's attraction for his mother and hostile attitudes toward his father. The Electra complex refers to the female's attraction for her father and hostile attitudes toward her mother.	The child identifies with the parent of the opposite sex and later takes on a love relationship outside the family. Encourage identity.
Latency	6 to puberty	Energy is directed to physical and intellectual activities. Sexual impulses tend to be repressed. Develop relationship between peers of the same sex.	Encourage child with physical and intellectual pursuits. Encourage sports and other activities with same sex peers.
Genital	Puberty and after	Energy is directed toward full sexual maturity and function and development of skills needed to cope with the environment.	Encourage separation from parents, achievement of independence, and decision making.

iii. Erikson Theory

Erik H Erikson (1902-1994) adapted and expanded Freud's theory of development to include the entire life span, believing that people continue to develop throughout life. He describes eight stages of development (Table 22.5).

Erikson envisions life as a sequence of levels of achievement. Each stage signals a task that must be achieved. The resolution of the task can be complete, partial, or unsuccessful. Erikson believes that the greater the task achievement, the healthier the personality of the person; failure to achieve a task influences the person's ability to achieve the next task. These developmental tasks can be viewed as a series of crises, and successful resolution of these crises is supportive to the person's ego. Failure to resolve the crises is damaging to the ego.

Erikson's eight stages reflect both positive and negative aspects of the critical life periods. The resolution of the conflicts at each stage enables the person to function effectively in

Table 22.5: Erikson's psychosocial stages of development				
Stage	*Age*	*Developmental crisis*	*Successful dealing with crisis*	*Unsuccessful dealing with crisis*
1. **Infant**	Birth to 1-year-old	**Trust versus Mistrust** Babies learn to trust or mistrust others based on whether or not their needs such as food and comfort are met	If babies' needs are met, they learn to trust people and expect life to be pleasant.	If babies' needs are not met, they learn not to trust.
2. **Toddler**	1 to 3 years old	**Autonomy versus Shame and Doubt**	If toddlers are successful in directing their own behavior, they learn to be independent.	If toddler's attempts at being independent are blocked, they learn self-doubt and shame for being unsuccessful.
3. **Preschool age**	3 to 5 years	**Initiative versus Guilt**	If preschoolers succeed in taking responsibility, they feel capable and develop initiative.	If preschoolers fail in taking responsibility they feel irresponsible, anxious, and guilty.
4. **School age**	5 to 12 years old	**Industry versus Inferiority** When children succeed in learning new skills and obtaining new knowledge, they develop a sense of industry, a feeling of competence arising from their work and effort.	When children succeed at learning new skills, they develop a sense of industry, at feeling of competence and self-esteem arising from their work and effort.	If children fail to develop new abilities, they feel incompetent, inadequate, and inferior.
5. **Adolescence**	12 to 18 years	**Identity versus Role Confusion** Adolescents are faced with deciding who or what they want to be in terms of occupation, beliefs, attitudes, and behavior patterns.	Adolescents who succeed in defining who they are and find a role for themselves develop a strong sense of identity.	Adolescents who fail to define their identity become confused and withdraw, or want to inconspicuously blend in with the crowd.
6. **Early adulthood**	18 to 25 years	**Intimacy versus Isolation** The task facing those in early adulthood is to be able to share who they are with another person in a close, committed relationship.	People who succeed in this task will have intimate relationships.	Adults who fail at this task will be isolated from other people and may suffer from loneliness.
7. **Middle adulthood**	25 to 65 years	**Generativity versus Stagnation**	Adults who succeed in this challenge will be creative, productive, and nurturant, thereby benefiting themselves, their family, community, country, and future generations.	Adult who fail will be passive, and self-centered, feel that they have done nothing for the next generation, and feel that the world is no better off for their being alive.
8. **Late adulthood**	65 years to death	**Ego Integrity versus Despair** The issue is whether a person will reach wisdom, spiritual tranquility, a sense of wholeness, and acceptance of his or in her life.	Elderly people who succeed in addressing this issue will enjoy life and not fear death.	Elderly people who fail will feel that their life is empty and will fear death.

society. Each phase has its developmental task, and the individual must find a balance between, for example, trust versus mistrust (Stage 1) or integrity versus despair (Stage 8).

When using Erikson's developmental framework, nurses should be aware of indicators of positive and negative resolution of each stage. If is also important to be aware that the environment is highly influential in development, according to Erikson. Nurses can enhance a client's development by being aware of the person's development stage and by helping the person develop coping skills relative to stressors experienced at that level. Nurses can strengthen a client's positive resolution of a developmental task by providing the individual with appropriate opportunities and encouragement. For example, a 10-year-old child can be encouraged to be creative, to finish schoolwork, and to learn how to accomplish these tasks within the limitations imposed by health.

Erikson emphasizes that people must change and adapt their behavior to maintain control over their lives. In his view, no stage in personality development can be bypassed, but people can become fixated at one stage or regress to a previous state under anxious or stressful conditions. For example, a middle-aged woman who has never satisfactorily accomplished the task of resolving identity versus role confusion might regress to an earlier stage when stressed by an illness with which she cannot cope.

iv. Peck Theories

Theories and models about adult development are relatively recent compared with theories of infant and child development. Research into adult development has been stimulated by a number of factors, including increased longevity and healthier old age. In the past, development was viewed as complete by the time of physical maturity, and aging was considered a decline following maturity. The emphasis was on the decremental aspects rather than the incremental aspects of aging. However, Robert Peck (1968) believes that although physical capabilities and functions decrease with old age, mental and social capacities tend to increase in the latter part of life.

Peck proposes three developmental tasks during old age, in contrast to Erikson's one (integrity versus despair).

1. ***Ego differentiation versus work-role preoccupation***: An adult's identity and feelings of worth are highly dependent on that person's work-role. On retirement people may experience feelings of worthlessness unless they derive their sense of identity from a number of roles so that one such role can replace the work-role or occupation as a source of self-esteem. For example, men who likes to garden or golf can obtain Body transact ego rewards from those activities, replacing rewards formerly obtained from his occupation.
2. ***Body transcendence versus body preoccupation:*** This task calls for the individual to adjust to decreasing physical capacities and at the same time maintain feelings of well-being. Preoccupation with declining body functions reduces happiness and satisfaction with life.
3. ***Ego transcendence versus ego preoccupation:*** Ego transcendence is the acceptance without fear of one's death as inevitable. This acceptance includes being actively involved in one's own future beyond death. Ego preoccupation, by contrast, results in holding onto life and preoccupation with self-gratification.

v. Gould Theories

Roger Gould is another theorist who has studied adult development. He believes that transformation is a central theme during adulthood: "Adults continue to change over the period of time considered to be adulthood and... developmental phases may be found during the adult span of life". According to Gould, the 20s is the time when a person assumes new roles; in the 30s, role confusion often occurs; in the 40s the person becomes aware of time limitations in relation to accomplishing life's goals; and in the 50s, the acceptance of each stage as a natural progression of life marks the path to adult maturity. Gould's study of 524 men and women led him to describe seven stages of adult development:

- Stages I (ages 16-18). Individuals consider themselves part of the family rather than individuals and want to separate from their parents.
- Stages 2 (ages 28-33). Although the individuals have established autonomy, they feel it is in jeopardy; they feel they could be pulled back into their families.
- Stages 3 (ages 22-28). Individuals feel established as adults and autonomous from their families. They see themselves as well-defined but still feel the need to prove themselves to their parents. They see this as the time for growing and building for the future.
- Stages 4 (ages 29-34). Marriages and careers are well-established. Individuals question what life is all about and wish to be accepted as they are, no longer finding it necessary to prove themselves.
- Stages 5 (ages 35-43). This is a period of self-reflection. Individuals question values and life itself. They see time as finite, with little time left to shape the lives of adolescent children.
- Stages 6 (43-50). Personalities are seen as set. Time is accepted as finite. Individuals are interested in social activities with friends and spouse and desire both sympathy and affection from spouse.
- Stages 7 (ages 50-60). This is a period of transformation, with a realization of mortality and a concern for health. There is an increase in warmth and a decrease in negativism. The spouse is seen as a valuable companion.

vi. Cognitive Theory (Piaget, 1896-1980)

Cognitive development refers to the manner in which people learn to think, reason, and use language. It involves a person's intelligence, perceptual ability, and ability to process information. Cognitive development represents a progression of mental abilities from illogical to logical thinking, from simple to complex problem solving, and from understanding concrete ideas to understanding abstract concepts.

The most widely known cognitive theorist is Jean Piaget. His theory of cognitive development has contributed to other theories, such as Kohlberg's theory of morel development and Fowler's theory of the development of faith.

PIAGET'S THEORY: FOUR STAGES OF COGNITIVE DEVELOPMENT

Early researcher Jean Piaget developed his theory from detailed observations of infants and children, most especially his own three children. Piaget made significant contributions to the understanding of how children think about the world around other, and shifted the view of children's thinking from heat of "little adults" to something quite different from adult thinking. Piaget believed that children from mental concepts or schemes as they experience new situations and events. For example, if Sandy points to a picture of an apple and tells her child, "that's an apple," the child forms a scheme for "apple" that looks something like that picture. Piaget also believed that children first try to understand new things in terms of schemes they already possess, a process called assimilation. The child might see an orange and say "apple" because both objects are round. When corrected, the child might alter the scheme for apple to include "round" and "red". The process of altering or adjusting old schemes to fit new information and experiences is accommodation.

Piaget also proposed that there are four distinct states of cognitive development that occur from infancy to adolescence, as shown in Table 22.6.

Table 22.6: Piaget's stages of cognitive development

Stage	*Cognitive development*
Sensorimotor Birth to 2 years old	Children explore the world using their senses and ability to move. They develop object permanence and the understanding that concepts and mental images represent objects, people, and events.
Preoperational 2 to 7 years old	Young children can mentally represent and refer to objects and events with words or pictures and they can pretend. However, they can't conserve, logically reason, or simultaneously consider many characteristics of an object.
Concrete Operational 7 to 12 years old	Children at this stage are able to conserve, reverse their thinking, and classify objects in terms of their many characteristics. They can also think logically and understand analogies but only about concrete events.
Formal Operational 12 years old to adulthood	People at this stage can use abstract reasoning about hypothetical events or situations, think about logical possibilities, use abstract analogies, and systematically examine and test hypotheses. Not everyone can eventually reason in all these ways.

The Sensorimotor stages: The sensorimotor stage is the first of Piaget's stages. It concerns infants from birth to age 2. In this stage, infants use their senses and motor abilities to learn about the world around them. At first, infants only have the involuntary reflexes present at birth to interact with objects and people. As their sensory and motor development progresses, they begin to interact deliberately with objects, by grasping, pushing, tasting, and so on. Infants move from simple repetitive actions, such as grabbing their toes to complex patterns such as trying to put a shape into a sorting box.

Near the end of this period, infants develop a sense of object permanence, the knowledge that an object exists even when it is not in sight. For example, the game of "peek-a-boo" is important in teaching infants that Mommy's smiling face is always going to be behind her hands. This is a critical step in developing language, as words themselves are symbols of things that may not be present. Symbolic thought, which is the ability to represent objects in one's thoughts with symbols such as words, becomes possible by the end of this stage, with children of 2 years capable of thinking in simple symbols and planning out actions.

The Preoperational stage: The preoperational stage (ages 2-7) is a time of developing language and concepts. Children, who can now move freely about in their world. No longer have to rely only on senses and motor skills but now can ask questions and explore their surroundings more fully. Pretending and make-believe play become possible because children at this stage can understand, through symbolic thinking, that a line of wooden blocks can "stand in" for a train. They are limited, however, in several ways. They are not yet capable of logical thought—they can use simple mental concepts but are not able to use those concepts in a more rational, logical sense. They tend to be overwhelmed by what they see, so when children of this age see Santa Claus in a book, on television, or at the mall, Santa Claus becomes real to them. It doesn't occur to them to think about how Santa might get to every child's house in one night or why those toys are the same ones they saw in the store just last week.

Another limitation is egocentrism, the inability to see the world through anyone else's eyes except one's own. For the preoperational child, everyone else must see what the child sees, and what is important to the child must be important to everyone else. For example, 2-year-old Vicki, after climbing out her crib for the third time, was told by her mother, "I don't want to see you in that living room again tonight!" So Vicki's next appearance was made with her hands over her eyes—if she couldn't see her mother, her mother couldn't see her. It would also be egocentric, but completely unselfish, if 4-year-old Kenny wants to give his grandmother an action figure for her birthday because that's what he would want.

Remember that children in this stage are also overwhelmed by appearances, as in the coin example. A child who complains that his piece of pie is smaller than his brother's may be quite happy once his original piece is cut into two pieces—now he think he has "more" than his brother. He has focused only on the number of pieces, not the actual amount of the pie. Focusing only on one feature of some object rather than taking all features into consideration is called centration. Centration is one of the reasons that children in this stage often fail to understand that changing the way something looks does not change its substance. The ability to understand that altering the appearance of something does not change its amount (as in the coin example), its volume, or its mass is called conservation.

Preoperational children fail at conservation not only because they centrate (such as the number of pieces of pie) but also because they are unable to "mentally reverse" actions. This feature of preoperational thinking is called irreversibility. For example, if a preoperational child sees liquid poured from a short, wide glass into a tall, think glass, the child will assume that the second glass holds more liquid. This failure to "conserve" (save) the volume of liquid as it takes on a different shape in the tall, thin glass is not only caused by the child's centration on the height of the liquid in the second glass but also by the inability of the child to imagine pouring the liquid back into the first glass and having it be the same amount again. Similar "reasoning" causes children of this age to assume that a ball of clay, when rolled out into a "rope" of clay, is now greater in mass.

Concrete Operations: In the **concrete operations stage** (ages 7-12), children finally become capable of conservation and reversible thinking. Centration no longer occurs as children become capable of considering all the relevant features of any given object. They begin to think more logically about beliefs such as Santa Claus and ask questions, eventually coming to their own more rational conclusions about the fantasies of early childhood. They are in school, learning all sorts of science and math, and are convinced that they know more than their parents at this point. In fact, they become so logical and focused on "the rules" that they find it difficult to alter rules—their thinking is set in "concrete".

The "concrete" thinking is the major limitation of this stage. Children in this stage are unable to deal effectively with abstract concepts. Abstract concepts are those that do not have some physical, touchable reality. For example, "freedom" is an abstract concept. People can define it, they can get a good sense of what is means, but there is not "thing" that they can point to and say, "This is freedom". Concrete concepts, which are the kind of concepts understood by children of this age, are about objects, written rules, and real things. Children need to be able to see it, touch it, or at least see it in their heads to be able to understand it.

Formal Operations: In the last of Piaget's stages, **formal operations** (age 12 to adulthood), abstract thinking becomes possible. Teenagers not only understand concepts that have no physical reality, but also they get deeply involved in hypothetical thinking, or thinking about possibilities and even impossibilities. "What if everyone just got along?" "If women were in charge of countries, would there be fewer wars?"

Piaget did not believe that everyone would necessarily reach formal operations. Studies show that only about half of all adults in the United States reach formal operations. That does not mean that they use a more practical kind of intelligence that suits their particular lifestyle. Successful college students, however, need formal operational thinking to succeed in their college careers, as most college classes require critical thinking, problem-solving abilities, and abstract thinking based on formal operational skills.

Educators have put Piaget's ideas into practice by allowing children to learn at their own pace, by "hands-on" experience with objects, and by teaching concepts to children that are at an appropriate cognitive level. But Piaget's theory has also been criticized on several points. Some researchers believe that the idea of distinct stages of cognitive development is not completely correct and that changes in thought are more continuous. Other point out that preschoolers is not as egocentric as Piaget seemed to believe and that object permanence exists much earlier than Piaget thought.

Piaget also focused on the child's cognitive development as if the other people in the child's world were not all that important to the acquisition of knowledge and the development of skills. This is not necessarily wrong; children are able to grasp many ideas and concepts through their own thought processes and interactions with objects, discovering basic principles and characteristics of objects in individual play. In contrast, Vygotsky theorized that other people, acting as teachers and mentors, were a crucial part of the cognitive development of the child.

According to Piaget (1966), cognitive development is an orderly, sequential process in which a variety of new experiences (stimuli) must exist before intellectual abilities can develop. Piaget's cognitive developmental process is divided into five major phases: the sensorimotor phase, the preconception phase, the intuitive thought phase, the concrete operations phase, and the formal operations phase.

A person develops through each of these phases; each phase has its won unique characteristics (Table 22.7). In each phase, the person uses three primary abilities: assimilation, accommodation, and adaptation. Assimilation is the process through which humans encounter and react new situations by using the mechanisms they already possess. In this way, people acquire knowledge and skills as well as insights into the world around them. Accommodation is a process of change whereby cognitive processes mature sufficiently to allow the person to solve problems that were unsolvable before. This adjustment is possible chiefly because new knowledge has been assimilated. Adaptation, or coping behavior, is the ability to handle the demands made by the environment.

Nurses can employ Piaget's theory of cognitive development when developing teaching strategies. For example, a nurse can expect a toddler to be egocentric and literal; therefore, explanations to the toddler should focus on the needs of the toddler rather than on the needs of others. A 13-year-old can be expected to use rational thinking and to reason; therefore, when explaining the need for a medication a nurse can outline the consequences of taking and not taking the medication, enabling the adolescent to make a rational decision. Nurses must remember, however, that the range of normal cognitive development is broad, despite the ages arbitrarily associated with each level. When teaching adults, nurses may

Table 22.7: Piaget's phases of cognitive development

Phases and stages	*Age*	*Significant behavior*
Sensorimotor phase Stages 1 use of reflexes Stages 2 primary circular reaction	Birth to 2 years Birth to 1 month	Most action is reflexive Perception of events is centered on the body. Objects are extension of self.
Stages 3 Secondary circular reaction	4 to 8 months	Acknowledges the external environment. Actively makes changes in the environment.
Stages 4 Coordination of secondary schemata	8 to 12 months	Can distinguish a goal from a means of attaining it.
Stages 5 Tertiary circular reaction	12 to 18 months	Tries and discovers new goals and ways to attain goals. Rituals are important.
Stages 6 Inventions of new 3 means	18 to 24 months	Interprets the environment by mental image. Uses make-believe and pretend play.
Preconceptual phase	2 to 4 years	Uses an egocentric approach to accommodate the demands of an environment. Everything is significant and relates to "me". Explores the environment. Language development is rapid. Associates words with objects.
Intuitive thought phase	4 to 7 years	Egocentric thinking diminishes. Thinks of one idea at a time. Includes others in the environment. Words express thoughts.
Concrete operations phase	7 to 11 years	Solves concrete problems. Begins to understand relationships such as size. Understands right and left. Cognizant of viewpoints.
Formal operations phase	11 to 15 years	Use rational thinking. Reasoning is deductive and futuristic.

become aware that some adults are more comfortable with concrete thought and solver to acquire and apply new information that are other adults.

vii. Moral Theories

Moral development, a complex process not fully understood, involves learning what ought to be and what ought not to be done. It is more than imprinting parents' rules and virtues or values on children. The term moral means "relating to right and wrong". The terms morality, moral behavior, and moral development need to be distinguished. Morality refers to the requirements necessary for people to live together in society; moral behavior is the way perceives those requirements and responds to them; moral development is the pattern of change in moral behavior with age.

viii. Kohlberg (1927-1987)

Lawrence Kohlberg's theory specifically addresses moral development in children and adults (Murray & Zentner, 2001).The morality of an individual's decision was not Kohlberg's concern; rather he focused on the reasons an individual makes a decision. According to Kohlberg, moral development progresses through three levels and six stages.

Levels and stages are not always linked to a certain development stage, because some people progress to a higher level of moral development than others.

At Kohlberg's first level, called the premoral or preconventional level, children are responsive to cultural rules and labels of good and bad, right and wrong. However, children interpret these in terms of the physical consequences of their actions, that is, punishment or reward. At the second level the conventional level, the individual is concerned about maintaining the expectations of the family, group or nation and sees this as right. The emphasis at this level is conformity and loyalty to one's own expectations as well as society's. Level three is called the postconventional, autonomous, or principled level. At this level people make an effort to define valid values and principles without regard to outside authority or to the expectation of others (Table 22.8).

ix. Gilligan Theory

After more than 10 years of research with women subjects, Carol Gilligan (1982) reported that women often consider the dilemmas Kohlberg used in his research to be irrelevant. Women scored consistently lower on his scale of moral development in spite of the fact that they approached moral dilemmas with considerable sophistication. Gilligan believes that most frameworks for research in moral development do not include the concepts of caring and responsibility.

Gilligan found that moral development proceeds through three levels and two transitions, with each level representing a more complex understanding of the relationship of self and other and each transition resulting in a crucial reevaluation of the conflict between selfishness and responsibility.

Stage 1: Caring for oneself. In this first stage of development, the person is concerned only with caring for the self. The individual feels isolated, alone, and unconnected to others. There is no concern or conflict with needs of other because the self is the most important. The focus of this stage is survival. The transition of this stage occurs when the individual begins to view this approach as selfishness and moves toward responsibility. The person begins to realize a need for relationships and connections with other people.

Stage 2: Caring for others. During this stage, the individual recognizes the selfishness of earlier behavior and begins to understand the need for caring relationships with others. Caring relationships bring with them responsibility. The definition of responsibility includes self-sacrifice, where "good" is considered to be "caring for others." The individual now approaches relationships with a focus of not hurting others. This approach causes the individual to be a more responsive and submissive to other's needs. A transition from goodness to truth occurs when the individual recognizes that this approach can cause difficulties with relationships because of the lack of balance between caring for oneself and caring for others. The woman makes decisions on personal intentions and consequences of actions rather than on how she thinks others will react.

Stage 3: Caring for self and others. During this last stage, a person sees the need for a balance between caring for others and caring for the self. The concepts of responsibility now includes responsibility for the self and for others people. Care remains the focuses on which decisions are made. However, the person recognizes the interconnections between the self and others and realizes that if one's own needs are not met, other people may also suffer.

Table 22.8: Kohlberg's stages of moral development

Level	*Stages*	*Average age*
I. Preconventional Person is responsive to cultural rules of labels of good and bad, right or wrong. Externally established rules determine right or wrong actions. Person reasons in terms of punishment, reward, or exchange of favors. **Egocentric focus**	**1. Punishment and Obedient Orientation** Fear of punishment, not respect for authority,is the reason for decisions, behavior, and conformity.	Toddler to 7 years
	2. Instrumental Relativist Orientation Conformity is based on egocentricity and narcissistic needs. There is no feeling of justice, loyalty, or gratitude. "I'll do something if I get something for it or because it pleases you".	Preschooler through school age
II. Conventional Person is concerned with maintaining expectations and rules of the family, group, nation, or society. A sense of guilt has developed and affects behavior. The person values conformity, loyalty, and active maintenance of social order and control. Conformity means good behavior or what pleases or helps another and is approved. **Societal focus**	**3. Interpersonal Concordance Orientation** Decisions and behavior are based on concerns about other's reactions; the person wants other's approval or a reward.	School age through adulthood (Most American women are in this stage)
	4. Law-and-Order Orientation The person wants established rules from authorities, and the reason for decisions and behavior is that social and sexual rules and traditions demand the response. ("I'll do something because it's the law and my duty").	Adolescence and adulthood (Most men are in his stage).
III. Postconventional The person lives autonomously and defines moral values and principles that are distinct from personal identification with group values. He or she lives according to principles that are universally agreed on and that the person considers appropriate for life. **Universal focus**	**5. Social Contract Legalistic Orientation** The social rules are not the sole basis for decisions and behavior because the person believes a higher moral principle applies such as equality, justice, or due process.	Middle-age or older adult. Only 20 percent or less of Americans achieves this stage.
	6. Universal Ethical Principle Orientation Decisions and behaviors are based on internalized rules, on conscience rather than social laws, and on self-chosen ethical and abstract principles that are universal, comprehensive, and consistent.	Middle-age or older adult. Few people attain or maintain this stage. Examples of this stage are seen in time of crisis or extreme situations.

Gilligan (1982 believes women often see morality in the integrity of relationships and caring, so that the moral problems they encounter are different from those of men. Men tend to consider what is right to be what is just, whereas for women what is right is taking responsibility for others as a self-chosen decision. The ethic of justice, or fairness, is based on the idea of equality: Everyone should receive the same treatment. This is the development path usually followed by men and widely accepted by moral theorists. By contrast, the ethic of care is based on the premise of nonviolence: no one should be harmed. This is the path typically followed by women but give little attention in the literature of moral theory.

In the development of maturity, according to Gilligan (1982), both viewpoints blend: in the realization that just as inequality adversely affects both perspectives in an unequal relationship, so too violence is destructive for everyone involved the blending of these two perspectives could give rise to a new view of human development and a better understanding of human relations.

Spiritual Theories

The spiritual component of growth and development refers to individual's understanding of their relationship with the universe and their perceptions about the direction and meaning of life.

x. Fowler's Theory

James Fowler describes the development of faith as a force that gives meaning to a person's life. He uses the term faith as a form of knowing, a way of being in relation to "an ultimate environment." To Fowler, "faith is a relational phenomenon; it is an active 'mode-of-being-in-relation' to another or other in which we invest commitment, belief, love, risk and hop" (Fowler and Keen, 1985). Fowler's stages in the development of faith are given in Table 22.9.

Fowler's theory and developmental stages were influenced by the work of Piaget, Kohlberg, and Erikson. Fowler believes that the development of faith is an interactive

Table 22.9: Fowler's stages of spiritual development

Stages	*Age*	*Description*
0. Undifferentiated	0 to 3 years	Infant unable to formulate concepts about self or other environment.
1. Intuitive projective	4 to 6 years	A combination of images and beliefs given by trusted others, mixed with the child's own experience and imagination.
2. Mythic-literal	7 to 12 years	Private world of fantasy and wonder; symbols refer to something specific; dramatic stories and myths used to communicate spiritual meanings.
3. Synthetic-conventional	Adolescent or adult	World and ultimate environment structured by the expectations and judgments of others; interpersonal focus.
4. Individuating-reflexive	After 18 years	Constructing one's own explicit system; high degree of self-consciousness.
5. Paradoxical-consolidative	After 30 years	Awareness of truth from a variety of viewpoints
6. Universalizing	May be never	Becoming an incarnation of the principles of love and justice.

process between the person and the environment. In each of Fowler's stages, new patterns of thought, values, and beliefs are added to those already held by the individual; therefore the stages must follow in sequence. Faith stages, according to Fowler, are separate from the cognitive stages of Piaget: they evolve from a combination of knowledge and values.

xi. Westerhoff Theory

Westerhoff describes faith as a way of being and behaving that evolves from an experienced faith guided by parents and others during a person's infancy and childhood to an owned faith that is internalized in adulthood and serves as a directive for personal action. For the client who is ill, faith-whether in a higher authority (e.g. God, Rama, Krishna), in the client's own self, in the health care team, or in a combination of all- provides strength and trust.

xii. Vygotsky's Theory

Russian psychologist Lev Vygotsky developed a theory of how children think that did not match the prevailing political ideas in Russia. After his death from tuberculosis in 1934, his ideas were suppressed by the government but kept alive by his students and later republished. Vygotsky's pioneering work in developmental psychology has had a profound influence on school education in Russia, and interest in his theories continues to grow throughout the world. Vygotsky wrote about children's cognitive development. Whereas Piaget stressed the importance of the child's interaction with objects as a primary factor in cognitive development, vygotsky stressed the importance of social interactions with other people, typically more highly skilled children and adults. Vygotsky believed that children develop cognitively when someone else helps them by asking leading questions and providing examples of concepts in a process called scaffolding. In scaffolding, the more highly skilled person gives the learner more help at the beginning of the learning process and then begins to withdraw help as the learner's skills improve.

Vygotsky also proposed that each developing child has a zone of proximal development (ZPD), which is the difference between what a child can do alone versus what a child can do with the help of a teacher. For example, if little Jenny can do math problems up to the fourth-grade level, her ZPD is two years. Suzi might be the same age as Jenny (and might even score the same on a traditional IQ test), but if Suzi can only work math problems at a fifth-grade level with the help of the teacher, Suzi's ZPD is not as great as Jenny's. This might be a better way of thinking about intelligence: It isn't what you know (as measured by traditional tests), it's what you can do.

Other researchers have applied Vygotsky's social focus on learning to the development of a child's memory for personal (autobiographical) events, finding evidence that children learn the culturally determined structures and purposes of personal stories from the early conversations they have with their parents. This process begins with the parent telling the story to the very young child, followed by the child repeating elements of the story as the child's verbal abilities grow. The child reaches the final stage at around age 5 to 6 when the child creates the personal story entirely-an excellent example of scaffolding. Vygotsky's ideas have been put into practice in education through the use of cooperative learning, in which children work together in groups to achieve a common goal, and in reciprocal teaching, in which teachers lead students through the basic strategies of reading until the students themselves become capable of teaching the strategies to others.

Information-processing theory: The information-processing theory, a theory that looks at the way people deal with information. Memory is one of the main focal points of the information-processing theory and is an important part of infant development.

Infants do have memory abilities because they can be operantly conditioned right after birth. In one classic study, for example, researchers found that newborns would suck on a pacifier harder to hear their mother's voice rather than some other woman's voice. Their mother's voice acted as reinforcement for sucking harder, implying that they had formed a memory for what had happened the last time they sucked hard.

Infants also habituate, or stop responding to a stimulus that is repeated and unchanging, just as adults do. This means that infants must be able to recognize that a certain stimulus is familiar from one time to the next. Habituation studies have allowed researchers to determine when infants can perceive color, changes in sounds, and so on.

Whereas infant memory is typically nonverbal, the preschool child is capable of using language to form memories. Short-term memory in the preschool years has a smaller capacity than it will in adulthood and is limited to about three items. To make matters worse, the typical preschool–year-old can only remember things for about 3 seconds. Preschool children do not yet know how to use strategies such as rehearsal to extend their short-term memories, nor do they know how to elaborate on information that should be stored in long-term memory. The long-term memories of children in the preschool years consist mostly of episodic (personal events) and procedural (skill) memories, with semantic memories (general knowledge) being limited to basic language concepts and word meanings.

As children grow up and go to school, they are directly taught by teachers and peers how to use memory strategies. They begin to learn how their own memories work, an understanding called metamemory. They learn control strategies such as rehearsal and organization, and their capacity for short-term memory approaches that of adults. They can, with effort, be taught the same kind of strategies that aid adults in storing and retrieving memories as their command of language grows.

Human Development Across the Life

In the context of life, human development is the scientific study of the changes that occur in people as they age, from conception until death. This chapter will touch on almost all of the topics covered in the other chapters of this text, such as personality, cognition, biological processes, and social interactions. But in this chapter, all of those topics will be studied in the context of changes that occur as a result of the process of human development.

A study in development is affected by the problem of age. In any experiment, the participants who are exposed to the independent variable (the variable in an experiment that is deliberately manipulated by the experimenter) should be randomly assigned to the different experimental conditions. The problem in developmental research is that the age of the people in the study should always be an independent variable, but people cannot be randomly assigned to different age groups.

There are some special designs that are used in researching age-related changes: the longitudinal design, in which one group of people's is followed and assessed at different times as the group ages; the cross-sectional design, in which several different age groups are studies at one time; and the cross-sequential design, which is a combination of the longitudinal and cross-sectional designs (Baltes et al., 1988).

The longitudinal design has the advantage of looking at real age-related changes as those changes occur in the same individuals. Disadvantages of this method are the lengthy amount of time, money, and effort involved in following participants over the years as well as the loss of participants when they move away, lose interest, or die. The cross-sectional design has the advantages of being quick, relatively inexpensive, and easier to accomplish than the longitudinal design. The main disadvantage is that one is no longer comparing an individual to that same individual as he or she ages; instead, individuals of different ages are being compared to one another. Differences between age groups are often a problem in developmental research. For example, if comparing the scores of 30 year-old to 80-year-old to see how aging affects intelligence, questions arise concerning the differing experiences those two age groups have had in educational opportunities that might affect IQ scores in addition to any effects of aging.

In studying human development, developmental psychologists have outlined many theories of how these age-related changes occur. There are some areas of controversy, however, and one of these is the issue of nature versus nurture.

Nature refers to heredity, the influence of inherited characteristics on personality, physical growth, intellectual growth, and social interactions. Nurture refers to the influence of the environment on all of those same things and includes parenting style, physical surroundings, economic factors, and anything that can have an influence on development that does not come from within the person.

So, is a person like Hitler born that way, or did something happen to make him the person he was? How much of a person's personality and behavior are determined by nature and how much are determined by nurture? This is a key question, and the answer is quite complicated. It is also quite important: Are peopling like Hitler, the infamous serial killer Ted Bundy, and Timothy McVeigh (the man responsible for the Oklahoma bombing of the Federal Building) the result of bad genes? Or was it bad parenting or life-altering experiences in childhood? Or are they the unique combination of both hereditary and environmental influences? After many years of scientific research, most developmental psychologists now agree that the last possibility is the most likely explanation for most of human development: all that people are and all that people become is the product of an interaction between nature and nurture.

This does not mean that the controversy one longer exists; for example, intelligence is still a "hot topic" with regard to how much is inherited and how much is learned. There are researchers and theorists who assume a large genetic influence and those who believe that culture, economics, nutrition in early childhood, and educational opportunities have a greater impact.

Behavioral genetics is a relatively new field in the investigation of the origins of behavior in which researchers try to determine how much of behavior the result of genetic inheritance is and how much is due to a person's experiences.

PRENATAL DEVELOPMENT

Any study of the human life span must begin with looking at the complex material contained in the cells of the body that carries the instructions for life itself. After discussing the basic building blocks of life, this text will discuss how the processes of conception and the development of the infant within the womb take place.

Chromosomes, Genes, and DNA Genetics is the science of heredity. Understanding how genes transmit human characteristics and traits involves defining a few basic terms.

Imagine a long, long ladder. Now imagine that the ladder is made of very soft rubber, and it is twisted around itself along its whole length. DNA (deoxyribonucleic acid) is a very special kind of molecule (the smallest particle of a substance that still has all the properties of that substance). DNA consists of two strands wind around each other in a spiral much like the two sides of the ladder wind around each other. Linking the two strands together are certain chemical elements called amines or bases arranged in a particular pattern. The rungs of the rubber ladder would be like these chemical links for realistic representation of DNA.

Because of DNA's unique shape, each molecule of DNA is linked end-to-end with the others, forming a very long strand. Sections of this DNA strand are linked by the amines, which are usually referred to by letters A, T, G, and C. Amines are organic structures that contain the genetic codes for building the proteins that make up organic life (hair coloring, muscle, and skin, for example) and that control the life of each cell. Each section of DNA containing a certain sequence (ordering) of these amines is called a gene. So a gene is nothing more than a section of the DNA strand that has the same sequence of amines. Genes are located on rod-shaped structures called chromosomes, which are found in the nucleus of a cell.

Humans have a total of 46 chromosomes in each cell of their bodies (with the exception of the egg and the sperm). Twenty-three of these chromosomes come from the mother's egg and the other 23 from the father's sperm. Most characteristics are determined by 22 such pairs, called autosomes. The last pair determines the sex of the person. These two chromosomes are called the sex chromosomes.

554 **Dominant and recessive genes:** The 46 chromosomes can actually be arranged in pairs, with one member of each pair coming from the mother and the other member from the father. Think about just one of these pairs for the moment. In this particular pair of chromosomes, assume that there is a gene for hair color on each chromosome. The actual color of the person's hair will be determined by those two genes, one gene from each parent. If both genes are for brown hair, the people will obviously have brown hair, right? And if both are for blond hair, the person's hair will be blond. Some genes that are more active in influencing the trait are called dominant. A dominant gene will always be expressed in the actual trait, in this case the hair color. A person with a dominant brown hair color gene will have brown hair, no matter what the other gene is, because brown in the most dominant of all the hair colors.

Some genes are less active in influencing the trait and will only be expressed in the actual trait if they are paired with another less active gene. These genes tend to recede, or fade, into the background when paired with a more dominant gene, so they are called recessive. Blond hair color is the most recessive color and will only show up in a person's actual hair color if that person has a blond hair color gene from each parent.

In reality, the pattern of genetic transmission of traits can be a little complicated. Almost all traits are controlled by more than one pair of genes in a process called polygenic inheritance. (Polygenic means "many genes"). Sometimes certain kinds of genes tend to group themselves with certain other genes, like the genes for blond hair and blue eyes. Other genes are so equally dominant or equally recessive that they combine their traits in the organism. For example, genes for blond hair and red hair are recessive. When a child inherits one of each from his or her parents, instead of one or the other controlling the child's hair color, they may blend together to form a strawberry-blond mix.

Genetic and chromosome problems: Several genetic disorders are carried by recessive genes. Diseases carried by recessive genes are inherited when a child inherits two recessive genes, one from each parent. Examples of disorders inherited in this manner are cystic fibrosis (a disease of the respiratory and digestive tracts), sickle cell anemia (a blood disorder), Tay-Sachs disorder (a fatal neurological disorder), and PKU (a problem with digesting a particular protein).

Sometimes the chromosome itself is the problem. Although each egg and each sperm are only supposed to have 23 chromosomes, in the creation of these cells a chromosome can end up in the wrong cell, leaving one cell with only 22 and the other with 24. If either of these cells survives to "mate," the missing or extra chromosome can cause mild to severe problems in development. Examples of chromosome disorders include Down syndrome, a disorder in which there is an extra chromosome in what would normally be the twenty-first pair. Symptoms include almond-shaped, wide-set eyes and mental retardation. Other chromosome disorder occur when there is an extra sex chromosome in the twenty-third pair, such as Klinefelter's syndrome, in which the twenty-third set of sex chromosomes is XXY, with the extra X producing a male with reduced masculine characteristics, enlarged breasts, obesity, and excessive height, and Turner's syndrome, in which the twenty-third pair is actually missing an X, so that the result is a lone X chromosome. These females tend to be very short, infertile, and sexually underdeveloped.

From conception to birth: Life begins at the moment of conception, the moment at which a female becomes pregnant. From conception to the actual birth of the baby is a period of approximately nine months, during which a single cell becomes a complete infant. It is also during this time that many things can have a positive or negative influence on the developing infant.

The zygote and twinning: When an egg (also called an ovum) and a sperm unite in the process of fertilization, the resulting single cell will have a total of 46 chromosomes and is called a zygote. Normally, the zygote will begin to divide, first into two cells, then four, then eight, and so on, with each new cell also having 46 chromosomes, because the DNA molecules produce duplicates of themselves before each division. Eventually, the mass of cell becomes a baby.

There are actually two kinds of twins, resulting from two different unusual occurrences. Twins who are commonly referred to as "identical" are monozygotic twins, meaning that the two babies come from one (mono) fertilized egg (zygote). Early in the division process, the mass of cell splits completely—no one knows exactly why-into two separate masses, each of which will develop into a separate infant. The infants will be the same sex and have identical features because they each possess the same set of 46 chromosomes.

The other type of twin is more an accident of timing and is more common in women who are older and who are from certain ethnic groups. A woman's body is only supposed to ovulate (release an egg from the ovary) once each monthly cycle. Sometimes something goes wrong, and her ovary releases more than one egg at the same time. If two of these eggs are fertilized, the woman may give birth to fraternal or dizygotic twins (two eggs), or possibly triplets or some other multiple number of babies. This is also more likely to happen to women who are taking fertility drugs to help them get pregnant.

Another form of dizygotic twins is the result of the woman's body releasing an egg in the next monthly cycle, even though the woman is already pregnant. Usually, once the woman is pregnant her body sends a signal to the brain, telling it that no more eggs need to be released. If that signal is too weak or is not sent, she will ovulate again and can become pregnant again. In this type of fraternal twin, one baby may be quite a bit larger than the other because the larger baby is actually older.

Twins provide developmental psychologists with another way to look at the contribution of nature and nurture to human development. Researchers may seek out identical twins that have been separated at birth; looking at all ways those twins are alike in spite of being raised in different environment.

The term Siamese twin is really not the most accurate way to describe identical twins that are physically joined together at some point on their bodies. The proper term is conjoined twins, and this condition occurs when the mass of cells begins to separate into two masses by remains linked at some particular point. Wherever that point is, the two infants will by physically "stuck" together, sometimes involving only soft tissues, like the original and truly Siamese twins, Chang and Eng, who were joined at the hip, and sometimes involving the sharing of certain body parts.

Dizygotic twins: Because identical twins come from one fertilized egg (zygote), they are called monozygotic. Fraternal twins, who come from different fertilized eggs, are called dizygotic.

Once fertilization has taken place, the zygote begins dividing and moving down to the uterus, the muscular organ that will contain and protect the developing infant. This process takes about a week, followed by about week during which the mass of cells, now forming a hollow ball, firmly attaches itself to the wall of the uterus. This two-week period is called the germinal period of pregnancy. The placenta also begins to form during this period. The placenta is a specialized organ that provides nourishment and filters away waste products from the developing baby. The umbilical cord also begins to develop at this time, connecting the organism to the placenta.

During the germinal period, the cells begin to differentiate, or develop into specialized cells, in preparation for becoming all the various kinds of cells that make up the human body-skin cells, heart cells, and so on. Perhaps the most important of these cells are the stem cells, which stay in a somewhat immature state until needed to produce more cells. Researchers are currently looking into ways to use stem cells found in the umbilical cord to grow new organs and tissues for transplant or to repair neurological damage.

The embryonic period: Once firmly attached to the uterus, the developing organism is called an embryo. The embryonic period will last from two weeks after conception to eight weeks, and during this time the cells will continue to specialize and become the various organs and structures of a human infant. By the end of eight weeks after conception, the embryo is about 1 inch long and has primitive eyes, nose, lips, teeth, little arms and legs, and a beating heart. Although no organ is fully developed or completely functional at this time, nearly all are "there".

Critical periods: As soon as the embryo begins to receive nourishment from the mother through the placenta, it becomes vulnerable to hazards such as diseases of the mother, drugs, and other toxins that can pass from the mother through the placenta to the developing infant. It is during this time of pregnancy that we most clearly see critical periods, times during which some environmental influence can have an impact-often devastating-on the development of the infant.

Prenatal hazards teratogens: Any substance such as a drug, chemical, virus, or other factor that can cause a birth defect is called a teratogen. Table 22.10 shows some common teratogens and their possible negative effects on the developing infant.

Table 22.10: Common teratogens

Teratogenic agent	*Effect on development*
Rubella	Blindness, deafness, heart defects, brain damage.
Marijuana	Irritability, nervousness, tremors; infant is easily disturbed, startles
Cocaine	Decreased height, low birth weight, respiratory problems, seizures, learning difficulties; infant is difficult to soothe
Alcohol	Fetal alcohol syndrome (mental retardation, delayed growth, facial malformation), learning difficulties, smaller than normal heads
Nicotine	Miscarriage, low birth weight, stillbirth, short stature, mental retardation learning disabilities
Mercury	Mental retardation, blindness
Syphilis	Mental retardation, deafness, meningitis
Caffeine	Miscarriage, low birth weight
Radiation	Higher incidence of cancers, physical deformities
High water temperatures	Increased chance of neural tube defects

The fetal period: The fetal period is the time from about eight weeks after conception until the birth of the child (now called a fetus) and is a period of tremendous growth. The fetus's length increases by about 20 times and its weight increases from about 1 ounce at 2 months to a little over 7 pounds. The organs, while accomplishing most of their differentiation in the embryonic period, continue to develop and become functional. Muscles begin to contract in the third month. In the fourth month, the mother will begin to feel this movement as a tiny "flutter" or "quickening" at first, and by the fifth month, the flutter will become a "kick".

The last few months continue the development of fat and the growth of the body, until about the end of the thirty-eighth week. At that time, the fetus is pushed out of the mother's body in the process of labor and childbirth and becomes a baby. Babies born before 38 weeks are called preterm and may need life support to survive. This is especially true if the baby weighs less than about five and a half pounds at birth.

The most likely time for a miscarriage, or spontaneous abortion, is the first three months, as the organs are forming and first becoming functional. Some 15 to 20 percent of all pregnancies end in miscarriage, many so early that the mother may not have even known she was pregnant. When a miscarriage occurs, it is most likely caused by a genetic defect in the way the embryo or fetus is developing that will not allow the infant to survive. In other words, there isn't anything that the mother did wrong or that could have been done to prevent the miscarriage.

INFANCY AND CHILDHOOD

Surprisingly, babies can do a lot more than researchers used to believe they could. At a lot of the early research on infants just after birth was done on babies who were still very drowsy from the general anesthesia that used to be give to their mothers during the labor process. Drowsy babies do not tend to respond well, as one might imagine. In the next few sections, it becomes obvious that infants accomplish a great deal throughout infancy, even in the first few days of life on the outside.

Physical development immediately after birth, several things start to happen. The respiratory system begins to function, filling the lungs with air and putting oxygen into the blood. The blood now circulates only within the infant's system because the umbilical cord has been cut. Body temperature is now regulated by the infant's own activity and body fat (which acts as insulation) rather than by the amniotic fluid. The digestive system probably takes the longest to adjust to life outside the womb. This is another reason for the excess body fat. It provides fuel until the infant is able to take in enough nourishment on its own. That is why most babies lose a little weight in the first week after birth.

Reflexes: Babies come into this world able to interact with it. Infants have a set of innate (existing from birth) involuntary behavior patterns called reflexes. Until an infant is capable of learning more complex means of interaction, reflexes help the infant to survive.

Pediatricians use these and other reflexes to determine whether or not an infant's nervous system is working properly.

Sensory development: Although most infant sensory abilities are fairly well-developed at birth, some require a bit more time to reach "full power". The sense of tough is the most developed, which makes perfect sense when one realizes how much skin-to-womb contact the baby has in the last months of pregnancy. The sense of smell is also highly developed. Breast-fed babies can actually tell the difference between their own mother's milk scent and another woman's milk scent within a few days after birth.

Taste is also nearly fully developed. At birth, infants show a preference for sweets (and human breast milk is very sweet), and by four months have developed a preference for salty tastes (which may come from exposure to the salty taste of their mother's skin). Sour and bitter, two other taste sensations, produce spitting up and the making of horrible faces.

Hearing is functional before birth but may take a little while to reach its full potential after birth. The fluids of the womb must clear out completely. From birth, newborns seem most responsive to high pitcher, as in a woman's voice, and low pitcher, as in a male's voice.

The least functional sense at birth is vision. The eye, is quite a complex organ. The rods, which see in black and white and have little visual acuity, are fairly well-developed at birth, but the cones, which see color and provide sharpness of vision, will take about another six months to fully develop. So the newborn has relatively poor color perception when compared to sharply contrasting lights and darks until about two months of age and has fairly "fuzzy" vision, much as a nearsighted person would have. The lens of the newborn stays fixed until the muscles that hold it in place mature. Until then the newborn is unable to shift what little focus it has from close to fat. Thus, newborns actually have a fixed distance for clear vision of about 7 to 10 inches, which is the distance from the baby's face to the mother's face while nursing. This focal distance may also be the reason adults almost instinctively hold a baby at about this distance from their own faces.

Newborns also have visual preferences at birth, as discovered by researchers using measures of the time that infants spent looking at certain visual stimuli. They found that infants prefer to look at complex patterns rather than simple ones, three dimensions rather than two, and that the most preferred visual stimulus was a human fact. The fact that infants prefer human voices and human faces makes it easier for them to form relationships with their caretakers and to develop language later on.

Motor development: Infants manage a tremendous amount of development in motor skills from birth to about two years of age. When looking at the ages listed, remember that these ages are averages based on large samples of infants. An infant may reach these milestones earlier or later than the average and still be considered to be developing normally.

An infant's normal development is related to many factors such as nutrition, care, and health. One important way to protect an infant's health is to make sure that immunizations against various illnesses are given at the appropriate times.

Cognitive Development

By the time average infants have reached age 1, triples its weight in the first two years, the brain is about 75 percent of its adult weight. By age 5, the brain is at 90 percent of its adult weight. This increase makes possible a tremendous amount of major advances in cognitive development, including the development of thinking, problem solving, and memory.

Stages of Language Development

The development of language is indeed a very important milestone in the cognitive development of a child because language allows children to think in words rather than just images, to ask questions, to communicate their needs and wants to others, and to form concepts. Early views of language development were based on Skinnerian principles of reinforcement. However, Noam Chomsky (1957) argued strongly against this. He proposed a LAD (language acquisition device), an innate "program" that contained a schema for human language. The children matched the language they heard against this schema and, thus, language developed in a well-researched sequence.

There are several stages of language development that all children experience, no more what culture they live in or what language they will learn to speak (Brown, 1973).

1. **Cooing:** At around 2 months of age, babies begin to make vowel-like sounds.
2. **Babbling:** At about 6 months, infants add consonant sounds to the vowels to make a babbling sound, which at times can almost sound like real speech.
3. **One-word speech:** Somewhere just before or around age 1, most children begin to say actual words. These words are typically nouns and may seem to represent an entire phrase of meaning. They are called holophrases (whole phrases in one word) for that reason. For example, a child might say "Milk" and mean "I want some milk!" or "I drank my milk!"
4. **Telegraphic speech:** At around a year and a half, toddlers begin to string words together to form short, simple sentences using nouns, verbs, and adjectives. "Baby eats," "mommy go," Doggie go bye-bye" are examples of telegraphic speech. Only the words that carry the meaning of the sentence are used.
5. **Whole sentences:** As children move through the preschool years, they learn to use grammatical terms and increase the number of words in their sentences, until by age 6 or so they are nearly as fluent as an adult, although the number of words they know is still limited when compared to adult vocabulary.

Psychological Development

The psychological and social development of infants and children involves the development of personality, relationships, and a sense of being male or female. Although these processes begin in infancy, they will continue in many respects well into adulthood.

Some children negative and whiny while others are sweet and good-natured.

Temperament: One of the first ways in which infants demonstrate that they have different personalities (long-lasting characteristics that make each person different from other person) is in their temperament, the behavioral and emotional characteristics that are fairly well-established at birth. Researchers have been able to identify three basic temperament styles of infants:

1. **Easy:** "Easy" babies are regular in their schedules of waking, sleeping, and eating and are adaptable to change. Easy babies are happy babies and when distressed are easily soothed.
2. **Difficult:** "Difficult" babies are almost the opposite of easy ones. Difficult babies end to be irregular in their schedules and are very negative about change of any kind. They are loud, active, and tend to be crabby rather than happy.
3. **Slow to warm up:** This kind of temperament is associated with infants, who are less negative, quieter, and more regular than difficult children but who are slow to adapt to change. If changes is introduced gradually, these babies will "warm up" to new people and new situations.

Of course, not all babies will fall neatly into one of these three patterns-some children may be a mix of two or even all three patterns of behavior. Even so, longitudinal research

strongly suggests that these temperament styles last well into adulthood, although they are somewhat influenced by the environment in which the infant is raised. For example, a "difficult" infant who is raised by parents who are themselves very loud and active may not be perceived as difficult by the parents, whereas a child who is slow to warm up might be perceived as difficult if the parents themselves like lots of change and noise. The first infant is in a situation in which the "goodness of fit" of the infant's temperament to the parents' temperament is very close, but the parents of the second infant are a poor fit in temperament for the less active child (Chess and Thomas, 1986).

A baby's temperament is going to be connected to how parents deal with many issues. Babies with easy temperaments allow parents to plan around their schedules, for example. Planning around the varying sleeping and eating behaviors of a difficult infant is much trickier. As children grow, their temperament and how well it matches a parent's own temperament becomes an issue in discipline and in the formation of emotional bonds to the parents or other caregivers.

Attachment: The emotional bond that forms between an infant and a primary caregiver is called attachment. Attachment is a very important development in the social and emotional life of the infant, usually forming within the first six months of the infant's life and showing up in a number of ways during the second six months, such as wariness of strangers and fear of being separated from the caregiver. Although attachment to the mother is usually the primary attachment, infants can attach to fathers and to other caretakers as well.

Many Ainsworth (1985), came up with a special experimental design to measure the attachment of an infant to the caretaker called the Strange Situation (exposing and infant to a series of leave-takings and returns of the mother and a stranger). Through this measurement technique Ainsworth and another colleague identifies four attachment styles:

1. **Secure:** Infants labeled as secure were willing to get down from their mothers' lap when they first entered the room with their mothers. They explored happily, looking back at their mothers and returning to them every now and then (sort of like "touching base"). When the stranger came in, these infants got upset. When the mother returned, the infants approached her, were easily soothed, and were glad to have her back.
2. **Avoidant:** In contrast, avoidant babies, although somewhat willing to explore, did not "touch base". They did not look at the stranger or the mother and reacted very little to her absence or her return, seeming to have no interest or concern.
3. **Ambivalent:** The word ambivalent means to have mixed feelings about something. Ambivalent babies in Ainsworth's study were clinging and unwilling to explore, very upset by the stranger regardless of the mother's presence, protested mightily when the mother returned, these babies would demand to be picked up, but at the same time push the mother away or kick her in a mixed reaction to her return.
4. **Disorganized-disoriented:** In subsequent studies, other researchers found that some babies seemed unable to decide just how they should react to the mother's return. These disorganized-disoriented infants would approach her but with their eyes turned away from her, as if afraid to make eye contact. In general, these infants seemed fearful and showed a dazed and depressed look on their faces.

If should come as no surprise that the mothers of each of the four types of infants also behaved differently from one another. Mother of secure infants were loving, warm, sensitive to their infant's needs, and responsive to the infant's attempts at communication. Mothers of avoidant babies were unresponsive, insensitive, and coldly rejecting. Mothers of ambivalent babies tried to be responsive but were inconsistent and insensitive to the baby's actions, often talking to the infant about something totally unrelated to what the infant was doing at the time. Mothers of disorganized-disoriented babies were found to be abusive or neglectful in interactions with the infants.

Attachment is not necessarily the result of the behavior of the mother along, however. The temperament of the infant may play an important part in determining the reactions of the mothers. For example, an infant with a difficult temperament is hard to soothe. A mother with this kind of infant might come to avoid unnecessary contact with the infant, as did the mothers of the avoidant babies in Ainsworth's studies.

Critics of Ainsworth's Stranger Situation research focus on the artificial nature of the design and wonder if infants and mothers would behave differently in the more familiar surroundings of home, even though Ainsworth's experimental observers also observed the infants and mothers in the home prior to the Strange Situation (Ainsworth, 1985). Other research has found results supporting Ainsworth's findings in home-based assessments of attachment. Other studies have also found support for the concept of attachment styles and stability of attachment over the first six years of life. Even adult relationships can be seen as influenced by the attachment style of the adult.

Evidence that similar attachment styles are found in other cultures demonstrates the need to consider attachment as an important first step in forming relationships with other's.

I've heard that you shouldn't pick a baby up every time it cries that if you do, it might spoil the baby. Unfortunately, a lot of people have not only heard this advice but also acted on it by frequently ignoring an infant's crying, which turns out to be a very bad thing for babies. When a baby under 6 months of age cries, it is an instinctive reaction meant to get the caretaker to tend to the baby's needs—hunger, thirst, pain, and even loneliness. Research has shown that babies whose cries are tended to consistently (that is the infant is fed when hunger, changed when wet, and so on) in the early months are more securely attached as late as age 1 than those infants whose caretakers frequently allow the infants to cry when there is a need for attention—hunger, pain, or wetness, for example. Erikson, a psychodynamic theorist who emphasized the importance of social relationships in the development of personality, would certainly disagree with letting a baby "cry it out," although allowing an infant who has been fed, changed, burped, and checked to cry on occasion will not damage attachment.

Erikson, who trained as a Freudian psychoanalyst but became convinced that social interactions were more important in development than Freud's emphasis on sexual development, believed that development occurred in a series of eight stages, with the first four of these stages occurring in infancy and childhood. Each stage is an emotional crisis, or a kind of turning point, in personality, and the crisis in each stage must be successfully met for normal, healthy psychological development.

Erikson focused on the relationship of the infant and the child to significant others in the immediate surroundings—parents and then later teachers and even peers. Summarizes the conflict in each of the four stages and some of the implications for future development.

Gender Role Development

Most children begin to realize the difference between girls and boys at about age 2, and most can say which one they are at that age. But knowing one's sex (the physical characteristic of being male or female) is not the same thing as knowing the different behavior expected of a male or a female (gender). The behavior that goes along with being male or female is heavily influenced by cultural expectations as well as biology, and is referred to as gender identity.

ADOLESCENCE

Adolescence is the period of life from about age 13 to the early twenties, during which a young person is no longer physically a child but is not yet an independent, self-supporting adult. In the past, adolescence was always defined as the "teens," from ages 13 to 19. But adolescence isn't necessarily determined by chronological age. It also concerns how a person deals with life issues such as work, family, and relationships. So although there is a clear age of onset, the end of adolescence may come early or late for different individuals.

Physical Development

The clearest sign of the beginning of adolescence is the onset of puberty, the physical changes in both primary sex characteristics (growth of the actual sex organs such as the penis or the uterus) and secondary sex characteristics (changes in the body such as the development of breast and body hair) that occur in the body as sexual development reaches its peak.

Puberty occurs as the result of a complex series of glandular activities, stimulated by the "master gland" or the pituitary gland when the proper genetically determined age is reached. Certain psychosocial and environmental factors such as stress, exercise, and nutrition may also have an impact on the timing of puberty. The thyroid gland increases the rate of growth, the adrenal glands and sex glands stimulate the growth of characteristics such as body hair, muscle tissue in males, and the menstrual cycle in girls, for example. Puberty often begins about two years after the beginning of the growth spurt, the rapid period of growth that takes place at around age 10 for girls and around age 12 for boys.

In addition to an increase in height, physic characteristics related to being male or female undergo rapid and dramatic change. In fact, the rate of growth and development in puberty approaches that of development in the womb. For females, breast tissue begins to enlarge, hips begin to widen, the uterus grows, and eventually the menstrual cycle begins. For boys, the penis and testicles increase in size, muscles become more defined, and the voice begins to deepen. For sexes, oily secretions increase (causing pimples and even acne in many teens), hair grows on the pubic area and under the arms, and body odor becomes more noticeable. After about four years, the changes of puberty are relatively complete.

Cognitive Development

The cognitive development of adolescents is less visible than the physical development but still represents a major change in the way adolescents think about themselves, their peers and relationships, and the world around them.

Adolescents, especially those who receive a formal high school education, move into Piaget's final stage of formal operations, in which abstract thinking becomes possible. This cognitive advance is primarily due to the final development of the frontal lobes of the brain, the part of the brain that is responsible for organizing, understanding, and decision making. Teenagers begin to think about hypothetical situations, leading to a picture of what an "ideal" world would be like. Many become convinced that such a world is possible to achieve for if only everyone else would just listen to the teenager.

Although headed into an adult style of thinking, adolescents are not yet completely free of egocentric thought. At this time in life, however, their egocentrism shows up in their preoccupation with their own thoughts. They do a lot of introspection (turning inward) and may become convinced that their thoughts are as important to others as they are to themselves. Two ways in which this adolescent egocentrism emerges are the personal fable and they imaginary audience.

In the personal fable, adolescents have spent so much time thinking about their own thoughts and feelings that they become convinced that they are special, one of kind, and that no one else has ever had these thoughts and feelings before them. "You just don't understand me, I'm different from you" is a common feelings of teens. The personal fable is not without a dangerous side. Because they feel unique, teenagers may feel that they are somehow protected from the dangers of the world and so do not take the precautions that they should. This may result in an unwanted pregnancy, severe injury or death while racing in a car, drinking and driving, and drug use, to name a few possibilities. "It can't happen to me, I'm special" is a risky but common thought.

The imaginary audience shows up as extreme self-consciousness in adolescents. They become convinced that everyone is looking at them and that they are always the center of everyone else's world, just as they are the center of their own. This explains the intense self-consciousness that many adolescents experience concerning what others think about how the adolescent looks or behaves.

MORAL DEVELOPMENT

Another important aspect in the cognitive advances that occur in adolescence concerns the teenager's understanding of "right" and "wrong". Harvard University professor Lawrence Kohlberg was a developmental psychologist who, influenced by Piaget and others, developed a theory of the development of moral thinking. Through looking at how

Table 22.11: Kohlberg's three levels of morality		
Level of morality	*How rules are understood*	*Example*
Preconventional morality (typically very young children).	The consequences determine morality; behavior that is regarded is right, that which is punished is wrong.	A child who steals a toy from another child and does not get caught does not see that action as wrong.
Conventional morality (Older children, adolescents, and most adults).	Conformity to social norms is right; nonconformity is wrong.	A child criticized his or her parent for speeding because speeding is a against the stated laws.
Postconventional morality (about 20 percent of the adult population).	Moral principles determined by the person are used to determine right and wrong and may disagree with societal norms.	A reporter who wrote a controversial story goes to jail rather than reveal the source's identity.

people of various ages responded to stories about people caught up in moral dilemmas. Kohlberg (1973) outlined three levels of moral development, or the knowledge of right and wrong behavior. Although these stages are associated with certain age groups, adolescents and adults can be found at all three levels. For example, a juvenile delinquent tends to be preconventional in moral thinking. Kohlberg's theory has been criticized as being male oriented, especially since he used only males in his studies. Carol Gilligan (1982) propped that men and women have different perspectives on morality: Men tend to judge as moral the actions that lead to a fair or just end, whereas women tend to judge as moral the actions that are nonviolent and hurt the fewest people. Researchers, however, have not found consistent support for gender differences in moral thinking.

Psychosocial Development

The development of personality and social relationships in adolescence primarily concerns the search for a consistent sense of self or personal identity. The psychosocial crisis that must be faced by the adolescent, according to Erikson, is that of identity versus role confusion. In this stage, the teenager must choose from among many options for values in life and beliefs concerning things such as political issues, career options, and marriage. From those options, a consistent sense of self must be found. Erikson believed that teens who have successfully resolved the conflicts of the earlier four stages are much better "equipped" to resist peer pressure and find their own identity during the adolescent years. Those teens who are not as successful come into the adolescent years with a lack of trust in others, feelings of guilt and shame, low self-esteem, and dependency on others. Peer pressure is quite effective on teenagers who desperately want to "fit in" and have an identity of some sort and who feel that others will not want to be with them unless they conform to the expectations and demands of other peer group. They play the part of the model child for the parents, the good student for the teachers and the "cool" juvenile delinquent to their friends and will be confused about which of the many roles they play is really their own identity.

Parent/teen conflict: Even for the majority of adolescents who end up successfully findings a consistent sense of self, there will be conflicts with parents. Many researchers believe that a certain amount of "rebellion" and conflict is a necessary step in breaking away from childhood dependence on the parents and becoming a self-sufficient adult. Self-sufficient:

able to function without outside aid; capable of providing for one's own needs. Although many people think that these conflicts are intense and concern very serious behavior, the reality is that most parent/teen conflict is over trivial issues—hair, clothing, taste in music, and so on. On the really big moral issues, most parents and teens would be quite surprised to realize that they are in agreement.

ADULTHOOD

Physical Development

Adulthood can be thought of as the period of life from the early twenties until old age and death. Exactly when adulthood begins is not always easy to determine. In some cultures, adulthood is reached soon after puberty. Some people feel that it begins after graduation from high school, whereas others would say adulthood doesn't begin until after graduation from college. Others define it as the point when a person becomes totally self-sufficient with a job and a home separate from his or her parents. In that case, some people are not adults until their late thirties.

Adulthood can also be divided into at least three periods: young adulthood, middle age, and late adulthood. Physical changes in young adulthood are relatively minimal. The good news is that the twenties are a time of peak physical health, sharp sense, and mature cognitive abilities. The bad news is that even in the early twenties, the signs of aging are already beginning. Oil glands in the neck and around the eyes begin to malfunction, contributing to wrinkles in those areas near the end of the twenties and beginning of the thirties. The thirties may not bring noticeable changes, but vision and hearing are beginning to decline and by around age 40, bifocal lenses may become necessary as the lens of the eye hardens, becoming unable to change its shape to shift focus. Hearing loss may begin in the forties and fifties but often does not become noticeable until the sixties or seventies, when hearing aids may become necessary.

In the forties, skin begins to show more wrinkles, hair turns gray (or falls out), vision and hearing decline further, and physical strength may begin to decline. In the fifties, these changes continue. Throughout middle age, weight may increase as the rate at which the body functions slows down but eating increases and less time is spent exercising. Height begins to decrease, with about half an inch of height lost for every 10 years past age 40, although people with the bone loss disease osteoporosis may lose up to eight inches or more. Although sexual functioning usually does not decline in middle age, opportunities for sexual activity may be fewer than in the days of young adulthood. Children, mortgages, and career worries can put a damper on middle-age romance.

For women, the forties are a time of great physical changes. At this time in life, a woman's reproductive organs become unreliable, as levels of the female hormone estrogen decline in preparation for the end of reproduction. The uterus slowly begins to get smaller in size, menstrual cycles become irregular, and some women begin to experience "hot flashes", a sudden sensation of heat and sweating that may keep them up at night. Interestingly, in some cultures, particularly those in which the diet contains high amounts of soy products, hot flashes are almost nonexistent. These changes are called the climacteric, and the period of five to ten years over which these changes occur is called per menopause. At an average age of 51, most women will cease ovulation altogether, ending their reproductive years. The cessation of ovulation and the menstrual cycle is called menopause.

Men also go through a time of sexual changes, but it is much more gradual and less dramatic than menopause. In males, andropause (Carruthers, 2001) may begin in the midtwenties with a decline in several hormones, primarily testosterone (the major male hormone). Physical symptoms are also less dramatic but no less troubling: fatigue, irritability, possible problems in sexual functioning, and reduced sperm count. Males, however, rarely lose all reproductive ability.

It is in middle age that many health problems first occur, although their true cause may have begun in the young adulthood years. Young adults may smoke, drink heavily, stay up late, and get dark tans, and the wear and tear that this lifestyle causes on their bodies will not become obvious until their forties and fifties.

Some of the common health problem that may show up in middle age are high blood pressure, skin cancer, heart problems, arthritis, and obesity. High blood pressure can be caused by lifestyle factors such as obesity and stress but may laud be related to hereditary factors. Sleep problems, such as loud snoring and sleep apnea (in which breathing stops for 10 seconds or more), may also take their toll on physical health. There is some evidence that high blood pressure and apnea are linked, although the link may be as simple as the common cause of obesity. The most common causes of death in middle age are heart disease, cancer, and stoke-in that order.

Intellectual abilities do not decline overall, although speed of processing (or reaction time) does slow down. Compared to a younger adult, a middle-aged person may take a little longer to solve a problem. However, a middle-aged person also has more life experience and knowledge to bring to bear on a problem, which counters the lack of speed. In one study, for example, older typists were found to outperform younger typists, even though they typed more slowly than the younger subjects. The older typists, because of years of practice, had developed a skill of looking farther ahead in the document they were typing, so that they could type more continuously without looking back at the document. This allowed them to complete their typing more quickly than the younger typists.

Changes in memory ability are probably the most noticeable changes in middle-age cognition. People find themselves having a hard time remembering a particular word or someone's name. This difficulty in retrieval is probably not evidence of a physical decline (or the beginning of Alzheimer's disease) but is more likely caused by the stresses a middle-aged person experiences and the sheer amount of information that a person of middle years must try to keep straight.

People who exercise their mental abilities have been found to be far less likely to develop memory problems and even senile dementias such as Alzheimer's in old age. "Use it or lose it" is the phrase to remember. Working challenging crossword puzzles, for example, can be a major factor in maintaining a healthy level of cognitive functioning. Reading, having an active social life, going to plays, taking classes, and staying physically active can all have a positive impact on the continued well-being of the brain.

In adulthood, concerns involve career, relationships, family, and approaching old age. The late teens and early twenties maybe college years for many, although other young people go to work directly from high school. The task of choosing and entering a career is very serious and a task that many young adults have difficulty accomplishing. A college student may change majors more than once during the first few years of college, and even after obtaining a bachelor's degree many may either get a job in an unrelated field or go on to a different type of career choice in graduate school. Those who are working may also change careers several times (perhaps as many as five to seven times) and may experience periods of unemployment while between jobs.

Forming Relationships

In young adulthood, Erikson saw the primary task to be finding a mate. True intimacy is an emotional and psychological closeness that is based on the ability to trust, share, and care, while still maintaining one's sense of self. Young adults who have difficulty trusting others and who are unsure of their own identities may find isolation instead of intimacy-loneliness, shallow relationships with others, and even a fear of real intimacy. For example, many marriages end in divorce within a few years, with one partner leaving the relationship and even the responsibilities of parenting- to explore personal concerns and those unfinished issues of identity.

Parenting

In middle adulthood, persons who have found intimacy can now focus outward on others. Erikson saw this as parenting the next generation and helping them through their crises, a process he called generativity. Educators, supervisors, health care professionals, doctors, and community volunteers might be examples of positions that allow a person to be generative. Those who are unable to focus outward but are still dealing with issues of intimacy or even identity are said to be stagnated. People who frequently hand the care of their children over to grandparents or other relatives so that they can go out and "have fun" may be unable to focus on anyone else's needs but their own.

Dealing with mortality: As a person's life enters the stage known as late adulthood, the reality of one's eventual death become harder and harder to ignore. Erikson (1980) believed that at this time, people look back on the life they have lived in a process called a life review. In the life review people must deal with mistakes, regrets, and unfinished business. If people can look back and feel that their lives were relatively full and come to terms with regrets and losses, then a feeling of integrity or wholeness results. Integrity is the final completion of the identity, or ego. If people have many regrets and lots of unfinished business, they feel despair, a sense of deep regret over things that will never be accomplished because time has run out.

THEORIES OF AGING

There are a number of theories of why people physically age. One theory states that the hormonal system gets out of balance, causing the immune system that keeps people healthy to start failing. But this theory fails to state why the hormonal system fails in the first place. Another has to do with the effect of outside influences, whereas two others have to do with biological influences.

Cellular clock theory: One of the biological based theories is the cellular clock theory (Hay flick, 1977). In this theory, cells are limited in the number of times they can reproduce to repair damage. Evidence for this theory is the existence of telomeres, structure on the ends of chromosomes that shorten each time a cell reproduces. When telomeres are too short, cells cannot reproduce and damage accumulates, resulting in the effects of aging. (Sounds almost like what happens when the warranty is up on a car, doesn't it?)

Wear-and-tear theory: The theory that points to outside influences such as stress, physical exertion, and bodily damage is known as the wear-and-tear theory of aging. In this theory, the body's organs and cell tissues simply wear out with repeated use and abuse. Damage tissues accumulate and produce the effects of aging. Collagen, for example, is a natural elastic tissue that allows the skin to be flexible. As people age, the collagen "wears out," becoming less and less "stretchy" and allowing skin to sag and wrinkle (Cua et. al., 1990). (This process is not unlike what happens to the elastic in the waistband of one's underwear over time).

Free radical theory: The free radical theory is actually the latest version of in the wear-and-tear theory in that it gives a biological explanation for the damage done to cells over time. Free radicals are oxygen molecules that have an unstable electron (negative particle). They bounce around the cell, stealing electrons from other molecules and increasing the damage to structures inside the cell. As people get older, more and more free radicals do more and more damage, producing the effects of aging (Hauck and Bartke, 2001).

Activity theory (Havighurst et. al., 1968) proposes that an elderly person adjusts more positively to aging when remaining active in some way. Even if a career must end, there are other ways to stay active and involved in life. Elderly people who volunteer at hospitals or schools, those who take up new hobbies or throw themselves full time into old ones, and those who maintain their friendships with others and continue to have social activities have been shown to be happier and live longer than those who withdraw themselves from activity. Contrary to the view of the elderly as voluntarily withdrawing from activities, the withdrawal of many elderly people is not voluntary at all. Others simply stop inviting elderly people to social activities and including them in their lives.

STAGES OF DEATH AND DYING

There are several ways of looking at the process of dying. One of the more well-known theories is that of Elisabeth Kubler-Ross, who conducted extensive interviews with dying person and their caretakers. Elisabeth Kubler-Ross theorized that people go through five stages of reaction when faced with death (Kubler-Ross, 1997). These stages are denial, in which people refuse to believe that the diagnosis of death is real; anger, which is really anger at death itself and the feelings of helplessness to change things; bargaining, in which the dying person tries to make a deal, with doctors or even with God; depression, which is sadness from losses already experienced (e.g. loss of a job or one's dignity) and those yet to come (e.g. not being able to see child grow up); and finally acceptance, when the person has accepted the inevitable something that cannot be avoided or escaped and quietly awaits death.

Obviously, some people do not have time to go through all of these stages or even go through them in the listed order. Some theorists do not agree with the stage idea, seeing the process of dying people, stating that the particular disease or condition and its treatment, the person's personality before the terminal diagnosis, and other life history factors make the process of dying unique and unpredictable. The danger in holding too strictly to a stage theory is that people may feel there is a "right" way to face death and "wrong" way, when in fact each person's dying process is unique.

APPLYING GROWTH AND DEVELOPMENT CONCEPTS TO NURSING PRACTICE

Different theories explain or more aspects of an individual's growth and development. Typically, theorists examine only one aspect of an individual's development, such as the cognitive, moral or physical aspects. The area chosen for examination usually reflects the researcher's academic discipline and personal interest. The theorists may also limit the population that is studied to a particular part of the life span, such as infancy, childhood, or adulthood.

Although such theories can be useful, they have limitations. First, the theory chosen may explain only one aspect of the growth and development process. Yet a person does not develop in fragmented sections but rather as a whole human being. Thus the nurse may find it necessary to apply several theories for an adequate understanding of the growth and development of a client.

Another limitation of some theories is the suggestion that certain tasks are performed at a specific age. In most cases, the child or adult does accomplish the task at the time specified by the guidelines. In other cases, however, the nurse may find that an individual does not accomplish the task or meet the milestone at the exact time suggested by the theory. Such individual differences are not easily defined or categorized by a single theory. Human development is a complex synthesis of physiologic, cognitive, psychologic, moral, and spiritual development. Nurses should expect individual variations and take these into consideration when applying these theories about growth and development. In so doing, they will be better able to understand a client's development and plan effective nursing interventions.

In nursing, developmental theories can be useful in guiding assessment, explaining behavior, and providing a direction for nursing interventions. An understanding of a child's intellectual ability helps a nurse to anticipate and explain certain reaction, responses, and needs. Nurses can then encourage client behavior that is appropriate for that particular developmental stage.

Theories are also useful in planning a nursing intervention. For instance, choosing the appropriate toy for a 3-year-old boy requires some knowledge of the physical and cognitive development of the child, as well as a sensitivity for individual preferences.

In adult care, knowledge about the physical, cognitive, and psychologic aspects of the aging process is a fundamental aspect of administering sensitive nursing care. For example, nurses can use their familiarity with the theories of development to help clients understand and anticipate the psychosocial changes that take place after retirement or the physical limitations that come with old age.

Understanding following points of growth and development help nurses to provide better care for their clients.

- Robert Havighurst believes that learning is basic to life and that people continue to learn throughout life. His theory describes six age periods with developmental tasks for each period.
- Psychosocial development refers to the development of personality. Psychosocial theorists include Freud, Erikson, Peck, and Gould.
- Cognitive development refers to the manner in which people learn to think, reason, and use language. The most widely known cognitive theorist is Piaget.
- Prenatal or intrauterine development lasts about 9 calendar months.
- The embryonic phase is the 9-week period during which the fertilized ovum develops into an organism with most of the features of the human.
- Monitoring the infant's weight, length, head and chest circumferences, fontanelle size and status, vision, hearing, smell and taste, touch, reflexes, and motor development are important indicators to the newborn's growth and health.

- Infants from birth to 12 months reveal marked growth is size and stature with appropriate nutrition and care. Birth weight doubles by 5 months and triples by 12 months.
- During infancy, motor development is notable: at 1 month infants can life their heads momentarily when prone; at 6 months they can sit unsupported; and at 12 months they can walk with help.
- Fulfillment of the infant's physiologic and psychologic needs is required to develop a basic sense of trust. Parents can enhance this sense of trust by reposing consistently to an infant's needs, providing a predictable environment in which routines are established, and being sensitive to the infant's needs and meeting those needs skillfully and promptly.
- Cognitive development, for the infant, is a result of interaction between an individual and the environment. The infant needs a variety of sensory and motor stimuli.
- The toddler group, ages 12 months to 3 years, develops from having no voluntary control to begin able to walk and speak. They also learn to control their bladders and bowels, and they acquire all kinds of information about their environment.
- During the preschool years, ages 4 to 5, physical growth slows, but control of the body and coordination increase greatly. The preschooler's world gets larger as they meet relative, friends, and neighbors.
- The school-age period starts when children are about 6 years of age, when deciduous teeth are shed. In general, this period from 6 to 12 years is one of rapid and dramatic change. Skills learned during this stage are particularly important in relation to work later in life and willingness to try new tasks.
- During psychosocial development, school-age children face Erikson's conflict of industry versus inferiority.

- School-age children begin to understand relationships and change from being egocentric to having cooperative interactions; according to Piaget, they are in the concrete operations phase of cognitive development.
- Rapid growth in height, development of secondary sexual characteristics, sexual maturity and increasing independence from the family are major landmarks of adolescence.
- Peer groups assume great importance during adolescence they provide a sense of belonging, pride, social learning, and sexual roles.
- Adolescents are at Fowler's synthetic-conventional stage of spiritual development.
- Adolescents between the ages of 11 and 15 begin the formal operations stage of cognitive development; they are able to think logically, rationally, and futuristically and can conceptualize things as they could be rather than as they are.
- The adolescent is at Kohlberg's conventional level of moral development, and some proceed to the postconventional or principled level.
- The four leading causes of adolescence death are motor vehicle crashes, homicide, suicide, and other unintentional injuries.
- Adults development is often divided into three phases: young adults (20–40 years), middle-aged adults (40–65 years), old (75–85 years), old-old (85–100 years), and the elite old (over 100 years).
- The young adult is essentially in a stable period physically, but psychological change is great. Choices must be made about education, occupation, marriage or an alternative lifestyle, child rearing, a place to live, civic roles, and so on.
- The middle-aged adult needs to adjust to an aging body, the increasing dependence of parents, and the incasing independence of children; however, new independent interests can be pursued.

- Both middle-aged men and women enter a midlife crisis in which they need to reexamine their purpose and reevaluate ways to use their energies and abilities.
- Older adults experience many physical changes associated with aging. All body systems undergo change: integumentary, neuromuscular, sensory/perceptual, pulmonary, cardiovascular, gastrointestinal, and genitourinary.
- Several theories have been proposed to account for the biologic aging process: wear-and-tear, rate of living, stress, endocrine, free-radical, genetic, programmed senescence, error catastrophe, collagen, cross-linking immunologic and autoimmune theories.
- Psychosocial theories about aging include the disengagement, activity, and continuity theories.
- The older adult has to adjust to possible psychosocial changes, including retirement (which necessitates financial and social adjustments), relocation, increasing dependence on others, and coping with losses and death.
- Cognitive development continues during young adulthood and the middle-aged years. Developments may extend beyond the formal operations phase of Piaget to one of post-formal operations thinking. The intellectual abilities of the healthy older adult undergo minimal change. In older adults, retrieval of information from long-term or recent memory.
- In the realm of moral development, most adults are in either Kohlberg's stage 4 (the law and order orientation) at the conventional level or in stage 5 (the social contract and legalistic orientation) at the postconventional level.
- Spiritual development of young, middle-aged, and older adults continues into Fowler's paradoxical-consolidative stage. Some adult enter the sixth stage of spiritual development, universalizing.
- Health problems of young adult include accidents, suicide, hypertensions (in African American males), substance abuse, sexually transmitted disease, abuse of women, and malignancies. Problems of middle-aged adults include accidents, cancer, cardiovascular disease, obesity, alcoholism, and mental health alterations. Health problems of older adults include accidents, chronic disabling disease, drug use and misuse, alcoholism, dementia, and abuse.
- Health promotion information for all adults needs to include positive health practice that can promote health and wellness. These include (a) recommended physical, visual, hearing, and dental assessments; (b) screenings for cardiovascular disease and tuberculosis; (c) breast and testicular self-examinations; (d) immunizations; (e) Papanicolaou smears for women; (f) safety precautions to prevent accidents; (g) the importance of appropriate nutrition and exercise; and (h) for older adults, the importance of measures to prevent constipation.
- When nurses have a good understanding of developmental tasks, their clients can be assessed more completely, and nurses can help them to maximize their potential and develop interventions that use resources to work on special needs. This becomes crucial in middle-aged and older adults as they experience many inevitable psychosocial and physical losses and changes.

23 CHAPTER

Psychology of the Group

Introduction

Group refers to any collection of human beings who are brought into social relationship with one another. There is reciprocal communication. Man lives in groups. Groups are universal aspects of human life.

The basic social environment is the group. Each individual is a member of many groups like the family group, the school group, the work group, the social club group, etc. within each group the individual assumes a "position" such as the child, the parent, the student, the teacher, etc. each of these positions in the group has an associated set of behaviors, attitudes and beliefs expected of an individual who occupies the position. Such a set of expectations is called a role.

An individual, as a member of a group, behaves quite differently than what he would otherwise do. As a member of the group he exhibits group behavior. Group behavior is not a mere sum total of the behavior of the individuals who constitute that group. Under the influence of group behavior, even the most disciplined and obedient students have been found indulging in the most coward, unsocial or irresponsible ones are found contribution significantly when observed to work in a group. Therefore it should be clearly understood that in a group; the behavior of the individuals rests on a different psychic level and thus psychology of the group should be considerably different from the psychology of the individuals. For understanding the psychology of the group or group behavior let us first try to understand the meaning of the term group.

Generally, a group is said to be a collection or aggregate of two or more objects or persons. But from the sociopsychological angle mere collection or aggregate of people does not form a group. A psychological group in the opinion of Kretch, Crutchfield and Ballachey may be defined "as two or more persons who meet the following conditions":

1. The relations among the members are interdependent—each members behavior influences the behavior of each of the others.
2. The members 'share an ideology'—a set of beliefs, values and norms which regulate their mutual conduct".

In this sense members of psychological group are said to be interdependent to some significant degree. They share common interests and aims and observe agreed rules of conduct and behavior. In more clear terms, the members of a psychological group must have a common psychology, i.e. they must feel, think and act together. *A group, therefore may be defined as the collection or aggregate of two or more interdependent individuals who usually feel, think and act together.*

A group is a collection or individuals who are in a cooperative interdependent relationship with one another. The term interdependent not only implies that there is "interaction" between the individuals, but also that the members share some common norms with regard to certain behaviors, attitudes, and beliefs and that there must be a system of interlocking 'roles' such that each member has certain expectations regarding how others behave towards him and how he ought to behave towards others in the group.

Moreover a sort of belongingness or we-feeling is essential for the formation of a psychological group. When the people say, we are teachers, we are nurse, we are laborers, etc. it means that they are the members of a psychological group. Under such feelings they can feel, act and think together and, therefore, can be called the members of psychological group. Hence the essential characteristics of a psychological group may be summarized in the following way:

1. It is the collection or aggregate of two or more individuals.
2. The members of the group have relations to one another that make them interdependent to some significant degree.
3. There is a feeling of belongingness or we-feeling in the members of the group.
4. It possesses a set of values or norms of its own that regulates the behavior of individual members to seek the common goal or purpose.
5. On account of group psychology, the members of psychological group merge their individualities and begin to feel, think and act together at least to a particular moment at a particular place.

Chief Characteristics of Group

To point out the characteristics of group of life is also a difficult problem. Even then some characteristic of group life can be described. They are as follows:

1. *Social relations:* The members of a group are related to each other—Simply a gathering of persons cannot be called a group. The members of the group should be interrelated. In fact, this social relation is called a group. Cuber has written, "A group is any number of human beings in reciprocal communication". Maclver and some other sociologists have also admitted the social relations to be fundamentals of the group life.
2. *Feeling of unity:* Group implies a feeling of unity—A feeling of unity is essential for every group. By virtue of such a feeling, members of a group treat each other as their own and a sense of sympathy between them develops.
3. *Sense of belongingness:* Members of a group have a sense of belongingness or 'we' feeling—By a sense of 'we' feeling the members of a group help each other in performing their duties; and they defend collectively against the harmful powers. They treat others as the outsiders and try to make their group prosperous and self-sufficient.
4. *Common interest:* The interests, ideals and values of the group members are common—A group includes those persons who are related to each other in such a way that they should be treated as one. For it, the interests, ideals and values of the persons of a group should tend to be common because this similarity promotes unity.
5. *Common behavior:* There is similarity of behavior in a group—As the interests, ideals and values of the persons of a group are common, similarly the behavior of the persons also tends to be similar. A social group is not merely a group of persons, but it is a continuation of their behavior.

6. *Social norms:* Control of group over the actions of the members—The main reason behind the similarity of behavior in group life is that actions of the members are controlled by the group. In each group there are some customs, norms and procedures which are acceptable to everyone and the members of the group give punishment. Even if the group fails to punish a person disobeying these, he shall be severely criticized by public. In this way, everyone has to obey the social norms. In fact, without some norms, the existence of group life is practically impossible.
7. *Social characteristics:* The members of a group are affected by its characteristics—Each group possesses some social characteristics which separate it from the similar and dissimilar groups. These characteristics affect the members constituting the group. The effect may be of different nature for different persons, but still all the members are affected by the group.

The above mentioned characteristics can be observed in a family group. In a family group, the members are related to each other by intimate relations such as husband-wife, father-son, brother-sister, etc. and all work together extending mutual help for the common good of the family and in the interest of the family. All members treat each other as their own and though their interests may be different, still ideals and interests tend to be similar. A family works as a separate unit by the virtue of this similarity of ideals and interests. All the members are controlled by the family and if they don't obey the family norms they are rebuked.

These characteristics of group life can be observed in other groups too though their quantity may be different.

Classification of Group

Every one of us is a member of some group that exists in the society. Various attempts have been made to classify these groups on one ground or the other. Some of these classifications are discussed head.

1. Summer's classification: WG Summer classifies the groups into two main categories:-

i. In group or we-group
ii. Out-group or others group.

In-group or we-group is the group with which we identify ourselves. The out group or others group is the group, the members of which are considered as outsides by us. Therefore, there are only two categories 'we' and 'they' and 'individual' might belong to either in-group or out-group. Those not members of the 'we-group' are of the 'they group'. Antagonistic feelings are often common between these groups. People do not try to understand the members belonging to out-group and show an attitude of indifference or scorn or even hate. In schools where segregation is observed, the girls or boys from two opposite groups. For the girls belong to in-group and boys are considered to be the members of out-group. Similarly boys consider the girls to be belonging to out-group.

2. Cooley's classification: The classification suggested by Cooley's is based on the degree of intimacy which the individual feels with other persons or groups or a we-feeling. On this basis groups may be classified as primary, secondary or tertiary. In primary groups there is an intimate face-to-face relationship and cooperation. We-feelings are found to a maximum degree among the members of such groups. Also they are bound with a mutual bond of interest. The family, play group of children and village community are some of the examples of primary groups.

In secondary groups the relationships are more or less casual. Here the relationships are usually marked by a single bond of interest. Examples of this type of groups are trade Unions. Professional associations, social organization and association, Lodges and clubs. In tertiary groups, the degree of intimacy or relationship is quite marginal and transient in character. The group of the audience in a cinema hall or passengers in a railway carriage, etc. are the examples of such groups.

3. Organized v/s spontaneous groups: Groups may be classified as organized groups and spontaneous group. In a spontaneous group, the individual belonging to it come together naturally without any previous planning or specific purpose. But organized groups exist for some specific purposes and are formed as a result of careful preplanning. The family, the army, the school, etc. are the examples of such organized groups.

4. Formal v/s informal groups: Psychological groups, according to another mode of classification, can be classified as formal and informal groups.

In formal groups the members of the group observe formalities and are bound by some specific rigid rules, values and norms; on the other hand in informal groups members are not bound by specification and are very information in their relationship and behavior.

Semiformal groups fall in between these two categories. The group of the students in a classroom is an example of a formal group. Various kinds of work organizations also belong to this category. In informal groups we can include family, play or peel group, hobby and recreational groups, etc. Under semiformal groups lodges, temples, social clubs can be considered.

By this sort of above classification it should not be concluded that individual is a member of only one group and he cannot belong to more than one group. An individual may belong to many groups and can be a member of many groups at a particular time. He may be the member of his family group, class or school group, play group, club and association and other so many primary, secondary or tertiary groups: formal and informal groups, spontaneous or organized groups, in-groups or out-groups, etc. Similarly it should also be considered that the classification of groups suggested above is rigid or static. The groups whatever their structure or composition may be, are always quite dynamic in nature. For example a formal group like participants in a seminar may turn into an informal group while taking tea or lunch. Similarly a spontaneous group that has been formed incidentally may take the shape of an organized group and secondary group like lodge or hostel may perform the function of the primary group.

School as a Group

School is a social group. All the students and teachers are its members. A school has a purpose, i.e. imparting education. It binds its members with its traditions and forces them to behave properly. The atmosphere of school persuades new members to join the group and continues making efforts to modify the behavior of elder members. The success of a school depends upon the fact that its members accept and follow its tradition.

Utility of school behavior in education. The school is a social group and educational institution. Hence group behavior is of utmost importance in education. This behavior helps the children is acquiring suitable education. The social aim of education depends on proper group behavior. Education aims at making such members of the society as are highly skilled, expert and useful. Training for this end in view can be given through group behavior in school.

Several types of conditions are essential for building up an organized school community. They are given below:

1. *Continuous existence of the community:* The school community is not like a crowd. It has stability. Teachers remain in the school for a long time. A large number of students study in the school and in this way it is stable. For its stability it is essential that the teachers do not change often and students do not leave it after studying for some time. Their stay at school for considerable time is necessary so that they may understand the value of school society and acquire its good virtues.
2. *Ideals of school:* The school should have some aims and ideals. It is necessary that the children should understand them. They should form a sentiment for the school. In order to achieve this purpose internal functions such as celebrations of national days, morning assembly, drama, prize distribution day, etc. should be organized. Activities of this type acquaint the students with the ideals of the school.
3. *Social feelings and pride in traditions:* The youngest student of the school feels proud of his school. The students of different schools compare the activities, etc. of their respective schools and each student tries to prove that his own school is the better one. Individuals competitions in debates, sports, games, one act plays, etc. develop love in the students for the school.

   Traditions of the school, results, sports, cultural activities of higher order, etc. produce a feeling of rivalry among the students.

   All the students wish to see their schools as winners. They are ready to do many a things to bring self-respect and glory to their alma mates. All these things help in the development of social feeling in them.

4. *Cooperative and creative atmosphere:* The school is an organized group. It is essential that the students work in cooperation with each other. In order to achieve this the teacher will have to lead them. As far as possible, individual competition should not be encouraged but group game, etc. should be organized, e.g. interclass game competition, etc.

   It is essential for the school environment to be creative and progressive. It should change with the time so that it remains the mirror of school. Its aims should be decided. It should lead the society. Such a thing is possible only in the creative atmosphere of a school.

Classroom as a Group

There are many kinds of groups in a school, e.g. club, team, literary societies, subject societies, classroom group, etc. Classroom group is the most important of all these groups.

Classroom as an instructional group helps its members to satisfy their needs and achieve the goals. In school program, the classroom group has a special place of importance. The classroom is especially important in the ways given ahead:

1. *To improve the behavior of students:* In a classroom group the students come into contact with each other and acquire appropriate type of education.
2. *To develop mental processes:* Some sort of exchange of thoughts goes on in the class group through which intellectual activities like reasoning, memory, judgment, decision, thinking and imagination develop.
3. *To develop the feeling of self-sacrifice:* The students in a classroom group remain in close contact with each other. Therefore so much love, goodwill and sympathy develop in

them in the time of need they do not hesitate to sacrifice themselves for the sake of others.

4. *To prepare for future social life:* Children in classroom group live together for pretty long time and try to adjust their thoughts, habits and viewpoints to others. Such a type of experience prepares them for future social life.
5. *To excite sympathy of numbers:* A student starts doing as other students do. This tendency is called sympathy of numbers.
6. *To develop qualities of leadership:* Students in classroom groups plan or organize a number of cocurricular activities. Thus qualities of leadership are developed in them.
7. *To acquire more knowledge:* In a classroom group the students learn the habits of completion and imitation and get an inspiration to acquire more knowledge.
8. *To develop the feeling of cooperation:* The teacher encourages all the members of a classroom group to work together and thus a feeling of cooperation is developed in them.

Social Distance in Groups

Groups possess strong likes and dislikes for other groups. Members of a group like to keep the members of other group and the group itself at a distance. This distance is named as social distance. In this way social distance as a team can be defined as the distance at which members of a particular group try to hold another group and its members. In the true sense this distance of social intimacy or understanding between the members of the different groups.

Social distance scales are helpful in measuring social distance of one group with the other. These scales differ from the scales of attitude measurement (like Thurstone or the Likert type) in the sense that they do not represent the exceptional attitude of a single number of any group towards other groups or its members but they represent the attitude or feeling of a group as a whole towards other groups or their members.

In India the attempts have been made to devise social distance scales for measuring social distance between different groups. B Kuppuswamy in 1951 devised a scale in which he asked his respondents, (the students in Madras State) to indicate to what extent they would admit Brahmins, Christians, Harijians, higher caste non-Brahmins, Muslims, Parsis and Sikhs to the following social relationships.

1. To kinship by marriage
2. To take food in your own dining room
3. As an intimate personal friend
4. As a guest in your house
5. As your neighbor
6. As an acquaintance.

In this way in the social distance scales we find two different types of the individual:

i. His relative willingness or unwillingness to be exposed to other group or their members.
ii. His relative willingness or unwillingness to be identified with other groups or their members.

The factors responsible for creating social distance. Social distance among various groups is the creation of the social condition and environment. The traditions, old beliefs, biased attitudes, discrimination or atrocities suffered by one group at the hands of others, and stereotypes all contribute towards widening the gulf between different groups and thus lengthen social distance. In brief, prejudices of any kind lead to social distance. It is the prejudice that manifests itself in an attitude unfavorable to the other group. The prejudiced keeps the other groups at varying distances depending upon the intensity of the unfavorableness of attitude towards that of the group. In this way prejudices are responsible for creating a huge social distance that is very persistent in nature. The examples of such social distance can be found in the social distance manifested between Harijians and Lower caste Hindus and between Muslims and Hindus.

Group Interaction

Groups are formed out of individuals. The mutual interdependence and interaction between and among the members of groups is responsible, to a great extent, in determining the nature, purpose and organization of the group. Every member of a group tries to influence the behavior of the other members of his group and in turn influenced by their behavior. Thus there is sort of give and take between the members of a group on the one hand and between different groups on the other. Such sort of give and take birth to the phenomenon of group-interaction. Borrowing the words of Brown it can be safely aid that group interaction is a two way process whereby each individual or group stimulates the other, and, in varying, degree modifies the behavior of the participants.

Thus the process of interrelations and associations within the group and between and among the different groups, is taken as group interaction and consequently it is supposed to include:

i. The influence or impact of the group on their individual members

ii. The influence or impact of individual members on other members or on the groups as a whole

iii. The mutual influence or impact of one group over the other.

In every society the groups, formal and informal, exert great influence over the behavior and conduct of their members. They persuade their members to conform to the norms established by them. Groups influence personal goals, interest, attitudes and thus mould the personality and character of their members. Moreover socialization of the individual takes place in the groups as interpersonal relationships is learnt in group membership. The family, childhood, gang, per group and other sociopsychological groups thus play a big role in grouping the personal and behavior of their members.

The behavior and personality characteristics of individual members of group affect the behavior of others and cast a significant impact or the functioning of the groups as a whole. The individuals sense on the group or on its members depends on his status, strengths and weakness. Leader of the group exerts a great impact on the group members and behavior of the group is molded by him accordingly. Powerful members other than their leader also influence decision of the group and can bring serious changes in the entire structure or functioning of the group. Sometimes a single member, by exceptionally bad or good personality characteristics and relationship within the group and outside the group may leave a mark on the group. Students, teachers or head of the institution as an individual member may bring a lot of change in the group life of the school and similarly in other walks of life, groups are formed, make progress or fail and die as a result of the effect on them of their individual members.

There is also a constant interaction between and among different groups. The structure, norms and values of one group exert influence on the other groups. For example family exercises great influence on the school life of the children. Peer-group relationships have impact upon the adjustment of children in other formal or informal groups. Community and its religious and social groups decide the working of the school as a group. On the other hand, school as a group also casts desirable impact on the community and society at large. In this way there is a constant give and take between the different formal or informal groups that exist in the society.

Group Mind

Group mind is a term in social psychology that has been used to express group psychology by sociologists and psychologist. Let see how this term has been used:

Firstly, we have sociologists like Lebon (A French man) who use this term for explaining the various characteristics of crowd behavior. Lebon asserted that individuals behave in a peculiar way when they are members of a crowd. Explaining the reason for such type of behavior he told that individuals as a member of crowd are in the grip of "Collective" or "group mind" and thus behave differently. At this time as a member of a crowd their conscious personality disappears and it is their unconscious personality moved by a group mind that is responsible for their peculiar behavior.

In the secondary category we have sociologists and psychologists like McDougall who use this term as a concept to explain the behavior of individuals and members of highly stable enduring groups like the army or some political and religious organizations. He asserted that members of these highly organized well-integrated groups behave differently in these groups as they would otherwise behave as an individual outside these groups. "The reason" he told, "is that as a member of these highly organized groups his behavior is directed by the Psychology of Group Mind, viz. he behaves as others behave".

In this way the concept of group mind has been made into use for explaining our peculiar behavior as a member of a crowd or a highly organized and integrated group. But there have been some difficulties in explaining the behavior of individuals in the group by this concept named as group mind. It has been now clearly admitted that the concept of group mind, a mind over and above the minds of the individual in that group is not necessary to explain the behavior of the individuals forming the group. The concept of group mind is now under attack. Kuppuswamy exposes this face in the following way:

"If we accept the concept of group mind we will have to speak of a Bengali mind or a Punjabi mind or Kerala mind and probably also of a *Brahmin* mind or a *Harijians* mind. Again we will have to speak of the mind of each area in the town or the city or even of each road or part of a road in a city. Thus the whole problem reduces itself into absurdity".

Therefore it is difficult to invent a new type of group mind for explaining the behavior of the individual, in the group. Moreover an individual is a member of different groups at the same time and behaves differently as the situations or conditions go on changing. In this way even for explaining the behavior of an individual as a member of different groups or the member of the same group in different situations we will have to invent a number of group minds.

Due to some of these practical difficulties this concept of group mind has been abandoned by the sociologists and psychologists. It has now been, replaced by a more comprehensive and general term 'group behavior'. Now it is understood that people behave differently as a members of a special group under the influence of 'group behavior'. We will study the factors affecting 'group behavior' afterwards in the present chapter.

Importance of Group Mind

1. *For the country.* A strong group mind elevates a country. The progress of Germany and Japan after the Second World War took place as a result of strong group mind.
   A weak group mind lowers a country. For this very reason, India is lagging behind other countries in the race of progress. In India we have many castes, subclasses, religions and groups. There cannot be one group mind in the country. In other words, we may say that there is diversity in the thoughts, feelings and actions of the country men which is great obstacle in the way of group mind.
2. *For the society.* A strong group mind elevates a society and a weak mind brings the downfall of a society.
3. *For the school.* A strong group mind makes if easier for a school to attain high position. On the contrary a school can reach a position of pride only by directing weak group mind and strengthening it.

Development of Group Mind in School

Group mind can be developed in the school in the following ways:-

1. Acquainting the students and teachers with the high traditions of the school. Every school should have some high traditions and the students and teachers should be fully acquainted with them.
2. Writing model sentences. Mottoes pertaining to group mind such as Union is strength, etc. should be written at important places in the school.
3. To organize functions. Some functions should be organized in the school, e.g. birthday celebrations of great leaders, annual function, prize distribution function, parents day. Meeting of Alumni (Old students) association.
4. To entrust jobs of responsibility to students. Students should be entrusted with jobs of responsibility in the school so that leadership traits and group mind may be developed in them.
5. To appoint teachers on permanent basis. Teachers should be appointed on permanent basis in the school. Only then they will take greater interest in the affairs of the school.
6. To keep the students in the school for many years. It is essential for development of group mind among the students that they continue their education in the school for a number of years. Development of group mind is possible in children every year.
7. To give opportunities of expression of feelings of rivalry and cooperations. At times the school should provide the students with opportunities of expression of feelings of rivalry and cooperation in play, cultural and other activities in class groups.
8. To develop the feeling of group consciousness. The feeling of group consciousness should be developed in the school in order to have a group mind.
9. To enroll the students as members of various groups. Students should be enrolled as members of many such groups as have own aims, traditions and methods.
10. To arrange for hostel accommodation. Hostel accommodation should be arranged in the school where the students may develop group mind by community living.

Group Behavior

The behavior of a person in a group is different from his individual behavior. In the individual behavior a person is free to think, feel and act but his freedom to do so is lost in a group. The individual is compelled to give up his individuality and his behavior is governed by social rules. Hence when a person is member of a club. Similarly when a person becomes the member of a crowd he is ready to do the meanest of actions. He indulges in actions which he would feel very shy of doing in an individual capacity. Individuality is lost in a crowd and the group dynamics becomes uniform. Here sympathy and suggestion play an extremely important part. This level of intelligence goes down in the case of a crowd. Here susceptibility to suggestion increases. This type of behavior seen in a group is called group behavior.

Characteristics of Group Behavior

1. *Common goals, interests, and ideals:* The goals, interests and ideals of a group are common. They do their best to achieve them.
2. *Similar behavior:* The members of a group show similarity of behavior because they have common aims, interests and ideals.
3. *Control of the group:* The actions of members are controlled by the group. All the members of the group follow the ideals and traditions of the group.
4. *Mutual obligation:* It is such a power as keeps not only the members of a group united but provides them with energy, e.g. the relationship between the parents and children in a family or the love of husband and wife. In spite of differences in many points, they have certain aims, ideal and values.
5. *Sense of oneness:* There is sense of oneness in the group because of similarity in interests. A member looks upon the others as related to him. In this way good feelings, devotion, faithfulness, adjustment, suggestion and imitation develop.
6. *Psychological relationship:* The behavior of one member of a group influences that of the other and in this way his own behavior too is influenced. This type of relationship is known as psychological relationship.
7. *Influence of group characteristics:* The characteristics or features of a group affect all its members.

Factors Affecting Group Behavior (Group Dynamics)

Man is social animal like the ant and the bee. He has an instinct of gregariousness which compels him to live in a group. He needs society and sociopsychological groups for the satisfaction of his biological, social and psychological needs. In fact the desire of satisfying various needs and motives brings people on the common platform and they join their hands to form different formal as well as informal groups. Later on the psychological factors work as a motivating force for sustaining these groups. People derive satisfaction from belonging to a group. In group life their tensions and anxieties are greatly reduced and development under proper care and suitable direction. For some people group life provides opportunity to satisfy their need of dominating over the leading others. In this way for the satisfaction of their instinctive and other basic needs the people prefer to form different groups. Interdependence of the members of the group, their common interests and purposes, and shared common experiences give birth to the group behavior. Now they begin to feel, think and act together. The individual of the group and leader, ideals and norms of the group and environment of situation in which it functions, are some of the factors that influence the structure of the group and its behavior at a particular time.

But most often, group behavior is motivated by different psychological functions as those of sympathy, suggestion, imitation and others as given below:

1. **Sympathy:** Sympathy influences the group behavior by arousing collective feelings. It enables an individual to perceive the psychological state of another person. He begins to feel as others feel without caring to know why others are feeling in such a way. In this way sympathy leads the individuals to feel together. In the playing group of the children when someone calls out snake and exhibits the emotion of fear, the others perceiving the psychological state of their fellow members begin to exhibit the emotion of fear. They are persuaded to feel collectively and share the common experience on account of the phenomenon of sympathy. And in this way, sympathy is said to influence the behavior of the group.
2. **Suggestion:** The phenomenon of suggestion influences the behavior of the group by making the individual members to think collectively. Suggestion make the individual think as others think. The thinking of an individual member in the group is merged with each collective thinking. In a group the members share the thought with each other. When someone puts an idea or solution of the problem then other in the group begin to think that way. Particularly, the suggestions put forward by the leaders of the group are readily accepted and thus suggestion plays a leading role influencing the group decisions and behavior. Moreover the group norms and rules of conduct and behavior are enforced through the phenomenon of suggestion. Through suggestion a person behaves in a group in accordance with the prepactices and ideals and in this way also the phenomenon of suggestion play a big role in influencing the group behavior.
3. **Imitation:** Phenomenon of imitation influences the behavior of the group by making the individual members act collectively. Imitation involves copying others. By imitating the behavior of the others, a member in the group does as other do and thus members of the group indulge in common action by imitating each other. Like suggestion and sympathy, imitation also proceeds unwittingly. The acts of a superior person in the group or of a leader are imitated blindly and thus individuals in the group exhibit uniformity in their behavior. They share the same conative experience through the help of the psychological phenomenon of imitation and in this way group behavior is said to be influenced by imitation.
4. **Individual and group goals:** All individuals and all groups have their goals. The personal goals of individuals can be satisfied in a group. So they willingly join groups. The goals in the classroom have been laid down in the form of goals of the curriculum. At present the students who do not come up to the mark of these goals from the majority of drop-outs, problem children, etc. and are punished. At teacher well-versed in group psychology would think of modifying these goals so as to make them acceptable to all and in order that the pupils as group members should develop strong bonds of interpersonal relationships.
5. **Cohesiveness:** The degree to which the members of a group wish to remain in the group is called cohesiveness. A cohesive group is one in which:
   1. There are common goals
   2. Members have similar background
   3. In spite of changing conditions it remains intact
   4. The members are concerned with their membership and have strong motivation for contributing to the groups welfare, to take part in its activities and to further its objectives.

Cohesiveness is influenced by the following factors:

1. *Goals:* Goals commonly accepted contribute to cohesiveness. Self-determined goals establish group unity more than imposed goals.
2. *Size of the group:* Group should be large enough to present diversity of views but small enough to make provision for all the members of the group to participate in its deliberation. The size of the group will be determined by the purpose, individual needs, leadership and the sensitiveness of the teaching in diagnosing group action.
3. *Discussion:* Zander (1950) discovered that there was less aggression and interpersonal resentment in groups which are discussion oriented.
4. *Effectiveness of subunit communication:* Sociometric groupings increase the solidarity and productiveness of the group. As a result, the members of the group like to live with one another in comfort.
5. *Participation and loyalty:* The cohesiveness of a group is directly proportional to the participation and loyalty.
6. *Spirit and interpersonal competition:* Twentieth century is the age of competition. It is in the fitness of things that in order to enable the pupils to meet the exigencies of life, it is desirable to inculcate in them the spirit of interpersonal competition. But excess of every thing is bad and much emphasis on competition inhibits effective group action.
7. *Democratic procedures:* These imply maximum participation and involvement of the group members in group activities, determining objectives, encouraging and reinforcing interpersonal contacts and relations, showing due regard for the individual specialists, employing the techniques of affection, warmth of feelings and persuasion.
8. *Satisfaction of common needs:* Group members have certain common needs on the existence of which depends group action.

Educational Implications of Group Psychology

Group psychology acquaints us with the nature and characteristics of group behavior. In the group students feel, think and act collectively. Their consciousness is centered about some common objects or purposes. They are more susceptible to suggestion, imitation and sympathy in group. They seek to satisfy their all instinctive and basic needs through formal as well as informal groups. Therefore, the school and teachers must pay due consideration to the group life. They should exploit the formal and informal groups in the society for the essential growth and development of their children.

Moreover, despite the individualistic tendencies advocated by modern psychology, it has been established that the proper development of the innate abilities and capabilities of an individual often takes place in the group. Group life presents a desirable proper learning environment where children consciously or unconsciously learn so many things by imitating the elders, superiors and leaders in the social groups. Group life presents an enormous opportunity for the physical, mental, emotional, social and esthetic development of an individual. He learns to get along well with himself and others. Also group life creates the feeling of solidarity, cohesiveness, loyalty, mutual love and cooperation, and other desirable habits among children and thus prepares them to lead a happy social life in the future. In short, art of successful living can be learnt well through group life.

Group psychology tells us why the individuals behave differently in groups. Students are made to achieve wonderful results if group psychology is exploited properly. The relationships and mutual interaction in the group can be maintained to a proper level and behavior of the group can be channelized into a productive and useful stream. The teacher can put the best example of group-achievement by organizing the class as a group under his able leadership. He can help children to form various other groups within the school boundary. Parental cooperation can also be secured to help the children in linking themselves with useful sociopsychological groups outside the school. Family relationship and atmosphere should produce a living example of a highly organized group. The child should be made to get along well with his family members, school and playing mates and other members of the society.

Actually group participation is essential for the proper development and adjustment in life. Therefore, isolates should be spotted out and helped in their proper adjustment. For imparting training to behave properly in the group a school can adopt various measures. It can provide enormous opportunities for the group participation through the help of cocurricular as well as classroom activities. The students may be encouraged to have interpersonal relationships. They should be made to feel, act and think together by encouraging cooperative work and group projects. They should be helped in sharing responsibilities and role playing. They must be helped to imbibe we-feeling and develop loyalty towards their respective groups, school and nation at large.

Leadership

Every group, whether formal or informal, spontaneous or organized has a leader. He is the person who manages the group activities and is responsible for intensifying feeling of belongingness and interdependence among the members of the group. He persuades the members to feel, think and act together, In fact, the leader is one of the members of a group who, by virtue of his exceptional qualities or unique position in the group rises to occasion, influences the behavior of the group and directs the energy of the group to any channel—desirable or undesirable.

The groups get integrated and flourish or get disintegrated or perish as a result of the efficient and inefficient leadership. A school in the able leadership of a headmaster can make tremendous progress while the unwise leadership may doom its future. Similarly the family, the class, playing group, hobby club and other so many groups can make progress or fail in their objectives as a result of the leadership they avail. Therefore, it is essential to know more about leadership and the characteristics of a good leader so that we can train children for effective leadership.

Types of leadership: Different authors have adopted different modes for the classification of leaders into various types. Some have classified them as political leaders, social leaders, religious leaders and intellectual leaders depending on the field of their activities. Writers like Prem Pasricha and Kuppuswamy assert to classify them into the following four different types:

- *Institutional leaders like head of the school, District collector, president of the country, manager of a factory, etc.* Their orders are obeyed through the hierarchies of ranks and the decisions are based on the established precedents.
- *Dominant leaders like Napolean, Stalin, Nasser, etc.* They lead the group due to an urge to dominate. They are autocrats and dictators.
- *Persuasive leaders like Gandhi, Lincoln and Nehru, etc.* They do not aim to dominate and dictate the group but to persuade the members to help them and follow them.
- *Experts:* They lead the group on account of their acquired proficiency and skill in science, art or any other sphere. They are recognized as the authorities in their respective fields

and have a line of followers among the people who are interested in that type of work.

The categories suggested above are not mutually exclusive and cannot be said to be sound classification. Therefore, a more appropriate ground is needed to classify the leaders. The behavior and the personality characteristics of the leaders or the way how they lead their groups should be made a criterion of classifying the leaders. On this ground, classification suggested by Kretch and Crutchfield, the leaders can be classified as Authoritarian and Democratic holds good.

i. Authoritarian leaders are very dominant and aggressive. They determine policy without consulting their followers and dictate every step and assign duties. They do not tolerate any debate and believe in action rather than planning and thinking. They typically forbid, direct communication or interaction among their followers. All communication and direction must flow through them. In this way they become indispensable to the followers and the group they lead. In their absence the group cannot function. All the autocrats and dictators belong to this category. It has been found that such type of leadership does not care for the wishes and ambitions of the members of the group or followers. Either they depend on him entirely and lose all initiative; or they feel frustrated and aggressive towards the leader. When practiced in the classroom by the teacher or headmaster such type of leadership makes the children quite dependent and submissive. In some cases it leads to the problematic behavior and maladjustment of children.
ii. Democratic leaders on the other hand, are very cooperative and accommodating. They do not dominate or dictate but persuade the members to follow them and share the power with other individuals in the groups. They win the hearts of their followers and identify themselves completely with the group they lead. They encourage group discussion and collective decision on matters of policy, allow members to choose their own work and also themselves actively participate in the work. They encourage freedom of thought and action and thus cultivate democratic values in the groups. Unlike the authoritarian leaders the democratic leaders are flexible. They bring desirable change in their ideas in the light of the needed group changes. They encourage interpersonal relationships and communications among the members and thus create a healthy group climate. They are able to generate maximum we-feeling and cooperation among the members and make them strive hard to achieve the desired objectives. Such type of leadership, if practiced in school may be very conducive and helpful in the proper growth and development of children.

Traits or Qualities of Leadership

Attempts have been made to discover the essential qualities or traits that different type of leaders possess. On this data, it has been tried to list the traits of leadership. Various mental, physical, emotional, social and moral qualities are thus generalized. But such generalization, however general it may be does not fit for all types of leaders. There is no single kind of skills and personally traits that will make a man always a leader. Leadership, besides the important trait of one's personality, is a function of the situation. Specific situations require specific qualities in a leader. However, the following few characteristics of traits are essential for becoming a successful leader:

1. *Identification with the group:* The leader must belong to the group he leads. He should have membership character in the group and should be able to make the members feel that he is one of them. He must share the values, attitudes and interest of the group and thus try to identify completely with the group.

2. *Superiority over the members of the group:* The leader, while identifying himself completely with group and perceiving the group members as one of them, must be able to show his superiority to the group members in the qualities esteemed by them. On account of his superior qualities and virtues, he can be able to exercise reflective control and coordination of work of the group. Moreover he can win confidence and cooperation of the members of the group if he is perceived as 'best of them' by the group members. But he apparently must not be too much superior or talented. In such a case group members do not consider him as one of them and thus do not accept his leadership.
3. *Knowing the psychology of the group:* The leader must have an adequate knowledge of group psychology. He should have a functional knowledge of the group mind or group behavior. Moreover he should be able to utilize his knowledge of group psychology for proper organization and working of his group.
4. *Dynamic and flexible:* The leader should be dynamic and flexible in his attitude, interests and other behavior patterns. In every case, he must fit his followers, expectations. He must be able to play democratic or authoritarian role depending upon the need of the situation. He should be able to bring change and lines of action according to the demands of situation and common wishes of his followers.

Training for Leadership

The notion that traits related with leadership are inherited and therefore, leaders are born and not made, is wrong. Similarly the belief that by mere training or education under suitable environment any person can be made to become a successful leader is also erroneous. The truth lies between these two extremes. Both heredity and environment coupled with adequate training or education is essential for helping children to become successful leaders. In this way the initial step, in any program of imparting leaders. In this way the initial step, in any program of imparting training for leadership to children, consist in the location of the would-be-leaders. Children, who exhibit the basic traits of leadership in the classroom as well as in other extracurricular group situations would be well-attended by the teachers and school authorities. The following few suggestions may work well in helping the potential leaders:

1. These children should be given opportunities for playing the role of leaders in curricular or extracurricular group situations. They can be made monitor of the class or assigned leadership role in the hobbies groups, games or other extracurricular group situations.
2. The biographies and autobiographies of National heroes, political, social and religious leaders and other great men educate and inspire the youngsters. Thus they should be encouraged and provided opportunities of reading stimulating and inspiring literature.
3. Example is better than precept. Therefore, the teachers and headmaster should produce a living example of successful leadership, before children. Student leader belonging to higher grades of the school may also stimulate and educate the would-be-leaders belonging to the lower grades.
4. Religious and moral education and the organization of social services may also help in the cultivation of proper social and moral traits as well as group tendencies among these children.
5. Cooperation of the parents and the organization of social services also be secured in the proper cultivation of desirable leadership traits among these children.

In this way school can play a big role in training the potential leaders by formal as well as informal techniques. In an advanced training program the potential leaders may be given an adequate knowledge of group psychology and the vicarious experiences for role playing can also be arranged. Teacher as well as other responsible elders can take a lead by putting self-examples and regulating the behavior of these trainees for acquiring the necessary skill, knowledge and other personality traits.

Group Dynamics

Group dynamics is relatively a new concept in sociopsychological field. It is in fact a new approach to the study of groups that has gained popular familiarity since World War II. Various attempts have been made to define the term 'group dynamics'. The attempt made by Cartwright and Zander seems to be more appealing. In their words 'group dynamics' should be defined as a field of inquiry dedicated to advancing knowledge about the nature of groups, the laws of their development, and their interrelations with individual, other groups and larger institutions".

Dynamics is derived from a Greek word meaning force. Hence group dynamics stands for the forces operating in a group.

Group dynamics implies an interactive psychology relationship in which members of a group develop a common perception based on feeling and emotions. This interstimulative relationships may be described by the term group dynamics.Good's dictionary.

Group dynamics implies changes that take place within groups.Kretch and Crutchfield.

In this sense group dynamics is that branch of knowledge that deals with the study of groups. It tries to answer the host of questions concerning the nature and working of groups. How are groups formed? What conditions are necessary for their growth and effective functioning? How do groups affect the behavior of individuals? In this way Group dynamics acquaints us with the human behavior and social relationships that exist in the group.

It is not easy to define or delimit the important area of group dynamics. From one point of view it represents a field of inquiry, a series of interrelated problems; from another it includes a set of techniques; from a third, a theory of the nature of groups and of interaction within groups.

In education and educational psychology, group dynamics is the study of the forces exerted by the individual on the group or by the group on the individual. The aspirations, attitudes, beliefs, character, emotions, personality and values of an individual are influenced by the group and *vice versa*.

The group helps a person to satisfy his fundamental needs and achieves the sense of accomplishment. It helps to transform the original nature of person to human nature. Expression of instincts and emotions, formulation of ambitions, attitudes, character, habits, and sentiments, values and the development of personality of the individual is influenced by interaction of an individual and group.

Basic Assumptions of Group Dynamics

They are given below:

1. Groups are inevitable and ubiquitous (omnipresent). Individuals from certain groups.
2. Groups mobilize powerful forces producing effects of utmost importance to individuals. The very sense of identify of a person is shaped by groups significant to him—his family, school, occupation and profession, church (in foreign countries). The position of a person

in a group may influence the way others behave towards him, his self-esteem and level of aspiration.

3. Groups may produce good as well as bad consequences. There is convincing evidence to show that groups are completely good and completely bad.
4. Correct understanding of group dynamics allows the possibility that desirable consequences from groups, can be knowingly increased. Through knowledge of group dynamics, groups can be made to serve better ends because knowledge gives power to modify human behavior and social institutions.

Educational Significance of Group Dynamics

According to AI Gates, group dynamics offers the best means available for the development of social skills essential for democratic living, better social understanding, and preparing the individual members of the group for democratic citizenship.

Group dynamics is an educational method which is being specially attempted to these days. Its aim is neither to produce leaders not to find ways in which a person can get work done by a group. Its purpose is to promote democratic activities. It is based on the assumption that only those persons can help in social progress who have learnt to make the most precious sacrifice for the welfare of the people and prepared to do the same. It is also supposed that qualitative as well as quantitative individual differences in the abilities of persons are present. Every member of the group takes active part in the activities of the group. It is for this reason that the total work done by a group is more than the sum of work done by them individually.

In the words of D Segel, the process by which one must consider other individuals in a group, and a problem at the same time, not only tends to increase understanding to the problem, but also creates a solution which the individual has practice in bringing about emotional balance.

The techniques used in group dynamics are such in which there is little mutual conflict. Conflict hinders in the proper working of group because it does not allow defining and having independent thinking for solving the problem. When we think alone we tend to accept our own thoughts. On the other hand, when we express own thoughts before a group, we have to give reasons for the way we think. With the help of this type of experience we come to know those thoughts and feelings of his about which he did not know earlier. We learn to think by paying more attention to facts and aims. It may not appear to be good in the beginning but exchange (give and take) is good for us.

When the members of a group develop familiarity and come closer, the feelings of enmity decrease and may even come to an end. Not only this, their place is taken up by new feelings of respect for others and others persons too start thinking about us in good terms. In this way group dynamics teachers us to solve with help of the others, the problems the groups is facing. More work is accompanied in a group than is done individually. This is the aim of group dynamics.

By a study of group dynamics teachers and counselors can make proper advantage of specific abilities of the students. The organizer should remember that he should not ignore individual's effects in the possibilities of group dynamics. The organizer and the supervisor should understand that each is important in its own place.

Besides focusing attention over the groups as the object of study, group dynamics pays attention to the questions concerned with dynamics of group life. It tells us what are the different centripetal and centrifugal forces that try to change the structure of the group?

How does an influential member, or a leader bring change in the composition or working of the group? What are the pressures that a group may exert in bringing uniformity of thinking, feeling and acting among its members? If a change of membership or leadership occurs in group which other features of the group will change and which will remain stable? What changes in group encourage creativity or heighten productivity? In what conditions does democratic structure of the group change into an autocratic one or *vice versa*? In what respect is the group structure and behavior influenced if there is change in the size of the groups or in the objective of the groups?

In this way there are a number of questions that relate to the enquiries made about the possible changes in the group life on account of some variations, interactions, inner communication and pressures that are experienced within the group or exercise by other groups or factors outside the group. In general it tries to answer the following types of questions related with the change that take place within the group:-

1. What kinds of groups tend to change?
2. Under what conditions do they change?
3. What is the direction of changes likely to be?

By imparting the answer of such questions and presenting a body of information and knowledge, group dynamics, thus, aims to make the groups serve better ends and to bring dynamic changes in them in order to attain their legitimate goals.

24 CHAPTER Mental Health

Introduction

People's health is an approach and perspective those focuses on the broad range of factors and conditions that have a strong influence on the health of population. The factors and conditions that are important considerations in people's health are determinations, which includes income and social factors. Social support networks, education, employment, working and living conditions, physical environments, social environments, biology and genetics endowment, personal health practices, coping skills, healthy child developments, health services, sex and culture, there determinant do not work independently of each other but form a complex system of interactions.

About 500BC, Pericles defined health as a state of moral, mental, and physical well-being, which enables a person to face any crisis in life with utmost grace of God and facility. Presently, World Health Organization defines, "Health as a state of complete physical, mental, social and spiritual well-being, not merely on absence of disease or infirmly". Since the complete well-being for all is unattainable goal, the US President Commission states that "Health is an optimal state of physical, mental and social well-being". Health is a dynamic state of physical, mental, social and spiritual well-being. This cannotes a state of dynamic equilibrium among various subsystem of a holistic person, i.e. it concern with the individual as a total system. So, it place emphasis on the positive state of well-being rather than focusing the lack of ability or disease or disaster. People in a state of emotional well-being or mental health, function comfortably within society and are satisfied with their achievement. Accordingly, health is a positive state of well-being, people are in a state of emotional, physical and social well-being, fulfills their roles and responsibilities, function effectively in daily life and are satisfied with their interpersonal relationships and themselves. A healthy person is not only physically healthy but also mentally healthy. Now health extends beyond the proper functioning of the body. It includes a sound, efficient mind and controlled emotions. Thus, health is a state of being hale, sound or whole in body, mind or soul. It means that body and mind are working effectively and harmoniously.

Health is a multidimensional process which includes physical, intellectual, developmental, emotional, spiritual and sociocultural components. Mental health is an integral part component of total health experiences. There is no clear singular definition of mental health. Bruck Baeur and Ward (1993) defines mental health is state of well-being often associates with happiness, contentment, satisfaction, achievement, optimism or hope. Mental health is a state of the individual mind, where individual can adjust and adapt to the situations in a harmonious manner, body and mind work together in some direction in order to lead a happy and productive life. It is a state of well-being which involves the adjustment of the individual to himself/herself satisfaction, cheerfulness and socially considerable/acceptable behavior and the ability if facing and accepting the realities of life. The attainment of level of health there will enable every individual to lead a socially and economically productive life.

Mental health is a dynamic or ever changing state, which is considered as an important aspects of individuals total health status. Mental health in a sound, efficient mind and controlled emotions. It is the total and harmonious functioning of the whole personality of an individuals for optimum functioning with maximum realization. It is the capacity of an individual to form harmonious relationships with others and to participate in or contribute constructively to changes in social environment.

Mental health is a state of balance between the individual and the surrounding world, a state of harmony between himself with others a coexistence between the realities of the self and other people and environment. A positive state of mental health shows an individual ability to cope with the present and to adjust satisfactorily in future. A state of compromise and adaptation to a situation in his/her life leads to better adjustment. His/ her responsibilities, function effectively and is satisfied with his/her interpersonal relationships and himself/herself.

One of the prerequisites of maintaining good mental health is to feel absolutely happy and satisfied with one's own work and achievement. Students are often apt to feel they have to study for the sake of passing the examination, or for the sake of pleasing their parents, or the sake of maintaining social prestige. These are not really good motives for study. In the long run individual will not be happy unless he/she have worked well and achieved their maximum possible credit. Their study and their work should be primarily viewed as the expression and development of them and unless individual develop him to the maximum possible extent individual will not be satisfied. Some day their are bound to feel unhappy and miserable.

Mental hygiene is a way of life in which the individuals makes to his environment is maintained intact. NE Cutts and N Moselay have also stressed the element of adjustment in mental hygiene. Accordingly mental health is that ability means of which people establish their adjustment with the difficult situations of life and mental hygiene is that means or tool which makes this adjustment possible. This definition also helps to reveal the relation between mental health and mental hygiene, as well as the difference between them. Mental hygiene is the means to mental health. In other words, mental hygiene is that science which studies the laws and means of achieving mental health, of maintaining it as well as doing away with mental ill health. Mental health is the end, and mental hygiene the means.

Characteristics of a Mentally Healthy Person

PV Lewkan has stated that a mentally healthy individual is one who is himself satisfied, lives peacefully with his neighbors, makes healthy citizens of his children, and even after performing these fundamental duties has enough energy left to do something of benefit to society. Possessing mental health, an individual can adjust properly to his environment, and can make the best effort for his own, his family's and his society's progress and betterment. KA Menninger has defined mental health as the adjustment of human beings to the world and to each other with a maximum of effectiveness and happiness ..... It is the ability to maintain an even temper, an alert intelligence, socially considerate behavior and a happy disposition. The chief characteristic of mental health, it is evident, is adjustment. The greater the degree of successful adjustment, the greater will be the mental health of the individual. Lesser mental health will lead to lesser adjustment and greater conflict. The healthy individual can interpret any new situation and adapt it to suit himself, or adapt himself to suit it. He maintains a healthy and benevolent attitude towards life. He is aware that difficulties visit everyone in life, so that running away from them is cowardice. They can be solved only by squarely facing up to them with courage.

In order to understand the full implications of mental health, it would be advantageous to know the characteristics of a person who enjoys mental health. Actually, mental health, like physical health, is also a condition. And this condition can be recognized by its characteristics features. To some extent, a mentally healthy individual would exhibit the following features:

1. *Self-evaluation:* A mentally healthy individual evaluating himself/ herself properly is aware of his/her limitations. He/she easily accepts his/her faults and makes efforts to rid himself/herself of them. He/she keeps an eye upon himself/herself so that he/she may be aware of his/her own tendencies and that he/she may be in a position to divert them in the desired directions. He/she introspects so that they may analyse his/her problems, prejudices, difficulties, and reduce them to a minimum.
2. *Adjustability:* One special characteristics of a mentally healthy individual is that he adjusts to a new situations with the least delay and disturbance. He/she is never disturbed of what might have been. He/she makes the fullest possible use of existing opportunities, and adjusts to every new situation that presents itself. He/she is aware of the fact that change is the law of life, he/she is ever prepared for change and always finds some suitable mode of adjustment. He/she has every desire to benefit the society, is even prepared to incur the wrath of society, with a show of intrepidity if its benefit lies that way. The weak individual becomes satisfied with circumstances, only to fall a prey to mental disturbances and disease. The great person loses his/her satisfaction with circumstances and strains every sinew to change them according to his/her own wishes. In fact, the most important aspect of adjustment is one's own mental condition rather than the external situation. A proper mental attitude gains a kind of immunity from the external situation affecting their peace and calm and balance.
3. *Maturity:* Intellectual and emotional maturity is another peculiar sign of mentally healthy individuals. The mature mind is constantly engaged in increasing his fund of knowledge, behaves responsibility, expresses his thoughts and feelings with clarity, and is prepared to sympathize with another's feelings and viewpoints. And in maturity, sexual maturity is very important. The healthy individual behaves like a balanced, cultured and sensible adult in matters relating to sex.
4. *Systematic habits and regulated life:* Habits are an important element in maintaining mental health. Forming proper habits in matters of food, clothing, the normal routine of daily life leads to their becoming systematic and regulated, which, in the long run, economizes upon energy and time. Many people are seen worrying over the most trifling things in their routine. Some women experience such acute difficulty in determining the sari and blouse that they should wear outside the house that it leads to considerable mental pain and complication. Some individuals are always conscious of the fact, erroneously, that their tie is not straight, and they spend much time in knotting it correctly, in spite of which they can be seen fiddling with it all the time. Such nervous behavior is not a sign

of mental health. Healthy persons perform most of the common functions of life with quick assurance and a show of naturality, without any bother and fuss. Their life is a model of regularity, balance and measured calculation.

5. *Absence of extremism:* An ideal man lacks excess in any and every direction, and the principle that excess of anything is bad is a golden rule as far as mental health is concerned. Whatever the instinct, if it is allowed to dominate an individual, it will bring him to harm and endanger his mental health. An unnecessarily courageous individual is often a prey to accident. Over-sexed individuals lose their health reserve very quickly. Excessive ambition is another treat that never lets its possessor rest. Hence, in order to maintain mental health, one's life should be integrated, interests should be wide and the personality balanced. Extremism is harmful to mental health.
6. *Social relationship:* It has been pointed out, from the point of view of mental health, a healthy individual maintains good adjustment with social situations, and is engaged in some or the other project intended to benefit society. And this is because in modern society the proper development of everyone's personality can take place only if there is mutual cooperation. Social relationship is a part of everyone's life. The greater the balance of these social relationships and the greater their simplicity, the better will be the individuals mental health. Improper conduct on the part of others can be the cause of both mental problems and diseases. Hence proper behavior and proper feelings are essential for everyone.
7. *Job satisfaction:* For mental health, it is essential that everyone should find satisfaction from his/her main occupation, his/her vocation. The individual who studies only to pass the examination and finds no pleasure in his/her works is neither a good student nor a healthy individual. A helpful professor teaches without worrying about the financial implications of his profession, a businessman trades and a laborer labors but with interest. Money is the result of work but if one works only for it, that much time is obviously a waste. If the work interests an individual, it will yield more money, but at the same time, a happiness. In fact, if one works for interests, one maintains it even in the event, of a loss in trade, or at least, the pain of loss is considerably lessened.

Complete mental health is an ideal. Any individual who possesses the greatest number of these qualities will be nearest the ideal.

Preservation of Mental Health by Institution

Institutions like family and school are having important role in preservation of mental health of an individual as given below:

i. *Role of family:* Family has the greatest role to play in importance in maintaining a condition of mental health, and within the family the greatest burden of responsibility is on the two parents. What is mostly needed in this connection is the creation of a suitable atmosphere in which the child's personality can adequately develop. A child's delicate and sensitive personality is influenced by the character of parents, their mutual behavior and relations, their behavior towards the children, the child's relations with brothers, sisters, and other relatives in the family. Hence, it is essential that these be healthy. There can be no hard and fast rule as to how the parents should behave towards the child under certain conditions; all that can be justifiably said is that they should consciously give the child every chance to develop his personality freely and without restraint. It is for them to prevent the child from treading the wrong path but they should not try to make him follow them in all things. The least they can do is to prevent any situation that causes repression in the child. All other things depend upon the parents insight into child and adolescent psychology, their patience, their labor and experience.

ii. *Role of school:* Following the family, the other institution that has responsibility of promoting mental health in children is the school. It is the school that has the greatest influence, after the home, in forming the child's personality. And even in school, the most important factor is the atmosphere existing there. In a healthy atmosphere the children adopt discipline and other qualities of their own. There is greater fear of some children being spoiled in school. Such children should be specially attended to and given definite and expect guidance. The greatest need is for providing each child with work adequate and proper to the needs of his personality. Hence, it is essential that the backward and the brilliant children should be given special treatment. Teachers present an ideal to the children in their charge, hence their character and conduct should be such as an profitably imitated by the children. Pupil personnel service should be introduced to remove the difficulties with which the children are faced from time to time in school.

In school, the teacher should keep the following factors vividly in mind if he is to preserve mental health, prevent mental disturbance and promote mental health among his students:

- *Maintaining discipline:* Maintaining good discipline in the school has an important influence upon the mental health of students. But this discipline should never be very hard since such conditions will lead to mental ill-health. Thus, discipline should be exercised not through creating fear of punishment but through arousing feelings of responsibility and the desire to be law-abiding among the students. True displace is self-discipline. And discipline in college or school should be maintained by selecting its guardians from among the students themselves. It develops feelings of responsibility among the students.
- *Showing affective behavior:* It is only too evident that affectionate behavior towards students on the part of teachers has good effect on the former's mental health. It will inspire him to obey the teacher, respect him to do nothing that may incur his displeasure. A teacher should maintain the same loving attitude towards all his students. Any discrimination in this treatment injures the feelings of students.
- *Providing facilities for play and recreation:* Mental disturbance and imbalance is created by the repressed motives surging in a student's brain. They can be given opportunities for healthy expression through games and other forms of recreation. Play and recreation have a cathartic effect.
- *Providing elementary sex education:* In adolescence, the morals of young boys and girls show alarming tendencies to proceed to degradation because of the sexual instinct, or alternately its repression leads to much mental distress. Teachers should make use of psychological weapons to remove any sexual deviations that may be embedded in the minds of students. And for this, the best way is to provide young boys and girls with the necessary elementary sex education. This will help them, on the one hand, to develop a healthy attitude towards sex and prevent them from forming harmful complexes, as well as assist in their physical, mental and emotional development, on the other; they can then later on become well-developed and integrated individuals.
- *Timely educational guidance:* In order to maintain a state of mental health, it is essential that they are given subjects that conform to their requirements and abilities, and their educational problems solved. Taking personal advice of a psychologist in this connection is called educational guidance. Timely education guidance help to maintenance mental health of the students.

- *Timely personal guidance:* Many of the problems that arise before the student are such that they cannot be solved by the student himself; hence he needs the personal guidance of the psychologist to solve them.
- *Timely vocational guidance:* Every individual is compelled to adopt some one or the other profession once his education is complete, and he begins to worry about it even while he is still engaged in his academic pursuit. The knowledgeable teacher can help his students in their choice of a suitable career.
- *Helps students in formation of good habits:* Mental health depends upon good habits. Hence it is desirable for the teacher to help students in the formation of good habits regarding a regular life, balanced diet and exercise, good behavior and high thinking, etc.
- *Develop and implement balanced curriculum:* The curriculum in school or college should be such as to develop all aspects of the students personality, to increase his fund of necessary knowledge, and to avoid all unnecessary strain on the mind. The integrated development of the students can be promoted through the organizing of the students can be promoted through the organizing of various kinds of extracurricular activities in the school and college.
- *Formulate balanced home assignment:* It is improper to think that if the child is given too much homework to do, he will not have the time to indulge in destructive and naughty pranks as he will be too busy. Loading them with too much homework only leaves them worried and anxious, with the worst influence upon their mind. Hence, the homework required of them should be carefully and sensibly formulated.

Finally, it may be stated that the prevention of mental imbalances is a problem of social and national importance. For this, efforts will have to be made to get rid of circumstances of social disorganization, exploitation, corruption, various tensions and conflicts, crimes, alcoholic effects, etc. The defects of urban life in the form of excessive crowding, unhealthy small houses, promiscuous mixing of the sexes, and noise will have to be provided, in addition to opportunities of health and recreation. It is only through efforts at the national level that proper and effective prevention of mental maladies can take place. And for this, cooperative effort on the part of government, teachers, social workers and sensible people in the public, will be necessary.

Mental Hygiene

Mental hygiene is approach to human adjustment and achievement which is related to the prevention of emotional maladjustment and preparation of the individual for skilled working. Mental hygiene is the science which studies the principles and practices or preventing mental disorders and promoting mental health. Accordingly "mental hygiene is that science which studies laws and means of curing and preventing mental disorders, personality disorders and complications it also discovers creative measures for the balancing adjustment, and healthy development of personality".

Mental hygiene means the science that maintains a condition of health in connection with mental functions. Just as physical hygiene discovers laws and means of maintaining healthy conditions of the body, mental hygiene discover laws and means of maintaining the mind in a healthy conditions. It not only insists on the curing of mental diseases, it also turns its attention to their prevention. Apart from the treatment of mental diseases, one important function of mental hygiene is the creation of favorable condition. In its negative sense, it means the more benevolent and skilful curing of mental patients. But in its positive implication, it means the discovery of mental aberration in their elementary stages, prevention of as many diseases of this kind as possible in society, and provision of a mentally healthy life in society for the greatest number of individuals. In this manner, while in its negative sense, mental hygiene implies nothing more than the curing of mental disease, in its positive aspect it includes all ways and means by which mental health is assured. The mental health, and in the functioning of mental hygiene, if he has insight into and a knowledge of human psychology. The child's mental health depends to quite an extent upon the conduct of his parents. In school, it is the teachers who casts much influence upon the mental processes of children. It is now understood that parents and teachers share the greatest responsibility for maintaining the child's mental health.

Mental hygiene is the art and science of preserving and maximizing the mental health. The means by which the process of mental health is realized, it is the way of life and involves that influences what one feels, says and does. It is the realization and maintenance of the mind, health and efficiency and it is a organized attempt to effect human adjustment through the application of principles and practice of living. It is concerned with the principle and practice in promotion, maintenance of the mental health and prevention of mental illnesses.

Mental hygiene as an art includes healthy practices for the promotion, preservation and maintenance of mental health. As a science which helps the individual to understand the ways that has to be followed to lead a peaceful life. Thus, mental hygiene is an art and science which deals with the application of scientific principles and practices for the promotion, preservation and maintenance of mental health and prevention of mental disorders, enjoys healthy practice to lead productive happy and contented life.

OBJECTIVES OF MENTAL HYGIENE

The objective of mental hygiene is not merely the prevention and curing of mental diseases, but the development of a personality in every individual in society that makes for good adjustment with the environment, that attains a proper synthesis between the intellectual, emotional and physical aspects, that is satisfied and optimistic, that experiences a minimum of tension and conflict in its conduct with other individuals in society. The aim of mental hygiene is the evolution and development of a properly adjusted and balanced personality. Its objectives may be as follows:

1. *Treatment and remedying of mental defects:* Mental hygiene, or the science of mental health is concerned with the prevention of inadequate adjustment or with those processes or methods which adjust the maladjusted individual. This statement of mental hygiene emphasizes its curative aspect. The main function of mental hygiene is the curing of mental ailments, defects and imbalances.
2. *Prevention of personality disorders:* This science prevents all kinds of personality disorders, since all mental diseases originate in them. Mental hygiene is that science which studies the human personality, and its deviations, from the curative standpoint. In this manner, another objective of mental hygiene is the curing or removal of abnormalities of the personality, since it is only in the absence of such aberration that the individual can be balanced. Abnormality lead to imbalance and all kinds of mental conflicts and diseases. Prevention of such diseases takes the form of curing them as well as prevention of further procreation from such parents since diseases are likely to be transmitted through heredity.

3. *Safeguard of mental health:* The most comprehensive function of mental hygiene is the safeguarding of mental health. Mental hygiene prevents mental aberrations and advances mental health. Mental hygiene consistently stresses the development or creation, of such qualities in the individual as optimism, confidence, cooperation, emotional adjustment and maturity, etc. It points out the means of improving the adaptability and efficiency of individuals.

Thus mental hygiene has three prominent aspects—curative, preventive and preservative. In its curative aspect, it indicates ways and means of curing mental deviations, defects and imbalances. Ways and means of preventing them or counteracting them are suggested by it under its preventive function while in its preservative guise it puts forward rules and suggestions by following which any and every individual can ensure his mental health.

Scope of Mental Hygiene

Mental hygiene is concerned with the principle and practice in promotion, maintainance of mental health and prevention of mental disorders. It is the science and art of preserving and maximizing mental health.

Mental hygiene comprehends the curing of mental defects, diseases, and abnormalities, as well as the prevention of such abnormalities, beside the active preservation of mental health, balance, pleasure and adjustment, etc. of the individual. Evidently, then, the scope of mental hygiene is very vast. It comprehends the entire life of the individual. Every individual stands in need of mental health. Young children, men and women experiences difficulty in adjusting to new circumstances which lead to mental complications and difficulties, that, in turn, endanger mental health. Hence, it is they who stand in greatest need of mental health and hygiene. In old age, when man is past his prime, his energy is on the decrease. There are very few ways in which he can pass his time; his children are busy in the affairs of their own families, while the young girls in the family have gone to their husbands. When retired from service, even the source of income is blocked. And one foot is already in the grave, as they say. Some or the other minor ailment of the body is always present; hence it is at such times that mental health is challenged the most. If, in such a state, one is to lose one's life partner, it is the last straw for the poor individual. What greater shock can there be for an individual to have his mother die at an early age, and the wife to die in old age? Hence mental hygiene is needed very greatly by the old and senile people. Besides children and senile folk, some adults in the prime of life also require mental hygiene since their mental balance is disturbed and personality can be recruited from lists of drunkards, confirmed alcoholics, gamblers, corrupt individuals and people who frequent prostitute homes, etc. They are themselves mentally diseased persons, but they are also potential threats to the mental health of society the social disorganization of society. And the list of sufferers is completed by people who have already lost their mental balance, who are prey to mental defects, diseases and aberrations. They require mental treatment and cure.

Curative and preventive aspects of mental hygiene have been depicted clearly in the foregoing description, but its preservative aspect remains to be delineated. Hence, even healthy individuals require mental hygiene as they stand to benefit by its preservative function. In other words, people who are healthy from the mental standpoint are also in need of mental hygiene. In fact, healthy and ill are words that are relative. In practical life, there is no individual who can be declared completely healthy. Secondly, even if he is healthy at some period of time, man's adjustment to the environment is not a static condition but rather a gradual dynamic process. The question of adjustment is forever present before the individual since man's condition is ever changing somewhat. Hence, there is no saying when an individual, who is at present manifesting the most perfect adjustment, may have cause to lose his mental balance. Consequently, he requires mental hygiene to see to it that he is not deprived of his mental bliss and happiness.

Thus it is evident that the scope of mental hygiene is not contained by any considerations of age since it is required by young, old, adolescent, man, woman, the healthy and the unhealthy alike. Its sphere extends from the home to school, factory, office, shop, market, meetings, society, in fact everywhere. It is needed in all human relationships and activities.

Value of mental hygiene: The meaning and scope of mental hygiene also help to clarify its value. Its value and efficacy consists not only in the curing and preventing of mental defects, diseases and imbalances, but also in preserving a state of mental health in the individual fortunately blessed with it. It is of value for young, old, men, women, boy, girl, healthy, insane, in fact for everyone. Just as every able-bodied being requires physical hygiene for its prolonged well-being, every living being with a mind needs mental hygiene. And for him, mental hygiene has its value and significance. Hence the requirement of mental hygiene in every sphere of human life—home, school, playground, office, profession, factory, mill, shop—is its value. And individuals who can be considered potential patients of mental hygiene are the senile, adolescents and the corrupt persons. Similarly, in the normal course of human life, mental hygiene is required wherever there are human relationships, yet it most essentially needed in the home and the school since these are the two institutions which are the greatest preservatives of mental health. Hence a complete comprehension of the value of mental hygiene can come only when one has understood its importance for the school and the home, as well as for mentally diseased persons, adolescents, senile people and corrupt persons.

Mental hygiene in family: Most experts are of the opinion that the influences that mould the personality of a child during the first five or six years of his life determine his conduct throughout his future existence. It is in the family that the child learns to express, control and refine or modify his emotions, thoughts, feelings and impressions. It is in the family that he develops the qualities of affection, sympathy, brotherhood, etc. His conduct towards his equals, his juniors and his seniors is moulded and formed in the family. Hence, if some situation or circumstance in the family affects him adversely his mental health is apt to suffer. Hence, it is evident that if the mental health of the future citizens of the nations is to be ensured, it is essential that mental hygiene be introduced into the family. It is not only as a child, but also as husband and father, wife and mother, that one is under family influence. Family, as an institution, is with an individual from the time he steps into the world to the time he steps out of it. Mental disease or ill health in even one member of the family has its repercussions on the other members. Hence it is as important to safeguard mental health in the family as it is to prevent and cure mental imbalances if it is present there. Without this, the peace and calm of family life becomes an ephemeral existent.

Mental hygiene in school: Following the family, another institution that casts important influence upon the child's development is the school. In school, the child's personality is influenced by his teachers and colleagues. It is in school that he learns lessons of self-dependence, self-confidence and self-reliance. Now he cannot seek protection in his mother's lap from the problems that confront him, neither can he look up to his father to save him. Hence he is compelled to conduct himself desirably towards all on his own initiative. And in this effort, it is only natural that he finds frustrations that endanger the balance of his personality with mental difficulties and complexes. Mental hygiene in school is important for preventing such unhealthy development and for preserving mental health.

Mental hygiene in adolescence: As it is mental hygiene is of importance throughout an individual life, but is assumes greatest importance during and adolescence. Adolescence is the most volatile stage in the development of personality. Mental, physical, and every other kind of development takes place at a rapid place during this stage. Young boys and girls manifest signs of approaching adulthood. The male member develops his beard, and his voice breaks. In girls, the breasts begin to develop, and various parts of the body begin to round out. This physical development is accompanied by mental development, due to which they do not appreciate being treated as children. They prefer to be counted among the adults. And in this fresh eagerness for adulthood, many boys are seen using the blade prematurely in an effort to acquire bread quickly. Imagination and emotionality are at their highest pitch while the adolescent is passing through this period. Interest in the other sex manifest itself in many peculiar adolescent is further anxious about his future and his livelihood, regarding which he develops ambitions and dreams constantly. From this vivid description of the various problems that confront the young folk during this stage of their life, it is evident that it is now that there is greatest need for preventing mental quirks and for ensuring mental health.

Mental hygiene in old age: It has been pointed out earlier that in old age, maintaining a sane outlook on life becomes something of a problem, hence the old men have much to gain from mental hygiene, its ways and means. Another class of men and women who stand to gain much from this science is that of the corrupt and evil-alcoholics, criminals, prostitutes and other antisocial elements. Many of their mental problems can be solved through the ways and means suggested by mental hygiene. In this manner, mental hygiene is an integral part of human welfare and life. It finds application everywhere, although reaping of the greatest possible benefit from it depends upon the skill of the person using it, and the ability with which he can control the circumstances. Mental hygiene is a science. It makes a study of the ways, means and rules that preserve mental health, prevent mental disturbance and cure mental diseases. Hence mental hygiene can benefit every sphere of life such as personal, family, social, national and international relationships, interrelations between various classes, sexes, age levels, communities, races and peoples. This is the value of mental hygiene, and it is not influenced by the very little benefit that is derived from it in practice. Being a science, it is neutral, and in no position to bestow gifts and benefits upon people of its own accord. It is for man to reap a rich harvest from it. Its value does not deteriorate if man chooses to neglect it, since its value is proved and beyond doubt.

Ethical Issues in Mental Health

Ethics as that branch of philosophy which is concerned with human character and conduct.

Ethics as a system of moral principles, the rules of conduct recognized in respect to a particular class of human actions or a particular group culture, etc.

Ethics as "a systematic study of ultimate problems of human conduct". Ethics deals with rightness and wrongness of certain actions and to the goodness and badness of the motives and ends of such actions. It relies on "judgment" and addresses itself to what ought to be.

EVOLUTION OF ETHICS IN HEALTH CARE

Much before Hippocrates laid down the rules of conduct contained in the oath, *Ayurvedic texts* gave a much more comprehensive and well-documented description of the codes of behavior for the teacher, for students of medical sciences, attendants, and various other activities connected with health care.

Guru used to administer the following oath to his students—

"A bachelor that you shall be, you shall abstain from all sex activities, anger, greed, attachment, pride, grandiosity, jealousy, roughness, back biting, immorality, idleness and defamation; you shall keep your head shaved and nails cut every fifth day; shall remain properly dressed, everyday to speak the truth and be respectful and obedient to the Guru". He warned his discipline that of the later acted otherwise, it would amount to immorality and he will loose all the powers gained through imparted knowledge. The "Guru" in turn used to take the following oath himself. "If you (disciple) keep to all the requirements worthy of a disciple student and if I do not systematically and fully impart the proper knowledge due to you, I shall be condemned to be a sinner for all times and will be bereft of all my knowledge". There was great importance attached to moral values and conduct. This was the bond of *Guru-Chela relationship (J.S. Neki, 1974).* Upon completion of their course, the practitioners were called upon "to treat Brahmins, gurus, poor, friends, saints and destitutes without distinction like ones own brethren". Long before the birth of Christ, medical codes were derived from prayers and oaths in a number of writings.

The main objectives of professional ethics are:

- To provide guidelines of conduct among the professionals themselves. It includes type of referral, commenting on opinion of another professionals, charging fee from coprofessionals and their families.
- To formulate guidelines in dealing with the client, e.g. maintaining dignity of the client; confidentiality, secrecy and privacy of information; providing competent and efficient advice, charging money, referral, etc.

ETHICAL ISSUES IN MENTAL HEALTH NURSING

The main ethical issues in mental health nursing involves the following areas:

I. Nurse Patient Relationship

There are many therapeutic processes involved in nurse patient relationship. They are as follows:

- ***Rapport:*** Conscious feeling of harmonious accord, sympathy, and mutual responsiveness between two or more persons.
- ***Empathy:*** The intellectual and emotional awareness and understanding of another person's state of mind. It involves the projection of oneself into another person's frame of reference.
- ***Transference:*** It is a process whereby the patient unconsciously projects his emotions, thoughts and wishes related to significant people in his past life onto people in his current life. It can be positive or negative.
- ***Counter transference:*** It is a process whereby psychiatrist unconsciously projects his emotions, thoughts, and wishes from his past life onto the patients personality or onto

the material is presenting, thus expressing unresolved conflicts and/or his own personal needs.

- ***Resistance:*** It is theoretical construct which reflects any attitude or behaviors which run counter to the therapeutic objectives to the treatment. It is of many types—Conscious, ego, id or superego resistance, manifested by many behaviors.
- ***Therapeutic alliance:*** It is a process whereby the patients mature, rational, observing ego, is used in combination with the psychiatrists analytic abilities to advance their understanding of the patient.

Essentially, the relationships is one of mutual trust and confidence. Nurse-patient relationship can be friendly, corporate, authoritarian, egalitarian, caretaker, parental, helper, etc. in addition nurses have to maintain confidentiality, privacy and privileged communication: Confidentiality involves the sharing of secrets and secrecy stands for tendency to conceal. The nurses responsibility is to safeguard the patients confidence within the constraints of law as it is in ethics. The only exception to this rule is when the patient is dangerous to others. It has been further clarified that where disclosure of a confidence is proper for instance, if compelled by a lawful court order or authorized by the patient, such disclosure should be limited to only that information which is relevant to a given situation, preferably with patients consent (i.e. privileged communication). Records of the patients should be strictly safeguarded but computerization of the records in hospitals may lead to some ethical problems as data can be deciphered by others. Confidentiality, secrecy and privacy should also be maintained in therapeutic procedures, e.g. psychotherapy, psychoanalysis, hypnosis, abreaction, etc. When the therapist communicates a case history or publishes a photograph, the patients informed consent should be taken.

II. INFORMED CONSENT

Consent means voluntary agreement, compliance or permission. To be legally valid, it must be given after understanding what it is given for, and of risks involved. The kinds of Consent may be: (1) Express, i.e. specifically stated by the patient, or (2) Implied. Express consent may be (a) Verbal, or (b) written.

'Therapeutic privilege' is an exception to the rule of "full disclosure". In these cases the doctor or nurse may exercise discretion as to the facts which he discloses.

Informed consent is the most complicated and important issue. The real problems come up when the patients are uneducated, unsophisticated and have little knowledge of science. They have confidence, trust and faith in their health care provider and medicines. Such patients may be shocked to learn that the health care provider is not sure about the medicine or the procedure, they are going to try. This creates a feeling of distrust and insecurity, leading to lingering suspicion. This may be appropriate in the western set up but may create iatrogenic suspicion. Thus a heavy moral and social responsibility lies on the health care provider when he takes the informed consent. There are several implications regarding informed consent.

i. Although the informed consent doctrine has substantive foundation in law, it is essentially and ethical imperative.
ii. Ethically valid consent is a process of shared decision-making based upon mutual respect and participation and not a ritual to be equated with reciting the contents of a form that details the risks of particular treatments.

iii. Though informed consent is portrayed as a highly rational process, implying thereby that it may be suitable for and applicable to well-educated, self-aware individuals, the desire for information, choice and respectful communication about decisions in universal (emphasis added).
iv. Incompetence as a disqualifying factor should be considered in only a minority of cases.
v. Information should not be withheld merely because it is unpleasant.
vi. Judicious attempts to involve family members in decision making for patients to understand information and in decision making. However, due regard must be given to privacy of patients and for the possibility of coercion.
vii. To protect the interests of those who lack decision-making capacity and to ensure their well-being and self-determination, decisions by other (relatives, friends or at least 2 treating physicians) should attempt to replicate the once patient would make if he/she were capable of doing so.

Setting up of ethics committees, developing clear guidelines for making decisions and reserving courts only for matters of substantive importance and provision of legal guidelines for advance directives can help improve the situations.

Three of the elements of the legal model of the decision making process are *voluntariness, competency and understanding.* All these three play an important role in mental disorders.

For understanding informed consent three variables namely provision of information, understanding and competence should be considered.

- **Provision of information:** Patients should be provided with information about the research before their decision considered valid. They must be informed of the risks, discomforts side effects, the anticipated benefits, available alternatives and likely consequences of failure to take part in research. This information should be provided in simple language.
- **Understanding:** Judicially it is not deemed necessary that the patient actually understand what he is told. The act of informing someone does not assure that one will understand the information that has been provided. It is therefore uncertain what obligation the researcher has to attempt to ascertain the level of understanding.
- **Competence:** Patients are presumed to have the capacity to comprehend the information with which they are provided. If a patient is not competent, any decision taken is not valid. Exactly what this means is not clear. There are several tests of competence may to be applied. There are basically five categories:
  1. Evidencing a choice
  2. "Reasonable" outcome of choice
  3. Choice based on 'rational' reasons
  4. Ability to understand
  5. Actual understanding.

Informed consent is also important in the following:

- *Admission or discharge of patient*: Telling the patient and informants about indications for admission, treatment modalities to be used, cost of therapies and admission and finally, likely complications and precautions after discharge.
- *Investigations to be used,* i.e. options, indications, advantages, cost, complications of an investigation.
- *Treatment methods:* Available options, advantages, disadvantages and costs of each treatment modality. Use of dependence producing drugs.

- *Research:* Revealing history, photographs, signs or diagnosis of patient or other family members using traumatic procedures, data collection, transfer and presentation of data.
- *Drug trials:* Using placebo or experimental drug with unknown side effects.
- *Medicolegal problems:* Role of informed consent is also important in issues of marriage, divorce, property dispute or criminal responsibility, revealing information to court, working place or relatives. When patient is not in a condition to give informed consent, informed consent from close relatives, friends, office colleagues or treating physicians (at least two, deciding in the interest of patient) is especially important. In remitting disorders, e.g. mood disorders, an informed consent may be obtained for future episodes.

The reasons for obtaining consent includes:

i. To examine, treat or operate upon a patient without consent is assault in law, even if it does not cause any harm or even if it is beneficial and done in good faith. The patient may recover damages.

ii. If a medical or nurse practitioner fails to give the requisite information to a patient before asking for his consent to a particular operation or treatment, he may be charged for negligence.

The rules of consent to be followed are given below:

1. Consent is necessary in every medical examination.
2. Written consent is not necessary in every case. However, it should be taken for proving the same in the court if necessity arises.
3. Any procedure beyond routine physical examination, such as, operation, blood transfusion.
4. The consent should be free, voluntary, clear, intelligent, informed, direct and personal. There should be no undue influence, fraud, misrepresentation of facts, compulsion and threat of physical injury death or other consequences.
5. The health care provider should inform the patient that he has right to refuse to submit to examination and that the result may go against him. Oral consent should be obtained in the presence of a disinterested third party, e.g. nurse.
6. The health care provider should explain the object of the examination to the patient, and he should be informed that the findings will be embodied in a medical report.
7. In criminal cases, the victim cannot be examined without his/her and he should be informed that the findings will be embodied in a medical report.
8. (A) When a person is arrested on a charge of committing on offence and there are reasonable grounds for believing that an examination of his person will afford evidence as to the commission of an offence, a registered medical practitioner can examine such person, even by using reasonable force if the examination is requested by a police officer not below the rank of sub-inspector.
   (B) In the case of a female, the examination should be made only by or under the supervision of a female registered medical practitioner.
9. In cases of drunkenness, the person should not be examined, and blood, urine or breath should not be collected without his consent.
10. A prisoner can be treated forcibly without consent in the interest of society.
11. Consent given for committing a crime or an illegal act, such as criminal abortion, is invalid.
12. A person above 18 years of age can give valid consent to suffer any harm which may result from an act not intended or not known to cause death or grievous hurt.

13. A person above 18 years of age can give valid consent to suffer any harm which may result from an act, not intended or not known to cause death done in good faith and for its benefit.
14. A child under 12 years of age and an insane person cannot give valid consent to suffer any harm which may occur from an act done in good faith and for its benefit.
15. A consent given by a person under fear of injury, or under a misconception of a fact is not valid. The consent given by an insane or intoxicated person, who is unable to understand the nature and consequences of that to what he give his consent, is invalid.
16. Any harm caused to a person in good faith, even without that person's consent is not an offence, if the circumstances are such that it is impossible for that person to signify consent, and has no guardian or other person in lawful charge of him from whom it is possible to obtain consent.
17. The health care provider should inform reasonably to the patient about the nature, consequences and risks of the examination or operation before taking the consent.
18. For contraceptive sterilization, consent of both the husband and wife should be obtained.
19. The consent of one spouse is not necessary for an operation or treatment of the other.
20. Consent of the inmates of the hostel, etc. is necessary if they are above 12 years.
21. It is unlawful to detain an adult patient in hospital against his will.
22. The nature of illness of patient should not be disclosed to any third party without the consent of the patient.
23. When an operation is made compulsory by law, e.g. vaccination, the law furnishes the consent.

24. Consent is not defense in cases of professional negligence.
25. Pathological autopsy should not be conducted without the consent of the guardian or legal heirs of the diseased.
26. If any person that donated his eyes to be used for therapeutic purpose after his death, the eyes can be removed only with the consent of the guardian or legal heirs.
27. A living adult person can give consent for donating one of his kidneys to be grafted into another person.
28. For organ transplantation, the organs of the deal person, such as heart, kidneys, liver, etc. should not be removed without the consent of the person having lawful possession of the body.
29. There is no special for obtaining written consent.

III. RIGHT TO TREAT AND TO BE TREATED

When a patient suffering from a serious cardiac illness needing intensive and urgent care refuses to go to a hospital or refuses any kind of treatment, no one can force him to do otherwise. In contrast when a seriously disturbed mentally ill does so, he is usually certified or forced to undergo treatment much against his will.

Right to treat and to be treated for raises ethical issues involving complex legal implications. Use of particular therapy when it is not called for also raises ethical issues. Health can be right or a privilege according to system prevalent in our country. The right to refuse treatment is complicated ethical issue both legally and psychiatrically. Compulsory hospitalization also involves ethical issues.

IV. SELFISH MOTIVES

Another crucial question on the ethical front requires some self-searching. How many of us are really interested in treating a patient selflessly, i.e. without regard to enhancement of our own interests, self-prestige, monetary advantage, research, publications, etc.

V. FRAUD AND ABUSE IN PSYCHIATRIC PRACTICE

The definitional problems of what is fraudulent or abusive makes it difficult to delineate and precisely determine what is inappropriate and illegal in the practice of psychiatry.

Towary and Sharfsten (1978) have enlisted a number of fraudulent and abusive practices.

i. ***Upgrading,*** i.e. billing for services more extensive than those actually provided.
ii. ***Ganging,*** i.e. billing for multiple services to the members of the same family on the same day.
iii. ***Touting,*** i.e. employing obstructive ways such as appointing agents, soliciting professional support, etc. for enhancing private practice.
iv. ***Self-advertisement*** and self-aggrandizement using audiovisual aids and mass media communication methods.
v. Unavailability of treating physician because of his absence (usually abroad) for participation in big conference.
vi. Calling pressmen to publish reports of the research work done.
vii. Doing unethical drug trials and giving false reports for receiving money from the pharmaceuticals.
viii. Missing lectures, teaching unprepared topics or passing or upgrading in examinations on approach.
ix. Not keeping one up to date with recent developments in the field of treatment and care of patients.
x. To practice quackery under the garb of modern medicine.
xi. To write unscientific drug combination to get favor from pharmaceuticals.
xii. Selling of samples.
xiii. Making addicts or sustaining them.
xiv. Billing for services not rendered.
xv. ***Ping-Ponging,*** i.e. Multiple referrals between psychiatrists or other professional brothers when there is no real necessity for these services.
xvi. Charging for physicians services actually provided by nonphysicians professionals not eligible for reimbursement.
xvii. Offering or receiving kickbacks.
xviii. Billing more than one part for the same services.
xix. Disturbing sample drugs indiscriminately to anyone who can pay.
xx. Making excessive profits from a legitimate treatment.
xxi. ***Steering:*** Directing patients to a particular pharmacy.

Some other unethical practices are:

i. Devoting much less than required time and effort in attending to outpatients and inpatients in hospitals.
ii. While away in hospital, gossiping or roaming about and not doing full duty during working hours.
iii. Prolonging the illness, creating relapses or exacerbation or wrongly treating the patients (intentionally).
iv. Sexual promiscuity, abuse or exploitation of patients.

v. Giving ineffective treatment or using treatment for indications not normally called for.
vi. Exploiting or blackmailing patients for privacy or secrecy.
vii. Giving wrong evidence in court (after receiving favor from a party).
viii. False medical certification.
ix. Duping the patients by administering of such procedures like injections of distilled water, IV glucose and tonics, etc. when not warranted.
x. Criticizing the prescription of specialists of one's own speciality to please the patients.
xi. Receiving gifts or economical status nonuniform fee from patients.
xii. Not referring the patient to other physicians when one knows that patient is not psychiatrically ill.
xiii. Not respecting the basic rights and humane nature of the patients.

Other Professional Misconducts

Infamous conduct (serious professional misconduct): It is defined as something which might reasonably be regarded as disgraceful or dishonorable by professional men of good repute and competence. It involves an abuse of professional position.

Medical ethics (Published by Medical Council of India (MCI) and by several State Medical Councils): Any one found guilty of any of the following offences mentioned in the warning notice issued by the Medical Council of India will be liable to have his name erased from the Medical Register.

i. (a) Adultery
ii. (b) Conviction, improper conduct or association with a patient or members of the patients family by a Court of Law for offences involving *moral turpitude.*
iii. Issuing a false, misleading or improper certificate in connection with sick benefit, insurance passport, attendance in court, public service, etc.
iv. Withholding from health authorities information of notifiable diseases.
v. Performing or enabling an unqualified person to perform any illegal procedure for which there is no indication.
vi. Contravening the provisions of the drugs.
vii. Selling *Act Scheduled* poisons to the public under cover of his qualifications, except to the patients.
viii. *Dichotomy or fee splitting,* i.e. receiving or giving commission or other benefits to a professional colleagues or manufacturer or traders in drugs or a chemist.
ix. Using of touts or agents for procuring patients.
x. Disclosing the secrets of a patient that have been learnt in the exercise of his profession, except in a court of law.
xi. Covering, i.e. assisting someone who has no medical qualification to attend, treat or perform a procedure on some person in respect of matters requiring professional discretion or skill.
xii. Association with manufacturing firms (i.e. personal ownership, receiving rebates or commission).
xiii. Advertising (unusual publication in lay press reports of cases treated publicizing scale of fees, unusually large sign boards or manufacturing firms) but he can write to lay press matter of public health, he can announce his availability schedule or can advertise the institution but not his name).

xiv. Professional association with bodies or societies of unqualified persons formed for the purpose of training unqualified practitioners.
xv. Running an open shop for sale of medicines or equipment.
xvi. Refusal to give professional service on religious ground.
xvii. Drunk or disorderly so as to interfere with proper skilled practice of medicine.

A Code of Ethics for Health professionals in Relation to Mental Health

Preamble

1. **Responsibility:** As a practitioner, the psychiatric nursing must know that they bears heavy social responsibility because he not only deals with disturbed human behavior but also has to contend with intimacies of life. As a scientist he/she would serve the society through observation, investigation and experimentation and well-planned and ethically carried out research.
2. **Competence:** The maintenance of high standards of professional competence is (the) responsibility of all nursing in the interest of both the public and the profession. Nurses are responsible for their own continuing education and should realize that their must be life-time learning. As members of the profession they will not violate ethical standards and, when such violation comes to their notice, will take steps to correct it.
3. **Benevolence:** The interests of the patient and his health will stand paramount with them in their professional practices. Personal interests would find but a secondary place. Financial arrangements will never contravene professional standards. Nurses will always safeguard the interests of the patient and the profession.
4. **Moral standards:** They will at all times be responsive to the moral codes and expectations of the community they serve, and will not let their behavior in anyway malign their profession.
5. **Patient welfare:** They will not treat a case that does not clearly fall within their competence. The patient's integrity and welfare as also that of the communities in which they work.

   They will terminate the clinical or consulting relationship with the patient when it is reasonably clear to them that the patient is no longer benefiting from it.

   In case of referral, they will continue to feel responsible for the patient's welfare until the responsibility has been formally transferred.
6. **Confidentiality:** They will safeguard information about a patient that they have obtained in the course of their clinical work, teaching or research in order to safeguard the patients interest and protect him from social stigma, discrimination and harm. They will treat this as a primary obligation and not reveal unto others any such information unless certain ethical conditions are met, or when there is clear and imminent danger to an individual or society and then only to the appropriate authorities or concerned coprofessionals. Confidentiality of the clinical record will be meticulously guarded and identity of the patients will not be revealed even in scientific communication.

No data about a patient shall be ordinarily revealed to any agency without the consent of the patient or his family.

Recommendations

1. Every person who has attained the age of majority and who does not appear to have lost the ability of reason shall be assumed to be capable of giving consent.

   A patient should be taken up for medical evaluation and treatment with his consent. In case a patient, because of his mental illness, is unable to express valid consent, the psychiatrist may undertake to treat him with the consent of a person close to him who appears to be clearly interested in the welfare of the patient. The only exception of treating without consent would be in an emergency situation involving an immediate threat to the life or health of patient or others. For purposes of research, the consent shall be contained on the lines indicated above after satisfying the following:

a. The consent is entirely voluntary
b. The patient can withdraw the consent at any stage
c. Withdrawal of the consent shall not affect the interest of the patient.

2. The decision to hospitalize a patient will essentially rest on the consideration of his welfare and will also take into consideration legal and administrative constraints as well as its social appropriateness.
3. Psychiatric treatment and nursing care shall be initiated only on clinical considerations and shall be in accordance with scientific knowledge and professional ethics. The patients welfare should be the primary factor determining the choice of the treatment modality, should the specific modality not fall within the patient to a competent colleague. The termination of therapy also shall be determined on clinical consideration. Treatment should not be permitted to continue unjustifiably or for material consideration.

   All treatment should be humane and never punitive. No psychiatrist shall refuse to treat in an emergency.
4. Gifts and gratifications from patients under treatment should not be accepted.
5. Any kind of sexual advances towards any patient during treatment.

6. In case of doubt or in situations where unconventional treatment procedures are contemplated, a second opinion must be obtained.
7. It is unethical to force a contract upon a patient during treatment.
8. Even when a patient has been referred by a legal or administrative authority or by the employer, welfare of the patient will remain of paramount consideration. The patient should be informed of the purpose for which he is to be examined.
9. Basic human rights of the mentally retarded should not be subjected to unethical abridgement. Due ethical discretion should be exercised when advising such procedures as sterilization.
10. In the interest of the patient and the society, drug abusers who refuse to give consent may be treated with the consent of their relatives. Effort has to be made to motivate them for accepting treatment voluntarily.

Legal Issues in Mental Health Nursing

Professional Negligence (Malpraxis): Malpraxis is defined as absence of reasonable care and skill, or willful negligence of a health care practitioner. Due care means such reasonable care and attention for the safety of patients as their mental and physical condition may require.

Civil negligence: The question of civil negligence arises (1) when a patient, or in case of death, any relative brings suit in a civil court for realization of compensation from his doctor, if he has suffered injury due to negligence. (2) When a doctor, brings a civil suit for the realization of his fees from the patient or his relatives who refuses to pay the same on the ground of professional negligence.

Liability for negligence arises if the following conditions are satisfied:
1. *Duty:* Existence of a duty of care by the doctor.
2. *Dereliction:* The failure on the part of the doctor or nurse to maintain care skill.
3. *Direct causation:* The failure to exercise a duty of care must lead to damage (proximate cause).
4. *Damage:* The damage which results must be reasonably foreseeable.
   The amount of damage done is a measure of the extent of the liability.

Criminal negligence: Criminal negligence occurs when the physician exhibits gross lack of competency, gross inattention, criminal indifference to the patient's safety, or gross negligence in the selection and application of remedies.

The following are some of the examples: (1) Gross mismanagement of the delivery of a woman, especially by doctor under the influence of drink or drugs.

Ethical malpraxis: Ethical malpraxis is the violation of the provisions of the Code of Medical Ethics. It evokes the condemnation of the doctor's professional brethren. In this, no financial compensation is payable unless there is also civil malpraxis.

Precautions Against Negligence

1. Never guarantee a cure.
2. Keep full and accurate medical records.
3. Employ ordinary skill and care at all times.
4. Do not fail to get written informed consent.
5. The diagnosis should be confirmed by laboratory tests.
6. Skiagrams should be taken in bone or joint injuries or when diagnosis is doubtful.
7. Immunization should be done whenever necessary, particularly for tetanus.
8. Sensitivity tests should be done before injecting preparations which are likely to produce anaphylactic shock.
9. When diagnosis is obscure consult a specialist.
10. In suspected cases of cancer all laboratory investigations should be done without delay to establish early diagnosis.
11. Do not criticize another practitioner.
12. The physician should not make a statement constituting or admitting fault on his part.
13. The doctor should refrain from over optimistic prognosis and should avoid promising too much to the patient.
14. The physician should advice his patient of any intended absence from practice and should recommend, or make available, a qualified substitute.
15. The doctor should frequently check the condition of his equipment and make use of available safety installation.
16. The drug should be identified before being injected or used otherwise.
17. The consent of the patient should be obtained.
18. The surgeon should obtain a written consent to use his discretion in obscure cases.
19. In a criminal wounding, operations should not be performed unless it is absolutely necessary.
20. No experimental methods should be adopted without consent.
21. No procedure should be undertaken beyond one's skill.

22. The doctor should keep informed the technical advances and use standard procedure of treatment.
23. Proper instructions should be given to the patient and proper postoperative care should be taken.
24. The patient must not be abandoned.
25. No female patient should be examined unless a third person is present.
26. It is dangerous to telephone a prescription, because of the possibility of error in transmission.
27. Anesthesia should be given by a qualified person. Only generally accepted anesthetic should be given after clinical and laboratory examination of the patient. The patient should be watched until he fully recovers from its effects.
28. In the case of death from an anesthetist should check the drugs to be given, bottles and cylinders, the apparatus to be used and take precautions to prevent statis electric explosion and fire.
29. Do not fail to exercise care in the selection of assistances and in the delegation of duties of them.
30. Do not leave a patient unattended during labor.
31. Do not fail to secure the consent of both husband and wife if an operation on either is likely to result in sterility.

Contributory negligence: Contributory negligence is any unreasonable conduct or negligence on the part of the patient which is the cause of the harm complained of, although the doctor was also negligent, e.g. if the patient fails to cooperate with his doctor in carrying out all reasonable and proper instructions, or refuses to take the suggested treatment, or fails to attend as requested for treatment.

Therapeutic misadventure: Therapeutic misadventure is a case in which an individual has been injured or had died due to some inadvertent, unintentional act by a doctor or agent of the doctor or hospital.

Some examples are hypersensitivity reactions, sometimes serious or fatal, may be caused by penicillin, aspirin, tetracycline, etc. Prolonged use of stilbesterol may cause breast cancer. Excessive admission of an antidote to a poisoned patient, who subsequently dies.

To avoid a therapeutic misadventure in prescribing drugs, the following points should be noted before prescribing any drug known to cause any adverse reaction, the doctor should make reasonable effort to determine if any adverse reaction is likely to occur.

The doctor should warn the patient of side effects which may occur while he is taking the drug.

Vicarious Liability (Liability for act of another)

The law holds that an employer is responsible not only for his own omissions and commissions, but also for the negligence of his employees in so far as such acts occur in the course of the principle of respondent superior (let the master answer).

Euthanasia (Mercy Killing): It means granting painless death to hopelessly noncurable disease.

Types: (1) Active or positive, (2) Passive or negative.

- **Active euthanasia** is a positive merciful act, taken deliberately to end futile suffering or a meaningless existence. It is an act of commission. Death is induced either by direct action to end the life or by indirect action, e.g. by giving large doses of drugs to hasten death.
- **Passive euthanasia** means discontinuing or not resorting to the use of extraordinary life-sustaining measures to prolong life in hopeless cases when such prolongation seems an unwarranted extension of suffering or unconsciousness. This includes acts of omission, such as, failure to resuscitation a terminally ill or hopeless incapacitated patient or a severely defective newborn infant. It is refraining from action that would probably delay death and permits natural death to occur.
- Voluntary euthanasia means at the will of the person and involuntary means against the will of the person, i.e. compulsory.
- Nonvoluntary refers to cases of persons incapable of making their wishes known, e.g. in persons with irreversible coma or severely defective infants.

Euthanasia advocates the administration of lethal doses of opium or other narcotic drugs. It has no legal sanction.

The ethics, being a concept like in iceberg that also changes with time and place of practice will always be on controversial grounds when applied to scientific endeavor.

25 CHAPTER

Ego Defense Mechanisms

Introduction

The term "defense mechanism" refers to the predominantly unconscious self-protective process that seeks to shield the ego from intense feelings or affect impulses. Additionally, these intrapsychic processes modify, nullify or convey painful affects or tendencies, so they can be tolerated consciously. Defense mechanism is a pattern of adjustment through which an individual relieves or decreases anxieties caused by an uncomfortable situation that threatens self-esteem.

The phenomena of stress and anxiety are remarkably interrelated. Stress produces enormous human strain, which consequently leads to inner conflict or anxiety. A response to stressful situation is primarily biologically, but psychosocial factors impact the perception of and number of stressors. Furthermore, coping skills, cultural factors, suggest systems and ego function (i.e. definite mechanisms) affects reactions to stress.

Ego defense mechanism is consciously or unconsciously operating device to keep conflictual issues out of consciousness of the individual to bring some protective measures.

These mechnisms are learned, usually during early childhood and are considered to be maladaptive when they become the predominant means of coping with stressors.

Defense mechanisms operate outside awareness in order to protect a person from feelings of worthless and inadequacy. They are legitimate strategies of adaption which are, in a complicated and often threatening society, regularly used by people to protect their sense of worth. They become problematic when used excessively or otherwise inappropriately. If the entire day is being spent defensive then the self is not allowing information to enter, which is a crucial factor in adaption to stress. From a nursing point of view, one can understand the importance of carefully assessing whether the clients use of defense mechanisms is essential to preserving self-image and sense of worth or whether it is maladaptive and nursing intervention might offer feasible alternatives to improve functioning.

Whenever man is faced with a situation that presents serious consequences for his mental balance, a state of conflict or injury, and he is not successful in achieving any direct adjustment with that situation, then in order to attain such an adjustment he has to take recourse to certain defensive or escapist reactions that satisfy the motive even without attaining the actual objective. These mental constructions are called mental mechanisms or defense mechanisms. Generally, the individual is not aware of their existence and purpose, and neither is he pleased to bother himself about their working. Yet, these mental mechanisms are to be found in normal individuals. Objectively, they reduce the shock of failures and maintain an internal balance and organization. If they were not present in him the human individual would have had to achieve adjustment with every situation on his own or otherwise he would soon have become a mental patient.

Anxiety and grief are two major, primary psychological response patterns to stress. *Anxiety* is defined as a diffuse apprehension that is vague in nature and associated with feelings of uncertainty and helplessness. Defense mechanism help to remove and also helps to deal with minor hurt, pain, anger, anxiety, sadness and self-devaluation. *Freud* noted that a major drive for most people is the reduction in tension and that major cause of tension was anxiety. Now, the ego has a difficult time satisfying both the id and the superego. The ego has some tools that it can use in its job as the mediator, tools that help defend the ego. These are called ego defense mechanisms or defenses or coping or adjustment mechanism. Everyone uses defense mechanisms. Their use does not imply mental illness or psychosocial imbalance. Defense mechanisms are only considered maladaptive, when they are the only way an individual responses to a threat or when they limit the individuals ability to function. So mental mechanisms help the individual in: protecting individuals from dangerous situations; to deal with minor hurt, pain, anger, anxiety, sadness and self-devaluation; removing anxiety and hurt; and plays an important role in normal adjustment mechanism.

Characteristics of Defense Mechanisms

1. The purpose of defense mechanism is to reduce anxiety.
2. Defense mechanisms are compromise solutions.
3. The pattern of defense mechanism depends on one's ability.
4. The same individual may use varied mechanisms as per his need.
5. Defense mechanisms may be used consciously but usually act at unconscious or subconscious level.
6. Defense mechanisms are healthy when one:
   - Uses them infrequently
   - Is able to form new acceptable behavior
   - Is able to change the external environment positively
   - Is able to modify his needs
   - Uses mechanisms like rationalization, sublimation, compensation, etc.
7. Defense mechanisms are unhealthy when one:
   - Do not develop ability to change or modify one's abnormal behavior
   - Retreats from the problem of reality
   - Repeatedly uses the specific mechanisms that may interfere with maintenance of self-image. E.g. in undoing, one repeatedly offers excuses but keeps making the same mistakes
   - Uses mechanisms like regression, denial, projection, etc.

Thus mental mechanisms lie between a state of health and disease, since their presence in the normal individual does not lead to any harm. However, when they develop to an excessive extent, mental health of the individual is endangered and abnormal traits appear. Adjustment is hindered by too many or over-developed mental mechanisms of his nature because the satisfaction attained by them is rather false and illusory than actual and real. A person with this affection is apparently healthy and well-balanced but in fact failures in his life are much greater. In fact, instead of running away from the problem taking refuge in such mental mechanism, an individual must make a constructive and definite effort to understand his situation and to arrive at some adjustment to it. Only then can he maintain mental health to sufficient extent. But such a happy state of affairs is not possible for every individual, nor is it possible even for one person at every stage of his varied and long life. Hence, mental mechanisms have sometimes to be resorted to. Normally, whenever the fulfillment of a person's requirement is hindered, and he is cognisant of the hindrance, then his first reaction is to increase his effort and achieve the end aimed at, but when further failures stop his footstep, then he compromises by lowering the objective somewhat to bring it within the pale of possibility. When even this measure fails to bring success then he turns to the other method of evolving a substitute goal, but when this line of approach also fails to bring home the bacon, as the saying goes, then he takes refuge in mental mechanisms, the fight has gone out of him and he has been reduced to hapless dejection. Some people are more precipitate in their activity and immediately the goal is some want to rise to fame as test cricketers, and they work hard to this end, but most of them fail by the wayside, for it is a long and arduous road to success. Now, some of them would compromise by trying to become the best players in their respective districts but when even this goal eludes them they will turn strenuously to the search for a lucrative post and means of employment. He that thinking that there is no fun in becoming even the best player at the district level since all the wealth and prestige is in a good post. He will come to the conclusion that anyway some cricket would not have fed him and he would have had to turn to job. This example exhibits a case of rationalizations as well as compensation.

People beset with too many mental mechanisms fail to achieve any adjustment with society, and the life of such people is often devoid of pleasure. Briefly, if mental mechanisms are used only for reducing the shocks of normal failure in life or as a purely temporary strategic retreat in the face of overwhelming forces, then mental mechanisms are healthy and they help in the adjustive process. In this position they are more in the form of means to an end but when they become ends in themselves, and the actual objective is substituted by them, then signs of abnormality develop in the individual.

Since defensive mechanisms are unconscious responses used by persons to protect themselves from internal conflicts and external stressors. A nurse skilled in therapeutic communication will notice when a client is using one or more mechanisms. When a nurse concludes that their clients is defense mechanism to avoid dealing with certain subjects, the nurse can use the knowledge to guide interactions, knowing that the defense mechanism indicates the presence of psychologically significant material. In interview the nurse may choose to pursue additional information on the topic, but the nurse will also realize that the client may not be able to answer direct questions about related issues.

It is now feasible to enter upon a brief account of the various mental mechanisms individually.

Types of Defense Mechanisms

All the mental mechanisms that have been described may be divided into two categories, the defensive and the escapist. The aim of defensive mechanisms, as is evident from the term, is to defend the individual from various harmful experiences and in this form they are very useful. On the other hand, the escapist mental mechanism has for its object the evasion of all circumstances and experiences that may cause pain or harm to the individual so that he is prevented from experiencing much pain, but, because he runs away from the situation, he sometimes falls prey to mental abnormality. Defensive mechanism help in the individuals adjustment while escape mechanisms only serve to hinder the adjustment sought to be established through them. In the mental mechanisms described earlier fantasy, identification, projection, rationalization, withdrawal, escape from reality and compensation are all escapist from some or the other kind of real situation and takes refuge in some imaginary and unreal world, as a result of which his trouble is temporarily solved but ultimately it devolves upon him with even greater urgency and catastrophic force. On the other hand, defense mechanisms are compensation, repression, suppression, inhibition, negativism, sublimation and reaction formation. Through their medium the individual protects himself from very injurious circumstances and this improves his adjustment. It need not be pointed out that among the two forms of mental mechanisms here discussed it would be more useful to resort to defense mechanisms.

These are commonly found among emotionally healthy adults and are considered the most nature, even though many have their origins in the immature level. However, these have been adapted through the years so as to optimize success is life and relationships. The use of these defenses enhances user's pleasure and feelings of mastery. These defenses help the users to integrate conflicting emotions and thoughts while still remaining effective. These include:

Altruism: This is constructive service to others that brings pleasure and personal satisfaction. Altruism is loving others as oneself, behavior that promotes the survival chances of others at a cost to ones own. In other words, it is self-sacrifice for the benefit of others. Altruism focuses on motivation to help others or a want to do good without reward, while duty focuses on a moral obligation towards a specific individual. Some individuals may feel both altruism and duty, while others may not. Pure altruism is giving without regard to reward or the benefits of recognition. The patriots, the God, the king, social workers, etc. are considered to be altruists. For instance, in Sikh religion, Guru Gobind Singh Ji (the Tenth Guru in Sikhism) was in war with the Mughul rulers to protect the people of different faiths.

Acting out: Direct expression of an unconscious wish or impulse without conscious awareness of the emotions that derives that expressive behavior. This behavior is very much common in children with temper tantrum, oppositional defiant disorder, truancy etc. Just as, a teenager gets mad at parents and begins staying out late at night.

Compartmentalization

It refers to separation of two incompatible aspects of psyche from each other to maintain psychological comfort, behavioral manifestation show the inconsistency.
Example: The person who attends temple regularly and is overtly religious conducts a business that includes handling stolen goods.

Condensatlon

It refers to reacting to a single idea with all of the emotions associated with a group of ideas, expressing a complex group of ideas with a single word or phase.
Example: The person says the word "CRAZY" as a shorthand expression for many types of mental illness and for feelings of fear and shame.

Conversion

It is the conversation of an emotional conflict through the development of a physical symptom, usually sensorimotor in nature. It refers to that unconscious conflicts are disguised and expressed symbolically by physical symptoms involving portions of the body, especially the five senses and motor areas. Symptoms are frequently not related to innervations by sensory or motor nerves.

Examples:
- A teenager forbidden to see X-rated movies is tempted to do so by friends and develops blindness and the teenager is unconcerned about the loss of sight.
- The person is under great pressure on the job awakes at 6 AM and is unable to walk but is unconcerned about the symptoms.

Compensation

It is the covering up of a real or perceived weakness by emphasizing a trait one considers more desirable. It is a defense against feelings of inferiority and inadequacy growing out of real or imagined personal defects or weaknesses as well as out of the individuals, inevitable failures and setbacks. It can lead to constructive deliberate, task-oriented behavior. In the over achievements in one area to offset deficiencies, real or imagined, or to overcome failure or frustration in another area.

Examples:
- Napoleon complex—diminutive man becoming emperor
- Nurse with low self-esteem work double shifts so her supervisor will like her
- The student who makes poor grades devotes much time and energy to succeed in music or sports
- Shri Chandrashekar (Karnataka), who was victim of poliomyelitis, paralyzed his one limb, struggled to become world known bowler in cricket.
- Kalidasa, who had been illiterate, became the famous epic poet, of Sanskrit, e.g. Abhigyanam, Shakuntalam.
- Socrates was an extremely ugly man who became a great philosopher.
- A handicapped boy who is unable to participate in sports compensates by becoming a great scholar.
- A young man who is shortest among members of his peer group views this as a deficiency and compensates by being overly aggressive and daring.

Denial

It is the refusal to acknowledge the existence of real situation or the feeling associated with it. This is the negation of reality of threatening situations, despite factual situations. An individual refuses to face reality. The person using denial is unaware of doing so. He/she fails to recognize an unacceptable impulse or undesirable, but obvious thought, fact, behavior, conflict or situation or its consequency or implications. It is failure to acknowledge an unbearable condition, failure to admit the reality situation or how one enables the problem continue.

It is protecting self from unpleasant reality by refusal to perceive it or face it. It is a defense mechanism in which a person is faced with a fact that is too painful to accept and reject it. The individual may deny the reality of the unpleasant fact altogether, admit the fact but deny its seriousness or admit both the fact and seriousness but deny responsibility. The concept of denial is particularly important to the study of addiction. When parents are informed of the death of a child, their first reaction is often of the form, "No! You must have seen some other child, you can't mean our child!" Many women deny that they any feelings about their abortion.

- In war, a mother receives word that her son has been killed, and yet refuses to believe it, still setting table for him, keeping his clothes and room current.
- At school, a student seeing a grade of 'C' next to their name and automatically assuming the professor made a grading error.
- Alcoholics and other substance abusers who refuse to admit they have a problem.

Examples:

- Diabetic eating chocolate candy.
- Spending money freely when broke or lost all in life.
- Waiting three days to seek help for severe abdominal pain.
- The client refuses to admit to anger, even though the situation warrants it and the clients voice indicates anger.
- The woman who miscarries denies that she has lost the baby and continues to wear maternity clothes.
- Individuals continue to smoke categories even though they have been told health risk is involved.
- The alcoholic person believes that he/she has no problem with drinking even though family and work colleagues observe the classic sign.
- A man who has been told that he had heart attack, that caused a great deal of damage to the heart muscle may deny that he has had a heart attack at all.

Denial generally operates as a healthy mechanism, protecting the individual from the immediate shock of reality. In time, denial usually diminishes and the person gradually begins the face, accept and deal with the harsh reality of the truth. Denial also may have treatment implications.

Delusional projection: Grossly frank delusions about external reality, usually of a persecutory nature. This defense mechanism is common feature of psychotic mental illnesses like schizophrenia, delusional disorder, etc. These delusions are the false beliefs of the person which are not shared by race, age, educational background, etc. Like, the person says that his family members are planning to kill him very soon.

Dislocation

It is dealing with emotional conflict by temporary attention in consciousness or identity. It refers to repression or splitting off from awareness of a portion of a personality or of consciousness. However, the repressed material continues to affect behavior (compartmentalization).

Examples:

- A client discussed a conflict laden subject and gas into a trance.
- Amnesia that prevents recall of yesterdays auto accident.
- An adult remembers nothing of childhood sexual abuse.

Distortion: A gross reshaping of external reality to meet internal needs. For example, mentally ill patients have no intact contact with reality. These patients are suffering with psychosis.

Dissociation: It is temporary drastic modification of one's personal identity or character to avoid emotional distress; separation or postponement of a feeling that normally would accompany a situation or thought. Dissociation is a state of acute mental decompensation in which certain thoughts, emotions, sensations and / or memories are compartmentalized because they are too overwhelming for the conscious mind to integrate. This subconscious strategy for managing powerful negative emotions is sometimes referred to as *splitting,* as these thoughts, emotions, sensations and/or memories are split off from integrated ego. This use of word 'splitting' here should not be confused with references to splitting mentioned with regard to borderline personality disorder or family relations theory.

For example, an adult relates severe sexual abuse experienced as a child but does it without feelings. She says that the experience was as if she were outside her body watching the abuse.

Displacement

Defense mechanism that shifts sexual or aggressive impulses to a more acceptable or less threatening target; redirecting emotion to a safer outlet; separation of emotion from its real object. If you ever had a bad day at college, then gone home and taken out your frustration on family and friends, you have gone home and taken out your frustration, feelings and impulses on people or objects that are less threatening. Displaced aggression is a common example of this defense mechanism. Rather than express our anger in ways that could lead to negative consequences (like arguing will our boss), we instead express our anger towards a person or object that possess no threat (such as our spouses, children, pets, or slamming a door instead of hitting the person).

It is the transfer of feelings reactions evoked by one topic or event to another that is less threatening. It is transfer of emotions from its original object to a substitute objects. Displacement refers to a release or redirection of feelings and impulses upon a safe object or person as a substitute for that which aroused the feeling.

Individuals who displaces feelings usually have no awareness of doing so. Later, they may look back on the events and realize that because they were angry with someone to whom they could not comfortably express the feelings, they took it out on another.

Displacement is a discharge of feelings on an object or person other than the one to which the feelings rightly belong. This involves shifting emotions toward a safer, less threatening person or object than the actual source of the feeling. For one more example Smt Asha has a very difficult day at her job. Her boss has been very critical of her efforts an important project. Although she did not express her frustration to her boss, when she arrived home, Smt Asha begins yelling at her husband and children.

Among the most noticeable occurrences of daily life that is that when an individual has been scolded and passed through the mill, as it were, by his boss, then he naturally takes it out on his nearest junior who cannot answer him back, and usually this unfortunate individual is his child or wife. There is no alternative since he cannot fire back upon the boss. This is an example of displacement, since, in it, one particular motive or emotion is turned from its natural objective on to some other object that is not in any way connected with the normal or natural one. And in many mental patients displacement is seen to an alarming extent. For example, the fear of suicide is expressed through fear of water or fear of knives. In this displacement the very notion of suicide passes out of the conscious mind but the emotion conjoined to that motive is manifested. Thus, displacement takes place when the normal expression of an emotion or motive is somehow inhibited. It is said that the burnt child dreads the fire, and this happens since the experience of burning is attached to the fire. This process of displacement takes place at some stage of life with everyone and generally it does not lead to much harm, but, as is usual with all these mental mechanisms any over-doing of it may very harmful.

Examples:
- The husband who is angry at his wife and yells at the family dog rather than dealing directly with his anger to his wife.
- A person angry with a superior at work or school may feel too threatened to confront that individual with anger, instead he or she may go home and vent the anger on a family member.
- The person punches a punching bag after an argument with boss.

Fantasy/Daydreaming

It is gratifying frustrated desires by imaginary achievement and wishful thinking to meet one's needs. Daydreaming or fantasy, is both escape and compensatory mechanism. It is means of tension, reduction and it helps the individual in imaginative planning invention, literature and arts. In a general sort of way, every individual is prone to make up for the failures and shortcomings of his life through his imagination to some extent. Consequently, fantasy as an adjustive mechanism is a normal one since it helps to reduce conflict and tension. One very vivid example of fantasy is daydreaming. Almost all adult individuals turn to daydreaming to some extent, and of college students two among every three are daydreamers, almost of the chronic type. The tendency to daydreaming is most pronounced in man during his adolescence and is comparatively less pronounced in infancy as well as in proper adulthood. One reason for the high degree of daydreaming during adolescence is that during this period the individual passes through a period of extensive mental conflicts and tantrums. Young boys and girls are on the threshold of their adult personalities towards which they are proceeding in this age, and their mental capabilities are becoming consciously developed. Sexual impulse develops very rapidly and occupies much of their thoughts. It manifests itself through the medium of self-love, homosexuality and heterosexual love. Imagination and sentimentality are rampant, a highly emotional sensibility is evident in adolescents. All these various factors combine and the individual is continually faced with novel problems that disturb and vex him. When they fail to find satisfactory solutions of these problems in their waking world, they turn to the domain of imagination and there work out their salvation. Fantasy controls and guides a persons desires and frustrations. Through its medium the individual finds more or less satisfaction for a motive that has been dissatisfied in the actual world, and the fantasy centers round the person seeing it, he being its sole hero. Fantasy helps the physically handicapped individual experience the satisfaction of having become a fine sportsman while the most ugly young lady finds her admirers in the fantasy even though not in actual life. The solitary reaper lives in the thickly populated world of his imagination, whose center she is. Fantasy conforms to the individuals age and position in life. Adolescent fantasy is more concerned with adventure, romance and success in future life while the older individuals relive their past lives with the help of this imagination. In this imaginary world, the fulfillment of motives is not faced with any insuperable obstacles. Generally speaking, if these fantastic imaging's do not take the place of actual action but remain sources of enjoyment and momentary pleasure, there is not much harm in them, instead there is positive good resulting from them since the moments of pleasure and contentment spent in the imaginary world renew a persons vigor and give him a new enthusiasm. Any new conflict to be overcome is met with new vigor and a more powerful resolve, but it becomes a chronic habit with the person to take leave of the actual world and spend much of his time in fruitless imagining then his adjustment with social life loses all reality. Any tendency to daydream too much is naturally considered despicable and harmful. Mental patients evince signs of very acute daydream tendencies.

Fantasy is gratifying frustrated desired by imaginary achievements. It is the defense mechanism involving tendency to retreat into fantasy in order to resolve inner and outer conflicts.

For example, imaging yourself beating up your boss with a chair after he is shouted at you is you fantasying to help make you feel better.

Humor: Overt expression of ideas and feeling (especially those that are unpleasant to focus on or too terrible to talk about) that gives pleasure to others. For example looking at the funny side of a situation can help you forget about the real situation.

Hypochondriasis: The transformation of negative feelings towards others into negative feelings toward self, pain, illness and anxiety, Hypochondrias (or hypochondria), sometimes referred to as health phobia refers to an excessive preoccupation or worry about having a serious illness. Often, hypochondria him/her that his/her concerns about symptoms do not have an underlying medical basis.

Identification

It is process by which a person tries to take on the characteristics of another admired individual. It is similar to and the result of intrajection. Unconscious modeling of another person so that basic values, attitudes and behavior are similar to those of a significant person or group, but overt behavior is manifested in an individual manner (Imitation is not considered as defense mechanism perse, but imitation usually precedes identification. Imitation consciously copying other's values, attitudes, movements, etc.). Identification is an attempt to increase self-worth by acquiring certain attributes and characteristics of an individual one admires.

Identification, as is evident from the term, consists in conjoining oneself to the achievement, success, and qualities of another individual or group, and feeling joy in these factors. The tendency towards such identification is evident in every individual to a greater or lesser extent. Fairly often, parents identify themselves with their children and find personal satisfaction in the fame and pleasure that their children acquire in the course of their life. In every country individuals are seen identifying themselves with the leaders in such various fields as politics, society, culture, etc. and they literally worship them. And at the root of the tendency to hero-worship is this inclination to identification. A majority of the youth are seen identifying themselves with various film personalities, copying their styles and mannerisms, imitating them and trying to emulate them in every respect. Sometimes this identification is so strong that the individual becomes oblivious to his own personality and behaves in conformity to the object with which identification is established. Again, different individuals identify themselves with their college, tuitions. Students are seen identifying themselves with their college, teams and groups while adults do the same in respect of clubs, professional organizations and highly sophisticated neighborhoods. It need hardly be pointed out that the sense of respect is conjoined to the object of identification, as a result of which the individual finds self-respect in its achievements.

Some people identify themselves with low, poor, suffering, cruel or characterless individuals because they suffer from a sense of guilt and want to punishment and pain upon themselves. In order to understand the significance of identification for mental disease it would be better to look at the following example.

Examples:

i. Mrs X was a woman of high social ambitions, but with limited means at her disposal. She very carefully pursued all the items of her local newspaper, and she knew the background, family life and members of every important family of her town. Names of such illustrations and famous people of her town were repeated in and out of her conversion, thereby creating the impression that she has intimate relations with all these families. She was invariably present at any occasion that may take place in any of these families, with her expression perfectly suiting the occasion and reflecting emotion, as if someone very near and dear to her was involved. It need not be pointed out that people of the kind of Mrs. X are to be seen by the dozen right around one if one looks at all carefully.
   The unconscious modeling of one's self upon another person's character and behavior. Some individuals try to resemble with another person's character, a lonely teenager begins copying the clothes and actions of a popular peer.
ii. Ms Jyothi, a college student begins to take and act like a Lecturer she admires.
iii. The adolescent's overtime manifests the assertive behavior and states ideas similar to those that she unaware that her behavior is similar.
   Identification is a modeling actions and opinions of influential others while searching for identity, or aspiring to reach a personal, social or occupational goal.
iv. Nursing student becoming ICU nurse because this is the speciality of an instructor she admires.
v. A teenage girl emulates the mannerisms and style of dress of a popular rock star.

Idealization: Subconsciously choosing to perceive another individual as having more positive qualities than he/she may actually have.

Intellectualization

It is avoiding unavoidable emotions by focusing on the intellectual aspects. It is separating from the emotional content of an event, focusing instead on the facts. Intellectualization protects gains anxiety by repressing the emotions connected with an event. Intellectualization works to reduce anxiety by thinking about events in a cold, clinical way. This defense mechanism allows us to avoid thinking about the stressful, emotional aspect of the situation and focus only on the intellectual component. For example, a person who has just been diagnosed with a terminal illness might focus on learning everything about the disease in order to avoid distress and remain distant from the reality of the situation.

It is the use of excessive reasoning rather than reacting or changing. For example, a woman attending an alcoholic anonymous meeting reports that she is a nurse and has conducted many such sessions. Through intellectualization, a person uses the intellectual powers of thinking, reasoning and analyzing to blunt or avoid emotional issues that are too threatening or painful. Feeling (personal) are often the heart of the issue in psychiatric mental health nursing, but facing them requires a degree of courage and confidence.

Intellectualization is an attempt to avoid expressing actual emotions associated with a stressful situation by using the intellectual processes of logic, reasoning and analysis. It is separation of the emotions of a painful events or situations from the facts involved, acknowledging the facts but not the emotions.

Examples:
- Person shows no emotional expression when discussing serious accidents.
- A wife who learns her husband is dying tries to learn all she can about the disease, prognosis, treatment options. By doing this she can help repress the emotional feelings of loss and anger which can accompany the death of a loved one.
- An alcoholic says, "Research shows I'm probably not an alcoholic/addict".

Introjection

It is identifying with some ideas or objects so deeply that it becomes a part of that person. It is complete acceptance of another's opinions and values as one's own.

Introjection refers to symbolic assimilation of or process of taking in attitudes, behavior, wishes, ideals or values of significant person into the ego and/or superego (a part of identification).

It is the internalization of the beliefs and values of another individual, so that they symbolically become a part of the self to the extent that feeling of separateness of distinctness is lost. It is accepting another person's attitudes, beliefs and values as one's own.

Introjection is one to the earliest mechanism developed, it is an increase form of identification which involves incorporation of another's qualities or values into one's self. It is incorporating, without examination or thought the qualities or attitudes of others.

Examples:
- A person who dislikes guns becomes an avid hunter, just like a best friend.
- Seven-year-old Savithri tells her younger brother "you must not spill your milk".
- The adolescent who takes on all the values and styles of an admired teacher.
  The client talks about how much he/she helps other people with their problems.
  An individual makes use of this mechanism, when he fears social retaliation and punishment.
- When an Indian officer enters into the enemy's land because he has lost his way, he introjects the enemy values and beliefs as a protection for himself.

Isolation

Isolation is the repression of the emotional component of a situation although the person is able to remember the thought, memory, or event dealing with problem, as interesting events that can be rationally explained but have no feelings attached.

It is separation of feelings from ideas and events. For example, describing a murder with graphic details with no emotional response. It is the separation of a thought or a memory from the feeling tone or emotions associated with it (emotional isolation).

Examples:
- The person talks about the spouse's death and details of the accident that caused it with an apathetic expression and without crying or signs of grieving.

- A young woman describes being attacked and raped by street gang. She displays an apathetic expression and no emotional tone.
- A physician is able to isolate his feelings about the eventual death of terminally ill cancer client, by his attention instead on the chemotherapy that will be given.

Negativism

Some children manifest the tendency to do the precise opposite of anything that they have been directed to do. Some examples follow:

- One young girl, relating her history, remarked that in her infancy she had been blamed for the mischief of her five brothers and sisters, and without heeding her pleadings her parents used to punish her for her alleged activity. She soon hit upon the idea of not answering the queries of her parents, and gradually developed and negative attitude towards any disciplinarian imposition upon her from whatever quarter it came. She always strongly objected to the anarchy of others and could never work well under the domination of others. She definitely and unequivocally contradicted each and every opinion expressed by her parents, so much so that she stopped meeting the person of whom her parents approved and that rejected any dress that her parents admired even if she herself linked it very much. This young girl had been brought up to a psychologist for treatment of obstinate and recalcitrant behavior.
- A young boy named Janakiram evinced much the same kind of reaction. When he was ten-year-old he with his sister went to live with his aunt after his parents had been divorced. His aunt was fond of girls but not of boys, and she was not reticent about hiding this aversion from the young boy. In reaction to this aversion Janakiram soon became so obstinate and naughty that it became necessary to put him in some concerned clinic for treatment.

It is quite evident from the above examples that normally negativity is manifested in reaction to very improper and highly prejudicial behavior, and takes the form of obstinacy and compulsive contradiction or negation. At the same time, it is also present in children who have been treated with too much love and are largely self-centered. Whenever some or the other desire of such children is thwarted, then they become obstinate, aggressive and violent. They are often ready to fight. They show much inclination to impose their will upon others and in adult life show very strong determination and obstinacy of a high order, not being very tractable. One very usual form of behavior in such persons is their thinking themselves superior to their colleagues and their constant endeavor to prove this superiority. It gives them much pleasure to be thought bigger and be asked for their advice in most matters, and in such things they are inclined to extend their heartiest cooperation. But, if one the contrary, some decision is reached without their cooperation being actively sought, they will very vigorously oppose even if it be the most appropriate and will be prepared to concoct all kinds of arguments in order to prove their point. In the political field, the tendency towards negativism is to be seen in many political leaders. It is an inclination found in all the great dictators of the world.

Projection

It is unconscious denial of unacceptable feelings and emotions in oneself while attributing to others. It is a primitive form of paranoia. It also reduces anxiety by allowing the expression of the undesirable impulses or desires without becoming consciously aware of them, e.g. when losing, an argument you state "You are just stupid". It is defense mechanism that involves taking our own unacceptable qualities or feelings and ascribing them to other people. For example, if you have a strong dislike for someone, you might instead that he or she does not like you. Projection functions to allow the expression of the desire or impulse, but in a way that the ego cannot recognize, therefore reducing anxiety. It is shifting one's unacceptable thoughts, feelings and impulses within oneself onto someone else, such that those same thoughts, feelings, beliefs and motivation are perceived as being possessed by the other.

Projection implies the act of recreating one's own motives and characteristics in another person. A student failing at the examination conveniently blames the teachers for his failure. This is an old practice, beginning with Adam in the garden of Eden where Adam blamed Satan for his downfall who immediately passed the responsibility on the snake. And right from that ancient day. The descendents of Satan and Adam are busy in passing the responsibility whenever is shows signs of settling on them. At the root of projection is the desire to protect one's self-respect from the terribly painful pangs of conscience as one's own faults are casually transferred to another person. Individuals who are constantly found complaining to others of their foolishness, selfishness and obstinacy never find cause to complain of the same shortcomings in their own mental make up, and thus they protect their self-respect from self-criticism. Thus, whenever you find some person constantly criticizing other people, you may take it for granted that at least some of the traits that he criticizes are certainly to be found in himself. This does not imply that people indulge in projection in order to conceal their own shortcomings. In fact, the process of projection is an unconscious one, and the person indulging in it is not aware that he is doing it. The truth of the matter lies in the fact that people who are aware of their own faults are rarely inclined to blame others for their failures. On the other hand, men ignorant of the real faults that lie embedded in their own personality are the ones most prone to this fault.

Examples of projection may be found more usually in fields in which personal relationships and laws are very avidly protected and respected. One such field is that of the family. Within the family the crude husband is seen projecting elements of crudity upon the wife while a crude wife does the same with her husband. Some husbands and wives blame their children for the domestic bliss that is lacking in their life. Unmarried mothers in particular are seen blaming their unwanted offspring for all infamy brought upon them, because had the offspring not been born, they could have retained respected place in society notwithstanding their immoral activities. Many patents who have themselves never been very good students in the classroom never tire in delivering long tirades on study to their unfortunate children. Many mothers whose own married life has never been at a very high level of success and contentment expect from their daughters that they will be very well-adjusted in their marriages. Baby has given example of the phenomenon of projection.

It is an unconscious blaming of unacceptable inclinations or thoughts of an external object. Protection involves displacing feeling, usually feeling, perceived, as negative, on to another individual. In projection attribution of one's own thoughts, impulses, wishes, or characteristics to another person. In other words, placing blame for own difficulties upon others or the attribution of one's own thoughts and feeling to another person in an effort to block awareness of their existence in one's self.

Examples:
- Man who has thought about same gender sexual relationship, but never had one, beats a man who is gay.
- A person with many prejudices loudly identifies others as bigots.
- A person feels guilty (or angry, dependent, aggressive, hostile) and this feeling is unacceptable, he or she may project it unto another rather than owning up to it.
- Woman unable to admit her own hostile feelings, remarks that other people are always getting angry at her.
- The student who fails an examination may feel that the teacher was unfair.

The following statements could indicate projection:
- "I am not attracted to him. My best friend is."
- "I am not angry, but she mad at me."
- "I do not have any bad feelings toward him, but he sure hates me."

Individuals with paranoid behavior frequently over uses projection. Projection is the attribution of feeling or impulses unacceptable to one's self to another person. The individual passes the blame for the undesirable feeling or impulses to another, thereby providing relief for the anxiety associated with them.

Rationalization

It is another commonly used mechanism. It is an attempt to justify unacceptable behavior through the use of socially approved or apparently logical explanations. It is intellectual explaining away of threatening circumstances. Rationalization refers to the substitution of acceptable reasons for the actual reasons that motivate behavior. Through rationalization, a person justifies behavior or conceals disappointments. In this excusing own behavior or conceals disappointment. In this excusing own behavior to avoid guilt, responsibility, conflict, anxiety or loss of respect.

One very prominent tendency in man is that he finds some or the other plausible and reasonable excuse even for his worst failures. And this clouding of one's motives, desires and failures is called rationalization. One's self-respect is maintained intact through this mechanism and one also avoids at the hands of others by convincing others of his helplessness in his failure. What is mainly worth noting in rationalization is the fact that the reasons for failure are all occurred, and the greater the number of arguments produced for one's failure, the more is evident that person's actual hollowness and lack of real profundity. Boys who are very much used to aimless wandering and loitering justify such activity by stating that it gives them inspiration for their study. Students who right from the school leaving stage to the university level never secure a good division, they talk in terms of accidental disease at examination time, or their matter, their lack of sufficient time to prepare for the examination or, for that matter, their lack of interest in the higher divisions instead of blaming their own lack of intelligence. Some say that it is devil who makes haste. But in fact proverbs of this kind are the outcome of lazy and docile genius as it is seen that people working faster and more precipitately are more successful and accurate as compared to those who take their time.

The mental mechanism of rationalization is not limited only to personal matters. Sometimes even responsible government heads are observed putting forward the most flimsy and meaningless pretexts for entering upon conflict with another nation. One such notable example came to notice that when China threatened India that it would attack, because some Indian soldiers had stolen some sheep belonging to them. There is hardly any need to point out the purely ridiculous nature of such a pretext for engaging in a long war. Much the same sort of rationalization is evident in the case of the preverbal fox who argued that the grapes were sour and so she would not try for them. Things that are outside reach are characterized in this manner as undesirable, and much of the pain accorded that they do not like the idea of serving under anybody and hence are not prepared to go into service. When a man is rejected by his beloved, he rationalizes upon the failure by saying that he does not want to marry her. One very important example of rationalization is evident in the philosophy that the world that we live in is the best of all possible worlds. Some extremely poor people are fond of saying that the pleasure in masticating a bit of rough bread is much greater than is to be found in the pleasures of the rich and the wealthy. Some people believe some of their successes to be the outcome of their other frustrations and it is possible of this kind who believe that there is some element of good concealed in every bad thing. And through rationalization of this kind the individual succeeds in making his faults his best qualities. An ugly girl satisfies herself by thinking that at least she is safe from the unwanted notice of wayside people. One young man was quite distressed by his out-size ears but he soon hit upon the scheme of claiming that because of these elongated appendages he was in a position to distinguish between the most subtle musical sounds. On the basis of this rationalization, however, he went to the extreme of taking training in music and succeeded in becoming a teacher of that subject.

Examples:

- Basant fails an examination and blames his ineffective instructor, rather than his lack of studying.
- Students blames failure on teacher being mean.
- Rationalization is the justification of behavior or offering a socially acceptable, intellectual and apparently logical explanation for an actor decision actually caused by unconscious or verbalized impulses. Behavior in response to unrecognized motive precedes reasons for it.
- Man says he beats his wife because she does not listen to him.
- A student fails a course but maintains that the course was not important and that the grade can be made up in another course.
- A student may say "the tests had too many trick questions, I really know all the material; our instructor was out to get me".
- The fox tried and did not get grapes, said grapes are sour.
- A woman with over-extended credit cards rationalized that she can use her savings to pay for a new dress she recently purchased.

Reaction Formation

Reaction formation is unacceptable impulses repressed, denied and reacted by opposite overt behavior. It is an expression of feelings that is the opposite of one's authentic feelings, or feelings that would be appropriate in the situation. Using reaction formation, a person acts in a way opposite to how he or she feels, because the feelings are unacceptable. It is acting the opposite to what one thinks or feels.

Converting unconscious wishes or impulses that are perceived to be dangerous into their opposites; behavior that is completely the opposite of what one really wants or feels; taking the opposite belief because the true belief causes anxiety. This defense can work effectively for coping in the short-term, but will eventually breakdown. Reaction formation reduces anxiety by taking up the opposite feeling, impulse, or behavior. An example of reaction formation would be treating someone you strongly dislike in an excessively friendly manner order to hide your true feelings. Why do people behave this way? According to Freud, they are using reaction formation as a defense mechanism to hide their true feelings by behaving in the exact opposite manner.

Reaction formation is the prevention of unacceptable or undesirable thoughts or behavior from being expressed by exaggerating opposite thoughts or types of behavior. In reaction formation, as is evident from the name, an undesirable tendency is not only prevented but in reaction to it an opposing or contradictory tendency is formed. It was Shakespeare who said that too vehement denial amounts to admission of guilt. People with very strong sexual tendencies become highly religious thought a defense reaction. In reacting to the repression of criminal tendencies many people become highly conscious of law and order, and abide by it religiously. Judges with these mentality award very rigorous punishments to criminal brought for trial for antisocial activity. A mother very conscious of and worried about her children's health administers her anger and hatred indirectly through extreme punishment. She gives them bitter medicines, does not permit them to eat certain kinds of foods, nor to play with other children, nor to move out of the house very much. Some very strong teetotalers are often those who have done much drinking in their younger days which they would probably like to forget. And among people who most vociferously carry on the campaign against various social vices are the ones who are actually victims to these very social evils. Men who wish to improve the morals of their society probably read pornographic literature as their positive contribution to the cause, and see immoral exhibition in order that they may justly criticize such activity.

From the above consideration on the nature of reaction formation, it should not be deduced that thereby the value of some such quality as social work, religiosity, spirituality or other trait is in any way reduced. On the contrary, reaction formation has considerable importance from the point of view of society because due to it many antisocial characteristics are turned into socially beneficial reactions and the individual's energy becomes engaged in constructive activity instead of antisocial work. Nevertheless, too much reaction formation in individuals is a sign of abnormality.

Examples:

- Women who never wanted to have children become a Superman.
- Person who despises the boss tells everyone what a great boss he is.
- A married woman who unconsciously disturbed by feeling sexually attracted to one of her husband's friends treats him rudely and keeps him at a safe distance.
- A client who brings gifts to the nurse at whom he is really mad.

In reaction formation, the person disguises unacceptable thoughts and feeling by developing attitudes and behavior patterns that are opposite to what is really felt or believed.

- A staff nurses in her word faces a fight with another staff member, and she goes to adjoining ward and shows exactly opposite behavior, i.e. laughing and talking pleasant events. Having a bias against a particular race or culture and then embracing that race or culture of the extreme.
- A staff nurse, has intense feelings of anger toward her Nurse Supervisor, she covers them up by being extremely polite.

- A person who feels aggressive or hostile toward another might behave very kindly and politely toward the object of those feelings.
- The person who uses reaction formation is not aware of the great disparity between feelings and actions.

Regression

Regression is returning to an earlier stage of behaviors when stress creates, problems at the present stage, involving less mature responses and usually lower level of aspiration.

It refers to retreat to a previous developmental level. It is a normal part of growth and development. It is a retreat from excessive stress through specific behavior characteristic of an earlier level of development. It is an immature way of responding to a stress and moving back to a previous development stage.

Say, sitting in a corner and crying after hearing bad news; throwing a temper tantrum when you don't' get your way. When confronted by stressful events, people sometimes abandon coping strategies and revert to patterns of behaviors used earlier in development. Anna Freud called this defense mechanism regression, suggesting that people act out behaviors for the stage of psychosexual development in which they are fixated. For example, an individual fixated at an earlier development stage might cry upon hearing unpleasant news. Behaviors associated with regression can vary greatly depending upon which stage the person is fixated at. An individual fixated at the oral stage might begin eating or smoking excessively, or might become very verbally aggressive.

Examples:

- A child starts to suck his thumb (after 2 years of not thumb sucking) when admitted to hospital.
- Four-year-old Kamala has been toilet trained for about one year. However, when her new baby brother is brought home from the hospital, she begins to wet her pants again.

In regression, adopting behavior characteristic of a previous developmental level; the ego returns to an immature but more gratifying state of development in thought, feeling or behavior.

- The person takes a nap, curled in a fetal position, upon arriving home after stressful day at work.
- The three-year-old child who begins wetting his pants after the birth of a new sibling.

Regression is the retreating to an earlier level of development and other comfort measures associated with this level of functioning.

- A person who is depressed may withdraw to his or her room, curl-up in fetal position on the bed, sleeps for long periods.

Fixation

A fixation at the anal stage might result in excessive tidiness or messiness.
It refers to immobilization of a portion of the personality resulting from unsuccessful completion of tasks in developing stage.

Examples:

- Never learning to delay gratification.
- Lack of clear sense of identity as an adult.

Repression

Repression is another well-known defense mechanism. Repression acts to keep information out of conscious awareness. However, these memories do not just disappear, they contribute to influence our behavior. For example, a person who has repressed memories of abuse suffered as a child may later have difficulty forming relationships. It is process of pulling thoughts into the unconscious and preventing painful or dangerous thoughts from entering consciousness, memory lapse or lack of awareness of one's own situation and condition. It is the complete memory loss of a painful event. In this case, your subconscious mind does not want you to remember what happened because it may negatively affect your mood. It is involuntary exclusion from consciousness of these ideas, feelings and situations, that are creating conflict and causing discomfort. After an accident, an individual don't want to talk about that accident.

Freud attributed repression to the mental conflict that occurs between the id, ego and superego. Repression is a kind of defence mechanism. It is based on the hedonistic principle. In it pleasure is accepted and pain summarily rejected. Immoral and antisocial desires that arise in the conscious mind of man are repressed by the superego. These repressed thoughts, desires and feelings are manifested through dreams, mental complexes, day-dreams, etc. Generally speaking, repression is not especially harmful but if it exceeds the normal limits then it may lead to mental disease and abnormality.

In the three forms of selective forgetting, repression, suppression and inhibition, it is quite apparent that selective forgetting is different from ordinary forgetting. Ordinary forgetting occurs through the gradual lessening of intensity in memories as time passes. While, on the other hand, selective forgetting is a defense mechanisms in which emotionally intense memories are unconsciously removed forcibly from the conscious sphere of man's thinking. This is not complete forgetting since psychoanalysis can help to recover such memories and bring them again to the conscious level.

In order to understand the nature of repression however, it is essential to understand inhibition. In the process of inhibition some motives, thoughts and desires are removed from active memory to be replaced by other motives, thoughts and desires that differ from them somewhat. Roughly speaking, repression and inhibition differ in the following respects:

1. While in inhibition the novel reactions are similar to the forgotten reactions, in repression these reactions are almost completely different, even to such an extent that the individual cannot recognize them.
2. Both in inhibition and repression motives, thoughts and desires are discarded and rendered obnoxious, but as compared with inhibition in repression the rejection and disgust is stronger and more intense. It has been pointed out that in repression the repressed motives is not even recognized.
3. The process of inhibition takes place at the conscious level while the repressive process in unconscious.
4. In inhibition the undesirably and unsuitably of motive is normal and bearable, while in repression it is very intense and unbearable.
5. Inhibition is essential for mental health, and it helps in the development of personality. On the other hand, repression is harmful for mental health and it leads to disorganization of personality. In this way inhibition is the tool of adjustment, repression is not.

There are two forms of inhibition as given below:

i. *Retroactive Inhibition:* Whenever we gain some new experience, many of our older memories are wiped out of the mind since the new experiences inhibit them. This is called retroactive inhibition.
ii. *Proactive Inhibition:* Sometimes it is some of the older experiences, that prove inhibiting to the new experiences, and this phenomenon is known as proactive inhibition.

It is often referred to as "selective forgetting". It is widely used mechanism in which unacceptable thoughts and feelings are unconsciously kept out of awareness. Requires considerable energy to keep material repressed. It is an automatic, involuntary exclusion of a painful or conflictual feeling, thought, impulse, experience or memory from awareness. The thought or memory of the event is not consciously perceived. It is unconscious blocking from awareness material that is threatening or painful. Repression is the involuntary blooding of pleasant feelings and experiences from one's awareness. Excluding emotionally painful or anxiety. Provoking thoughts and feelings from conscious awareness.

Examples:

- Woman has no memory of the mugging she suffered yesterday.
- "I never got angry at my father, our family lived in harmony and love" (when such description of the family, life would not fit with any one else, interpretation of events).
- A woman cannot remain being sexually assaulted when she was 15-year-old.
- The married woman who expresses hostility toward a male coworker to avoid dealing with her sexual attractions, to him.
- A woman has no memory before age seven when she was removed from abusive parents.
- The mother seems unaware of the date or events surrounding her child's death and shows no emotions when the death is discussed.

Reality Evasion

One simple method, that of the ostrich, is simply to close one's eye in trying to evade the painful and bitter experiences arising out of the environment. Many people are immune to any and every criticism for the simple reason that they are not prepared to listen to it, and keep their ears turned to a different wavelength. Almost all their difficult decisions are left for a tomorrow, and tomorrow, and tomorrow. Many senile people do not find it agreeable to accept that their mental and physical powers are continuously on the decline as they advance in age. Backward students do not find any reliability in intelligence tests. When some very near and dear one in the family dies, some people try to keep up the pretense that he is alive, and for this they resort to various tricks such as keeping the deceased person's belongings and room in perfect order, in the manner in which he used to maintain it during his life-time. At the dining table his place is left vacant, and they are sometimes even seen holding imaginary conversations with him. All such examples amount to reality evasion. Through this mental mechanism an individual refuses to grant the factual occurrence of certain events that are undesirable and painful in order that he may forget them. Its serious development may lead to the occurrence of mental disease and a high degree of abnormality in the individual.

Resistance

Overt or covert antagonism toward remembering or processing anxiety producing information.

Example: Nurse it too busy with tasks to spend time talking to a dying patient.

Selective Forgetting

One simple method of avoiding pain of distressing circumstances is the forgetting of them, and most people do use the method. This forgetting is selective. Experiments have proved that painful experiences are forgotten sooner than soothing and pleasurable experiences. And, usually one forgets the promises that one does not want to remember or fulfill. Selective forgetting has been classified into the following two type—suppression and repression.

a. *Suppression:* Intentional and forcible ejection of painful tendencies and memories from the field of consciousness is called suppression. For example if a young student causes a serious accident through momentary lapse of caution, the memory of this accident will pinch him occasionally. Hence, he tries to concentrate on other subjects consciously and thus tries to remove this memory from his consciousness. This is the process of suppression.
b. *Repression:* Contrary to the process of suppression, that of repression is unconscious, and in it painful experiences, memories, tendencies and thoughts are pushed from the conscious mind into its unconscious recesses, and are prevented from re-entering into the conscious one by creating an obstacle wall. Memories that are repressed are often of a traumatic kind. In treating mental patients Freud saw that most of the patients have recourse to repression in order to throw undesirable emotions and thoughts out of the conscious mind. Repression has the effect either of attaining a complete forgetfulness with regard to these memories or at least of reducing their intensity and immediacy. The process of repression was discovered by Freud during his treatment of a hysteric patient. He found that many patients exhibit signs of paralysis and approaching blindness but that neither of these diseases have any physical basis. These patients were incapable of remembering their fatal experiences and only after mental therapy could they recall them.

In the example of suppression if the student forgets the memory of the accident unconsciously and cannot recall it even upon conscious effort, then it is a state of repression. Repressed memories, thoughts and experiences may be recalled through analysis. The aim of repression is the removal of all mental conflict. It at least helps to clear the conscious sphere of mental conflict.

Suppression

It is an intentional exclusion of material from consciousness. In this conscious or unconscious attempt to keep threatening material out of consciousness or conscious or deliberate forgetfulness of painful or undesirable thoughts and ideas.

Examples:

- A rape victim attempts to forget the incident and fails to report it to the proper authorities.
- Failure to remember a significant childhood event such as death of a grandmother.
- Suppressions occurs when certain anxiety producing thoughts and feelings re-consciously excluded from consideration. A person deciding to "put something out

of mind" or "not worry about it until tomorrow in using suppression". The classic example of suppression found is "Gone with the Wind"/ when Scarlett 'O' Hara faces insurmountable odds with the words "I won't think about that today. I'll think of it tomorrow".

Suppression: It is the conscious process of pushing thoughts into the preconscious, able to later access uncomfortable or distressing emotions and accepts them. It is voluntary exclusion from consciousness of those ideas, feelings and situations that are creating conflict and causing discomfort. For example, more concentrating on examination by suppressing friends argument. The postabortive woman is consciously pushing down negative or painful feelings as they begin to surface.

Sublimation

It refers to substitution of a socially acceptable behavior for an unacceptable sexual or aggressive drive or impulse. This is channelizing of socially unacceptable impulses into socially acceptable activity. It is a normal form of dealing with undesirable feelings or thoughts by keeping them in an acceptable context.

The transformation of negative emotions or instincts into positive actions, behavior or emotion is sublimation. Sublimation is a defense mechanism that allows us to act out unacceptable impulses by converting these behaviors into a more acceptable form. For example, a person experiencing extreme anger might take up kick boxing as a means of venting frustration. Freud believed that sublimation was a sign of maturity that allows people to function normally in socially acceptable ways.

The process of sublimation is constructive, not negative. It consists in the change in directions of the motives. And, even as it is, some sublimation of the child's impulses is always taking place during his socialization. And it is only because of sublimation that very many normal people have succeeded in achieving great heights in the field of intellectual, esthetic and spiritual endeavor. Sublimation is a healthy solution of problems that arise in a persons social adjustment, and in civilized society it is required all the more because every expression of an individuals impulses has been shackled by rules and laws. Sublimation succeeds not only in achieving satisfaction of the drive but also much fame for the individual through very valuable social work and through manifestations of constructive tendencies. Thus, the psychologists suggest sublimation for everyone.

For example, sublimating your aggressive impulses toward a career as a boxer; becoming a surgeon because of your desire to cut; lifting weights to release 'pent-up' energy to satisfy hidden needs of violence. An artist attracted to a married person may rechannel sexual energy into creating a beautiful statue of the person.

Examples:

- Person who has quit smoking sucks on hard candy when the urge to smoke arises.
- The woman who is unable to bear children begins working in a preschool.
- A young man who is dealing with aggression by playing football.

Sublimation is the rechannelizing of drives or impulses that are personally or socially unacceptable (aggressiveness, anger, sexual drive) into activities that are more tolerable and constructive.

It is the mechanisms by which a primitive or unacceptable tendency is redirected into socially constructive channels. An individual selects substitutes for satisfaction that is healthy. Here the transformation of energy associated with unacceptable urges into socially approved pursuits. This is thought to be one of the more important mechanism in the precise of learning.

Example: Mr Chandrappa has an extremely aggressive nature. He is able, tough to transfer energy associated with his aggressive impulses to becoming a star tackle on his high school football team.

Substitution

Replacing the desired gratification with one that is more readily available.

Example: Woman who would like her own children, opens a day care center.

Symbolization

It is use of an object, idea or act to express emotion that is not expressed directly. In which, one object or act unconsciously represents a complex group of objects and acts, some of which may be in conflict or unacceptable, to the ego, external objects or acts stand for any internal or repressed in desire, idea, attitude of feeling. The symbol may not overtly appear to be related to the repressed ideas or feelings.

Examples:
- A client who leaves the nurse a flower rather than directly saying she cares about the nurse.
- The husband sends his wife a bouquet of roses which ordinarily represents love and beauty. But roses have thorns, his beautiful wife is hard to live with, but he consciously focuses on her beauty.

Undoing

It refers to exhibiting acceptable behavior to make up for negating unacceptable behavior. It is an act of symbolically negating or cancelling out a previous action or experience that one finds intolerable. Is an act, communication or thought that cancels the significance or partially negates a previous one; treating an experience as if it had never occurred.

Examples:
- The husband purchases a gift for his wife after a quarrel the previous evening.
- When a child commits a mistake, he apologies to his parents and thinks that he can start all over again with a clean state and with renewed parental approval. As a consequences of such early learning, people commonly develops methods of undoing their misleads and methods to avoid punishments and self-devaluation.
- A man pills some salt on the table, then sprinkles some over his left shoulder to prevent back luck.

Withdrawal

Whenever an individual suspects he is likely to be criticized, ridiculed or disgraced on account of some prior unfortunate experience or failure, then he resorts to what is known as withdrawal. This tendency of withdrawal is to be seen in the form of a shy, solitude-loving and frightened nature. Such a person is always seen avoiding all hard work and exclaiming that he cannot do this, he cannot do that. Burnham has elucidated the condition of 'pseudo-feeble-mindedness' in his examples of very acute withdrawal. It is more often to be seen in weak individuals, and the policy that they adopt is that nothing attempted nothing done, such a policy cannot win them any punishment, criticism and frustration. Hence, they do not take any interest in their work and do their best to avoid it. Sometimes the weapon of withdrawal has the worst effect inasmuch that positively intelligent youngsters and adults are branded idiots and morons on account of their inclination to avoid work though if they are trained and encouraged they may prove quite useful and often very intelligent.

Passive aggression: Aggression towards others expressed indirectly or passively. Passive aggressive defenses create a disorder known as passive aggressive personality disorder (also called negativistic personality disorder) is said to be marked by a pervasive pattern of negative attitude and passive, usually resistance in interpersonal or occupational areas. This is said to stem from a specific childhood stimulus (e.g. overbearing parental figures, or alcohol/ drug addicted parents). These persons show certain behaviors such as ambiguity, avoiding responsibility by claiming forgetfulness, blaming other, chronic lateness and forgetfulness, complaining, do not express hostility or anger openly (e.g. express it instead by leaving notes) fear of authority, competition, dependency and intimacy.

26

CHAPTER

Adjustment

Introduction

The word 'adjustment' means 'to fit', make suitable, adapt, arrange, modify, harmonize, correspondence with. Whenever we make an adjustment between two things, we adapt or modify one or both of them to correspond to each other.

Primary interest of everyone is human adjustment, must have a thorough background in physiology. He must know something about the organs of adjustment, especially the brain and nervous system and the wonderfully complex, interacting endocrine gland system. Here an overview of these systems will be given as a background for the understanding of many of the specifies of human behavior, for without these structures there could be no human behavior or conscious experience.

Adjust means to alter (something) slightly in order to achieve a correct or desired result or adopt or becomes used to a new situation. The word, adjustment means to fit, make suitable, adapt, arrange, modify, harmonize, corresponds with, whenever an adjust between two things. People adapt or modify one or both of them to correspond to each other. It is the establishment of satisfactory relationship, as representing, harmony, conformance, adaptation, etc. It is a continual process in which a person varies his behavior to produce a more harmonious relationship between himself and his environment. So it is process of findings and adapting modes of behavior suitable to the environment or changes in the environment. Adjustment is said to be adequate, wholesome or healthful to the extent that he has established harmonies relationship between himself and the conditions, situation and individuals who compromise his physical or social environment.

The person purposefully applies efforts and energy to accommodate perfectly to the society and to the environment to fulfill individuals total needs and to lead a happy social life. The adjustment is highly selective and a specialized process. The adjustment of a civilized man is less stable and more dynamic. However, he is capable of readjustment with new environment and there is remarkable mobility in the process of adjustment.

Adjustment is the process by which a living organism maintains a balance between its needs and the circumstances that influence the satisfaction of these needs (Laurence F Shaffer). Accordingly, the process of adjustment has two main elements: the needs of the living organism, and the circumstances that influence those needs. These needs may be biogenic, sociogenic, personal or communal, or arising from any other conceivable source. On the other hand, the circumstances influencing these needs also can either be inside the individual or outside him. Factors within the individual that influence these needs are his physical and mental states, capacity, attitudes, interests, etc. For example, most weakly constituted individuals cannot fulfill their own psychological motives, and thus their needs are definitely effected by their lack of strength. Factors existing within the environment are usually geographical conditions, social conditions, political and cultural influences. And, these conditions and circumstances may help as well as deter the fulfillment of the individuals requirements. In this manner, the nature of influences upon the person's needs can be of two kinds—favorable and unfavorable. Positive or favorable influences help in the fulfillment of needs while unfavorable influences hinder their satisfaction.

Thus, adjustment refers to an interactions between a person and his environment by which he adapts depend upon his personal characteristics and circumstances of a situation producing a more hormones relationship between himself and environment.

DEFINITIONS OF ADJUSTMENT

- According to Warren (1934), any operation whereby an organism becomes more favorably related to the environment or to the entries situation, environmental and internal.
- According to Webster (1951), it is the establishment of satisfactory relationship, as representing, harmony, conformance, adaptation, etc.
- According to Gates and Jersild (1948), a continual process in which a person varies his behavior to produce a more harmonious relationship between himself and his environment.
- According to Cater V Good (1959), the process of finding and adopting modes of behavior suitable to the environment or the changes in the environment.
- According to Crow and Crow (1956), an individuals adjustment is said to be adequate, wholesome or healthful to the extent that he has established harmonious relationship between himself and the conditions, situations, and persons who compromise his physical or social environment.
- Vonhaller (1970) says that adjustment is psychological survival.

Thus, adjustment is defined as an interaction between a person and his environment by which he adapts depends upon his personal characteristics and circumstances of a situation producing a more harmonious relationship between himself and his environment.

MAN AS A IN ADJUSTING LIVING BEING

Since man as an organism—a living being made up of interdependent parts (organs) which, working together, enable it to meet demands made on it. Psychology is concerned with the adjustive behavior through which man meets these demands, whether they derive from his biological needs or those of social origin. If an individual is thirsty, he may seek a drink of water, if he is badgered by his mother, he may rebel. Both responses are adjustive. Because activity may be initiated by conditions outside his a body or within his own tissues and physiological processes, psychologists distinguish between his external environment and his internal one, though of course no sharp line can be drawn between organism and environment.

Adjustment to inner and outer demands is a continuing and never-completed process: as long as a person lives, he is adjusting. Sometimes he adjusts by changing his surrounding, as when he builds a house for shelter or moves to another town to find a better job. Sometimes he adjusts by changing himself, and when he goes to night school to improve his opportunities for promotion. Whatever form adjustment takes, it always involves a complex relationship between the individuals and individuals needs, the opportunities provided by his particular environment, and his competence in using the resources available to him.

Normally many activities are going on at once in the human organism. Yet man behaves as a whole in the sense that, even though he may be reacting to an intricate pattern of conditions, he does not one main thing at a time. For example, as a person drives along in a car he may at the same time be mentally reviewing for an examination or thinking about last night's date. Other secondary activities, such as breathing, sweating, and hearing surrounding noises, are also taking place. But still he obeys the traffic signals, for he is doing one main things at a time—driving a car.

The secondary activities, if they are to persist, must either support the main thing that is being done or at least not seriously interfere with it. When an activity is antagonistic to the one main thing, it tends to be suppressed, or inhibited. Under normal conditions all of one's activities are smoothly integrated. Man functions as a whole.

The organs of the human body are classified into two chief groups, according to whether they (1) function internally to maintain the individuals health and growth or (2) function in the individual activities in the environment as he overcomes obstacles to the satisfaction of his needs. The first group, called the organs of maintenance, includes the heart and blood vessels, the lungs, the alimentary canal and its digestive glands, and the liver. The second group, known as the organs of adjustment, includes the muscles, the skeleton, and certain glands. The organs of adjustment enable the organism to carry on such activities as finding food, mating, and working. The organs of maintenance and adjustment are coordinated and regulated by the endocrine glands, which work through the circulatory system, and by the central nervous system.

STIMULUS, ORGANIZATION, RESPONSE AND FEEDBACK

The word stimulus (plural stimuli) comes from the Latin word meaning 'goad'. In psychology a stimulus is regarded as some form of radiant, chemical, or other energy which, if sufficiently strong, acts on a specially sensitive tissue in the eye, ear, skin or other sense organs, setting off nerve impulses. Thus a doorbell is a stimulus object, and the sound waves it emits are stimuli that enter a person's ear and create the sensation of hearing—perhaps leading to the response of going to the door.

A very brief and inadequate formula for adjustive behavior is S→R, where S stands for stimulus and R stands for response. Early experimentation inspired by this oversimplified model consisted, for the most part, of varying stimuli in systematic ways and observing the changes in response, in an attempt to discover consistent relationships between stimulus conditions and given reponses. Such relationships are not invariable, because consequences of past behavior and the presence of various processes within the organism, especially in the brain and nervous system can influence the behavior that follows a given stimulus.

It is generally assumed that when a response (behavior) is observed, there must have been a stimulus to produce it. If no stimulus is apparent, an internal one has been postulated. Studies have shown that in some cases an internal stimulus may be applied directly to a nerve cell rather than to a sensory receptor cell. The organism is never immobile and passive in the absence of external stimulation to arouse it to action. Instead it is constantly active, scanning its surroundings, monitoring its own actions, seeking certain conditions and avoiding others. Stimulation may serve as a goad to action but external stimulation is not essential for action. Such stimuli may serve only to guide behavior—as a source of information to be used in improving an ongoing action or stored for later use.

The Gestalt psychologists have been the severest critics of the S→R formula. Most psychologists today prefer the S→O→R model, where the O inserted between the S and the R symbolizes the internal conditions and organizing processes which, although difficult or impossible to observe at times, are logical constructs essential to our understanding of the behavior we see. One more term must be introduced in the picture of the organism as an adjusting system to round out the picture. Both the S→R and the S→O→R formulas give the impression that a unit of behavior is terminated by the muscular or glandular response, R. This is far from the case. Typically the response produces some change in the environment which, in turn, leads to further action. While driving, you hear an automobile horn honking—S. Past experience causes you to seek an explanation—O. You glance in the review mirror—R—but your response does not stop at that point. You see another car following closely, and you respond by pressing harder on the accelerator. Your response of looking in the mirror supplied sensory feedback, which served as a new stimulus. Thus, we see that our formula will not be really adequate unless we add the element of sensory feedback.

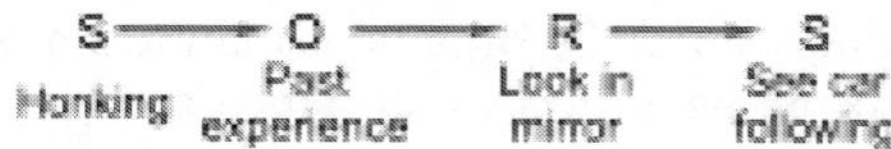

Sensory feedback, since it aided in adjustment, can be expected to affect the tendency to look in the mirror when an aid to adjustment is needed in a similar situation in the future.

PROCESS OF ADJUSTMENT

Human situation is a constantly changing one. New conditions and problems are constantly besetting the individual right from his infancy to his death-bed, and he is invariably engaged in trying to find a satisfactory and pleasurable solution to them by employing his intelligence and other gifts of the mind and body. In other words, life is the name of this unceasing process, the process of adjustment.

An analysis of the process of adjustment will reveal the presence of the following main elements:

1. *Motive:* The process of adjustment in the living being is set in motion by the presence within him of some motive or need.
2. *Thwarting conditions:* When the environment does not present any thing that tends to become obstacle in the fulfillment of these needs, then the adjustment is natural, facile and effortless, and no problems arise. But if circumstances create obstacles in the path of such fulfillment, then the process of adjustment continues.
3. *Varied responses:* Once the fulfillment of a need has been obstructed, the individual indulges in various actions whish are a reaction to the obstacle such a reaction made by normal jut as much as it may be abnormal.
4. *Solution:* As a result of these reactions and responses the individual achieves a degree of adjustment with the circumstances. The problem of adjustment is thereby solved.

All these various component elements of adjustment may be well-understood with the aid of concrete example. A student is actuated by a strong desire to stand first in his class, and to do so by scoring very well. He works extremely hard but fails to achieve his objective because he has not the necessary mental equipment. Lack of the requisite intelligence forms an obstacle to the satisfaction of this motive, and hence, as a result, the student condescends to lower his aim somewhat by aiming at securing a second division. In order to accommodate this change of objective the student changes his mode of study. A change of response, a suitable modification of the objective, and the objective is achieved with satisfaction. The adjustment problem is also solved. Such a process of adjustment is a universal phenomenon, and it is to be seen at every level of life, at various times and under most conditions.

PROCESS OF MALADJUSTMENT

The process of maladjustment is the same as the process of adjustment. It involves motives, thwarting and maladjusted activities which will be explained in sequence as given below:

1. *Motivation:* The process of adjustment may be set in motion by any motive, for example, our physical needs are constantly being manifested in the form of adjustive behavior patterns. But from the point of view of abnormal psychology these needs do not have much importance, for firstly they are easily satisfied, and secondly, in the event of their dissatisfaction life itself ceases in the organism, thus obviating all further adjustment activity. Social motives and needs have greater importance for the adjustment process. Social motives are developed within a cultural environment. Individuals of different cultures have different motives. For example, our society requires the development and encouragement of such motives as self-respect, self-realization, acceptance, security, love, sympathy, etc. and these social motives naturally have definite influences upon sex and other biological needs. Just as social motives have greater importance than physiological needs, in the same manner the process of adjustment places greater emphasis upon motives that are stronger than others. Inability to satisfy strong motives, once they have been excited only leads to further dissatisfaction, and this tension does not end till the objective has been attained.
2. *Thwarting:* It has been remarked earlier that an important element in the process of maladjustment is the presence of conditions that thwart the satisfaction of motives. Many are the forms that this thwarting can take and one form is frustration. If, for example, a person failed to catch a train and reach his destination because his wrist watch was not functioning properly, then he has to face frustration that has its roots in the external environment. This frustration can also be present in the individual himself. Another form of thwarting is because of conflict. A state of conflict is precipitated when the individual is actuated by more than one motive arising simultaneously. And in the throes of these various motives he cannot decide upon the direction of action that he should adopt. Frustration and conflict, the two forms of thwarting are closely related. Normally, when frustration results from some obstruction, the organism involved is seen adopting aggressive and violent behavior towards the obstacle. Such aggressive behavior can be direct as well as indirect. In children and unintelligent people it takes a direct from while in the case of most adults and intelligent people it takes a more indirect manifestation. Now, if the child's normal expression of aggression and violence resulting from some form of frustration is curbed and restricted, then it is actually prevented, but at the same time it becomes repressed and gives rise to feelings of fear and insecurity. Thus, some people become violent on being faced with some frustrating feeling of fear and insecurity as a result of the curb on their aggressive behavior. As to the mode of behavior that should be adopted in dealing with obstacles that cause frustration, an individual learns through trial and error. Different situations and circumstances find

him behaving differently, and the patterns of behavior that satisfy him are repeated while the patterns that cause him displeasure are discarded and replaced. And, the various reactions concerning the adjustment to different frustrations gradually take on the form of habits. Hence, adult individuals display permanent individual differences in the patterns of adjustment.

3. *Maladjusted reactions:* Any state that contradicts that of adjustment is called maladjustments. In this condition contradicting that of adjustment, the individual organism fails to maintain a balance between his needs and the circumstances that influence the satisfaction of them. And, in this condition one observes reactions that are tendentious towards further imbalance. Reactions of this kind include all those behavior patterns which can be called abnormal. For example, all kinds of mental illness will be cited as maladjusted individuals fails to attain to a state of adjustment with his circumstances, and instead of trying to face the situation, he runs away from it. Abnormal fears and mental formations are to be seen in the individual. Even his mistakes are construed as no mistakes, and he rationalizes upon them. Instead of working to achieve something of his own accord, he identifies himself with the achievement of others and thereby satisfies himself. He has very little capacity to cooperate with others, and he finds it difficult to live with them. He prefers solitude and loves to wander in an imaginary world. Extreme daydreaming is a maladjusted reaction. Another example of it is the projection of one's faults upon another and holding him responsible for one's own frustrations. Similarly, many apparently adult individuals are seen behaving in a markedly childish manner; this too is a form of maladjusted reaction. Briefly, maladjusted reactions include all such reaction that prove obstacles to adjustment.

GENERAL CRITERIA OF ADJUSTMENT

The implication of adjustment is the balance between an individuals needs and the circumstances that satisfy them. Hence the evaluation of the adjustment achieved by a person will require the knowledge of two things firstly, the requirements of this person and secondly the conditions and circumstances that influence the satisfaction of his needs. Once these two are known it will be necessary to find the balance that is struck between them. If the balance is good and desirable, then the individual can be said to be properly adjusted, but if the balance is distruebd then the person will be considered maladjusted. Evidently, this adjustment will differ from individual to individual, since their needs and the conditions that satisfy them need not be common. In this manner, the criterion of personality adjustment is relative to the individuals requirements and the cultural and social complex of circumstances in which he lives. In other words, the criterion changes when these conditions change. For example, in a culture that encourages the combative and aggressive spirit men have greater need for this motive in their adjustment. On the other hand, in a culture that places very great stress upon amiability, the adjustments of personality will depend upon this motive, and it will have great influence upon the criterion of adjustment. Adjustment itself is relative to the individual and his circumstances. Thus, the traits that are required for adjustment to a particular society and culture cannot be considered efficacious in every society and culture.

Despite the fact that have above limitation are operative every where, certain tentative and general criteria of adjustment may be established. Main criteria would be the following:

1. *Integration of personality:* One criterion of adjustment is the integration of personality. Personality is a complex of psychophysical traits. In an integrated personality the various

mental reactions and processes of intelligence and sentiment, desire and determination, etc. do not subsist in any disorder but rather in a proper organized system of functioning. Conflict is quite absent form them. Evidently, the proper integration of the personality is an ideal at which one and all should aim. It is only in such a state that persons can have internal peace and total welfare. The integrated personality is flexible, determined and organized. McDougall calls it the organization of character and intelligence. The higher the degree of organization in an individual's personality the better will be the degree of his adjustment, since in the absence of adjustment the personality cannot be integrated and organized. On the other hand, permanent adjustment is not possible in the absence of personality integration. The individual with an adjusted and organized personality maintains a balanced and practical outlook on life. Failures and frustration do not disturb him unduly, and he persists in looking calm and the master of the situation. His emotions, needs, thinking and other mental activities are adequately balanced and systematic. On the other hand, the personality of a maladjusted person is disintegrated, his life is disturbed, without any peace, and he also tends to disturb the peace of everyone else.

2. *Reduction in tension:* Another criterion of personality adjustment is the reduction or decrease in tension, such as consequent upon the fulfillment of his needs, irrespective of whether the fulfillment is achieved through socially acceptable or objectionable modes. It is a psychological fact that whenever some one or the other need of a person remains dissatisfied it creates a state of tension. And this tension is removed only when the object satisfying that need is obtained. Absence of adjustment results in the increase of tension while adjustment helps in reducing tension. In other words, a person's adjustment may be evaluated in terms of tension existing in his mind.

3. *Harmony between need and environment:* It has been mentioned earlier the adjusted personality can be recognized from a harmony between his needs and his environment. Greater the degree of such harmony, the better will be his adjustment, while on the other hand his personality will be considered less adjusted if this harmony is not of a high order. An adjusted individual has the capacity and energy to accommodate his needs and motives according to his environment, as also to mould this environment to suit his own needs and motives. In this manner, maximum satisfaction and pleasure is to be had in the mutual adjustment and harmony of both environment and requirement. Persons who fail to make an adjustment of their motives and needs to the environment in which they are placed cannot be happy even in the best of circumstances, and are always to be found complaining of the adversity of conditions. Failure of this kind also meets the individual who has not within him the power and capacity to mould conditions according to his own add spice to its otherwise dull fare. There is hardly any, if any at all, individual who is never in his life called upon to face a situation that promises conflict, promises him frustration and anger. If such conditions are present then the enterprising individual bends himself to varying and modifying them to suit his own requirements and thus achieves adjustments or otherwise makes changes in his own requirements and needs. For example, it is commonly noticed that some people succeed in making their ends meet very facilely even on a low income, and they give every appearance of being happy and contented. Contrary to such are people who are incessantly complaining of the paucity of their means even when they have a reasonable income. There is a condition of unhappiness, since there is a wide gap between their income and their expenditure, their needs are never even temporarily completely

fulfilled. In such a condition the adjustment of personality is liable to be disturbed from two sides, first in case the needs of the person do not conform to circumstances, and in the second case when the conditions are not propitious to the fulfillment of the needs. Hence, adjustment requires the balance between these two, even if modification and alteration is essential in both.

COMMON MODES OF REACTIONS TO DIFFICULTIES

Every individual has certain definite needs, and every individual lives in certain specific conditions. It is within these conditions that his needs are fulfilled. When the conditions are favorable no particular difficulty arises in such fulfillment, but for every individual this is not always possible. A condition that is not propitious for the fulfillment of some need is common in the life of every individual and such circumstance and conditions always prove obstacles in the satisfaction of that need, thus creating problems. Difficulties refer to the conditions that prove obstacles to the satisfaction of persons needs. As it is, one finds great individual differences in the manner of reacting to these difficulties, but even then there are certain modes of reaction that can be seen in every pattern of reaction behavior. These methods are roughly the following:

1. *Constructive adjustment:* One very general form of reaction to difficulties is the mode of constructive adjustment, and examples of this mode of behavior are to be seen everywhere in life. Students in educational institutions are constantly faced with situations that become obstacles to the achievement of their educational and vocational objectives, praise and knowledge of self needs that are basic to them. Most students have resource to constructive adjustments in order to overcome these situations, such as putting in longer hours of study or consulting numerous books and teachers in order to overcome their academic obstacles. Similarly, when a trader is faced with some problem of his trade, he resorts to some constructive adjustment to solve that problem. If person is in financial difficulty then the simplest constructive adjustment would before him to exercise economy in his expenditure. The constructive adjustment characteristically offers an opportunity of facing the situation rather than running away from it, and of making efforts that solve the problem instead of merely postponing it.
2. *Substitute adjustment:* All individuals do not have the ready wit and wisdom to achieve constructive adjustment and thus retain their mental balance in the face of difficulties. A very large number of individuals have recourse to substitute adjustments when faced with difficult situations. This, also, is a common and usual method of reacting to difficulties. For example, in a large number of cases, when students fail to pass at an examination, then instead of urging themselves to work harder, they take it upon them to blame to teachers in particular to work harder, they take it upon them to blame the teachers in particular and the entire educational system in general, and daydream themselves into success in future. Some students start avoiding school when they fail while other more enterprising though more censured are the ones who leave home. The question that now arises is whether these reactions are activities of adjustment, since they do not tend to solve the problem inherent in the situation. A close observation will reveal are activities of adjustment, since they do not tend to solve the problem inherent in the situation. A close observation will reveal that even through such reactions the individual is trying to satisfy needs that in other individuals are solved through constructive and positive adjustment and activity. A student failing in an examination is usually defamed and this obstructs his social ambitions and motives. Tensions that

are created through this obstruction he tries to end by his activity of running away or by transferring the blame on the teachers or by daydreaming of success. Thus, for this reason are these reactions to difficulties called substitute reactions. Even though no direct satisfaction is forthcoming from such activity, yet the unsatisfied motive is indirectly and momentarily pacified, and in this manner adjustment is improved through decreases in tension. It must be noticed that adjustment is not a question of successful results, but one of satisfaction of motives, irrespective of the methods that are adopted, be they normal or originating in disease and mental deficiency. It is often remarked that weak, lean and thin individuals usually walk with a swagger and an imposing style. The psychological reason for this is that in weak and lean individuals the motive of self-respect is suppressed, and in order to overcome this repression, instead of resorting to some form of constructive adjustment is equal to the satisfaction caused by a substitute adjustment. The facts of the matter are other than this. Reaction of substitute adjustment usually with scorn and ridicule for the person practicing them, from other members of society, and this further causes suppression of the person's desire for social acceptance. A person running to solitude away from this life's ignoble strife can save his desire for competition from being dejected, but then his motives of security and sociability are frustrated. Hence, it is evident that the substitute adjustment usually results only in more frustration and suppression. On the other hand, these modes of adjustment are also usually harmful for the individual. For example, certain normally ugly individuals are seen trying to attract female attention through undesirable activity since they cannot win it in the normal course, and this usually results in great inconvenience to other more reasonable members of society. One characteristic of proper and constructive adjustment is that only the individual but entire society benefits from it, besides improving the individuals social relationships.

3. *Mental mechanisms:* Another mode of reacting to difficulties is that of mental mechanisms, main among them being projection, compensation, rationalization, etc. As a general rule the consequence of these mechanisms is not good either for the individual or for society. Yet, in some degree or other all or some of these mechanism are to be found in every individual, hence no individual can be declared abnormal on their account. It is only when one of them develosp out of proportion that symptoms of abnormality may be pointed out. Normally, a tendency to overlook one's own fault and to blame others for one's failures is only naturally present in men, but if a person is found doing this all the time and unduly regarding everyone else as his enemy, then his behavior will undoubtedly be classed as abnormal. These mechanisms are also called the tools of adjustment, since they aim at the attainment of adjustment through various methods. Chapter 25 deals the details of mental mechanisms.

The above exposition makes it clear that adjustment process may be complete or partial, proper or improper. It will be relevant here to throw some more light on adjustive, partially adjustive and maladjustive reactions:

1. *Adjustive reactions:* Adjustive reactions, as is evident by the name, are those that achieve an adjustment between the individual and his circumstances. In this manner constructive adjustment reactions are included in adjustive reactions. As a general rule the simplest method available to a person to satisfy his motives when conditions exist to frustrate them is to redouble his efforts to achieve his satisfaction and to do so with patience and persistence. When poverty besets the normal individual, he does his best to overcome it by earning wealth, working hard and laboriously, and normally he meets with reasonable

success. His economic position improves, and most of his motives arrive at a stage of satisfaction. On the other hand there are other individuals who avoid a condition of stress and conflict by controlling emotions and motives in a manner that leads to a reasonable adjustment and compromise with circumstances. Consequently, much of their existence is free from frustration. Hence, the class of adjustive reactions includes all action and behavior that aim at the control and delimiting of his motives or the adjustment of circumstances so that some equilibrium between motives and the conditions of their satisfaction is attained. One very important feature of adjustive reaction is that is benefits the individual organism as well as the community of organisms, or at least is not harmful to such a community.

2. *Partially adjustive reactions:* All reactions aimed at facing obstacles so as to satisfy motives are not completely and entirely successful in achieving their objective. Some of them succeed only in attaining a practical adjustment. Simple examples of such partially successful adjustive reactions are daydreaming as well as other forms of escape from troublesome situations. For example, a majority of poor individuals, instead of making constructive efforts to ameliorate their condition, indulge in making constructive efforts to ameliorate their condition, indulge in making castles in the air, with the result that their poverty fails to pinch them as it would otherwise do. People of this kind are of a very optimistic bent of mind, and even though they never try they are seldom frustrated, always with the hope that their days will turn, that every dog has his day, that some relative will leave them a legacy or that they will win a pool. Some partial and temporary adjustment of a kind is definitely achieved by this escapist dreaming, but no individual adjustment. Evidently, reactions of this kind do not achieve any considerable adjustment.

3. *Nonadjustive reactions:* Nonadjustive reactions as a class activities that do not bring about any adjustment at all between the individual and his conditions. For instance, some people do not attend to some motive even when it is persistently and continually being frustrated, and they continue in activities that do not bring satisfaction for this motive, their activities can only be classed as nonadjustive. Poverty, to take an oft-repeated example, is painful for everyone, but some individuals ignore its demands and pass their days in scholarly and academic pursuits. And, these activities in the pursuit of knowledge prove nonadjustive reactions for all those motives that are frustrated because of the individuals financial poverty since he makes no effort to satisfy them. Sex impulse is commonly repressed, and when this happens, some people, instead of doing something to satisfy it, only choose to repress it all the more, but such efforts are only nonadjustive reactions, as they no real adjustment at all.

4. *Maladjustive reactions:* Maladjustive reactions, do succeed in achieving some adjustment but a type that is of a wrong kind, it harms the individual organism as well as the community of organisms. This class of reaction includes all kinds of mental mechanisms. Frustration is to some extent avoided and postponed by the individual when he succeeds in convincing himself that someone else is to be blamed for his failure, but doing so only endangers his mental relationships, and ultimately he and others come to harm. Besides, the person who finds satisfaction in the achievements of other individuals by identifying himself with them gives some appearance of being adjusted, but he neither himself progresses nor does he afford assistance to others in their progress and development. Individuals who choose to satisfy their desire and overcome their frustrations through daydreaming are not likely to succeed in practical affairs of life and waste their time to no end. Excessive repression that takes place in individuals who

cannot find other means of satisfying their motives and drives usually leads to the development of common errors of daily life, abnormal behavior and mental illness or even derangement. Consequent upon such a condition is much embarrassment for themselves as well as for others. Society glares at and vociferously criticizes people who have recourse to maladjustive reactions, and ultimately it causes them much pain and discomfort.

From the above description it is fairly evident that maladjustive reactions differ essentially from adjustive and partially adjustive reactions in this that while they do lead to some sort of adjustment they also jeopardize the person's social relationships. Secondly, reactions of this kind are the origin of many forms of abnormal behavior and mental disease. Consequently, people with such tendencies require expert treatment and advice.

ADJUSTMENT AND NURSING

Since adjustment helps to maintain harmonious and active relationship between structural components of society. Nurses need to have good interpersonal relationship while dealing with their clients. So adjustment helps to provide a good interpersonal relationships and to perform functions effectively in relation to their culture, customs, values and beliefs. Knowledge and understanding of adjustment play an important role in performing academic work both curricular and cocurrence activities or helps to understanding of social needs and requirement of living in school, college, home, culture and community. Nurses adjustment in the setting of health care institutions helps the patient and their significant ones while hospitalization and at proper regular checkups. This helping the patients to adjust to hospital environment and find out the causes for maladjustments, i.e. orienting them towards equipments and staff involved in health care.

For nurses adjustment needed for their all walks of life including career nursing, i.e. Develop interpersonal relationships with patients and staff, promote character building, render better nursing services, and to lead a harmonious social life, etc. As well-adjusted person nurses—

- Knows their capabilities, strength, weaknesses and limitations
- Has self-respect and respects other, as person
- Has their level of aspirations according to their own strengths and abilities
- Feels reasonably secure and maintain their self-esteem by satisfaction of their basic needs.
- Has flexibility, adapt themselves to changes in environmental by making necessary changes in their behavior.
- Has the will and courage to resist and fight the difficulty.
- Will have control over their environment possess the capacity to deal with adverse conditions.
- As realistic understanding and perception of the universe, are always plans, thinks and act, pragmatically.
- Feels satisfied with their surroundings.
- Has a balance or positive philosophy of life.

When dealing with nurse should understand the human adjustment in following reactions.

Human adjustment is a never ending process of dealing with frustration, which may be environmental or personal in nature or may involve a conflict of motives. Four kinds of conflict are possible: approach-approach, avoidance-avoidance, approach-avoidance and double approach-avoidance. Frustration and the resultant stress often play an important role in motivation, adding to the original drive. Sometimes, however, the best solution is to withdraw from the frustrating situation. The most painful frustrations are usually those which are ego involving. To protect the self-concept against such frustrations, a number of behavioral devices known as defense mechanisms are employed. These may be classified as aggressive reactions, flight or withdrawal reactions, or compromise reactions.

Aggressive reactions to frustrations do not always take the form of direct attack. Instead, aggression may be displaced onto some person or object less threatening or more accessible than the one responsible for the frustration. The most common forms of displaced aggression are scapegoating, free floating anger, and threatened or attempted suicide. Although the threat of punishment can be effective in controlling some kinds of aggressive behavior, actual punishment, which is itself frustrating, may increase aggression. A better method of controlling aggressive tendencies is through controlled expression—release of hostile feelings verbally or in other harmless or even constructive ways.

Withdraw reactions include repression, the exclusion from consciousness of painful thoughts or feelings; flight into fantasy, as in daydreaming; nomadism, aimless wandering from place to place; the beatnil reaction of withdrawal from conventional modern life and regression to childish modes of adjustment.

Compromise reaction to frustration include sublimation, the indirect expression of needs (usually of the sexual urge) in socially acceptable ways, and substitution, in which the conscious quality of the desire is not fundamentally changed and the means of expression are usually undesirable and accompanied by guilt feelings. Another compromise mechanism is reaction formation, by which the individual develops conscious attitudes that directly oppose repressed thoughts and desires. In projection, he convinces himself

that others have toward him the very thoughts and feelings he has repressed. Compensation is an attempt to disguise or hide an undesirable trait by emphasizing a desirable one. It ceases to be of value if it gets out of control and becomes overcompensation. Three basic mechanisms of compromise through intellectualization are rationalization, finding false reasons for unacceptable behavior; isolation, separation of conflicting attitudes into 'logic-tight' comments, and undoing, ritualistic cleansing behavior. Sometimes individuals in a weak position attempt to destroy a threat to their self-esteem by identification with the aggressor.

The difference between normality and abnormality is one of degree only, but it is usual classify behavior as normal when the individuals defensive reactions become exaggerated and disorganized so that they hinder rather than help. Abnormal reaction patterns are classified either as neuroses (disturbances that may be either mildly or seriously incapacitating but seldom require hospitalization) or as psychoses (very severe disturbances characterized by partial or complete loss of contact with reality).

Typically, neurotic disorders are based primarily upon anxiety—generalized feelings of worry and apprehension. Specific symptoms vary a great deal in kind and severity. Typical neurotic reactions include phobias, which are irrational fears; obsessions (persistent irrational thoughts) and compulsions (bizarre actions, usually symbolic or ritualistic in character); and dissociative reactions, which may take the form of amnesia (loss of memory), fugue (loss of memory accompanied by physical flight), or multiple personality (the attention of two or more separate 'personalities').

A neurotic reaction less common today than formerly is conversion reaction (hysteria) in which anxiety is converted into physical symptoms which have no organic basis. Closely related to hysteria but less severe is asthenic reaction, in which the patient suffers constant weariness and mild unpleasant sensations such as palpitation of the heart. Extreme preoccupation with bodily activities and health, known as hypochondria, is another frequent form of neurosis, as is the neurotic depressive reaction, in which the significance of frustrations is overestimated.

Psychotic reactions are usually characterized by bizarre and sometimes violent symptoms but not by the anxiety found in neurotic disorders, since psychotic individuals have to a greater or lesser degree lost contact with reality. Insanity, a legal concept applied to any mental condition that renders the individual incapable of knowing right from wrong, may include severe neuroses as well as psychos. Organic psychoses are related to neural damage caused by injury or illness. Functional psychoses, on the other hand, are apparently precipitated primarily by psychological stress. They are classified as schizophrenic, paranoid, affective and involutional psychotic.

The most common symptoms of psychotic behavior, occurring either singly or in combination, are delusions (strong beliefs opposed to reality—such as delusions of grandeur, of reference, or of persecution); hallucinations (sensory impressions of external objects in the absence of an appropriate stimulus); and emotional distortion. The latter may be character of emotional responsiveness. In the schizophrenic reaction known as catatonia the patient suffers extreme stupor or apathy, remaining motionless for hours. In manic-depressive psychoses the patient may alternate between extreme elation and deep gloom.

Studies indicate that heredity may play a part in the development of functional psychoses, probably through the inheritance of a predisposition to the psychosis, which appears only under conditions of extreme frustration. Recent experiments have also indicated that differences in body chemistry play a part, but the relationships between cause and effect has not yet been established. The drugs mescaline and lysergic acid diethylamide (LSD) produce temporary symptoms of mental illness in healthy persons and, while they are useful in research, are dangerous in the hands of amateurs. Environmental factors such as parental rejection insecurity can also predispose an individual to mental illness in adulthood.

Only recently has experimental analysis of abnormal behavior in human beings been attempted. A technique (based upon operant conditioning methods) which makes use of machine similar to a candy dispenser has shown promise as a method of measuring the severity of psychoses and also of determining the effectiveness of drugs used in treatment.

Alcoholism, drug addiction, and compulsive gambling are also used as means of escape from the frustrations of life. Although the first two involve some physiological factors, all three are usually rooted in emotional problems which can be solved most effectively by psychotherapy. Alcoholics Anonymous, Gamblers Anonymous, and Synanon, a therapeutic community which uses similar techniques with drug addicts, are effective in bringing about rehabitation in many cases.

27 CHAPTER
Guidance and Counseling

Definitions of Guidance

Guidance may be defined as the process of helping the individual in selecting, preparing, entering and progressing in the behavioral patterns which comprise human activities in the educational, vocational, recreational fields as well as connection with community service groups.

Hamrin and Erikson define guidance as "that aspect of educational program which is concerned especially with helping the pupil to become adjusted to his present situation and to plan his future in line with his interests, abilities and social needs".

According to Crow and Crow, "guidance is not direction. It is not making decisions for an individual which he should make for himself. It is not carrying the burden of another's life. Rather, guidance is assistance made available by competent cousellor to an individual of any age to help him direct his own life, develop his own points of view, make his own decisions and carry his own burdens". Guidance is assistance made available by personally qualified and adequately trained men or women to an individual of any age to help manger his own life activities, develop his points of view, make his own decisions and carry his own burdens.

- *CE Skinner defined:* Guidance is a process of helping young person's learn to adjust to self, to others, and to circumstances.
- *James A J (1951) defined:* Guidance is the help given by one person to another in making choices and adjustments and in solving problem that confront him in the attainment of goals.
- *Secondary education committee (1953) defined:* Guidance involves the different art of helping boys and girls to plan their own future wisely in the full light of the factors that can be mastered about themselves and about the world in which they are to live and work.
- *Stoop and Wahlquist defined:* Guidance is the continuous process of helping the individual development in the maximum of their capacity in the direction most beneficial to himself and to society.
- *JM Brewer defined:* Guidance is the process through which an individual is able to solve their problems and pursue a path suited to their abilities and aspiration.

So guidance may be defined as assisting the individual to prepare, for his future life, to fit him for place in society.

Characteristics of Guidance

Guidance offers all-round assistance to individual in all aspects of his or her development whenever required. Thus, guidance connotes the function of giving the needed enlightenment particularly in unknown areas. Guidance makes use of the science of psychology to determine the aptitudes, interests, intelligence, personality, attitudes, etc. and the discipline of education for providing the right and suitable assistance. Guidance has the following characteristics.

- **It is a process:** As a process, it helps every individual to help himself, to recognize and use his inner resources to set goals, to make plans and to work out his own problems of development.
- **It is a continuous process:** It is needed right from early childhood, adolescence, adulthood and even in the old age.
- **Choice and problem points are the distinctive concerns of guidance:** Guidance operates in the zones in which the individuals own unique world of perceptions interacts with the external order of events in his life context.
- **Guidance is the assistance to the individual in the process of development rather than a direction of that development:** The aim of guidance is to develop the capacity for self-direction, self-guidance and self-improvement through an increased understanding of one's problems, resources available to solve the problems and limitations to solve the problem.
- **Guidance is a service meant for all:** It is a regular service, which is required at every stage for every student, not only for awkward situations and abnormal students. It is a positive program geared to meet the needs of all students.
- **Guidance is both generalized and a specialized service:** It is a generalized service because everyone teachers, parents, advisors—play a part in the program. It is a specialized service because specially qualified personnel such as counselor, psychiatrists and psychologists render their services needed to help the individual to get out of his problem.
- **Guidance is an organized service and not an incidental activity of the school:** It is broad based and has a definite purpose. It makes use of the entire facilities available in the school to achieve its objectives and if needed brings about changes in the guidance program in order to meet new demands or challenges.
- **Guidance is not a branch of any discipline:** Even though it draws insights and methods from psychology, sociology, anthropology, philosophy, economics, it is not a branch of any of these disciplines.
- **Guidance is not a branch of any discipline:** It has limits to what it can accomplish.
- **Guidance is more an art than science:** While guidance should always utilize the tested results, guidance practice most often makes decisions on the basis of best judgment in the absence of complete scientific verification.
- **Guidance has its roots in the education system:** Guidance program followed in a particular country must be based on the broad educational objectives of that country.
- Above all, guidance is centered around the needs and aspirations of students.

Meaning of Counseling

Counseling is a process of enabling the individual to know himself and his present and possible future situations in order that he may make substantial contributions to the society and to solve his own problems through a face to face personal relationship with the counselor. Thus, counseling is an enabling process. Counseling is also a learning oriented process carried on in a social environment in which the professionally competent counselor attempts to assist the counselee using appropriate procedure to become a happy and productive member of the society by formulating realistic and purposeful goals for attaining total growth.

In the educational context, counseling is a method of intervention when the teacher observes that a student under her care or supervision exhibits a problem that may be affecting his role performance. Ideally, counseling is a therapeutic process, wherein a student seeks the teacher's help is assisted to clearly identify his problem and to find methods of resolving his problem by utilizing all the resources available to him.

DEFINITION OF COUNSELING

Stone and Shertzer define student counseling as an interaction process that facilitates meaningful understanding of self and environment and result in the establishment and/ or clarification of goals and values for future behavior.

Roges writes of effective counseling as a definitely structured permissive relationship which allows the client to gain an understanding of himself to a degree which enables him to take new positive steps in the light of his new orientation.

Counseling is a specialized service of guidance and basically an enabling process designed to help individual come to terms with his or her life and grow to as greater maturity through learning to take responsibility and to make decisions for himself or herself.

- Wren states that Counseling is a dynamic and purposeful relationship between two people, who approach a mutually defined problems with mutual consideration of each other to the end that the troubled one or less machine aided to a self-determined resolution of his problem.
- According to Cormier and Hackney Counseling is a helping relationship that includes someone seeking helps, someone willing to give help who is capable or trained to help in a setting that permits help to be given and received.
- Vedanayagam states that Counseling is an accepting, trusting and safe relationship in which client learn to discuss freely what upset them, to define their goals, to acquire certain essential skills and to develop the courage and self-confidence to implements desired behavior.

Characteristics of Counseling

Analysis of the above definitions reveal the following characteristics of counseling.

- Counseling involves two individuals one seeking help and the other a professionally trained person who can help the first. The one who seeks the help is known as the counselee and the one who provide the help is the counselor.
- There should be a relationship of mutual respect between the two individuals. The counselor should be friendly and cooperative and the counselee should have trust and confidence in the counselor.
- Counseling is aimed at bringing about desired changes in the individual for self-realization and providing assistance to solve problems through an intimate personal relationship.
- The counselor discovers the problems of the counselee and helps to set up realistic goals and guide him through difficulties and problems.

- If the counselee is a student, counseling helps him to take a decision, make a choice or find a direction in matters related to an educational program or career.
- It helps the counselee acquire independence and develop a sense of responsibility. It also helps him explore and fully utilize his potentials and actualize himself.
- It is more than advice giving. Solution emerges through the thinking that a person does for himself rather than through solutions suggested by the counselor.
- It involves something more than offering an assistance to find a solution to an immediate problem. Its function is to produce changes in the individual thereby enabling him to deal with the difficulties in a more productive and independent manner.
- Counseling is democratic. Counseling takes place in a nonthreatening and democratic atmosphere, which allows the counselee to think independently with the counselor and not under the counselor.
- Counseling concerns itself with attitudes as well as actions.
- Emotional rather than purely intellectual attitudes are the raw materials of the counseling process. Information and intellectual understanding have their place in the counseling, but it is the emotionalized feelings which are most important.
- Counseling is a body of techniques that helps individuals to grow up normally through guided learning. It helps an individual to know himself better, gives him confidence, encourages his self-directiveness and provides him with new vision to grow and flourish.
- In the educational context, counseling is centered around the needs and aspirations of students.

Guidance and Counseling Differentiation

Very few terms have been more freely or interchangeably used than the terms 'guidance' and counseling'. Guidance is mainly preventive and developmental, whereas counseling is remedial as well as preventive and developmental. Intellectual attitudes are the raw materials of the guidance process but emotional rather than purely intellectual attitudes are the raw materials of the counseling process. Thus, in guidance, decision making operates at intellectual level, whereas in counseling it operates at emotional level.

As far as education is concerned, the counseling service is one among various services offered by the guidance program. Thus, in education, our goal is guidance and our technique among others is counseling. Counseling is called the crux, heart, essence or pivot of the guidance program. The success or failure of the guidance program is determined by counseling service. This importance has helped the counseling to outgrow all other services of the guidance program and to achieve a status more or less equal to the guidance. Thus, in strict sense, mentioning guidance and counseling instead of guidance. In the educational context is just like mentioning central nervous system and brain.

Aims of Guidance

According to National Guidance Association of America, the aims of guidance can be stated as follows: (a) to help the schools adapt to the needs of the pupils and the community and to make sure that each child obtains the equality of opportunity which is the duty of the schools to provide, (b) to assist individuals in choosing, preparing for, entering upon and making progress in occupation, (c) to provide knowledge regarding the characteristics of the common occupations and problems of the occupational world, (d) to secure help for the worker to understand his relationships to workers in his own and other occupational settings and to society as a whole, (e) to secure better cooperation between schools on the one hand and the various commercial, industrial and professional pursuits on the other hand and (f) to encourage the establishment of courses of study in all institutions of learning that will harmoniously combine the cultural and practical studies.

Humphrey and Traxler state that the aims of guidance are to help the individual: (a) to understand himself, (b) to make the most of his capacities, interests and other qualities, (c) to adjust himself satisfactorily to the varied situations within his total environment, (d) to develop the ability to make his own decisions and (e) to make his own unique contributions to society to the finest possible extent.

Principles of Guidance

According to Hollis and Hollis, there are eight principles on which any guidance program should be based. They can be modified in order to meet the requirement of the local context where guidance is carried out. The principles are:

a. The dignity of the individual is supreme.
b. Each individual is different from every other individual.
c. The primary concern of guidance is the individual in his social setting.
d. The attitudes and personal perceptions of the individual are the basis on which he acts.
e. The individual generally acts to enhance his perceived self.
f. The individual has the innate ability to learn and can be helped to make choices that will lead to self-direction consistent with social improvement.
g. The individual needs a continuous guidance process from early childhood through adulthood.
h. Each individual may at times need the information and personalized assistance best given by competent professional personnel.

According to Crow and Crow there are fourteen significant guidance principles. They are:

a. Every aspect of a person's complex personality pattern constitutes a significant factor his total displayed attitudes and forms of behavior. Guidance services which are aimed at bringing about desirable adjustment in any particular area of experience must take into account the all-round development of the individual.
b. Although all human beings are similar in many respects, individual differences must be recognized and considered in any efforts aimed at providing help or guidance to a particular child, adolescent or adult.
c. The functions of guidance is to help a person:
    1. Formulate and accept, stimulating, worthwhile and attainable goals of behavior.
    2. Apply these objectives in the conduct of his affairs.
d. Existing social, economic, and political unrest is giving rise to many maladjustive factors that require the cooperation of experienced and thoroughly trained guidance workers, counselors and the individual with a problem.
e. Guidance should be regarded as a continuing process of service to an individual from young childhood through adulthood.
f. Guidance service should not be limited to the few who given observable evidence of its need, but should be extended to all persons of all ages who can benefit there from either directly or indirectly.

g. Curriculum materials and teaching procedures should evidence a guidance point of view.
h. Although guidance touches every phase of an individuals life pattern, the generally accepted areas of guidance include—concern with the extent to which an individuals physical and mental health interfere with his adjustment to home, school and vocational and social demands and relationships or the extent to which his physical and mental health are affected by the conditions to which he is subjected in these areas of experience.
i. Parents and teachers have guidance appointed responsibilities.
j. Specific guidance problems of any age level should be referred to persons who are trained to deal with particular areas of adjustment.
k. To administer guidance intelligently and with as thorough knowledge of individual is possible, program of individual evaluation and research should be conducted and accurate cumulative records of progress and achievement should be made accessible to guidance workers. Through the administration of well-selected standardized tests and other instruments of evaluation, specific data concerning degree of mental capacity, success of achievement, demonstrated interest and other personality characteristics should be accumulated, recorded and utilized for guidance purposes.
l. An organized guidance program should be flexible according to the individual and community needs.
m. The responsibility for the administration of guidance program should be centered in a personally qualified and adequately trained chairman or head of guidance, working cooperatively with his assistants and other community welfare and guidance agencies.
n. Periodic appraisals should be made for existing school guidance programs. The success of its functioning should rest on outcomes that are reflected in the attitudes towards the program of all who are associated with it—guider, guide, etc. and in the displayed behavior of those who have been served through its functioning.

NEED OF GUIDANCE AND COUNSELING IN EDUCATION AND NURSING

The problems of students must be properly tackled with an intention to solve them. Unresolved problems may affect not only the academic performance of students but also their personality development. Guidance and counseling help teachers to solve the students problems with their active involvement. They also assist the teacher in creating a healthy climate in the institution by ensuring harmonious and integrated personality development of students.

The need for counseling and guidance can be summarized as follows:

a. To help in the total development of students.
b. To assist students in leading a healthy life by abstaining from whatever is deleterious to health.
c. To help in the proper selection of educational programs.
d. To help in the selection of careers according to their interests and abilities.
e. To help the students in vocational development.
f. To develop readiness for changes and to face challenges.
g. To minimize the mismatching between education and employment and help in the efficient use of man power.

h. To help fresher's establish proper identity.
i. To identify and motivate the students from weaker sections of society.
j. To help students to overcome the period of turmoil and confusion.
k. To identify and render help to students who are in need of special help.
l. To ensure proper utilization of time spent outside the classrooms.
m. To help in tackling problems arising out of student explosion and coeducation.
n. To make up the deficiencies at home.
o. To minimize the incidence of indiscipline.
p. To motivate the youth for self-employment.
q. To assist the needy students in availing financial assistance from appropriate organizations.

The need for guidance and counseling in nursing education is very obvious. Different from their past learning experiences, nursing students are exposed to a situation where errors are detrimental and commitment is the way of life. Many students who have joined for nursing are unaware about the realities waiting for them as nursing students. They opted nursing just because of a promising future ensured by the nursing career. Guidance and counseling will assist them in developing proper attitude, commitment, dedication and other qualities required for a successful nursing practice. Moreover, emerging and re-emerging diseases, technological advancements in the patient care, evolving of new specialists, especially in the clinical areas, changing role of nurses in the health care sector, impact of Consumer Protection Act, etc. underlines the need of a viable guidance and counseling service in all nursing institutes. The need for guidance and counseling in nursing education can be summarized as follows:

a. To help students adjusting with the new environment of the nursing institute
b. To help in developing qualities required for a successful nursing practice
c. To help students in getting adjusted with the clinical environment
d. To help students keeping in touch with the latest trends in nursing and to reap benefits from the trends
e. To help students in developing positive learning habits, especially in skill learning so that they can retain and transfer the learned lessons in a better way
f. To help in the development of appropriate coping strategies in order to deal with stress in a productive manner
g. To help nursing students in establishing proper identity
h. To help them to develop a positive attitude towards life
i. To help them to overcome periods of turmoil and confusion
j. To help students in developing their leadership qualities
k. To motivate them for taking membership in professional organizations after completing their studies
l. Help them to make advantages of the technological advancements in the patient care
m. Help them to develop readiness for changes and to face challenges both in the personal as well as professional life
n. Help them to carry out the responsibilities as a worthwhile health team member
o. Help them in the proper selection of careers both in India and abroad
p. Motivate them to do higher studies according to their abilities and interest
q. To assist the needy students in availing financial assistants from appropriate organizations.

Classification of Guidance

Classification According to Problems

As has been pointed out, an individual has to turn to the psychologist, in the latter's role of specialist, for personal advice when he fails to solve the problems that confront him. This personal advice is guidance. How this guidance can take effect depends on the fact that it be given in the context of some problem the solution of which is being sought. As a matter of fact it is no easy matter to recount all the possible problems that arise in a various spheres of human life, but some psychologists have attempted a classification of them. For example, Jones has divided the problems of life into eight spheres on the basis of their nature:

1. Related to health and psychological development
2. Related to house and family
3. Related to time for recreation
4. Concerned with personality
5. Religious
6. Educational
7. Social
8. Vocational or occupational.

Having achieved the classification of problems it becomes possible to classify the kinds or forms of problems it becomes possible to classify the kinds or forms of guidance that is to be given correspondingly. For example, vocational guidance is required in connection with profession and educational guidance in the field of education. Psychologists have professed many and various kinds of guidance. For example, Myers has mentioned the following eight kinds of guidance:

1. Vocational guidance
2. Educational guidance
3. Recreational guidance
4. Civic guidance
5. Community service guidance
6. Social and moral guidance
7. Health guidance
8. Leadership guidance.

Classification According to Mode of Guidance

The above classification that we have been viewing is made on the basis of problems for which guidance is required. If the mode of guidance is taken into consideration guidance can be classified in the following manner:

1. Individual guidance
2. Group guidance.

Before going on to a detailed description of educational, vocational and personal guidance, it would be advisable to comprehend this classification of guidance made on the basis of its modes.

1. Individual guidance method—In the individual guidance method the person to be guided and his guide, the psychologists, are in direct and personal contact with each other. He invades the ill person's house and makes a study of his family conditions, and

for this purpose he interviews the various members of the individuals' household. Besides the family background, the individual's social, financial, and cultural background is also investigated so that no possible source of information is left untapped. And for this it becomes essential to study his neighborhood and to collect as many facts of his life as are possible so as to build up a fairly complete case history. The schools and colleges that he has attended are contracted in order to gaining formation concerning his behavior and scholastic attainments there. His teachers too, are consulted on the matter.

Study of this type and the collection of all possible information concerning the individual is followed by testing of the individual himself. He is made to take of intelligence, specific mental abilities, interests, attitudes and personality. Interview is another weapon that is used to uncover much information and, incidentally, to learn the patient's opinion of himself. Accordingly, then, in individual guidance the following information concerning the individual is gathered.

1. Information concerning his intelligence, mental abilities, interests, attitudes and personality.
2. Information concerning family conditions.
3. Information concerning the social, financial and cultural background.
4. Other relevant information.

Having gathered all this information it is subjected to close and intelligent scrutiny, and then curative measures are introduced to remove the problems which have made this guidance necessary. Among these efforts are logical arguments, suggestions, psycho-analysis, etc.

The individual guidance method has the following qualities:

1. It renders almost complete information concerning the individual. Hence a proper cure can be effected.
2. Cures in this method are simpler and more effective.

Despite these advantages, the method suffers from the following drawbacks:

1. It consumes much time, with the result that a very large number of psychologists are required if there is a big number of patients.
2. Accordingly, this method is extremely expensive also.
3. It needs highly trained and specialist psychologists.

2. Group guidance method—These short comings of the individual guidance method are not found in group method because in this a number of people are guided simultaneously. Group guidance should not be interpreted to imply that it involves guiding the group. Actually, the guidance is aimed at the individual because it consists of the personal assistance rendered by a psychologist. In the group guidance technique a complete group is guided. But this guidance is intended to help the individual members of the group to solve their own problems, the sole differences being that the group is comprised of individuals facing more or less the same problems. Evidently, then, there is no need to waste money and time in giving individual guidance to individuals who are facing similar problems and the advice is likely to be the similar. Hence there can be no questioning of the importance of the group guidance technique. It economies upon time and money.

Nevertheless, group guidance technique lacks all the advantage that accrues from an application of the individual guidance method. Due to the smaller degree of personal contact between the psychological and his subjects, the cures are not quite so effective as in the case of individual guidance. When group guidance is administered it is also not possible to gather the same amount of authentic information concerning the subject as is feasible in the individual guidance method. Hence, it may be tentatively concluded that group guidance method can be of value only in circumstances in which the problems faced are similar to a degree without wide individual differences and are also not particularly complex.

GUIDANCE AREAS

Guidance help students to make proper adjustments with the environment which they are living and also make the best possible contributions commensurate with one's strengths and limitations. Every individual, at sometime or other needs help to become happier, more creative and better adjusted in his family and society. There are several areas where student require assistance. These areas can be classified into education, vocation, personal, social, avocation, health, moral, religion and financial. Let us see each area in detail with special emphasis to nursing education.

One of the most important areas in education which has acquired considerable importance and received much attention in recent years is guidance and counseling. Present day teachers have to acquire some specialized knowledge regarding guidance and counseling in order to guide the students tactfully in his highly competitive world. As students are living in a materialistic and consumer driven society under the influence of media, the possibility of deviating from the healthy lifestyle is more than ever before, making guidance and counseling an integral part of the modern education system. Guidance and counseling ensures a healthy climate in the institution, which is essential for the harmonious and integrated personality development of students. Let us see in detail regarding guidance and counseling with special reference to nursing education.

In the educational context, guidance means assisting students to select courses of study appropriate to their needs and interests, achieve academic excellence to the best possible extent, derive maximum benefit of the institutional resources and facilities, inculcate proper study habits and satisfactorily participate in curricular and extracurricular activities or in other words, guidance is a process of assisting or helping the students in developing their potentialities, in solving their immediate or future problems and in planning their own future wisely thereby enabling them to lead a successful personal and social life.

Vocational Guidance

Vocational guidance is an assistance rendered by an individual to another in the latters solving problems related to his progress and vocational selection, keeping in mind the individuals peculiarities or special abilities and their relations with his occupational opportunity (ILO 1954).

Vocational guidance is the assistance provided for selection of a vocation and preparation for the same. It is concerned with enabling students to acquire information about career opportunities, career growth and training facilities. For organizing an effective vocational guidance program, the teacher has to consider the students goals, needs, interests and emotional characteristics.

The functions of vocational guidance are:

a. Enabling the students to discover information about themselves—their abilities interests, needs, ambitions and above all what is expecting from them.

b. Providing them information regarding the dynamic nature of the modern world, the advantages and disadvantages of different occupations and educational courses, the qualifications necessary for entry into them and the range of opportunities available to them.
c. Provide them with a frame of reference in which to see themselves in relation to these educational and vocational opportunities, to orient them to the helping agencies available to them to implement those plans.
d. Promote self-understanding and to develop educational and occupational plans.
e. Providing placement services to help them to implement those plans.
f. Providing follow up service to help them; if necessary, when faced with future decision making situations.
g. Train students for entrepreneurship. This function is very important in the light of the new world order where money is not a problem for starting a new venture. Individuals with adequate knowledge and commitment can easily convert their knowledge into money by starting new ventures with the help of financial institutions.

The process of vocational guidance has two aspects study of the individual and study of the occupational or professional sphere. Before any vocational guidance can be rendered to an individual, it is essential that adequate information concerning his education, level of intelligence, mental abilities, aptitude, interests, physical development, health, nature, personality characteristics and economic status be gathered, because variations in any and having collected all the necessary and desired information regarding the individual consideration it is necessary to professional or occupational sphere. Occupations have been classified in different ways according to the view point adopted in doing so. Classification is beneficial because the individual comes to know all the profession from one point of view and select from among there. This has two fold advantage of narrowing down the range from which the selection is to be made while at the same time it provides a number of alternatives. It will be advantageous to glance various profession or occupation.

After gathering information regarding profession from one or more from various source it is possible to select ones profession but before committing oneself finally has been pointed out before, the following thing must be taken into consideration and made of note of, i.e. nature of work, working conditions, necessary personality traits (Nature, behavior, leadership), level of intelligence, mental activities, interests and aptitudes, necessary education and training, income, chances of promotion and permanency of work procedure for entrance, necessary physical development and health, social prestige and demand of the job.

Vocational Guidance in Nursing Education: The functions of vocational guidance in nursing education are (a) Provide a clear picture regarding the latest trends in nursing service and nursing education like changing roles of nurses, emerging new specialties, especially in the clinical areas, etc. (b) Help the nursing students to find a suitable career either in the nursing education or service according to their skills, abilities and interests. (c) Orient them to the abroad opportunities and assist them in preparing for the qualifying examinations like CGFNS, NHS exams, etc. (d) Since good English is the key to success around the world, provide them an idea regarding the English language tests conducted in various countries like, TOFEL, IELTS, OET, etc. (e) Guide students in preparing curriculum vitae or biodata and conduct mock interviews to prepare them for the upcoming interviews. (f) Conduct placement services in association with reputed man power consultants and do the follow up services. This function can be carried out easily due to the advancements in the communication and information technology. Many nursing institutes have tie-ups with well known man power consultants, which will help them in ensuring promising careers to the students either in India or abroad. (g) Another important function is to collect opinions and suggestions from the passed out students regarding the various aspects of the educational program. Guidance service should also try to get a feedback from the institutions regarding the performance of the passed out students place through it. Valuable suggestions from the passed out students and employers should be handed over the curriculum committee for further actions. This will also help in the curriculum revision.

A vocational guidance is the assistance to be provided to students to spend their available leisure time profitably. Activities and programs outside the formal classrooms provide many opportunities for the blossoming of talents of students.

Functions of vocational guidance in nursing education are (a) Help students to prepare for the monthly educational and cultural programs conducted by SNA. (b) Assist students to conduct programs related to World Health Day, Nurses Day, etc. (c) Assist students to participate in the activities of national service scheme, drugs bank, blood donors forum, etc. (d) Help students to use their leisure time to increase their vocabulary by reading English periodicals, newspapers and hearing English news. (e) Help students who are spiritually inclined to meet their spiritual needs. (f) Help students to develop hobbies related to nursing care like collecting drug literature.

An increasing global demand for qualified nurses and the emergence of various specialists in nursing in order to meet the challenges of the modern health care system has given a facelift to this area of guidance in nursing education. More than ever before nursing institutions are giving much consideration to vocational guidance. Some institutes even renamed their guidance and counseling services into guidance, counseling and placement services to show their commitment towards vocational guidance. Even though placement service is a part and parcel of vocational guidance, the word placement is separately mentioned with an intention to highlight the help rendered to the students by the institute in the matter of finding a promising career. Of course, this renaming doesn't carry any sense except some cosmetic advantages, but it is a clear indication of the elite status grabbed by this area of guidance.

Educational Guidance

According to Jones A J Educational guidance is concerned with assistance given to pupils in their choices and adjustment with relation to 'schools', curriculum, course and school life.

According to Myers GE Educational guidance is a process concerned with bringing about between an individual pupil with his distinctive characteristics on the one hands, and differing groups of opportunities and requirements on the other, a favorable setting for individual development or education.

Educational guidance help the students to get maximum benefit out of education and to solve their problem related to education. The emphasis is on providing assistance to students to perform satisfactorily in their academic work, choose the appropriate course of study, overcome learning difficulties, foster creativity, improve levels of motivation, utilize institutional resources optimally such as library, laboratory, etc. The function of guidance in this area are (a) to help the students make educational plans consistent with their abilities, interests and goals and to select appropriate courses and cocurricular activities which will enable them to join careers of their choice. They also need to be guided for developing good study habits, prepare for examinations properly and face examinations with confidence, (b) help the students to explore educational level. They need to be guided in selecting subjects for specialization and additional courses of studies. They also need to be made familiar with the various fellowships, scholarships, competitive examinations, etc. so that their journey ahead becomes smooth and profitable, (c) provide help at crisis points of students in their academic and personal life, (d) monitor academic progress of students and help the students who are not studying as expected, (e) identify special learners such as academically backward, gifted and creative and provide help in meeting their educational needs, (f) diagnose the learning difficulties of students in different subjects and assist them to overcome the difficulties and (g) help students in their adjustment to curricular and cocurricular demands of the educational programs.

So educational guidance is a process of rendering help to the students in their proper educational development and adjustment. The reason for the justification of educational guidance includes the following:

- Need of checking the wastage and stagnation in education
- Need of realizing the aims and objectives of education
- Need of making right educational choices
- Need of proper educational adjustment.

The nature of educational guidance has following facts:

- It is administered to students
- It is intended for educational selection
- It is rendered for adjustment in education.

Objectives of educational guidance: The objectives of guidance in respect of education is the solution of education problems, helping his students select his curriculum and to impart him the activity to adjust to school or college surroundings and conditions. The following are the main objectives of educational guidance.

- Selection of curriculum according to ability and capability
- Improvement in the methods of study
- Arrangement of a special method of education for the backward child
- Creation of special education programs for the gifted children
- Consideration and solutions of failure at examinations
- Encouraging the child inspiration to study
- Removing weakness in particular subjects.

Principles of Educational Guidance: The strategies that teachers adopt to plan and implement educational guidance must be appropriate to the problems for which they are needed. The following are some of the principles on which educational guidance must be based. (a) They should be based on clear cut objectives. (b) Every student is capable of achieving the best of his ability. (c) Individual differences in academic achievement of students must be recognized. (d) The strategies adopted must be student oriented. (e) The strategies must take into consideration the resources and facilities to the students. (f) Educational guidance is not meant for a few students only; they need to be provided to all.

Educational Guidance in Nursing Education: In nursing education, guidance must perform the following functions in the educational area.

a. Provide a orientation regarding the aim and philosophy of nursing education.
b. Help them to differentiate between previous learning experiences and the learning experiences they are going to receive in the nursing institute.
c. Help them to develop an awareness regarding the qualities required for a successful nursing practice.
d. Help students to develop a realistic educational planning.
e. Help them to make an objective analysis regarding their own abilities and interests.
f. Help students in developing positive learning habits, especially in skill learning so that they can retain and transfer the learned lessons in a better way.
g. Provide an orientation regarding the clinical area and the methods of teaching employed there with special reference to the student's role in terms of active participation.
h. Help them to utilize institutional resources such as clinics, library, various labs, etc. to the maximum extent possible.
i. Provide knowledge regarding the latest trends in nursing education and nursing service. This will help them to plan their career and higher education.
j. Motivate them to do higher studies and help in choosing specialization according to their needs and interests. This can be done by providing information regarding higher education such as qualifying examinations, fellowships, etc.
k. Assist them in preparing for the internal assessments and university exams.

The process of educational guidance to students involves three phases which includes:

- Collecting information or data of the students
  1. Scholastic achievement
  2. Level of intelligence
  3. Aptitude, interest
  4. Personality characteristics
  5. Health and physical develops
  6. Family background and economic conduct
- Rendering guidance on the basis of this information
- Follow-up programs.

Personal Guidance

Personal guidance in the guidance which is rendered to a person for solving his personal problems. It constitute the personal and individual advice offered by the guide to a individual for the solution of latters personal problems. This helps the person adjust to circumstances in his life.

Personal guidance refers to the guidance offered to students for enabling them to adjust themselves to their environment so that they become efficient citizens. Adolescent behavior, to a great extent, depends upon the moods and attitudes of the adolescent. Emotional inability is a characteristic of adolescents and this is often the cause of many of their personal problems. Personal guidance will help them to solve these problems. Severe competition and irrational expectations of the parents also lead to personal problems.

Students may find it difficult to follow the lectures, especially when exposed to a new medium of instruction. Difficulty in understanding in turn leads to disliking of teachers and ultimately results in poor achievement. Guidance needs to be provided to such students to enable them to adjust to the situation which they cannot change.

The function of personal guidance can be summarized as follows:

a. Help students to improve mental health
b. Assist students in becoming progressively responsible for their own development
c. Assist students to understand and resolve their emotional problems
d. Assist students in exploring various mechanisms of adjustment
e. Assist students to get control over emotions
f. Assist students to deal with the difficulties of personal as well as academic life
g. Help students to develop interpersonal skills
h. Help students to accept themselves and others
i. Help students to solve the problems of coeducation
j. Help students to maintain healthy heterosexual relationships
k. Assist students to deal with the stress in a productive manner
l. Assist students to overcome the times of turmoil and confusion
m. Help students to find suitable accommodation if needed and to adjust with the hostel life.

Generally human problems of a personal nature can be of two kinds—Personal or individual and social.

Individual problems may be physiological problems (Health, disease, developmental and concerned problems) and Family welfare.

Taking all such aspects into consideration Personal Guidance may be found to cover all the problems and aspects concerning the developments and adjustment of a person. It is a very comprehensive and wild meaning. Crow and Crow emphasize such broad meaning in their attempts of making correct interpretation of this term. In their words, "Personal Guidance refers to help given to an individual towards a better adjustment in the development of attitudes and behavior in all areas of life". Thus, in its wider sense, Personal Guidance may be interpreted to include all kinds of guidance that may be rendered to a person.

Personal Guidance in Nursing Education: Since a large number of students opt nursing without prior knowledge regarding nursing education, personal guidance has to play a vital role in nursing education. In addition to the above listed functions, personal guidance has the following functions in the nursing education: (a) Assist students to deal with homesickness: Many nursing students are staying in the hostel for the first time in their life and this creates a lot of homesickness. A well-planned interaction with the parents by the teachers in presence of students, assigning a teacher guardian for every group of ten students, arrangements for a comfortable hostel stay and a well-organized orientation program in an informal atmosphere will reduce their homesickness within a short period of time. (b) Protect students from the ragging: Nowadays ragging is not a problem in a civilized campus, even then precautions should be taken to avoid any incident of ragging. Even though prevention of ragging is an administrative aspect, many institutes seek the help of guidance and counseling service to prevent it. Ragging can be prevented by constituting an antiragging committee with the active participation of senior students, motivating first year students to report any incidents of ragging, educating all students regarding the consequence of ragging and conducting surprise visits to the hostel where first year students are staying. (c) Assist students to develop proper attitude required for a successful nursing practice: In addition to the routine teaching sessions, personal guidance also contributes to the proper development of attitudes among students. Personal guidance helps the students to differentiate between empathy and sympathy and contributes to the nurturing of the former. In the presence of empathy, compassion and commitment will naturally develop the needed extent. (d) Assist students to adjust with the new learning experiences and to overcome learning difficulties: Personal guidance help students to adjust with the new learning experiences, especially those provided in the clinical areas, special help should be rendered to students in the matter of developing mastery in English. Maintaining a wall magazine for displaying literary works in English, insisting to speak in English rather than the local language, encouraging to read English periodicals and newspapers and placing a vocabulary board outside the library to display meaning of five words per day will help them in developing fluency in English. This will also help them in scoring high grades in the future qualifying examinations like TOFEL, IELTS, etc. (e) Help students to develop emotional maturity: In the clinical area, nurses have to face many situations which may cause an emotional breakdown in the case of freshers. Helping students to develop empathy rather than sympathy, teaching them to analyze events in the clinical area with a rational basis, teaching them the healthy ways to ventilate emotions and above all, educating them regarding the role of a nurse in the critical situations will help to develop emotional maturity. (f) Assist students to cope with the stress: In fact, nursing students are the only student group who are forced to bear the responsibility of staff nurses to look after the patients. This immature shouldering of responsibility creates enormous stress among nursing students. Unfortunately, in many of the case, nursing faculty are helpless and only thing they can do is to equip the student to convert this stress laden situation into an opportunity oriented one. Teaching relaxation techniques, ensuring the availability of teachers round the clock to help students in the crisis situations, constituting peer groups and assigning senior students to look after juniors are some of the ways to deal with the stress among nursing students. (g) Help students to achieve balance between personal and professional life: From the very beginning itself students should be taught how to achieve balance between personal and professional life and the danger of giving more importance to professional life at the cost of personal life and *vice versa*. Equal importance should be given to both and there should be clear cut demarcation between the two for a successful life. Students should be instructed to concentrate on other responsibilities after returning from the clinics instead of being preoccupied with the matters related to patient care. (h) Help students to develop a healthy interpersonal relationship with other health team members, patients and others related to patient care.

The following steps are involved in a personal guidance program:

1. **Collection of all the information or data:** First of all, the essential information or data concerning the individual, who needs personal or psychological guidance, should be collected. It may be concerned with his physical, intellectual, social and emotional development, academic achievement, personality characteristics, interests and aptitudes family and school background and other environment conditions. Thus an adequate picture of the background and personality make-up an individual should be drawn in the mind for the solution of the problems, faced by the individual.
2. **Diagnosis of the causes of the problems:** Now the problem of the individual is analyzed in relation with the collected information. The causes lying within the individual or his environment are detected. For having a correct diagnosis, a personal interview or other techniques may also be adopted and more information, if needed, may also be acquired.

3. **Thinking about the remedial measure:** In view of the detected possible causes, the remedial measures are chalked out. The guidance worker, now thinks about the personal guidance that may be provided for the individual in getting rid of his trouble.
4. **Rendering personal guidance:** By establishing proper rapport, the Guidance personnel makes the individual realize the main cause of his difficulty or trouble. Sometimes, on this basis he is made to realize or even think about the possible change in his behavior or attitude. For this purpose so many valuable techniques like suggestion, imitation, sympathetic, affectionate advice, sublimation or catharsis, psychoanalysis or other psychological therapy can be adopted. The sole purpose of such guidance is to help asset the individual in getting rid of his difficulty either by modifying his behavior or brining some changes in his environment.
5. **Follow-up service:** After rendering personal guidance to an individual, it is essential to evaluate the progress or outcome of such guidance through personal interview, contact or any other suitable technique. It is such follow-up program that helps in knowing the strength and weakness of the administered personal guidance. It may also suggest the need of further guidance to him or any alteration in the proposed guidance.

The knowledge about the above mentioned process of personal guidance is not only needed by guidance personnel specially appointed in the school, but the headmaster and teachers should also make themselves acquainted with it. Teachers with their unique position in the school, are able to develop close contacts with children and may be able to know the real causes of a trouble. With a little training, they can learn they are of rendering personal guidance to their students. Therefore our schools are required to play their due role of this direction. In every school, the Head of the institution should try to organize a personal guidance program with the active help of his staff and cooperation of the parents and State guidance services.

Social Guidance

Social guidance enables the student to make substantial contributions to the society, assume leaderships, confirm to the social norms, work as team members, develop healthy and positive attitudes, appreciate the problems of society, respect the opinions and sentiments of fellow human beings, acquire traits of patience, perseverance and friendship. Its main purpose is to enable the student to become an efficient citizen.

Social Guidance in Nursing Education: In nursing education, social guidance has to perform the following: (a) *Train students for leadership and followership qualities:* Since nursing is experiencing a shortage of capable leaders, this function of guidance deserves special attention. Various leadership development programs should be conducted under the guidance service in cooperation with the student nurses association to promote leadership qualities among nursing students. (b) *Help students to carry out their responsibilities as a responsible health team member:* Nurses constitute fifty percent of the total health care workers and to a certain extent success of any health team is determined by how well the nurses render their service. So special care should be taken to inculcate a sense of accountability and responsibility among nursing students. (c) Assist them in acquiring desirable set of values and developing a positive life philosophy. (d) Motivate students to become a responsible member of professional organizations. (e) Social guidance also help students to develop a healthy interpersonal relationship with other health team members, patients and others related to patient care. (f) Motivate students to contribute towards bridging the gap between nursing education and nursing service.

Health Guidance

Health guidance implies the assistance rendered to students for maintaining sound health. Sound health is a prerequisite for participating in curricular and cocurricular activities. This type of guidance focuses on enabling students to appreciate conditions for good health and take steps necessary for ensuring good health, maintaining sound physical and mental health.

The functions of health guidance in nursing education are: (a) Conduct periodic health checkup of students and maintain the health records, (b) insist students to take universal precautions strictly, especially when posted in infectious departments, (c) alert students to take vaccines correctly, (d) motivate students to take food regularly, especially breakfast for maintaining good health, (e) motivate students to seek help of the faculty members when they are under stress, (f) ensure the availability of faculty members round the clock to help students in matters related to health, (g) motivate students to seek medical help in the initial stage of disease itself, (h) supervision of college facilities such as hostels and canteen to see that healthful conditions are maintained.

Financial Guidance

The function of financial guidance is to help the needy students in determining the financial assistance they need in the light of the expected expenses and to get it from financial organizations after completing the formalities. Earlier financial guidance was included along with the personal guidance. Nowadays, a new guidance area namely finance and welfare is also mentioned along with other areas of guidance. Some students are hard-pressed for finances. They need to be guided regarded freeships, fee concessions, scholarships, stipends, etc. available in the institution or offered by other welfare agencies and how and when to apply. The provision of financial assistance has to be ensured so that no meritorious student is denied education for lack of financial assistance. In this era of liberalization, securing an educational loan is not a big task. Any talented can pursue education by seeking hassle free, easily repayable educational loans. Nursing students also require financial guidance just like other students.

Glossary

Abnormal: Maladaptive behavior detrimental to the individual and of the group.

Abreaction: Expression of pent-up emotions.

Absolute rating scale: A method of rating in which the judge assigns scores to each individual by comparing him to a standard independent of the group being rated.

Absolute savings score: Difference between amount of practice required for original learning of a given task and the amount of practice required to relearn it. Original learning score; this is the relative savings score.

Absolutely refractory period: Period immediately following a nerve impulse, during which the nerve is incapable of responding to even very strong stimuli.

Accommodation: Process by which the lens of the eye increases in thickness to focus on near objects and flattens for distant vision.

Acromegaly: An overgrowth of certain portions of the skeleton (notably the hands, arms, jawbone, and chest), caused by an over secretion of the pituitary growth hormone in adolescence or adulthood.

ACTH: See corticotrophin

Action potential: Activity in the nerve cell which can be measured; it is an electric potential change rather than a current.

Action therapies: Therapies, usually based on learning theory, which seek primarily to eliminate symptoms and change behavior. Also called behavior therapies.

Acting out: Defense mechanism in which individual reduces anxiety, hostility, or other unpleasant emotions by permitting their expression in overt behavior.

Activation (arousal): Energy mobilization required for organism to pursue its goals and meet its needs.

Actualization strivings: Strivings toward growth and fulfillment.

Actuarial approach: Application of probability statistics to human behavior, as in insurance.

Acute: A disorder of sudden onset and relatively short duration.

Acute alcoholic hallucinosis: State of alcoholic intoxication characterized by auditory hallucinations.

Adaption: Adjustment of the receptors to stimulation or lack of stimulation.

Adaptability: Flexibility in meeting changed circumstances or demands.

Addison's disease: Disease of the adrenal glands characterized by an anemic, emaciated conditions an brownish coloration of the skin.

Additive color mixture: The mixing of lights, in which different wavelengths are added together.

Adequacy feelings: Feeling of being confident or capable.

Adjective behavior: Behavior by which the individual attempts to deal with stress and meet his needs, including efforts to maintain harmonious relationships with the environment. Or activities by men or the lower animals attempt to meet the demands made upon them by biological and social needs.

Adjustment: Outcome of the indicia's efforts to deal with stress and meet his needs.

Adrenal androgens: Hormones secreted by the adrenal cortex which regulate the development of secondary sex characteristics associated with masculinity.

Adrenal cortex: Outer layer of the adrenal glands; secretes the adrenal steroids and other hormones.

Adrenal glands: Endocrine glands located at the upper end of the kidneys; consist of inner adrenal medulla and outer adrenal cortex, which secrete the hormones adrenaline and noradrenaline during strong emotion, and outer adrenal cortex, which secretes the adrenal androgens and other hormones that influence maturation.

Adrenaline: Hormone secreted by the adrenal medulla in strong emotion; causes such bodily changes as an increase in blood sugar, a rise in blood pressure, and a more rapid pulse rate. Or hormone secreted by the adrenal medulla during strong emotion; causes such bodily changes as an increase in blood sugar and a rise in blood pressure. Also called epinephrine.

Affective: Experience of emotion or feeling.

Affective reaction: Psychosis characterized by extreme fluctuations of mood.

Afferent neuron: Neuron which carries messages toward the central nervous system from a receptor cell; also known as a sensory neuron.

After discharge: Process whereby, because of self-exciting circuits and impulses traveling through long-circuit chains, a single stimulus can cause a motoneuron to discharge for several seconds or minutes.

Afterimage: See Negative after sensation and positive after sensation.

After care: Follow-up therapy after release from a hospital.

Age regression: Inducing a hypnotized subject to evidence behavior of an earlier life period.

Aggression: A response that delivers hurtful stimuli to another object or person.

Aggressive reaction: A response to frustration in which the source of frustration or some substitute is attacked.

Agitated depression: Type of psychotic depressive reaction characterized by both severely depressed mood and hyperactivity.

Agitation: Marked restlessness and psychomotor excitement.

Agoraphobia: Morbid fear of large, open places.

Alarm reaction: First stage of the general-adaption-syndrome characterized by the mobilization of defenses to cope with a stressful situation.

Agnosia: A disorder of perception in which sensations are felt but cannot be organized into normal perceptions.

All-or-none principle: Principle that if a nerve fiber responds at all, it responds with full strength.

Alpha rhythm: The electrical rhythm typical of the brain during normal wakefulness.

Alcoholic deterioration: Personality deterioration, including impaired judgment, associated with alcoholism.

Alcoholic intoxication: State reached when alcohol content of blood is 0.1 percent or above.

Alcoholism: Dependence on alcohol to the extent that it seriously interferes with life adjustment.

Anglophobia: Irrational fear of pain.

Alienation: Lack or loss of relationships to others.

Alpha waves: Brain waves having a frequency of 8 to 12 cycles per second and accompanied by a state of wakeful relaxation.

Alzheimer's disease: A prehensile dementia.

Ambivalence: Experiencing both positive and negative feelings toward the same person or object. Or simultaneous existence of contradictory emotional attitudes toward the same person, e.g. love and hate.

Ambulatory schizophrenic: Mild schizophrenic who is not hospitalized and continues to live and function in the community.

Amnesia: Total or partial loss of memory especially of part personal experiences.

Amphetamine: One type of drug that produces a psychologically stimulating and energizing effect.

Amplitude: Height of light waves, determining brightness; intensity of sound waves, determining volume.

Ampullae: Swellings at the base of the semicircular canals; contain hair cells which are the chief receptors for accelerating or decelerating motion.

Amygdala: Area in the rhinencephalon whose destruction causes excessive sexual behavior and a cessation of rage and savageness.

Anal period: In psychoanalytic theory, stage of development during which bowel control is achieved and the focus of pleasure is the eliminative processes.

Anal personality: Personality characterized by miserliness and obsessive orderliness, traits which, according to psychoanalytic theory, are related to unsatisfied cravings during the period of preoccupation with elimination.

Anal stage: In psychoanalytic theory, stage of psychosexual development in which behavior is presumably focused on anal pleasure and activities.

Analgesia: Insensitivity to pain without loss of consciousness.

Analysis of covariance: A complex procedure involving a blend of analysis of variance and correlation; used to achieve statistical control.

Analysis of variance: Technique for determining the statistical significance of differences among the dependent variable means of different experimental groups.

Analytical psychology: The personality theory of Jung, which emphasizes the purposive aspect of personality and regards the integration of the conscious and unconscious parts of the personality into a unified self as the individual's highest goal. The school or system of psychology developed by Carl Jung.

Anatomical method: Method of studying brain functions by tracing nerved pathways in nonliving tissue under a microscope.

Androgen: Male hormone which regulates sexual development; some androgens are produced by the testes and others by the adrenal cortex. Hormones associated with the development and maintenance of male characteristics.

Anesthesia: Loss or impairment of sensitivity (usually to touch but often applied to sensitivity to pain and other senses as well).

Anomie: State of deregulation of social norms and values.

Anorexia nervosa: Loss or severe diminishment of appetite.

Anoxia: Lack of sufficient oxygen.

Antabuse: Drug used in the treatment of alcoholism.

Anterograde amnesia: Loss of memory for events following trauma or shock.

Antianxiety drugs: Drugs which are used primarily to elevate mood and relieve depression.

Antidepressant drugs: Drugs which are used primarily to elevate mood and relieve depression.

Antisocial (psychopathic) personality: Personality disorder involving a marked lack of ethical or moral development.

Anxiety: Generalized feelings of fear and apprehension.

Anxiety attack: Acute episode of intense anxiety.

Anxiety hierarchy: Ranking of anxiety-eliciting situations utilized in systematic desensitization therapy.

Anxiety neurosis: Type of neurosis characterized by chronic anxiety and apprehension.

Anomic: Loss of the sense of personal identity.

Anoxia: Lack of sufficient oxygen.

Anxiety: Generalized feelings of apprehension; a symptom of many neuroses and psychosis.

Aphasia: Impairment of ability to use or understand language, even though hearing and speech mechanisms are unimpaired. Or loss or impairment of ability to communicate and understand language symbols-involving loss of power of expression by speech, writing, or signs, or loss of ability to comprehend written or spoken language-resulting from brain injury or disease.

Applied science: Study which seeks and uses scientific knowledge for some practical purpose.

Approach-approach conflict: Form of conflict frustration in which the individual must choose between two desirable but mutually exclusive goals.

Approach-avoidance conflict: Form of conflict frustration in which the individual is at the same time attracted and repelled by the same goal. In other words it is a type of stress situation involving both positive and negative features.

Apraxia: Loss of ability to perform purposeful movements.

Aptitude tests: Instruments designed to measure capacity to learn or perform certain tasks.

Arousal: General energizing component of motivation; involves organs controlled by both central and autonomic nervous system.

Ascending reticular system: System of ascending nerve fibers over which impulses go to the cortex from the subcortical areas. See also Reticular formation.

Assimilation effect: Tendency to misperceive a trusted speaker's stand as being closer to the subject's own stand on an issue than it really is.

Association areas: Areas of the cerebral cortex which serve to correlate and integrate the functions of the sensory and motor areas.

Associationistic theories of learning: Theories which regard learning as a process of forming associative bonds or connections.

Asthenic reaction: Neurotic reaction in which the individual feels tired all the time and suffers from mild physical symptoms in the absence of known organic pathology. Formerly called neurasthenia.

Astigmatism: Visual defect caused by unequal curvature of the cornea and/or lens. Producing unfocused, fuzzy vision in one dimension.

Arteriosclerosis: Degenerative thickening and hardening of the walls of the arteries, occurring usually in old age.

Assertive training: Behavior therapy technique for helping individuals become more self-assertive in interpersonal relationships.

Astasia-abasia: Inability to stand or walk without the legs wobbling about and collapsing, although the person has normal control of legs while sitting or lying down; no associated organic pathology.

Asthma: A respiratory disorder.

Ataxia: Muscular incoordination, particularly of the arms and legs. See locomotor ataxia.

Atmospheric perspective: Difference in clarity between near and far objects; an aid in depth perception.

Attention: The process of psychological selectivity by which we select, from a vast number of potential stimuli, only those which are related to present interests and needs.

Attitude: A relatively stable, learned, emotionalized predisposition to respond in some consistent way toward an object, person, or situation.

Atrophy: Wasting away or shrinking of a bodily organ.

Attitude: A consistent, learned, emotionalized predisposition to respond in a particular way to a given object, person, or situation.

Auditory area: Cortical area in the wall of the fissure of Sylvius on each temporal lobe, to which fibers from both ears are connected.

Auditory nerve: Nerve which transmits impulses from the organ of Corti to the brain.

Aura: Subjective sensations, such as a peculiar odor, preceding an epileptic seizure.

Autism: Disorder beginning in infancy characterized by inability of child to relate to others or form normal self-concepts.

Autistic thinking: Thinking as an end in itself and not a means to an end; determined primary by individual's needs or desires, as in daydreaming.

Autokinetic movement: The apparent movement of small stationary point of light in a dark room.

Autonomic nervous system: That part of the nervous system which regulates bodily activities not subject to voluntary control, including the visceral changes that occur. During emotion; composed of the sympathetic and parasympathetic division. Or the section of the nervous system that regulates the internal organs; consists primarily of ganglia connected with the brainstem and spinal cord and may be subdivided into the sympathetic and parasympathetic systems.

Automation: The use of machines to control machines.

Autonomic reactivity: Individual's characteristic degree of emotional reactivity to stress.

Autonomy: Self-reliance; the sense of being an individual in one's own right.

Autosome: Any chromosome other than those determining sex.

Aversion therapy: Form of behavior therapy in which punishment or aversive stimulation is used to eliminated undesired responses.

Aversive conditioning: Use of noxious stimuli noxious stimuli to punish unwanted behavior.

Aversive stimulus: A stimulus that elicits psychic or physical pain.

Avoidance conditioning: Form of conditioning in which the subject learns to behave in a certain way in order to avoid an unpleasant stimulus. Or instrumental aversive conditioning in which the organism can prevent an unpleasant stimulus by making an appropriate response in time.

Avoidance-avoidance conflict: Form of conflict frustration in which the individual cannot avoid one alternative without encountering the other.

Axon: Long fiber leading from the cell body of the neuron, terminating in end brushes.

"bad trip": An unpleasant or traumatic experience while under the influence of a hallucinogenic drug, such as LSD.

Barbiturate: Type of commonly used synthetic sedative drug.

Basilar membrane: Membrane in the cochlea on which is located the organ of Corti; varies in width and responds selectively to impulses of lower frequency as it becomes wider.

Behavior: Isolated reactions and organized, goal-directed patterns of reaction which can be observed objectively and internal processes such as thinking and emotional reactions, which can only be observed introspectively or inferred from external behavior.

Behavior control: Shaping and manipulation of behavior by drugs, persuasion, and other techniques.

Behavior modification: See Behavior therapy.

Behavioral contract: A contact, often between family members, stipulating privileges and responsibilities.

Behavioral sciences: The various interrelated disciplines, including psychology, sociology , and anthropology, that focus on human behavior.

Behavior therapy: Action therapies. Therapeutic procedures based primarily on application of principles of respondent and operant conditioning.

Behavioral science: A coordinated discipline in which psychologists, sociologists and anthropologists work together on the problem of developing valid generalizations about human behavior.

Behaviorists: School of psychologists who restricted their study to man's overt behavior, believed to be determined by stimulus-response connections.

Behaviorism: School of psychology which formerly restricted itself primarily to study of overt behavior.

Behavior sampling: Technique for measuring personality traits; the examiner observed the subject's behavior in a specified situation, without the subject's knowledge.

Benign: Of a mild, self-limiting, nature; not malignant.

Bestiality: Sexual relations with animals.

Beta waves: Brain waves having a frequency of 18 to 30 cycles per second and associated with problem solving and feelings of tensions.

Between variance: The variability between samples; an estimate of the population variance based upon the variation due to the independent variable as well as that due to random effects.

Bilateral symmetry: Condition in which the two halves of an object or organism are essentially alike.

Biochemical disorders: Disorders involving disturbances in metabolic processes.

Biofeedback: Feedback information concerning blood pressure and other bodily processes under control of the autonomic nervous system.

Biogenic amines: Chemicals that serve as neurotransmitters or modulators.

Biographical method: Technique by which the psychologist seeks to understand behavior by analyzing the records of men's lives.

Biological drives: Innate drives resulting from basic tissue needs.

Biological clocks: The 24 hour rhythmic fluctuations in metabolic processes of plants and animals. Also called circadian cycles.

Bisexual: A person sexually attracted to the both females and males.

Bipolar cells: First neurons in the visual pathway; conduct messages from the rods and cones to ganglion cells.

Bit: Unit of information; amount of information which, when put into a system, reduces the number of alternatives by half.

Blind spot: Region of the retina where nerve fibers leave the eye: no rods or cones are found here.

Blur point: Distance from eyes at which print becomes blurred, as it is moved closer to the eyes.

Blocking: Involuntary inhibition of recall, ideation, or communication (including sudden stoppage of speech).

Body image: A persons image of his or her body in terms of attractiveness and other characteristics.

Brain pathology: Diseased or disordered condition of the brain.

Brain potentials: Brainwaves; minute oscillations of electrical potential given off by the cerebral cortex; measured by the electroencephalograph.

Brainstem: Term used to designate all the structures the lie between the cerebrum and the spinal cord.

Brain storming: A technique for stimulating creativity in group or individual problem solving, consisting of a "green light" stage in which solutions are suggested and a "red light" stage in which they are evaluated.

Brain washing: Intensive form of propaganda, often conducted under emotional stress but typically without corporal punishment. It is an extreme form of thought modification and control.

Brain waves: Minute oscillations of electrical potential given off by neurons in the cerebral cortex and measured by the electroencephalograph.

Brain-wave therapy: The appempt to use alpha or other brain waves for psychotherapeutic purposes.

Brightness: Quality of color determined by the amplitude (height) of the light wave, greater amplitude causing a brighter (lighter) color.

Broca's area: Area in frontal lobe of cerebral hemisphere above the fissure of Sylvius; important for speech.

Butch: Slang term for lesbian, particularly one who assumes a masculine appearance.

Cardiovascular: Pertaining to the heart and blood vessels.

Case study: Assessment information on a specific individual.

Castrating: Refers to any source of injury to or deprivation of the genitals, or more broadly, to a threat to the masculinity or feminity of the individual.

Catalepsy: A condition in which the muscles are waxy and semirigid, tending to maintain the limbs in any position in which they are placed.

Catatonic schizophrenia: Type of schizophrenia characterized by periods of extreme excitement and extreme withdrawal.

Catatonia: Schizophrenic reaction characterized by motionless, unresponsive stupor.

Catharsis: The discharging of emotional tension by "talking out" or otherwise expressing troubled emotions; important in most psychotherapy.

Cell body: Thickened portion of cell, containing nucleus.

Centiles: Points which divide a distribution of measurements into 100 equal parts; sometimes called percentiles.

Central nervous system: The brain and spinal cord.

Central value: A statistic which represents the average or typical value of a series of measurements; common central value measures are the mean, the median, and the mode.

Centralist theories: Cognitive learning theories, which emphasize the importance of organizing processes as central to learning.

Centrifugal impulse: "wrong-way" impulses which go from the sense organs toward the brain centers; "right-way" impulses.

Cerebellum: The part of the brain that controls the coordination of movements necessary for balance in sitting, walking, and manipulation.

Cerebral cortex: A thin, grayish rind of tissue covering the cerebrum; active in conscious experience and higher mental processes.

Cerebral dominance: Control of a function of both sides of the body by one side of the cerebrum.

Cerebral syphilis: Syphilitic infection of the brain.

Cerebral thrombosis: The formation of a clot or thrombus in the vascular system of the brain.

Cerebrovascular accident (CVA): Blockage or rupture of large blood vessel in brain leading to both focal and generalized impairment of brain function. Also called stroke.

Cerebrum: Main part of brain; divided into left and right hemisphere.

Central nervous system (CNS): The brain and spinal cord.

Cerebral arteriosclerosis: Hardening of the arteries in the brain.

Cerebral concussion: Mild head injury that disrupts brain functions.

Cerebral contusion: Brain damage resulting from head injury severe enough to shift brain and compress it against skull.

Cerebral cortex: The surface layers of the cerebrum.

Cerebral hemorrhage: Bleeding into brain tissue from a ruptured blood vessels.

Cerebral laceration: Tearing of brain tissue associated with severe head injury.

Character disorder: See antisocial personality.

Chemical senses: The senses of smell and taste.

Chemotherapy: Use of drugs in the therapy. Use of drugs in treatment of mental disorders.

Child advocacy: Movement or agencies concerned with protecting rights and ensuring well-being of children.

Chlorpromazine: One of the major tranquilizing drugs.

Chorea: A pathological condition characterized by jerky, irregular, involuntary movements.

Choroid coat: Middle layer of coating of the eye.

Chromatin body: Macroscopic structure found in cells of female organisms, which takes a deep stain while male cells will not.

Chromosomes: Chain-like structures within cell nucleus that contain genes. They are small bodies, found in pairs, which contain the genes responsible for hereditary traits; half an individual's chromosomes come from the mother, half from the father, making a total of 46 in normal human cells.

Chronic: Referring to relatively permanent maladaptive pattern or condition.

Circadian rhythms: Regular biological cycle of sleep and activity characteristic of each species.

Civil commitment: Procedure whereby an individual certified as mentally disordered can be hospitalized, either voluntarily or against his will.

Clairvoyance: Form of extrasensory perception in which the subject supposedly becomes aware of an external object without the use of his sense organs.

Classical conditioning: See Conditioning.

Claustrophobia: Irrational fear of small enclosed places.

Client-centered psychotherapy: A nondirective approach to psychotherapy developed chiefly by Carl Rogers and based on his personality theory.

Client-centered therapy: A nondirective technique of psychotherapy based on the theory that many individuals can work through their own problems by "talking them out" in a permissive and supportive atmosphere.

Clinical method: A method of studying human behavior in which the life history of the individual is reconstructed on the basis of all available information, usually in an effort to discover the cause of some maladjustment.

Climacteric: The life period associated with the menopause in women and various related glandular and bodily changes in men.

Clinical picture: Diagnostic picture formed by observation of patient's behavior or by all available assessment data.

Clinical psychology: Field of psychology concerned with the understanding, assessment, treatment, and prevention of maladaptive behavior.

Clinical psychologist: Nonmedical psychologist who practices psychotherapy.

Closure: Perceptual process by which we "close" gaps in a figure so that we see it as whole figure.

Cochlear canals: Canals of the inner ear, containing fluid which is set in motion by vibrations of the oval window and which in turn stimulated the basilar membrane.

Cocaine: A stimulating and pain-reducing psychoactive drug.

Cognitive dissonance: Condition existing when new information is contradictory to one's assumptions.

Cognitive dissonance theory: Principle that dissonant (unbalanced or incongruous) cognitions tend to become more congruous, better balanced.

Cognitive learning theories: Learning theories which regard learning as a process of making new differentiations and discriminations or reorganizing material into new patterns.

Cognitive map: See Frame of reference.

Cognitive process (cognition): Mental processes, including perception, memory, and reasoning, by which one acquires knowledge, solves problems, and makes plans.

Cohabitation: A male and female living together without being married.

Coitus: Sexual intercourse.

Collaterals: Branches of neurons.

Collective unconscious: Term used by Carl Jung to refer to that portion of the unconscious which he considered common to all humanity. In Jungian theory, racial unconscious or storehouse of racial memories with which every person is thought to be endowed.

Color solid: Double cone which classifies colors three dimensionally, with points along the vertical axis representing degrees of brightness, points along any radius representing degrees of saturation, and points around the circumference representing the different hues.

Coma: Profound stupor with unconsciousness.

Community mental health: Application of psychosocial and sociocultural principles to the improvement of given environment.

Community psychology: Use of community resources in dealing with maladaptive behavior. It tends to be more concerned with community intervention rather than with personal or individual change.

Compensation: Type of ego-defense mechanism in which an undesirable trait is covered up by exaggerating a desirable trait.

Commissures: Connecting fibers between the two hemispheres of the brain.

Compensation: Attempt to disguise the presence of a weak or undesirable trait by emphasizing a desirable one. See also Overcompensation.

Complementary colors: Two colors located opposite each other on the color wheel; complementary colors combine to give gray.

Complementary tastes: Tastes which tend to neutralize each other if mixed.

Complex: Group of emotionally toned attitudes, desires, or memories which are partially or totally repressed.

Compulsion: An irrational and repetitive impulse to perform some act.

Computer assessment: Use of computer to obtain or interpret assessment data.

Computer model: Use of computer to simulate group functioning.

Compromise reaction: A response to frustration in which the individual partially gives into the frustrating obstacle but without entirely relinquishing his original goal.

Compulsion: Bizarre action which the individual himself does not understand but nevertheless feels impelled to perform; usually symbolic in nature.

Concept: Abstract idea derived from the grouping of objects in terms of some common property.

Conceived values: The individual's conception of the ideal values.

Concept: General idea based on similarities among different objects, events, etc.

Concordance: Similarity in diagnosis or other traits in a twin pair.

Concussion: See cerebral concussion.

Conditioned reinforce: A reinforce that derives its value from basic unconditioned reinforces.

Conditioned inhibition: Process by which the organism becomes conditioned not to respond; occurs when a conditioned stimulus and a neutral stimulus are presented together and not followed by reinforcement. The neutral stimulus becomes the suppressor. This is not the same as simple extinction because the CS alone still elicits the CR.

Conditioned response (CR): A learned response to a stimulus not originally capable of arousing the response.

Conditioned stimulus (CS): A previously neutral stimulus which has become capable of evoking a particular (conditioned) response.

Conditioning: A basic form of learning in which conditioned responses are established. In classical conditioning, a response comes to be evoked by a previously neutral stimulus when this stimulus is paired for a number of tails with the (unconditioned) stimulus which normally elicits the response. In instrumental conditioning, no eliciting stimuli are presented; the subject is placed in a situation where he learns to make an instrumental response leading to reward or, in aversive conditioning, one which terminates or prevents an unpleasant stimulus.

Cones: Retinal receptor cells sensitive to both hue and brightness responsible for color vision.

Confabulation: The filling in of memory gaps with false and often irrelevant details.

Confidentiality: Commitment on part of professional person to keep information he obtains from a client confidential.

Conflict: Simultaneous arousal of opposing impulses, desires, or motives.

Congenital: Existing at birth or before birth but not necessarily hereditary.

Confidence interval: An interval of measurements with a known probability of containing a parameter.

Conjugate movements: Simultaneous movements of the eyeballs in changing the fixation from one equidistant points to another; comprise jump and pursuit movements.

Connectors: Biological structures which connect receptors with organs of response; used primarily with reference to the nervous system, but also including the bloodstream and certain chemical substances.

Conscience: The functioning of an individual's system of moral values in the approval or disapproval of his own thoughts and actions. Equivalent to Freudian concept of superego.

Consciousness: Awareness of inner and/or outer environment.

Constitution: The relatively constant biological makeup of the individual, resulting from the interaction of heredity and environment.

Consummatory response: Action which represents the completion of goal-seeking activity.

Contiguity theory: Learning theory which emphasizes the role of temporal contiguity of stimulus and response, holding that learning occurs regardless of whether reinforcement is given, so long as the conditioned stimulus and the response occurs together; espoused by Guthrie and Watson.

Contingency: Relationship, usually causal, between two events in which one is usually followed by the other.

Continuous reinforcement: Reward or reinforcement given regularly after each correct response.

Continuous reinforcement: Reinforcement given regularly after each conditioning trail.

Contrast effect: In persuasive communications, tendency to displace a speaker's message away from the subject's own stand on an issue; occurs when the speaker arouses negative feeling in the subject. In taste, tendency of relatively sour things to taste more sour if sweet things are tasted first. See also Simultaneous brightness contrast and simultaneous hue contrast.

Control group: Group of subject for which the experimenter holds the independent variable under control either by keeping it constant or by removing it from the situation entirely.

Convergence: In the nervous system, distributing process whereby impulses from many neurons or receptor cells reach the same neuron or effectors; makes it possible for the same muscle fiber to take part in many different reflexes. In vision, process by which the eyes turn toward each other when focusing upon objects closer than about twenty feet so that both eyes fixate the same point in space; a cue in depth perception.

Conversion reaction: Neurotic reaction to stress in which psychological distress is converted into bodily symptoms; formerly called hysteria.

Convulsion: Pathological, involuntary, muscular contractions.

Corpus callosum: Nerve fibers that connect the two hemisphere of the brain.

Correlational studies: Studies dealing with the extent to which two or more variables covary.

Cornea: Transparent portion of the protective coating of the eye, in front of the lens.

Corpus callosum: Massive bundle of fibers connecting the two hemispheres of the brain.

Correlation coefficient: A statistic which summarizes the relationship of two sets of measurements taken on the same sample.

Corticotrophin: A pituitary hormone which interacts with the secretions of the adrenal cortex—an important factor in rheumatoid arthritis and other disorders; also called ACTH.

Corticovisceral control mechanism: Brain mechanisms that regulate autonomic and other bodily functions.

Counseling psychology: Field of psychology that focuses on helping person with problems pertaining to education, marriage, or occupation.

Counter conditioning: Relearning by using particular stimulus to establish a new (and generally more adaptive) response.

Counter culture: Subculture in conflict with established culture in a given society.

Counter transference: Arousal by the client of feelings of transference on the part of the analyst during the course of psychoanalytic therapy.

Convert trial and error: Trial and error in which alternatives are eliminated by thought instead of action.

Covert: Concealed, disguised, not directly observable.

Crazy: Mentally disordered (term not used in scientific circles).

Cretinism: Condition arising from thyroid deficiency in early life and marked by mental retardation and distinctive physical characteristics.

Criminal responsibility: Legal question of whether an individual should be permitted to use insanity as a defense after having committed some criminal act.

Crisis: Stress situation which approaches or exceeds adaptive capacities of individual or group.

Crisis intervention: Various methods for rendering therapeutic assistance to an individual or group during a period of crisis.

Critical period: Period of development during which organism most needs certain inputs or is most ready for acquisition of a given response.

Cretinism: Retarded development of the skeletal and nervous systems caused by thyroid deficiency during infancy or early childhood; often accompanied by low intelligence.

Critical ratio: A ratio whose numerator is the difference between an obtained statistic and the parameter expected under the null hypothesis, and whose denominator is the standard error of the statistic if the null hypothesis is assumed; used to test statistical significance.

Critical region: That part of a sampling distribution into which a statistic must fall if the null hypothesis is to be rejected at a given level of statistical significance.

Cross-sectional approach: Method of studying the effects of age on various traits by grouping a large number of subjects according to their ages and using one set of tests for all.

Cultural bias: Use of assessment criteria which are biased in favor of a given group.

Cultural-familial mental retardation: Mental retardation resulting from lack of needed environmental stimulations, with no evidence of brain pathology.

Culture-free test: Test designed to eliminate the effects of cultural differences on performance.

Cushing's syndrome: An endocrine disorder resulting from over secretion of cortisone and marked by mood swings, irritability, and other mental symptoms.

Cue function: Indication of the direction of appropriate activity.

Curve of decreasing returns: Graphic representation of learning situation in which the greatest improvement in performance occurs during the early trials; the most commonly obtained learning curve.

Curve of equal returns: Graphic representation of a learning situation in which early trials yield the same amount of improvement as later trials; essentially a straight line.

Curve of increasing returns: Graphic representation of a learning a learning situation in which improvement is greater in later trials than in early trials.

Cutaneous senses: Sense of pressure, pain, warmth, and cold, located primarily in the skin.

Cybernetics: Science of control and communication in the organism and machine.

Cyclofusional movement: Independent rotation of each eye about its axis so that light from an object strikes corresponding points onto the two retinas.

Cyclothymiac (affective) personality: Personality type characterized by extreme mood swings-alternating periods of depression and elation.

Day hospital: A community-based mental hospital where the patients are treated during the day, returning to their homes at night.

Dark adaptation: Process by which the eyes become more sensitive so that they can see under low illumination; usually requires about half an hour of darkness.

Davis-Eells Games: An intelligence test designed in such a way, it was hoped, as to be culture fair, with problems whose content is not limited to the experience of any socioeconomic level. Such tests are low in reliability and validity.

Daybook method: A form of the life-history method of obtaining data usually employed in observing children; the individual's development is carefully observed and recorded day-by-day.

Decibel: Unit of measurement of the intensity of sound.

Decompensation: Ego personality disorganization under excessive stress.

Defense mechanism: See Ego-defense mechanism.

Defense-oriented reaction: Reaction involving one's feelings of adequacy and worth rather than objective handling of the stress situation.

Deficiency motivation: Motivation directed primarily toward maintaining or restoring physiological or psychological equilibrium rather than toward personal growth.

Defense of freedom (df): Number of independent observation jupon which an estimate of a parameter is based.

Delayed reaction: Introduction of a brief waiting interval after a stimulus before a previously learned response can be made; a measure of ability to carry images or symbols in the memory.

Delirium tremens: Organic psychosis with visual hallucinations, resulting from severe alcoholism.

Delusion: A strong belief opposed to reality and maintained in spite of logical persuasion and evidence to the contrary; symptom of psychosis. Three main types; delusion of grandeur (belief that one is being plotted against), and delusion of reference (belief that chance happenings and conversation concern oneself).

Delusion of persecution: False belief that one is being mistreated or interfered with by one's enemies. Often found in schizophrenia.

Delusion system: An internally coherent, systematized pattern of delusions.

Dementia: Severe mental disorder involving impairment of mental ability; not congenital.

Dementia praecox: Older term for schizophrenia.

Denial of reality: Ego-defense mechanism by means of which the individual protects himself from unpleasant aspects of reality by refusing to perceive them.

Deoxyribonucleic acid (DNA): Principal component of the genes.

Dendrites: Highly branched, usually quite short fibers at the receiving end of the neuron.

Dependency: A class of responses capable of eliciting positive attending and ministering responses from others; may be task-oriented or person-oriented.

Dependent variable: In an experiment, the factor which the hypothesis predicts will change with changes in the independent variable.

Depersonalization: Loss of sense of personal identity, often with a feeling of being something or someone else.

Depression: Emotional state characterized by extreme dejection, gloomy ruminations, feelings of worthlessness, loss of hope, and often of apprehension.

Depressive neurosis: Neurotic reaction characterized by persistent dejection and discouragement.

Depressive reaction: Neurotic reaction in which the individual reacts to a frustrating situation or a loss with greater sadness and for a longer time than the normal person would.

Depressive stupor: Extreme degree of depression.

Desensitization: Therapeutic process by means of which reactions to traumatic experiences are reduced in intensity by repeatedly exposing the individual to them in mild form, either in reality or in fantasy.

Detoxification: Treatment directed toward ridding the body of alcohol or other drugs.

Deterrence: The premise that punishment for criminal offenses will deter that criminal and others from future criminal acts.

Development task: A competency that is considered essential to master during a particular life period, e.g. learning to talk during infancy.

Deviant behavior: Behavior which deviates markedly from the average or norm.

Diagnosis: Determination of the nature and extent of a specific disorder.

Didactic group therapy: Group therapy consisting of more or less formal group lectures and discussions.

Directive therapy: Type of therapeutic approach in which the therapist supplies direct answers to problems and takes much of the responsibility for the progression of therapy.

Discrimination learning: Learning to interpret and respond differently to two or more similar stimuli.

Descriptive statistic: A number which stands for a series of measurements collected on a group.

Dichromat: Person who has normal vision for only two primary colors, usually yellow and blue.

Difference limen: Smallest detectable difference in stimulus intensity. See also Weber's law.

Dimension: A characteristic which can be measured and expressed in numerical terms.

Diplopia: Double vision; may be caused by hereditary weakness of eye muscles or by disease, poison, or (temporarily) alcohol.

Directive counseling: Least complicated type of psychotherapy, in which the therapist supplies reassurance, suggestions, or direct solutions.

Discrimination learning: Learning in which the task is to distinguish between two or more stimuli or between stimulus and not stimulus.

Disinhibition: Temporary reappearance of a conditioned response which has been extinguished, in response to an extraneous stimulus different from the conditioned stimulus; inhibition of an inhibition.

Displaced aggression: Transfer of hostility from the object or person actually causing frustration to some other object or person or to the self.

Dissociative reaction: Neurotic reactions to extreme stress in which entire episodes of life are repressed from consciousness, as in amnesia, fugue, and multiple personality.

Distributed practice: Use of spaced learning periods.

Divergence: Distributing process in the nervous system whereby impulses from a single neuron or receptor cell reach many neurons or muscles.

Dominant gene: Gene of an opposing pair which takes effect to produce a hereditary trait.

Double alternation test: Test of ability to learn a sequence, as: left, left, right, right, left, left, right, right; used as a measure of thinking ability.

Double approach-avoidance conflict: Form of conflict frustration in which both alternatives have attractive and undesirable features.

Double-blind technique: Method of studying the effectiveness of drugs or other treatments in which neither the subjects nor the individuals evaluating the results know which ones received which treatment.

Diseases of adaptation: Stomach ulcers and other disease condition resulting from the stresses of life.

Disintegration: Loss of organization or integration in any organized system.

Disorganization: Severely impaired integration.

Disorientation: Mental confusion with respect to time, place, or person.

Displacement: Ego-defense mechanism in which an emotional attitude or symbolic meaning is transferred from one object or concept to another.

Dissociation: Separation or "isolation" of mental processes in such a way that they become split off from the main personality or lose their normal thought-affect relationships.

Dissociative reaction: Psychoneurotic reaction characterized by amnesia, fugue, somnambulism, or multiple personality.

Dizygotic (fraternal) twins: Twins that develop from two separate eggs.

DNA: Deoxyribonucleic acid, principal component of genes.

Dominant gene: A gene whose hereditary characteristics prevail in the offspring.

Double-approach conflict: Type of conflict in which individual is confronted with choosing between two or more desirable alternatives.

Double-avoidant conflict: Type of conflict in which individual is confronted with choosing between two or more aversive alternatives.

Double-blind: Situation in which an individual will be disapproved for performing a given act and equally disapproved if he does not perform it.

Down's syndrome (mongolism): Form of mental retardation associated with chromosomal anomalies.

Dream analysis: Psychoanalytic technique involving the interpretation of the patient's dreams.

Drive: Internal condition directing organism toward a specific goal, usually involving biological rather than psychological motives.

Drive: Complex of internal conditions directing the organism toward a specific goal; a motive.

Drug abuse: Use of a drug to extent that it interferes with health and/or occupational or social adjustment.

Drug addiction (dependence): Physiological and/or psychological dependence on a drug.

Drug therapy: See Chemotherapy.

Dual personality: See Multiple personality.

Dwarfism: A condition of arrested growth and very short stature. In this underdevelopment of the bones caused by a deficiency of the pituitary growth hormone early in life.

Dyad: Two-person team or a two person group.

Dysfunction: Impairment or disturbance in the functioning of an organ.

Dyslexia: Impairment of the ability to read.

Dyspareunia: Painful coitus in male or female.

Dysrhythmia: Disturbance in rhythm.

Dissocial personality: Behavior pattern characterized by criminal values but good ego strength.

Eardrum: Thin membrane which separates the external ear from the middle ear; made to vibrate by the pressure impulses of sound waves.

EGG: See Electroencephalogram.

Echolalia: Meaningless repetition of words by an individual, usually of whatever is said to him.

Echopraxia: Repetition of another person's actions or gestures.

Ecology: Relation or interaction between organisms and their physical environment.

Economy, principles of: Theory that the individual meets stress in the simplest way possible.

Eco-spasm: Term used by Toffler to refer to the breakdown of industrial civilization on Earth, accompanied by the initial fragmentary appearance of a new type of civilization.

Effectors: The organs (muscles or glands) which perform the actual response functions.

Efferent neuron: Neuron which carries messages from the central nervous system to an organ of response; also known as motoneurons.

Ego: In psychoanalytic theory, the rational aspect of the personality; regulates the impulses of the id in order to meet the demands of reality and maintain social approval and self-esteem. More generally, the individual's concept of self. In other words theory, the rational subsystem of the personality which mediates between id and superego demands and reality. More generally, the individual's self-concepts.

Ego-defense mechanism(reaction): Type of reaction designed to maintain the individual's feelings of adequacy and worth rather than to cope directly with the stress situation; usually unconscious and reality distorting.

Ego-ideal (self-ideal): The person of "self" the individual thinks he could and should be.

Ego involvement: Perception of a situation in terms of its importance to the individual. Or perception of a situation in terms of its potential effect on one's self concept.

Egocentric: Preoccupied with one's own concerns and relatively insensitive to the concerns of others.

Ejaculatory incompetence: A male's inability to ejaculate.

Electra complex: In psychoanalytic theory, and excessive emotional attachment (love) of a daughter for her father.

Eidetic imagery: Mental imagery, usually visual, which is almost like actual perception in its clarity and accuracy; rare but most often found in children.

Effect low of: Theory holding that satisfying events strengthen S-R connections and annoying events weaken them; proposed by Thorndike.

Electroconvulsive shock: Form of therapy for mental illness; electric current passes through the brain produces instant unconsciousness and convulsions.

Electroencephalogram (EEG): Recording of the minute electrical oscillations of the cerebral cortex known as brain potentials or brain waves.

Electroconvulsive therapy (ECT): Use of electricity to produce convulsions and unconsciousness; also called electroshock therapy.

Electroencephalogram (EEG): A recording of the brain waves by an electroencephalograph.

Elicited behavior: In conditioning, a response already in the organism's repertoire which is initiated by some recognizable physical stimulus.

Electrotherapy: Methods of therapy which involve the influence of electric current on the central nervous system.

Embolism: Lodgment of a blood clot in a blood vessels to small to permit its passage.

Embryo: The organism between conception and birth or hatching. In humans, the organism from the second to the eighth week after conception.

Emergency reaction: The alarm reaction stage of the general-adaption-syndrome.

Emitted behavior: Behavior which appears without the use of an external stimulus to initiate it; basis of instrumental conditioning.

Emotion: A strong feeling accompanied by physiological changes. Complex state of feeling involving conscious experience, internal and overt physical responses, and power to motivate the organism to action.

Emotional insulation: Ego-defense mechanism in which the individual reduces the tensions of need and anxiety by withdrawing into a shell of passivity.

Empathy: Ability to understand and to some extent share the state of mind of another person.

Encephalization: Increasing concentration of neural components in the head region, eventually constituting a brain, in ascending forms on the evolutionary scale.

End brushes: Tiny fibers at end of an axon.

End plates: Structures at the end of the axons of motoneurons, corresponding to end brushes.

Encephalitis: Inflammation of the brain.

Encounter: Term applied to the interaction between client and therapist (in existential therapy) or between patients (in encounter-group therapy).

Endocrine glands: Ductless glands which secrete hormones directly into the lymph or bloodstream.

Energizer: Drug which has a stimulating effect.

Engram: Hypothesized physiological changes in nervous system thought to be responsible for memory.

Entrophy: Deterioration and eventual disintegration or death of a living system.

Enuresis: Bed-wetting; involuntary discharge of urine.

Environmental psychology: Field of psychology focusing on the effects of environmental setting on an individual's feelings and behavior.

Enzyme: Catalyst regulating metabolic activities.

Epidemiology: Study of the distribution of physical or mental disorders in a populations.

Energetic: Variability in the intensity of responding; one of the two basic but interacting characteristics of human and animal behavior. See also Plasticity.

Energizer: Drug which stimulates the patient, making him feel more energetic.

Engram: Memory trace; formed and temporarily stored during learning but must be stored through a process of consolidation or it is rapidly lost.

Environment: The totality of conditions within and surrounding the organism that serves to stimulate behavior or act to bring about change of behavior.

Epidemiology: Study of the incidence, distribution, and control of physical or mental disease.

Epilepsy: Group of disorders varying from momentary lapses of consciousness to generalized convulsions.

Epinephrine: Hormone secreted by the adrenal medulla; also called adrenaline.

Equilibrium: Steady state; balance.

Erotic: Pertaining to sexual stimulation and gratification.

Escape learning: Condition response in which the subject learns to terminate or escape an aversive stimulus.

Essence: Existential term referring to the fact that one's existence is given but what is made of it is up to the individual and becomes his essence.

Essential hypertension: High blood pressure, presumably of a psychological or emotional origin.

Escape conditioning: Instrumental aversive conditioning in which the organism can stop an unpleasant stimulus by making the appropriate response.

Estrogens: Female hormones produced by the ovaries; promote growth in the reproductive organs and other body parts important to childbearing and motherhood.

Estrus: Period when a female lower mammal is highly receptive or even aggressive in sexual behavior, a signal that she is in readiness for pregnancy; popularly called heat.

Eustachian tube: Tube leading from the middle ear to the throat; provides for the maintenance of equal air pressure on both sides of the eardrum.

Ethnic group: Group of people who are treated as distinctive in terms of culture and group patterns.

Ethnocentrism: Belief that one's own country and race are superior to other countries and races.

Etiology: Causation; the systematic study of the causes of disorders.

Eugenics: The application of methods of selective breeding of human beings with the intent of improving the species.

Euphoria: Exaggerated feeling of well-being and contentment.

Evoked potentials: Electrical responses made by the brain to specific sensory stimuli.

Exacerbate: Intensify.

Excitation: Process whereby activity is elicited in a nerve.

Excitatory postsynaptic potential (EPSP): Potential change which occurs in a neuron when a nerve impulse is approaching it from a synaptic knob; not subject to all-or-none law; when it builds to certain size, an impulse is set up in the neuron.

Exhibitionism: Public display or exposure of genitals for conscious or unconscious purpose of sexual excitement and pleasure.

Existential anxiety: Anxiety concerning one's ability to find a satisfying and fulfilling way of life.

Existential neurosis: Disorder characterized by feeling of alienation, meaninglessness, and apathy.

Existential therapy: Therapy based on existential concepts, emphasizing the development of a sense of self-direction and meaning in one's existence.

Existentialism: A view of human beings that emphasizes the individual's responsibility for becoming the kind of person he should be. Or a philosophy which emphasizes the importance of existence as primary, with man himself responsible for the kind of person he shall be; a personality theory which emphasizes a sort of self-actualization, although not generally optimistic.

Exogenous: Originating from or due to external causes.

Expanded consciousness: Sensation caused by psychedelic drugs or meditation in which individual feels his mind is opened to new types of experience.

Experimental method: Rigorous scientific procedure by which hypotheses are tested.

Experimental control: In the experimental method, holding constant all variables other than the independent variable which might affect the outcome.

Experimental extinction: Gradual disappearance of a conditioned response when the conditioned stimulus is repeated without being reinforced.

Experimental group: Group of subjects for whom the experimenter alters the independent variable whose influence he wishes to study. Cf. Control group.

Experimental method: The most highly formalized scientific method, in which hypotheses are tested under precisely specified conditions.

Extinction: See Experimental extinction.

Extirpation method: Method of studying brain functions in animals by systematically destroying part of the brain and observing behavioral changes.

Extrasensory perception (ESP): Becoming aware of objects or ideas without use of the sense organs; comprises the phenomena of mental telepathy, clairvoyance, and incorporeal personal agency; not definitely established as a reality.

Experimental neurosis: Neurotic behavior produced in animals by inescapable conflicts and other types of stress.

Extinction: Gradual disappearance of conditioned response when it is no longer reinforced.

Extrapunitive: Characterized by a tendency to evaluate the source of frustrations as external and to direct hostility outward.

Extraversion: Personality type oriented toward the outer world of people and things rather than concepts and intellectual concerns. Or orientation toward the external world of things and people; the extravert tends to enjoy social contacts.

F distribution: The sampling distribution expected from a large number of F ratios.

F ratio: The ratio of the between sample variance to the within sample variance.

Factor analysis: The statistical technique of identifying and measuring the relative importance of the underlying variables, or factors, which contribute to a complex ability, trait, or form of behavior.

Factorial design: Experimental design in which the independent variables are studied in all possible combinations.

Fantasy: Withdrawal reaction in which the individual escapes from frustration through daydreaming.

Fabrication: Relating imaginary events as if they were true without intent to deceive; confabulation.

Familial: Pertaining to characteristics which tend to run in families and have a higher incidence in certain families than in the general population.

Family therapy: Form of interpersonal therapy focusing on relationships within the family.

Fantasy: Daydream; also, an ego-defense mechanism by means of which the individual escapes from the world of reality and gratifies his desires in fantasy achievements.

Feedback: Knowledge of results of one's behavior; used in judging appropriateness of one's responses and making corrections where indicated. Or error-correcting information returned to the control center of a servomechanism or to the nervous system and brain of a living organism, enabling it to offset deviations in its course toward a goal.

Feeble-mindedness: See Mental retardation.

Fetishism: Maladaptive sexual deviation in which an individual achieves sexual gratification by means of some inanimate object or part of the body.

Fetus: The unborn human organism from the eighth week after conception until birth.

Field-study method: Research technique in which the investigator observes the subjects under their usual environmental condition without attempting to control the conditions and often without the subject's knowledge that they are being observed.

Field theory: The systematization of psychology by analogy with fields of force in physics, maintaining that all experience has field prosperities which makes the total experience (or total field) greater than the sum of its parts.

Fissure of Rolando: Deep, nearly vertical furrow or groove on the side of each cerebral hemisphere, separating the frontal and parietal lobes; also known as the central sulcus.

Fissure of Sylvius: Deep horizontal groove on the lateral surface of each cerebral hemisphere, separating the temporal from the frontal and parietal lobes; also known as the central sulcus.

Fixed interval schedule: Schedule by which reinforcement is given regularly at the end of a certain period of time, such as every two minutes.

Fixed ratio schedule: Schedule by which reinforcement is given regularly at the end of a certain period of time, such as every two minutes.

Field properties: Characteristics of the environment surrounding a living system.

Fixation: Unreasonable or exaggerated attachment to some person or arresting of emotional development on a childhood or adolescent level.

Fixed-interval schedule: Schedule of reinforcement based on fixed period of time after previous reinforced response.

Fixed-ratio schedule: Schedule of reinforcement based on reinforcement after fixed number of nonreinforced response.

Flashback: The recurrence of a drug experience, usually in a negative manner, without further ingestion of the drug.

Flight of ideas: Rapid succession of ideas without logical association or continuity.

Flooding: Anxiety-eliciting technique used in implosive therapy.

Folle a deux: A psychotic interpersonal relationship involving two people; e.g. husband and wife both become psychotic with similar symptomatology.

Follow-up study: Research procedure in which individuals are studied over a period of time or are recontacted at a late time after initial study.

Forensic psychiatry: Branch of psychiatry dealing with legal problems raised by mental disorders.

Forced-choice method: Method of reducing faking on self-inventories and rating devices in which the rater must choose from alternatives of equal desirability.

Form board: A board with recesses into which the subject must fit blocks of the proper size and shape as quickly as he can; used as a performance test to measure intelligence.

Fovea: Area in center of retina with greatest density of cones and complete absence of roads; area of clearest daytime vision.

Frame of reference: The reality, ethical and possibility assumptions which form the individual's "cognitive map" for interpreting and coping with his world.

Fraternal twins: Dizygotic twins; fertilized by separate germ cells, thus not having same genetic inheritance. May be of the same or opposite sex. Or twins which, unlike identical twins, develop from two separate fertilized eggs and do not resemble each other any more closely than other brother and sisters. Also called dizygotic twins.

Fraudulent interpersonal contract: Violation of rules or norms governing healthy interpersonal relationships.

Free-floating anxiety: Anxiety not referable to any specific situation or cause.

Free association: Principal procedure used in psychoanalysis to probe the unconscious; patient lets his mind wander freely, giving a running account of every thought and feeling.

"free-floating" anger: Chronic reaction pattern in which anxiety becomes generalized and patient feels a sense of impending doom for no specific reason; may become fixed on specific objects in the form of phobias.

Frequency distribution: A distribution showing the number of times each measurement value occurs in a sample.

Frequency theory: See Telephone theory.

Frigidity: Inability to experience sexual pleasure or orgasm on the part of the female.

Frontal lobe: Portion of the brain active in reasoning and other higher thought processes.

Frustration: Thwarting of a need or desire.

Frontal lobe: Portion of each half of the cerebrum located in front of the fissure of Rolando and above the fissure of Sylvius.

Frustration: Denial or thwarting of motives by obstacles which lie between organism and goal; may be environmental, personal, or the result of conflict.

Fugue: Loss of memory accompanied by actual physical flight. Dissociative reaction in which the individual leaves his present life situation and establishes a somewhat different mode of life in another locale. Although he is amnesic for his past life, his other abilities are unimpaired and he appears normal to those around him.

Functional explanation: Explanation of an event in terms of its use or purpose.

Functional fixedness: Inability to see a new use for a familiar tool.

Functional psychosis: Severe mental disorder precipitated primarily by psychological stress.

Functionalists: School of psychologists who define mental phenomena in terms of their function or activity in adjusting to the environment.

Funneling: Process by which, through a ring of inhibition around a core of excited fibers, auditory sensations are sharpened; fibers on the periphery contribute to other intensity of the sensation but do not change the frequency, which is that of the tone conducted by the central fibers.

Furor: Transitory outbursts of excitement or anger during which the individual may be quite dangerous.

Future shock: Condition brought about when social change proceeds so rapidly that the individual cannot cope with it adequately.

Galvanic skin response (GSR): Increase in voltage and/or change in electrical resistance of the skin during emotion as a result of action of the autonomic nervous system on the sweat glands. Also called psychogalvanic response.

Gamete: Male or female germ cell; contains only half the number of chromosomes found in the other cells of the body.

Ganglion (pl. ganglia): A collection of nerve cells and synapses located outside the central nervous system.

Gating: Process of inhibiting certain stimuli and "opening the gate" so that one at a time can pass through, making attention possible; performed by the "wrong way" or centrifugal nerve fibers.

Gay: Synonym for "homosexual".

Gender identity: Individual's identification as being male or female.

General-adaptation-syndrome: The body's reaction under continued stress, consisting of the alarm reaction, during which the body makes a number of complicated physiological changes in response to a stressor; the stage of resistance, during which the organism, with the aid of increase secretions of the adrenal glands, is able to withstand the stressor for a time without showing symptoms; and the stage of exhaustion, in which the organism can no longer resist the stressor and may die if stress does not cease.

General paresis: Mental disorder associated with syphilis of the brain.

General systems theory: A comprehensive theoretical model embracing all living systems.

Generalization: Tendency of a response that has been conditioned to one stimulus to become associated with other similar stimuli.

Generalized reinforce: Reinforce such as money which may influence a wide range of stimuli and behaviors.

Genes: Ultramicroscopic areas of DNA which are responsible for transmission of hereditary traits.

Genetic code: Means by which DNA controls the sequence and structure of proteins manufactured within each cell and also makes exact duplicates of itself.

Genetic counseling: Counseling prospective parents concerning the probability of their having defective offspring as a result of genetic defects.

Genetics: Science of heredity.

Genes: Ultramicroscopic areas within the chromosomes; the real bearers of heredity.

Genetic explanation: Explanation of an event in terms of a description of the sequence of major events leading up to it.

Genital stages: In psychoanalytic theory, the final stage of psychosexual development involving shift from autoeroticism to heterosexual interest.

Genitalia: Organs of reproduction, especially the external organs.

Genotype: Genetic characteristics inherited by an individual.

Geriatrics: Science of the diseases and treatment of the aged.

Germs cells: Reproductive cells (female ovum and male sperm) which unite to produce a new individual.

Gerontology: Science dealing with the study of old age.

Germ cells: Reproductive cells (male sperm and female ovum) which unite to produce a new individual.

Germinal period: First two weeks of prenatal development, during which the zygote develops by division into a hollow sphere of cells.

Gestalt psychology: School of psychology which emphasizes patterns rather than elements or connections, taking the view that the whole is more than the sum of its parts.

Gestalt therapy: Type of psychotherapy emphasizing the wholeness of the person and integration of thought, feeling, and action.

Gigantism: Overgrowth of the skeletal structure caused by over secretion of the pituitary growth hormone early in life. Or abnormally tall stature resulting from hyperfunctioning of the pituitary.

Gonads: The sex glands.

Goal: Some substance, objects, or environmental condition capable of reducing or temporarily eliminating the complex of internal conditions which initiated action on the part of an organism. Also called reward, incentive, or reinforcement.

Gonads: The sex glands (testes in the male and ovaries in the female); produce gametes and also secrete hormones which influence bodily development and behavior.

Grand mal epilepsy: Type of epilepsy characterized by generalized convulsive seizures.

Grief work: Necessary period of mourning for an individual to assimilate his loss into his self-structure and view it as an event of the past.

Group therapy: Form of psychotherapy in which a group of persons discuss their problems under the guidance of therapist; usually nondirective.

Guidance center: Clinic or agency where individuals may be helped with problems of adjustment.

Gustatory area: Area of the brain responsible for taste sensations is not yet located in man; may be in the somesthetic area near the centers controlling the tongue.

Guilt: Feelings of culpability arising from behavior or desires contrary to one's ethical principles. Involves both self-evaluation and apprehension growing out of fears of punishment.

Habit: Any product of learning, whether it is a customary or transitory mode of response.

Habituation: Process whereby an individual's response to the same stimulus lessens with repeated presentations.

Habit strength: In Hull's theory of learning, a learned connection between stimulus and response (an intervening variable), represented by the symbol Hr.

Halfway house: Facility which provides aftercare following institutionalization, seeking to ease the individual's adjustment to the community.

Hallucination: Sense perception for which there is no appropriate external stimulus. Sensory impression of external objects in the absence of any appropriate stimulus in the environment.

Hallucinogens: Drugs or chemicals capable of producing hallucinations.

Halo effect: Tendency, when interviewing or rating an individual on a particular trait, to be influenced by one's opinion of some other trait or by the individual's personality as a whole.

Harmonics: See Overtones.

Hashish: The strongest drug derived from the hemp plant; a relative of marijuana.

Hebephrenic schizophrenia: Type of schizophrenia characterized by severe personality decompensation of disintegration.

Homophobia: Pathological fear of blood. Also called hematophobia.

Hemiplegia: Paralysis of one lateral half of the body.

Heredity: Genetic transmission of characteristics from parents to their children. Or the totality of biologically transmitted factors that influence the structure of the body and thus limit behavior.

Hemianopia: General terms for blindness in one half of the field of vision of one or both eyes.

Heterozygous: Possessing two unlike genes for a particular trait.

Hermaphroditism: Anatomical sexual abnormality in which an individual has well-developed sex organs of both sexes.

Heterosexuality: Sexual interest in a member of the opposite sex.

Hierarchy of needs: The concept that needs arrange themselves in a hierarchy in terms of importance or "prepotence", from the most basic biological needs to those psychological needs concerned with self-actualization.

High-risk group: Group showing great vulnerability to physical or mental disorders.

Higher-order conditioning: Process by which, once a conditioned response has been established, the conditioned stimulus may in turn function as an unconditioned stimulus in setting up a conditioned response to a third stimulus.

Hippocampus: A subcortical structure of the brain which is crucial for recent memory.

Holistic theories: Cognitive learning theories, so-called because of their emphasis on the importance of the whole in shaping the parts.

Holistic: A systematic approach to science involving the study of the whole or total configuration; the view of human beings as unified psychobiological organisms inextricably immersed in a physical and sociocultural environment.

Homeostasis: Tendency or organisms to maintain conditions making possible a constant level of physiological functioning. It is the complex process of maintaining stability in the internal and external environment so that the body's chemical balance can be maintained and personality needs can be satisfied; homeostasis on the physiological level is largely automatic.

Homozygous: Possessing two identical genes for a particular trait.

Hermetic traits: Direct motivational aspects of the person, which depend upon both tissue needs and the kinds of experience the individual has had.

Homosexually: Sexual preference for member of one's own sex.

Hormones: Chemicals released by the endocrine glands that regulate activity in various bodily organs.

Hostility: Emotional reaction or drive toward the destruction or damage of an object interpreted as a source of frustration or threat.

Hue: Quality of color sensation determined by the wavelength of the light waves.

Human engineering: Planning of work space and equipment in accordance with the sensory capacities, strength, and body dimensions of the worker, so as to bring about maximum efficiency while maintaining maximum safety and comfort of the operator; also called engineering psychology.

Humanistic-existential therapy: Type of psychotherapy emphasizing personal growth and self-direction.

Human potential movement: Movement concerned with enrichment of experience, increase sensory awareness, and fulfillment of human potentials.

Huntington's chorea: Incurable disease, presumably of hereditary origin, which is manifested in jerking, twitching movements and mental deterioration.

Hydrocephalus: Organic condition associated with brain damage and mental retardation.

Hydrotherapy: Use of hot or cold baths, ice packs, etc. in treatment.

Hyper: Prefix meaning increase.

Hyperkinetic (hyperactive) reaction: Disorder of childhood characterized by over activity, restlessness, and distractibility.

Hypertension: High blood pressure.

Hyperventilation: Rapid and deep breathing associated with intense anxiety.

Hypoesthesia: Partial loss of sensitivity.

Hyperalgesia: Exceptional sensitivity to pain.

Hyperopia: Far-sightedness, caused by the lens being unable to bulge out enough for close vision; image comes into focus behind the retina.

Hypnosis: Artificially induced state of extreme suggestibility; used in psychotherapy primarily as an aid in uncovering repressed or forgotten experiences.

Hypnosis: Trancelike mental state induced in a cooperative subject by suggestion.

Hypnotherapy: Use of hypnosis in psychotherapy.

Hypnotic regression: Process by which a subject is brought to relive, under hypnosis, early forgotten or repressed experiences. Or a process by which a subject vividly relives, under hypnosis, early experiences which he has forgotten or repressed.

Hypnotic suggestion: Process of inducing acts, thoughts, or feelings in the subject while hypnotized. See also Posthypnotic suggestion.

Hypo: Prefix meaning decreased.

Hypochondriacal delusions: Delusions concerning various horrible disease conditions, such as the belief that one's brain is turning to dust.

Hypochondriacal neurosis: Condition dominated by preoccupation with bodily processes and fear of presumed disease.

Hypochondria: Neurotic preoccupation with the body's activities and the state of one's health.

Hypomania: Mildest form of manic reaction, characterized by moderate psychomotor over activity.

Hypothalamus: Key structure at the base of the brain; important in emotion and motivation.

Hypothesis: Statement or proposition, usually based on observation, which is tested in an experiment; may be denied or supported by experimental results but never conclusively proved.

Hysteria: Older terms used to include conversion and dissociative neurotic reaction; involves the appearance of symptoms of organic illness in the absence of any related organic pathology.

Hysterical neurosis: Disorder characterized by involuntary psychogenic loss of motor or sensory function.

Hysterical personality: Personality pattern characterized by excitability, emotional instability, and self-dramatization.

Id: In psychoanalytic theory, the primitive part of the unconscious, composed of instinctive organic cravings and characterized by unrestrained pleasure-seeking impulses. Or the reservoir of instinctual drives; the most inaccessible and primitive stratum of the mind.

Identical twins: Twins which develop from a single fertilized egg. Also called monozygotic twins.

Identification with the aggressor: Defense mechanism by which the frustrated individual incorporates into his own personality structure the qualities of those who threaten him.

Identification: Ego-defense mechanism in which the individual identifies himself with some person or institution, usually of an illustrious nature.

Ideology: System of beliefs.

Idiographic: Approach to personality study in which the unique aspects of an individual's personality are of chief importance.

Idiot: Older term referring to severe and profound degrees of mental retardation (IQ below 24).

Idiot savant: A mental retarded who can perform unusual mental feats, usually involving music or manipulation of numbers.

Illusions: Misinterpretation of sensory data; false perception,

Imbecile: Former classification of individual with IQ of 25 to 50. See Mental retardation.

Implicit speech: Tiny muscular contractions, in the speech mechanism and elsewhere, which occur during thought.

Implosive therapy: Form of action therapy developed by Stampfl; extinction occurs as frightening stimuli are imagined; called implosive because the frightening stimuli produce an inner explosion-an implosion –of panic.

Imprinting: A form of learning which occurs very early in life and determines the form which behavior will take, as in the case of ducklings which follow the first moving object they see and remain closely attached to it.

Implosive therapy: Type of behavior therapy in which desensitization is achieved by eliciting a massive "flood" or implosion of anxiety.

Impotence: Inability of male to achieve orgasm.

Impulse: Tendency to action.

Incentive: External inducement to behave in a certain way.

Incest: Sexual relations between close relatives such as father and daughter or brother and sister.

Incidental learning: Ability to notice and remember things which are not immediately relevant to the task at hand; also called *latent learning*.

Inclusiveness: Factor by which we use up all the elements in perceiving a pattern.

Incus: The second of three hinged bones in the ear which together transmit vibrations from the eardrum to the oval window; also called the anvil.

Independent variable: Factor whose effects are being examined in an experiment; it is changed in some systematic and predetermined manner while the other variables are held constant.

Index case: In a genetic study, the individual who evidences the trait in which the investigator is interested. Same as proband.

Inferiority complex: Strong feelings of inadequacy and insecurity which color an individual's entire adjustive efforts. Or deep rooted but concealed feelings of inferiority which, according to Adlerian theory often lead to a lust for domination over others as a means of compensation.

Information: In information theory, a reduction in uncertainty

Information theory: The study of communication system and the principles that make for understanding, control, and predictability in communication.

Inhibition: Suppression or restraint of behavior; term has many specific meanings.

Inhibitory postsynaptic potential (IPSP): Potential change occurring in a neuron which suppresses the development of a nerve impulse.

Infantile autism: See Autism.

Inhibition: Conscious restraint of impulse or desire.

Innate: Inborn.

Inner controls: Reality, value, and possibility assumptions which serve to inhibit dangerous or undesirable behavior; could also apply to conditioned avoidance reactions.

Innervations: The excitation of a muscle or gland by a nerve.

Input: In cyber metrics, the stimuli which initiate the activity of a machine or an organism.

In patient: Hospitalized mental patient.

Insanity: Legal term for mental disorder, implying lack of responsibility for one's acts and inability to manage one's affairs.

Insight: In Gestalt theory, the apparently sudden appearance of the solution to a problem. In psychotherapy, the understanding of one's own behavior, motives, feelings and attitudes. Awareness of key relationships, not always sudden.

Insight therapy: Therapy: Type of psychotherapy focusing on helping the patient achieve greater self-understanding with respect to his motives, values, coping pattern, and so on. Or form of psychotherapy which seek to enable the patient to find his underlying conflict or problem and gain insight into it.

Instinct: Behavior pattern whose underlying biological pattern is produced by maturation rather than learning and which appears fullblown upon the first occasion that an adequate stimulus is presented, without the organism's having previous opportunity to learn; common in lower animals but very rare in man.

Insomnia: Difficulty in sleeping.

Instinct: In born tendency to particular behavior patterns under certain conditions in absence of learning; characteristics of species.

Instrumental act: Act directed toward achieving specific goals and meeting needs.

Instrumental (operant) conditioning: Type of conditioning in which the subjects is reinforced for making a predetermined response, such as pressing a lever.

Integration: Organization of parts (Psychological, biological functions) to make a functional whole.

Integrity therapy: A form of psychotherapy developed by mowrer; regards neuroses as forms of moral failure and advocates taking the consequences of one's actions and being more faithful to moral values.

Integrative properties: Tendency of living systems to maintain their organization and function integrity.

Intellectualization: Ego-defense mechanism by which the individual achieves some measure of insulation from emotional hurt by cutting off or distorting the emotional charge which normally accompanies hurtful situations. In other words, a defensive compromise reaction in which the individual attempts to divest his problems of painful feelings by pushing them into the realm of the intellect through rationalization, isolation, or undoing.

Intelligence: Complex mental ability includes such primary abilities as verbal comprehension, space visualization, reasoning ability, numerical ability, and others; operationally defined, intelligence is what intelligence tests measure. Pertaining to ability to learn, reason and adapt.

Intelligence quotient (IQ): Measure of intelligence obtained by dividing the individual's mental age (MA), as determined by his performance on standardized test items, by his chronological age (CA) and then multiplying by 100. An IQ of 100 is considered to be average.

Intensity deafness: Inability to hear faint sounds or, in more severe cases, loud sounds.

Interaction: Influence by some other variable upon the effect of changing the independent variable.

Interdisciplinary (multidisciplinary) approach: Integration of various scientific disciplines in understanding, assessing, treating, and preventing mental disorders.

Intermittent reinforcement: Reinforcement give intermittently rather than after every response.

Interneurons: Nerve cells with many short dendrites and a short axon, the latter often giving off branches called collaterals; can connect a sense organ with many effector neurons and many muscles.

Interpersonal accommodation: A reciprocal process give and take ment to promote satisfactory interpersonal relationships.

Intrapsychic conflict: Psychoanalytic concept referring to conflict between id, ego, superego.

Interval scale: Scale of measurement in which equal differences between measurements stand for equal differences in the amount of the attribute which is being measured.

Intervening variable: A logical construct to account for a process intervening between the variables controlled by the experimenter and the observed changes which take place in the dependent variable; this term is ordinarily applied only to logical constructs which are quantitative in nature or at least constant in form.

Introjection: Incorporation of qualities or values of another person or group into one's own ego structure with a tendency to identify with them and to be affected by what happens to them.

Intromission: Insertion of the penis into the vagina or anus.

Intropunitive: Responding to frustration by tending to blame oneself.

Introspection: Observing (and often reporting on) one's inner experiencing. Or a technique of observing conscious processes and states, such as thinking and emotion, which go on within oneself.

Introversion: Orientation toward the subjective, inner world of thought and feeling; the introvert tends to avoid social contacts. Or direction of interest toward one's inner world of experience and toward concepts rather than external events and objects.

In vivo: Taking place in a real-life situation as opposed to the therapeutic or laboratory setting.

Involutional melancholia (involutional psychotic reaction): Depressive psychotic reaction characterized by depression, agitation, and apprehension.

Involutional psychotic reaction: Psychosis characterized by abnormal anxiety, agitation, delusion, and depression; occurs in late years, without previous history of psychosis; may be characterized chiefly by depression or can center around paranoid ideas.

Iris: Colored portion of the eye immediately surrounding the pupil; adjusts in size to regulate amount of light entering the eye.

Irradiation: Mass action; the sluggish, irregular, widespread movement characteristic of the spontaneous movements of the fetus process whereby, as more sensory fibers are activated by a stronger stimulus more motoneurons are stimulated and a larger part of the body reacts.

Isolation: Avoidance of conflict between two opposed desires or attitudes by kepping them apart in "logictight compartments" in consciousness.

Item analysis: Method for determining the extent to which the responses to each item in a test differentiate between two groups.

Ionizing radiation: Form of radiation; major cause of gene mutations.

Isolation: Ego-defense mechanism by means of which contradictory attitudes or feelings which normally accompany particular attitudes are kept apart, thus preventing conflict or hurt.

James-Lange theory: Theory that emotion consists of the bodily changes which occur in response to an exciting event, holding that we feel sad because we cryrather than *vice versa*.

Jump movements: Series of short conjugate movements made by the eyes in looking at motionless objects.

Juvenile delinquency: Legally prohibited behavior committed by minors.

Juvenile paresis: General paresis in children usually of congenital origin.

Klinefelter's syndrome: Type of mental retardation associated with sex chromosome anomaly.

Korsakoff's psychosis: Usually associated with chronic alcoholism and characterized disorientation gross memory defects, and confabulation

Kinesthetic sense: Sense of active movement.

Labyrinth: Inner ear; contains cochlea, vestibule and semicircular canals.

Labyrinthine sense: Sense of passive movement.

Latent content: Hidden content of a dream which indicates the individual's true wishes; changed to manifest content by dream work.

Labeling: Assigning an individual to a particular diagnostic category, such schizophrenia.

Lability instability: Particularly with regard to affect.

Latent content: In psychoanalytic theory repressed wishes indirectly expressed in the manifest content of dreams.

Latent learning: Learning that becomes evident only after an incentive is introduced.

Latent periody: Delay between the presentation of a stimulus and the beginning of a response; consists of time required for sensory nerve ending to be aroused, for impulse to be conducted through nerves, and for responding muscles to begin contracting the more synapses involved the longer the period.

Law of effect: Principle that responses,that have rewarding consequences are strengthened and those that have aversive cosequences are weakened or eliminated.

Learning: Modification of behavior as a consequence of experience. Or a process which brings about a change in the individual's way of responding as a result of contact with aspects of the environment.

Learning curve: Graphic device for showing the amount or quality of subject's performance after successive units of practice.

Learning set: A readiness to respond in a certain way to a learning situation: learning how to learn.

Leniency error: Tendency on the part of judge to rate nearly all persons near the top of a rating scale; may be corrected by the use of forced-choice scales.

Lens: Structure of the eye which focuses the light rays on to the sensitive retina.

Lesion: A portion of the brain (or other tissue) destroyed by an experimenter, by accident, or by disease.

Lesbian: Female homosexual.

Lethality scale: Criteria used to assess the likelihood of an individual's committing suicide.

Level of aspiration: Standard by which the individual judges success or failure of his behavior.

Libido: In Freudian theory, the instinctive pleasure–seeking drive which is the source of energy underlying all human behavior.

Lie detector: Collection of instruments to measure the intensity of visceral responses during questioning.

Life-history methods: Techniques of psychological observation in which the development of particular forms of behavior is traced: include daybook method, clinical method, and biographical method.

Life crisis: Stress situation that approaches of exceeds the individual's adjustive capacity.

Life-style: The general pattern of assumptions, motives, cognitive styles, and coping techniques that characterize the behavior of a given individual and give it consistency. In Adelerain theory, the unique manner in which each individual strives for the basic goal of superiority.

Light adaptation: Adjustment of the eye to light.

Linear perspective: Phenomenon of objects appearing both smaller and closer together as they become more distant.

Labotomy: Drastic form of psychosurgery rarely used at present. It involves cutting the nerve fibers that connect the frontal lobes to the thalamus.

Locomotor ataxia: Muscular in coordination usually resulting from syphilitic damage to the spinalcord pathways.

Logic-tight compartments: Form of intellectualization in which contradictory desires or attitudes are "sealed off" in separate areas of consciousness.

Logical construct: A quality, substance, or event whose existence is postulated by the experimenter as an aid in explaining how the independent variable operates on the dependent variable; sometimes called a hypothetical construct.

Logotherapy: School of existential analysis which focuses upon the individual's need to see meaning in his life; emphasizes spiritual and ethical values.

Long-conducting neuron: Nerve cell with a long axon or long dendrites; all sensory and motor fibers are of this type.

Longitudinal method: Method of studying effects of age on various traits or abilities by testing and retesting (or otherwise observing) the same individuals over a period of time.

Lysergic acid diethylamide (LSD): Drug capable of bringing on symptoms of mental disease in normal individuals; used legally in mental therapy only by medical prescription. A potent hallucinogen.

Lunacy: Legal term roughly synonymous with insanity.

Lycanthropy: The delusion of being a wolf.

Macro-factor: A general factor such as socioeconomic status, as opposed to specific, more precisely defined micro-factors.

Macrocephalic: Having an abnormally large cranium.

Madness: Nontechnical synonym for mental illness.

Maintaining cause: Environmental rein forcers of contingencies that tent of maintain maladaptive behavior.

Maintenance strivings: Strivings directed toward maintenance of physiological and psychological equilibrium and integration.

Major tranquilizers: Antipsychotic drugs, such as the phenothazenes.

Maladaptive (abnormal) behavior: Behavior which is detrimental to well-being of the individual and/or group.

Maladjustment: A more or less enduring failure of adjustment; lack of harmony with self or environment.

Malinger: To fake illness of disability symptoms consciously.

Mania: Suffix denoting a compulsive or morbid preoccupation with some impulsive or activity; e.g. compulsive stealing is called kleptomania.

Malleus: The first of three hinged bones in the ear which together transmit vibrations from the eardrum to the oval window; also called the hammer.

Manic-depressive reactions: Psychotic reactions characterized by alternation between periods of extreme elation (manic episodes) and periods of extreme depression.

Manic-depressive psychoses: Group of psychotic disorders characterized by prolonged periods of excitement and over activity (mania) or by periods of depression and under activity (depression) or by alternation of the two. Manifest content. In psychoanalytic theory, the apparent meaning of a dream; masks the latent content.

Manifest content: Surface content of a dream, which we remember; masks the emotionally painful latent content.

Manipulandum: In operant conditioning devices, a response mechanism which must manipulate to obtain reinforcement.

Mannerism: Recurring stereotyped gesture, posture, or movement.

Marathon encounter group: Intensive group experience lasting for 2 or more days with only brief breaks for sleep.

Marijuana: Drug derived from the plant cannabis indica; often used in cigarettes called "reefers" or "joints".

Maritalschism: Marriage characterized by severe chronic discord which threatens continuation of marital relationship.

Marital skew: Marriage maintain relationship.

Marital therapy: Therapy directed toward impressing. Communication and interaction between marital partners.

Masked disorder: of underlying depression or other emotional disturbance by delinquent behavior or other patterns seemingly unrelated to the basic disturbance.

Masochism: Sexual deviation in which an individual obtains sexual gratification from having pain inflicted upon him.

Mass action: Sluggish, irregular, widespread movement characteristic of the spontaneous movements of the fetus; also called irradiation.

Massed practice: Use of concentrated learning periods.

Mass hysteria: Group outbreak of hysterical reactions.

Masturbation: Self-stimulation of genitals for sexual gratification.

Maternal deprivation: Lack of adequate care and stimulation by the another or mother surrogate.

Maturation: Process of development and bodily change resulting from heredity acting over a period of time; independent of learning but may be hampered by a subnormal environment.

Mean: Measure of central value, more familiarly known as the average; obtained by adding a group of measurements together and dividing the sum by the number of measurements; also called the arithmetic mean.

Measurement: Assigning numbers to persons, objects, or events according to certain rules.

Median: Measure of central value; the measurement which splits an ordered distribution exactly in half.

Megalomania: Delusions of grandeur.

Melancholia: Mental disorder characterized by severe depression.

Memory drum: Instrument used in experiments on vertim learning.

Memory span: Amount of material which can be mastered from a single presentation; usually about six to eight digits or letters presented orally.

Mental age (MA): Degree of mental development as measured by standardized intelligence test; based on ate at which average children make a given score; used of determing 10. A scale unit indicating level of intelligence in relation to chronological age.

Meninges: Membranes which envelop the brain and spinal cord.

Mental deficiency: Synonym for mental retardation; the latter term is now preferred.

Mental disease: Mental disorder associated with an organic disease of the nervous system.

Mental disorder: Entire range of abnormal behavior patterns.

Mental health movement: Movement started by Clifford Beers shortly after 1900; seeks to create public awareness of the importance of psychological prophylaxis and psychotherapy.

Mental illness: Once used synonymously with mental disorder but now ordinarily restricted to psychoses.

Mental retardation: Below normal intelligence. Includes mildly retarded (IQ range from 50 to 70), moderately retarded (IQ 35 to 50), severely retarded (IQ20 to 35), and profoundly retarded (IQ below 20).

Mental relepathy: Form of extrasensory perception involving the alleged passage of awarness from one mind to another without intervention of the sense organs.

Mescaline: Drug which can bring on symptoms of mental illness; also used in therapy, primarily to induce regression to childhood experiences. It is one of the hallucinogenic drugs.

Mesmerism: Theories of "animal magnetism" (hypnosis) formulated by Antom Mesmer.

Methadone: An orally administered narcotic which kills the craving for heroin and paves way for rehabilitation of heroin addicts.

Metabolism: Chemical changes taking place in all living tissue by which energy is provided to carry on the life processes.

Metrazol: Drug used for shock therapy, producing violent convulsions; seldom used today.

Micro-factor: Relatively specific, precisely defined factor, as opposed to more general macro-factors.

"Middle man" hormones: Secretions of the pituitary gland which act directly upon other encocrine glands to stimulate their functioning.

Microcephaly: Form of mental retardation characterized by abnormally small cranium and retarded development of brain.

Migraine headache: Type of psychosomatic disorder characterized by recurrent headaches, usually on one side of head only, and associated with emotional tension.

Milieu: Therapy, attempt to make the institution as a whole a therapeutic community for the mentally ill.

Mind-body problem: Classical question of how the mind relates to the body.

Minimal brain dysfunction (MBD): Controversial term referring to various "soft' neurological signs presumably indicative of malfunctioning of brain.

Minor tranquilizers: Antianxiety drugs such as the meprobramates.

Model: An analogy that helps a scientist order his findings and see important relationships among them.

Model psychoses: Psychotic like states produced by various hallucinogenic drugs such as LSD.

Modeling: Form of learning in which individual learns by watching someone else (the model) perform the desired response.

Modus operandi: Manner or mode of behavior; a criminal's typical pattern of performing his crimes.

Modes of appearance: Characteristics of visual sensations other than those of hue, brightness, and saturation; include glow, luster, and bulk.

Mongolism: See Down's syndrome.

Monozygotic twins: Identical twins, developed from one fertilized egg.

Moral nihilism: Doctrine which denies any objective or real ground for moral beliefs, and holds that the individual is not bound by obligation to others or society.

Moral therapy: Therapy based on provision of kindness, understanding, and favorable environment; prevalent during early part of 19th century.

Morbid: Unhealthy, pathological.

Morita therapy: Treatment of neuroses involving deprivation of external stimulation and other procedures.

Moron: Term formerly used to refer to mild degrees of mental retardation. Former classification of individual with IQ from 50 to 70: now more often called mildly retarded.

Mood: An emotional state that is drawn out over a period of hours or days and is usually less intense than an "emotional outburst" such as anger.

Morphine: Addictive opiate drug.

Motivation: Often used as a synonym for drive or activation; implies that the organism's actions are partly determined in direction and strength by its own inner nature.

Motivational selectivity: Influence of motives on perception and other cognitive processes.

Motive: Internal condition which directs action toward some goal; term usually used to include both the drive and the goal to which it is directed.

Morphology: Method of judging personality from physical appearance.

Motivational research: Qualitative advertising research concerned with determining the underlying the and presumably unconscious motives which cause people to buy certain products.

Motor areas: Areas of the brain involved in controlling body movements; primary motor area is in front of the fissure of Rolando and body surface is projected onto this area in reverse. Secondary motor area is near fissure of Sylvius, and supplementary motor area is in front of secondary area on midline of brain.

Motor primacy: The principle that the neuromuscular structures of the body must reach a certain stage of development (maturation) before they are capable of responding to stimulation.

Motor skill learning: Learning in which performance involves primarly the use of the muscles.

Multiple personality: Extreme dissociative reaction in which the individual develops two or more distinct personalities which alternate in consciousness, each personality being based on sets of motives which are in conflict with those of the others.

Muscle spindle: Specialized group of muscle fibers wrapped with afferent nerve endings; involved in postural reflexes.

Multiple personality: Type of dissociative reaction characterized by the development of two or more relatively independent personality systems in the same individual.

Mutant gene: Gene that has undergone some change in structure.

Mutation: Change in the composition of a gene, usually causing harmful or a abnormal characteristics to appear in the offspring.

Mutism: Refusal or inability to speak.

Myxedema: Disorder due to thyroid deficiency in adult life, characterized by mental dullness.

Myelin sheath: Fatty white covering which surrounds the axons and collaterals of large diameter in the nervous system.

Myclination: Process by which certain nerve axons become surrounded by the myelin sheath; necessary before they can function.

Myopia: Near-sightedness, caused by the lens bulging out too far so that the image comes into focus slightly in front of the retina and appears fuzzy.

Narcoanalysis: Brief form of narcosis in which sleep-producing drugs are administered in amounts sufficient to cause a state of "twilight sleep" rather than deep unconsciousness; while in this state, the patient is encouraged to talk about emotionally painful experiences.

Narcosis: Technique of therapy which uses sleep-producing drugs; in prolonged narcosis, now used only for severely agitated patients, the patient may be kept asleep for fifteen or more hours a day for one or two weeks.

Narcissism: Self-love.

Narcolepsy: Abnormal reaction characterized by transient, compulsive states of sleepiness.

Narcotherapy (narcoanalysis, narcosynthesis): Psychotherapy carried on while the patient is in a sleep like state of relaxation induced by a drug such as sodium pentothal.

Narcotic drugs: Drugs such as morphine which lead to physiological dependence and increased tolerance.

Need: Biological or psychological condition whose gratification is necessary for the maintenance of homeostasis or for self-actualization.

Need achievement score (n Ach): A measure of the individual motivation to achieve, obtained from a modified form of the Thematic Apperception Test; not a unity factor.

Need-integrative therapy: A brief form of psychotherapy which focuses on the basic present need that is behind the maladjustive behavior.

Negative after sensation: Perception of a complementary hue after original stimulation ceases.

Negative transfer: See Proactive inhibition.

Negativism: Form of aggressive withdrawal which involves refusing to cooperate or obey commands, or doing the exact opposite of what has been requested.

Neologism: A new word; commonly coined by persons labeled as schizophrenic.

Neonate: Newborn infant.

Neoplasm: Tumor.

Nervous breakdown: Refers broadly to lowered integration and inability to deal adequately with one's life situation.

Neurasthenic neurosis: Neurotic disorder characterized by complaints of chronic weakness, easy fatigability, and lack of enthusiasm.

Neurology: Field concerned with study of brain and nervous system and disorders thereof.

Neo-Freudians: Modern psychoanalysts who believe that therapy must be aimed at understanding the patient's present situation as well as his unconscious processes and childhood experiences.

Neonate: Newborn infant.

Nerve: Nerve trunk.

Nerve fiber: Axon.

Nerve impulse: Electrochemical excitation propagated along a chain of nerve cells.

Nerve tract: Nerve pathway; bundle of nerve fibers which have a common place of origin and destination.

Nerve trunk: Nerve; nerve tract connecting the central nervous system with other parts of the body.

Neurasthenia: See Asthenic reaction.

Neurologist: Holder of an MD who specializes in the diagnosis and treatment of mental abnormalities caused by disease or injury to the brain and nervous system.

Neuron: Individual nerve cell.

Neuropsychiatrist: MD who specializes in the treatment of mental illnesses, including those caused by damage to the brain and nervous system.

Neurosecretion: Formal of a hormone in the nuclei of neurons; occurs, for example, in the hypothalamus.

Neurosis: Abnormal reaction pattern which lowers efficiency but seldom required hospitalization; the neurotic usually retains contact with reality. Or an emotional disturbance characterized by exaggerated use of avoidance behavior and defense mechanisms against anxiety.

Neurosyphilis: Syphilis affecting the central nervous system.

Neurotic nucleus: Basic personality characteristics underlying neurotic disorders.

Neurotic paradox: Failure of neurotic patterns to extinguish despite their self-defeating nature.

Neurotransmitters: Chemical substances which transmit information from one neuron to another.

Night hospital: Mental hospital in which an individual may receive treatment during all or part of the night while carrying on his usual occupation in the daytime.

Nihilistic delusion: Fixed belief that everything is unreal.

Nomadism: Withdrawal reaction in which the individual continually attempts to escape frustration by moving from place to place or job to job in an attempt to get away from frustrating situations.

Nominal scale: Lowest scale of measurement, consisting only of classification; measurement on the nominal scale distinguishes between two or more mutually exclusive categories of persons, objects, or events, but imparts no quantitative information.

Nomothetic: Approach to personality study which attempts to describe certain psychological elements presumed to be common to all individuals.

Nondirective therapy: An approach to psychotherapy in which the therapist refrains from advice or direction of the therapy. See also Client-centered psychotherapy.

Noradrenaline: Hormone secreted by the adrenal nodulla during emotion; brings emotion; brings about a number of bodily changes, including constriction of the blood vessels near the body's surface.

Norepinephrine: Hormone secreted by adrenal medulla. Also called noradrenaline.

Norm: Standard based on measurement of a large group of persons; used for comparing the scores of an individual with those of others in a defined group.

Normal: Conforming to the usual or norm. Healthy.

Normal distribution: Tendency for most members of a population to cluster around a central point or average with respect to a given trait, with the rest spreading out to the two extremes. A mathematical model often used in psychology to describe the form of the distribution of measurements in a population; if the mean and standard deviation of a normal distribution are specified, it is completely described; it yields a symmetrical, bell-shaped curve with the greatest number of measurements concentrated around the mean, tapering off toward the extremes.

Nucleus: Specialized protoplasm of a cell, important to cell physiology and reproduction. A group of cell bodies located within the central nervous system of Ganglion.

Null hypothesis: The hypothesis that is contradictory to the one which is to be tested; is rejected when the sample mean falls in the critical region.

NREM sleep: Stages of sleep not characterized by the rapid eye movements that accompany dreaming.

Objective observation: Observation of overt behavior and the conditions under which it occurs.

Objectivity: In a test, the degree to which two or more persons can score a subject responses and get the same results; more generally, freedom from bias.

Obsession: Persistent and irrational idea, usually unpleasant, that comes into consciousness and cannot be banished voluntarily.

Obsessive-compulsive reaction: An abnormal reaction characterized by the presence of anxiety, with persisting unwanted thoughts accompanied by the compuling.

Obsession: Persistent idea or thought which the individual recognizes as irritation but cannot get rid of.

Obsessive-compulsive neurosis: Disorder characterized by persistent intrusion of unwanted desires, thoughts or actions.

Obsessive-compulsive personality: Personality disorder characterized by excessive concern with conformity and adherence to ethical values.

Occipital lobe: Portion of cerebrum concerned with visual function.

Occupational therapy: Use of occupational training or activity in psychotherapy.

Occipital lobe: Portion of the cerebrum located at the back of the brain; location of the visual center.

Old brain: Portions of brain which developed first in evolution; comprises the cerebellum, the thalamus, and the hypothalamus.

Oedipus complex: Desire for sexual relations with parent of opposite sex, specifically that of a boy for his mother.

Olfactory hallucinations: Hallucinations involving the sense of smell, as of poison gas.

Olfactory area: Anterior (front) portion of the rhinencephalon is associated with olfaction, as are parts of the hindbrain.

One-tailed test: A test of statistical significance in which the critical region lies at one or the other extreme of the sampling distribution.

Operant behavior: Behavior which is emitted by the organism and operates on the environment.

Operant conditioning: Form of conditioning in which the organism becomes progressively more likely to respond in a given situation with that response which previously has brought a reward, such as a reward of food for pressing a lever. Or a form of learning in which the correct response is reinforced and becomes more likely to occur.

Operational definition: Defining a concept on the basis of a set of operations that can be observed and measured.

Oplum: Narcotic drug which leads to physiological dependence and the building up of tolerance; derivatives are morphine,heroin paregoric, and codeine.

Opponent-process theory: Theory of color vision which postulates three pairs of neural processes yellow, blue, red-green, and white-black each of which is capable of two modes of response that are opposed in nature.

Optic chiasma: Point at which optic nerves leading from each retina form a partial cross at the base of the brain.

Optic nerve: Nerve which carries impulses from the retina to the brain.

Oral period: In psychoanalytic theory, stage of development when satisfactions center around sucking, biting, chewing, etc.

Oral stage: First stage of psychosexual development in Freudian theory, in which mouth or oral activities are primary source of pleasure.

Organic brain syndromes: Mental disorders associated with organic brain pathology.

Organic viewpoint: Concept that all mental disorders have an organic basis.

Ordinal scale: Scale of measurement in which persons, objects, or events are ranked according to the amount of some attribute that they possess.

Organ of Corti: Thickening of the basilar membrane at the floor of the cochlear duct; contains hair cells which are stimulated by motion of the fluid in the cochlear canals; impulses pass from nerve fibers associated with the hair cells to the auditory nerve and thence to the brain.

Organic psychosis: Mental disorder resulting from injury to the nervous system of from such conditions as glandular deficiency or poisons.

Organism: Living being composed of a group of interdependent organs which work together to carry on life activities.

Organismic theory: Personality theory which stress the orderly unfolding of the inherited potentialities of the organism and its unity; based on field theory.

Organs of adjustment: Organs which function to help the individual adjust to his environment and overcome obstacles to the satisfaction of his needs.

Organs of maintenance: Organs (such as the heart, stomach, and lungs) which function to maintain the individual's health and growth.

Orgasm: Peak sexual tension followed by relaxation.

Outcome research: Studies of effectiveness of psychotherapy.

Outpatient: An ambulatory patient who visits a hospital clinic for examination and treatment, as distinct from a hospitalized patient.

Oval window: Membrane separating the middle from the inner ear; receives vibration from the hammer, anivil and stirrup bones and in turn forces movement of the fluid in the cochlear canals.

Ovaries: Female gonads.

Overanxious reaction: Disorder of childhood characterized by chronic anxiety, unrealistic fears, sleep disturbances, and exaggerated autonomic responses.

Overarousal: Excessive physiological mobilization or response to stimulus.

Overcompensation: Extreme or socially unacceptable attempt to counterbalance actual or felt inferiority.

Overt behavior: Activities which can be observed by an external observer.

Overtones: The fainter tones produced by the vibration of fraction of a vibrating wire or reed in a musical instrument and heard along with the fundamental tone; give a distinctive timber to the sound of each instrument, also called partials or harmonics.

Overloading: Subjecting organism to excessive stress, e.g. forcing the organism to handle or "Process" an excessive amount of information.

Overprotection: Shielding a child to the extent that he becomes too dependent on the parent.

Overbehavior: Activities which can be observed by an outsider.

Ovum: Female gamete or germ cell.

Oviduct: Tube leading from the ovary to the uterus, through which the mature egg travels.

Ovulation: Time when a mature egg cell is released down the oviduct to the uterus.

Ovum: Female gamete or germ cell.

Paired-associated learning: Learning in which the subject must respond with oneword or syllable when presented with another word or syllable.

Panic: Severe personality disorganization involving intense anxiety and usually either paralyzed immobility or blind flight.

Paradigm: A model or pattern; in research, a basic design specifying concepts considered legitimate and procedures to be used in the collection and interpretation of data.

Paraconditioning: Occurrence during conditioning experiments of changes in behavior that do not qualify as conditioning but may easily be confused with true conditioning.

Paradoxical cold: Sensation of cold aroused by a warm object; obtained when cold-sensitive spots are stimulated by objects with a temperature above 110 degrees Fahrenheit.

Paradoxical warmth: Sensation of warmth obtained when warmth-sensitive spots are stimulated by objects with temperatures well below the psychological zero point.

Parameter: A number which represents a certain property of a population; usually estimated from a statistic computed on a sample from the population.

Parasympathetic division: Division of the autonomic nervous system which controls most of the vital functions of life, such as digestion; its action is antithetic to that of the sympathetic division in most cases; its nerves orginate from the lower segments of the spinal cord and from the brainstem. Also called cranio-sacral division.

Parietal lobe: Portion of the cerebrum above the fissure of Sylvius and back of the fissure of Rolando.

Partial reinforcement: Reinforcement given only intermittently rather than regularly on every conditioning trial.

Paranoia: Psychosis characterized by a systematized delusional system.

Paranoid personality: Individual showing behavior characterized by projuction (as a defense mechanism), suspiciousness, envy, extreme jealousy and stubbornness.

Paranoid schizophrenia: Type of schizophrenia in which delusions and hallucinations are usually prominent.

Paranoid state: Transient psychotic disorder in which the main element is a delusion, usually persecutory or grandiose in nature.

Paraphasia: Garbled speech.

Paraprofessional: Individual who has been trained in mental health services, but not at the professional level.

Parasympathetic nervous system: Division of the autonomic nervous system that controls most of the basic metabolic functions essential for life.

Paresthesia: Exceptional sensations, such as tingling.

Paresis: See General paresis.

Parkinson's disease (Paralysis agitans): Progressive disease characterized by a masklike, expressionless face and various neurological symptoms.

Partial reinforcement: Intermittent reinforcement of a response.

Passive-aggressive personality: Personality pattern characterized by passively expressed aggressiveness.

Pathogenic: Pertaining to conditions which lead to pathology.

Pathological intoxication: Servere cerebral and behavioral disturbance in an individual whose tolerance to alcohol is extremely low.

Pathology: Abnormal physical or mental condition.

Partials: See Overtones.

Partiles: Points which divide a distribution of measurements into a number of equal parts.

Pederasty: Sexual intercourse between males via the anus.

Pedophilia: Sexual deviation in which an adult engages in or desires sexual relations with a child.

Peer group: Social group of equivalent age and status.

Perception: Interpretation of sensory input.

Perceptual filtering: Processes involved in selective attention to aspects of the great mass of incoming stimuli which continually impinge on organism.

Perception: Process of becoming aware of events that stimulate the sense organs, and of determining the relationships among them.

Perceptual defense: Selective perceiving by which an individual unconsciously screens out perceptions which are unpleasant or threatening to him.

Performance test: Test in which muscular responses rather than verbal ones are required.

Peripheral nervous system: Nerve fibers passing from the receptiors to the central nervous system or from the central nervous system to muscles and glands.

Peripheral nervous system: Nerve fibers passing between the central nervous system and the sense organs, muscles, and glands.

Persevaration: Persistent continuation of a line of thought or activity once it is under way clinically, inappropriate repetition.

Peripheralist theories: Associationistic learning theories, which emphasize the importance of stimulation and reinforcement from the environment.

Person-oriented dependency: Dependence upon other persons for support, approval, affection, etc.

Personality: The whole person, including his external appearance and behaviot (social stimulus value), his inner awareness of self as a permanent organizing force in his life, and his particular pattern of measurable traits.

Personnel psychology: Selection and classification of personnel and analysis of job structure; motivation and training of workers.

Personality: The unique patterns of traits which characterizes the individual.

Personality disorder: See Psychopathic personality.

Perversion: Deviation from normal.

Petit mal: Relatively mild form of epilepsy involving a temporary partial laps of consciousness.

Phallic-Oedipal stage: In psychoanalytic theory, stage of development (between third and fifth year) when genital manipulation and exploration occurs and there is a strong attraction for the parent of the opposite is a strong attraction for the parent of the opposite sex, with jealousy toward the same-sexed parent.

Phallic stage: In psychoanalytic theory, the stage of psychosexual development during which genital exploration and manipulation occur.

Phallic symbol: Any object which resemble the erect male sex organ.

Phenomenological: Referring to the immediate perceiving and experiencing of the environment by the individual.

Phenylketonuria (PKU): Type of mental retardation resulting from a metabolic deficiency.

Phenomenal field: In Regerian personality theory, private world of individual experience.

Phobic: Irrational fear resulting from the displacement of free-floating fear onto some environmental object or situation other than the original cause of the fear.

Phobia reaction: Process of displacing free-floating fear onto some environmental object.

Phobia: Irrational fear; the individual may realize its irrationality but nevertheless be unable to dispel it.

Phobic neurosis: Disorder characterized by intense fear of an object or situation which the individual consciously realizes poses no real danger to him.

Phrenology: The false belief that the personality consists of " faculties", each located in a specific area of the brain, and evidenced through "bumps" on the skull.

Physical psychiatry: Use of drugs, shock therapy or other physical therapy by the psychiatrist, usually in order to prevent extreme acts or to make the patient more receptive of psychotherapy.

Physiognomy: An invalid method of judging personality from facial characteristics.

Physiological gradient: A line of decreasing intensity of reaction to stimulation, lying along the central vertical axis of the organism, with reaction being greatest at the head. Maturation follows the physiological gradient, proceeding from the head to the feet and from the center outward.

Physiological limit: Point beyond which further practice no longer improves performance.

Physiological sensitivity: Degree to which our sense organs are capable of responding to stimuli.

Physiological dependence: Type of drug dependence involving withdrawal symptoms when drug is discontinued.

Pineal gland: Small gland at the base of the brain which helps regulate body's biological clock and may also pace sexual development. A small endocrine gland at the base of the brain, now thought to translate cyclic nervous activity generated by light into hormonal messages.

Pitch: Quality of sound produced by the frequency of the sound wave; expressed in cycles per second.

Pituitary gland: The most important endocrine gland associated directly with growth; secretes pituitary growth hormone and a number of "middle man" hormones which act upon other endocrine glands.

Pituitary growth hormone: Secretion of the pituitary gland which controls the growth of the skeleton, muscles, and various internal organs.

Placebo: An inactive substance administered in such a way that the patient believes he is receiving an active drug.

Plasticity: Modifiability; one of the two basic but interacting characteristics of human and animal behavior. See also Energetics.

Plateau: Period of no apparent learning, as measured by performance; appears as a flat place on a learning curve.

Play therapy: Use of play activities in psychotherapy with children. The counterpart for adults is recreational therapy.

Pleasure principle: In psychoanalysis, the demand that an instinctual need be immediately gratified regardless of reality.

Point of indifference: See Psychological zero point.

Population: Whole group in which a researcher is interested, from which samples are drawn for study. Also called universe.

Positive after sensation: Sensation of the original hue after stimulation ceases.

Positive transfer: See Proactive facilitation.

Positive rein forcer: A rein-forcer that increases the probability of recurrence of a given response.

Posthypnotic amnesia: Subject's lack of memory for the period during which he was hypnotized.

Posthypnotic suggestion: Suggestion given during hypnosis to be carried out by the subject after he is brought out of hypnosis.

Postpartum disturbances: Emotional disturbances associated with child birth.

Posttraumatic disorders: Residual symptoms following traumatic experience.

Precipitating cause: The particular stress which triggers a disorder.

Predisposing cause: Factor which lowers the individual's stress tolerance and paves the way for the appearance of a disorder.

Predisposition: Likelihood that an individual will develop certain symptoms under given stress conditions.

Proactive facilitation: The more ready learning of a new task because of prior learning of another task; also known as positive transfer.

Proactive inhibition: Interference of a prior learning task with the learning and recall of a new task; also known as negative transfer.

Probability of response: Criterion of learning often used for group learning; percentage of the group who make the correct response is the measure used.

Proband: In a genetic study, the individual who evidences the same trait in which the investigator is interested. Same as index case.

Process-reactive: Dimensions of schizophrenia referring to gradual of acute onset of symptoms.

Prognosis: Prediction as to the probable course and outcome of a disorder.

Programmed learning: Method of instruction or learning in which the student is guided through the subject matter step by step.

Profile: See Psychograph.

Progesterone: Female hormone secreted by the ovaries; produces changes in uterus tissues so that they can support fetal life.

Programmed instruction: Instruction in which material is presented in a sequence of steps, or frames, each ending with an item which the student must answer correctly before proceeding to the next.

Projection: Defense mechanism by which the individual unconsciously convinces himself that others have the undesirable thoughts and motives which he actually has himself.

Projection: Ego-defense mechanism in which individual attributes his own unacceptable desires and impulses to others.

Projective techniques: Methods of measuring personality traits in which the subject is presented with a standardized set of ambiguous or neutral stimuli and is allowed to interpret freely what he sees in them; also called depth techniques. Or any psychological technique for the diagnosis of personality organization utilizing relatively unstructured stimuli which reveal the individual's basic attitudes, conflicts, and so on.

Prophylaxis: Use of precautionary methods to prevent physical or mental illness.

Prostitution: Sexual intercourse for financial gain.

Pseudocommunity: Delusional social environment develop by a paranoiac.

Pseudomutuality: Relationship among family members that appears to be mutual, understanding, and open, but in fact is not.

Pseudoconditioning: Phenomenon by which behavior similar to conditioned behavior is obtained without the typical pairing of stimuli which is the essence of true conditioning; usually reflects a heightened state of excitement in which the organism makes the same response to whatever stimulus is introduced.

Psilocybin: Psychoactive drug derived from a mushroom.

Psychedelic drugs: "Mind expanding" drugs, such as LSD, which often result in hallucinations.

Psychiatric nursing: Field of nursing primarily concerned with mental disorders.

Psychiatrist: Medical doctor who specializes in the diagnosis and treatment of mental disorders.

Psychiatry: Field of medicine concerned with understanding, assessing, treating, and preventing mental disorders.

Psychic pain: Synonym for anxiety.

Psychic trauma: Stressful psychological experience of a severely traumatic nature.

Psychoactive drug: Any drug that markedly affects psychological functioning.

Psychiatric social worker: The holder of a master's degree in social work who works with psychiatrists, psychologists, and other mental health workers, especially in providing data about the social aspects of a client's often practices limited psychotherapy.

Psychiatrist: Medical doctor who specializes in the diagnosis and treatment of mental disorders.

Psychic trauma: An experience in which emotional relationship bring pain; thought to lead to physical disorders such as cancer later in life.

Psychoanalysis: School of psychology, originated by Freud, which emphasizes the study of unconscious mental processes; also a theory of personality and a method of psychotherapy which seeks to bring unconscious desires into consciousness and make it possible to resolve conflicts which usually date back to early childhood experiences.

Psychoanalyst: Therapist who uses the special system of theory and practice called psychoanalysis; required by organized psychoanalysts, though not by law, to have an MD degree.

Psychobiology: Eclectic approach to therapy aimed at an understanding of all factors biological, psychological, and social involved in a disorder.

Psychodiagnosis: Total study of an individual to determine his present psychological functioning in relation to past events and to predict the outcome of remedial measures.

Psychodrama: Form of psychotherapy in which the patient acts out life situations that are related to his difficulties.

Psychogalvanic response: See Galvanic skin response.

Psychograph: Chart showing an individual's standing on a group of objectively measured or rated traits; the traits are listed on one axis of the chart and the centimes or other values for each trait are marked at the appropriate points along the other axis, the points often being connected so as to show a profile of the individual's traits.

Psychological feedback: Process whereby the individual gains information concerning the correctness of his previous responses in order to correct errors; knowledge of results.

Psychological motives: Drives resulting from such needs as those for social approval, self-esteem, economic security, and greater knowledge; probably acquired as the result of experience.

Psychological primaries: Red, yellow, green, and blue, so called because they appear psychologically irreducible.

Psychological selectivity: See Attention.

Psychological zero point: Point at which neither warmth sensitive spots nor cold sensitive spots are stimulated; also known as point of indifference; usually about 90 degrees Fahrenheit.

Psychology: Science of the behavior of organisms.

Psychometrist: Specialist in psychological measurement.

Psychogenic: Of psychological origin; originating in the psychological functioning of the individual.

Psychological autopsy: An analytical procedure used to determine whether or not death was self-inflicted.

Psychological need: Need emerging out of environmental interactions, e.g. the need for social approval.

Psychological test: Standardized procedure designed to measure the subject's performance on a specified task.

Psychomotor: Involving both psychological and physical activity.

Psychomotor epilepsy: State of disturbed consciousness in which the individual may perform various actions, sometimes of a homicidal nature, for which he is later amnesic.

Psychomotor retardation: Slowing down of psychological and motor functions.

Psychomotor abilities: Abilities which require strength, coordination, and dexterity.

Psychopathic personality: Personality characterized by inability to envision results of one's actions or to care about results; tends to be incapable of deep emotional feelings and indifferent to social customs and ethics; "moral imbecile".

Psychopathic (antisocial) personality: Sociopathic disorder characterized by lack of moral development and inability to show loyalty to other persons or groups.

Psychopathology: Mental disorder.

Psychopharmacological drugs: Drugs used in treatment of mental disorders.

Psychophysics: A science concerned chiefly with determining the relationships between the physical qualities of stimuli and the sensations they produce; the direct forerunner of experimental psychology.

Psychophysiology disorders: See Psychosomatic disorders.

Psychosexual development: Freudian view of development as involving a succession of stages, each characterized by a dominant mode of achieving libidinal pleasure.

Psychosis: Severe personality disorder involving loss of contact with reality and usually characterized by delusions and hallucinations. Hospitalization is ordinarily required.

Psychosomatic disorder: Physical symptoms, often including actual tissue damage, that may result from the continued mobilization of the body during a sustained emotional disturbance.

Psychosocial: Pertaining to personality makeup or characteristics of the individual and to interpersonal interactions and relations which influence the individual's development and or behavior.

Psychosocial deprivation: Lack of needed stimulation and interaction during early life.

Psychosomatic (psychophysiology) disorders: Physical symptoms, which may involve actual tissue damage, resulting from continued emotional mobilization under stress; usually involve single organ system under autonomic nervous system innervation.

Psychosurgery: Brain surgery used in treatment of functional mental disorders. Also broadly used to refer to any from of brain surgery used to correct brain pathology resulting in a mental disorder.

Psychotherapy: A general term to describe treatment of personality and behavior disorders by psychological methods.

Puberty: Stage of physical development when reproduction first becomes possible.

Punishment: Application of aversive stimulation in response to behavior considered undesirable.

Pupil: Opening in the iris of the eye through which light enters the eye.

Papillary reflex: Automatic contraction of the pupil of the eye in response to excessive light.

Pupillometrics: Method of measuring changes in pupil size during emotion. The pupil of the eye dilates in response to stimuli which arouse a favorable reaction in the subject and contracts in response to distasteful stimuli.

Pure science: Scientific study in which understanding is sought as an end in itself.

Purkinje effect: Phenomenon experienced at nightfall, when the hues at the violet or short-wave end of the spectrum appear brighter than other colors; caused by the fact that during dark adaptation the eye loses sensitivity first to red and yellow and later to blue and green.

Pursuit movements: Conjugate gliding movements made by the eyes in following moving objects.

Pursuit rotor: Apparatus used in studies of motor learning; subject must keep the point of a hinged stylus in contact with a revolving brass target.

Pyriform cortex: Layer of cortex on the underside of the temporal lobe which aids in control of sexual impulses; lesions cause extreme sexuality in animals.

Q-sort test: A personality inventory in which subject, or someone evaluating him, sorts a number of statements into piles according to their applicability to the subject.

Qualitative classification: Grouping of items into categories on the basis of some characteristic which cannot be measured in a quantitative manner.

Quantitative classification: Classification of items into categories on the basis of some characteristic which can be measured on a mathematical scale.

Quartiles: Points which divide a distribution of measurements into quarters.

Racism: Prejudice and discrimination directed toward individuals or groups because of their racial background.

Random sample: Sample drawn in such a way that each member of population has equal chance of being selected; hopefully representative of population from which drawn.

Radial motion: Movement directly toward or away from the observer.

Random sampling: Method of drawing a sample so that each member of the population has an equal chance of being selected, and so that the probability of each member being selected is independent of whether or not any other member is selected.

Randomization: A form of experimental control in which subjects are assigned to experimental groups by chance or at random so as to eliminate any selective factor which might affect the results.

Range: Simplest measure of variability; the difference between the highest and lowest measurements.

Rape: To force sexual relations upon another person.

Rapport: Interpersonal relationship characterized by a spirit of cooperation, confidence, and harmony.

Rapid eye movement (REM) sleep: Type of sleep during which dreams occur.

Rating scale: Device for recording the rater's judgment of himself or others on defined traits. On relative rating scales, the rater ranks the subjects in order from highest to lowest in the group on the trait in question. On absolute rating scales, the judge assigns an absolute value or score to the individual on each trait being rated.

Rational-emotive therapy: Form of psychotherapy focusing on cognitive and emotional restructuring to foster adaptive behavior.

Ratio scale: Highest scale of measurement; has both equal units and an absolute zero; equal ratios between measurements stand for equal ratios of the amount of the attribute being measured.

Rational psychotherapy: Form of brief psychotherapy developed by Albert Ellis, which encourages the patient to substitute rational for irrational ideas in the inner dialogue which he constantly holds with himself.

Rationalization: Ego-defense mechanism in which the individual thinks up "good" reasons to justify his actions. Defense mechanism by which seemingly logical explanations are devised to explain and justify behavior which might otherwise result in loss of social approval and self-esteem; a form of intellectualization.

Raw score: Numerical score obtained on a test; cannot be compared with scores from other tests until all have been converted into common terms.

Reaction formation: Defense mechanism in which the individual's conscious attitudes and overt behavior patterns are the opposite of his unconscious wishes, which have been repressed.

Reaction time: Time that elapses between a stimulus and an individual's response to it.

Reality assumptions: Assumptions which relate to the gratification of needs in the light of environmental possibilities, limitations, and dangers.

Reality principle: Awareness of the demands of the environment and adjustment of behavior to meet these demands.

Reality testing: Behavior aimed at testing or exploring the nature of the individual's social and physical environment; often used more specifically to refer to the testing of the limits of permissiveness of his social environment.

Reality therapy: Form of therapy based on assumption that emotional difficulties arise when an individual violates his basic sense of right and wrong.

Recall: Most widely used method of measuring retention; with a bare minimum of cues, subject must reproduce a response learned earlier.

Recessive gene: Gene which is effective only when paired with an identical gene.

Recidivism: A shift back to one's original behavior (often delinquent or criminal) after a period of treatment or rehabilitation.

Reciprocal inhibition: Technique of desensitization used in behavior therapy in which responses antagonistic to anxiety are paired with anxiety-eliciting stimuli.

Receptive field: Area of retina from which impulses travel to a given neuron; always round for retinal ganglion cells, elongated for cortical cells. If center is excitatory, surround (periphery) is inhibitory and *vice versa.*

Receptors: Structures in the nervous system which are sensitive to stimuli and set up nerve impulses in the sensory nerve fibers.

Recessive gene: Gene which is ineffective unless paired with another gene just like it.

Reciprocal inhibition: Technique of psychotherapy developed by Wolpe in which the positive response invoked in the patient-therapist relationship combine with, and then inhibit, the patient's anxiety responses; a modification of the use of conditioning in therapy.

Reciprocal innervation: Process by which the excitation of one of an antagonistic pair of muscles is accompanied by the inhibition of the motoneurons supplying the other.

Recognition: Method of measuring retention in which subject identifies previously learned items from among a list in which they are interspersed.

Recommendations: Increase in integration or inner organization. Opposite of decompensation.

Reduction division: Special kind of cell division which occurs in the development of the gametes, causing them to contain only half the number of chromosomes contained in other body cells.

Reentry: Return from the openness of an encounter group to the real world, which is presumably less open and honest.

Referral: Sending or recommending an individual and or family for psychiatric assessment and or treatment.

Reflex: Specific, automatic response involving only a part of the body, such as the knee jerk or the grasping reflex of an infant.

Reflex arc: See Sensory-motor arc.

Regression: Defense mechanism in which the individual seeks to return to an earlier, more secure period of his life. Ego-defense mechanism in which the individual retreats to the use of less mature responses in attempting to cope with stress and maintain ego integrity.

Rehabilitation: Use of reeducation rather than punishment in dealing with criminal offenders.

Reinforcement: In classical conditioning, the process of following the conditioned stimulus by the unconditioned stimulus; in instrumental conditioning, the rewarding of the learner for adequate responses: In both cases, the response to a stimulus is strengthened.

Rejection: Lack of acceptance of another person, usually referring to such treatment of a child by his parents.

Relative rating scale: A method of rating in which each person's position on the scale is relative to that of other subjects in the group being considered.

Relatively refractory period: Period during which a very strong stimulus is needed to produce a response in the nerve fiber; follows absolutely refractory period.

Relearning: Most sensitive method of measuring retention; the subject relearns the original task under the original conditions, the difference in amount of practice needed to reach the original point of mastery providing the measure of retention.

Relevant variable: A variable which might produce changes in the dependent variable and therefore must be controlled throughout the experiment.

Reliability: The degree to which people earn the same rank or score each time they take the same test or an equivalent but different form of it; one characteristic of a good measuring instrument.

Reminiscence: Ability to remember a larger amount of incompletely mastered material at a later date than was recalled immediately after the cessation of practice.

REM sleep: Stage of sleep involving rapid eye movements (REM), associated with dreaming.

Remission: Marked improvement or recovery appearing in the course of a mental illness; may or may not be permanent.

Replication: Repetition of an experiment under the same conditions to see if the same results are obtained. In a factorial design, each of a number of representations of the same combination of independent variables.

Representative sample: A group of individuals selected from a larger in such a way that they accurately represent the characteristics of the larger group; essential for accurate results in an opinion poll or survey.

Repression: Defense mechanism in which painful or guilt-producing thoughts, feelings, or memories are excluded from conscious awareness; such repressed material may remain active at an unconscious level, resulting in bizarre behavior.

Representative sample: Small group selected in such a way as to representative of the large group from which it is drawn.

Reserpine: Tranquilizing drug widely used in the treatment of mental patients.

Resistance to extinction: Criterion of learning based upon the persistence of a conditioned response during extinction trials. Tendency of a conditioned response to persist lack of reinforcement.

Resistances: In psychoanalysis, inability or unwillingness to discuss certain ideas, desires, or experiences during free association.

Resistance: Tendency to maintain symptoms and resist treatment or uncovering of repressed material.

Respondent conditioning: See Classical conditioning.

Resonance theory: See Place theory.

Respondent behavior: Behavior which is elicited or evoked by events in the environment.

Response: Any reaction, usually a muscular or glandular process, that depends upon stimulation.

Response generalization: Use of a response similar to the correct one in conditioning.

Reticular activating system (RAS): Fibers going from the reticular formation to higher brain centers and presumably functioning as a general arousal system.

Reticular formation: Mass of neural nuclei and fibers in the brainstem just above the spinal cord; important in arousing and alerting the organism and also in controlling attention and perceptual discrimination.

Retina: Inner layer of the eye, containing the light-sensitive rods and cones.

Retinal disparity: The slight difference in the retinal image which the two eyes get from the same object; helps make depth perception possible.

Retroactive facilitation: Greater case of remembering caused by the nature of activity which intervenes between learning and recall.

Retroactive amnesia: Loss of memory for events immediately prior to a blow on the head or an electroshock convulsion, with no impairment of more permanent memories; explained by two-stage memory process.

Retrograde degeneration: Deterioration occurring in the nerve cell body when the long axon is cut; entire cell does not die.

Retrograde amnesia: Loss of memory for events during a circumscribed period prior to brain injury or damage.

Retrospective study: Research approach which attempts to retrace earlier events in the life of the subject.

Reverse tolerance: Situation in which a decreased amount of some psychoactive drug brings about the effects formerly achieved by a larger dose.

Reward centers: Clumps of cells in the brain, stimulation of which is sought by animals and inferred to give satisfaction.

Rhinencephalon: Area in the brainstem consisting of primitive cortex and complicated subcortical structures which have both olfactory and emotional centers; oldest part of the cerebral hemispheres; the "nose brain".

Rigid control: Coping patterns involving reliance upon inner restraints, such as inhibition, suppression, repression, and reaction formation.

Rigidity: Tendency to follow established coping patterns, with failure to see alternatives or extreme difficulty in changing one's established patterns.

Risky shift: Tendency for a group to be willing to take greater risks than its individual members would take on their own.

RNA: Ribonucleic acid, a cellular molecule similar in structure to DNA and regarded by some scientists as being responsible for encoding memory traces in the brain.

Rods: Receptor cells of the retina capable of producing sensations of white, gray and black but not of hues; effective in both day and night vision.

Rote learning: Verbatim learning, without regard for meaning.

Role: See Social role.

Role distortion: Violation of expected role behavior in an undesirable way.

Role obsolescence: Condition occurring when the ascribed social role of a given individual is no longer of importance to the social group.

Role playing: Form of psychotherapy in which the individual acts out a social role other than his own or tries out a new role for himself.

Rorschach test: Projective personality test making use of inkblots to elicit assessment data from the subject.

S-shaped curve: Graphic representation of an entire learning process; indicates a period of increasing returns from practice during early trials, a period during which the rate of improvement remains constant, and finally a period of decreasing improvement.

Saccule: Sac-like chamber in the vestibule at the base of the semicircular canals of the ear; contains receptors which respond to the static force of gravity and to straight line motion.

Sadism: Sexual deviation in which sexual gratification is obtained by the infliction of pain upon others.

St. Vitus' dance: Hysterical chorea of common occurrence during the middle ages.

Sample: Group upon which measurements are taken; should normally be representative of the population about which an inference is to be made.

Sampling distribution: A distribution of statistics, each based on a sample.

Saturation: Quality of color determined by the complexity of the light waves emanating from an object. More complex waves decrease the saturation, resulting in a grayish color.

Scapegoating: Process of displacing aggression into some object or person not the cause of the frustration. Or displacement of aggression onto some object, person, or group other than the source of frustration.

Schedule of reinforcement: Program of rewards for requisite behavior.

Schizo-affective psychosis: Disorder characterized by schizophrenic symptoms in conjunction with pronounced depression or elation.

Schizoid personality: Personality pattern characterized by shyness, oversensitivity, seclusiveness, and eccentricity.

Schizophrenia: Psychosis characterized by the breakdown of integrated personality functioning, withdrawal from reality, emotional blunting and distortion, and disturbances in thought and behavior.

Schemat: a. Persistent, deep-rooted, well-organized classifications of situations and of kinds of behavior appropriate in those situations; influence our perceptions.

Sclera: Outer protective layer of the eye; sclerotic coat.

Score: A number expressing quantitatively the results of a measurement.

Scotoma: Temporary or permanent blind spot; may be caused by excessive use of tobacco or alcohol, by overexposure to light, or by certain diseases.

Secondary cause: Factor which contributes to a mental illness but which in and of itself would not have produced it, as distinct from the primary cause.

Secondary gain: Indirect benefit from neurotic or other symptoms.

Secondary impotence: Condition in which male is capable of successful intercourse but manifests impotence 25 percent or more of the time.

Secondary prevention: Preventive techniques focusing on early detection and correction of maladaptive patterns within context of individual's present life situation.

Secondary process: Reality-oriented rational processes of the ego.

Secondary reinforcer: Reinforcement provided by a stimulus that has gained reward value by being paired with a primary reinforcing stimulus.

Secondary reinforcement: Reward which, although it does not directly satisfy a need, has come to be satisfying in itself, usually because of previous association with primary reinforcements.

Security: Maintenance of conditions necessary to need gratification.

Sedative: Drug used to reduce tension and induce relaxation and sleep.

Self (ego): The integrating core of the personality which mediates between needs and reality.

Self-acceptance: Being satisfied with one's attributes and qualities while remaining aware of one's limitations.

Self-actualization: Man's constant striving to realize his full inherent potentials, regarded by Goldstein, Rogers, Maslow, and others as the most fundamental goal of the human personality. Fulfillment of one's potentialities as a human being.

Self-concept: The individual's awareness of his continuing identity as a person; develops gradually from an infant's discovery of the parts of his own body and comes to include all an individual's thoughts, feelings, attitudes, values, and aspirations. It is the individual's sense of his own identity, worth, capabilities, and limitations.

Self-devaluation: Lowered feelings of worth and self-esteem.

Self-differentiation: Degree to which the individual achieves a sense of unique identity apart from the group.

Self-direction: Basing one's behavior on inner assumptions rather than external contingencies.

Self-esteem: Feeling of personal worth.

Self-exciting circuit: Arrangement of neurons whereby when one neuron discharges, the nerve impulse passes down the main axon into a collateral which connects with a second neuron which, in turn, transmits the impulse to the original cell, exciting it a second time. Self-exciting circuits make possible the prolongation of excitation.

Self-evaluation: Way in which the individual views himself-his worth, adequacy, etc.

Self-fulfillment: Living a meaningful, actualizing, and fulfilling life.

Self-ideal: See Ego-ideal.

Self-identity: Individual's delineation and awareness of his continuing identity as a person.

Self-inventory: Instrument for measuring personality traits by having the individual give information about himself; validity limited by subject's lack of self-understanding and by his desire to make himself appear better than he really is.

Self-recrimination: Self-condemnation and blame.

Self-reinforcement: Reward of self for desired or appropriate behavior.

Self-theory: Personality theory which utilizes the self-concept as the integrating core of personality organization and functioning.

Self-worth: The individual's evaluation of himself.

Semicircular canals: Canals in the bony labyrinth of the inner ear forming three loops extending in three different planes; site of the labyrinthine receptors, which keep the organism informed of position and movement in space.

Semistarvation neurosis: Psychological symptoms which appear as a result of prolonged periods on a markedly insufficient diet; characterized by apathy, depression, and irritability.

Senile: Pertaining to old age.

Senile dementia: A form of psychosis caused in part by deteriorative brain changes to aging.

Sensate focus training: Training to drive pleasure from touching one's partner and being touched by him or her; used in sexual therapy to enchance sexual feelings and help overcome sexual inadequacy.

Sensitivity training group (T-group): One type of small group designed to provide intensive group experience and foster self-understanding and personal growth.

Sensory awareness: Openness to new ways of experiencing and feeling.

Sensory deprivation: Restriction of sensory stimulation below the level required for normal functioning of the central nervous system.

Sensitization: Process by which emotional arousal increases general sensitivity so that a weaker stimulus than usual will elicit a response or a stronger response.

Sensory aphasia: Inability to recognize spoken words; "word deafness", can occur in persons who can hear simple sounds.

Sensory deprivation: Minimal sensory stimulation, sometimes achieved by eliminating all visual and auditory stimulation as nearly as possible, sometimes by depriving subject of structured stimulation; may lead to hallucinations and delusions.

Sensory feedback: Information supplied by the sense when a response is made to a stimulus; this information, in turn, acts as a new stimulus.

Sensory motor arc: Functional unit of the nervous system; a chain containing a receptor neuron, one or more interneurons in the spinal cord or brain, and an effector neuron; also called a reflex arc.

Sensory neuron: See Afferent neuron.

Sentence-completion test: Form of projective technique utilizing incomplete sentences which the subject is to complete.

Separation anxiety: Intense fear experienced when individual is separated from someone on whom he feels dependent.

Septal region: Area of the brain along the dividing line between the two hemispheres, just below the front bend of the corpus callosum; active in control of rage and savageness.

Serial learning: Learning in which the subject learns a series of words or syllables one at a time so that on successive showings he can anticipate the item that comes next.

Serial position effect: Tendency for the early items in a series to be easier to recall than later items and for the last items to be easier to recall than the middle ones.

Servo control: Use of external sources to maintain body temperature, as distinguished from the control maintained by internal homeostatic mechanisms.

Servomechanism: Machine which is intrinsically purposeful or goal seeking.

Set: Readiness to respond in a particular way to some stimulus situation for which there are a variety of possible responses. See also Learning set.

Sequelae: Symptoms remaining as the aftermath of a disorder.

Sexual deviate: Individual who manifests nonconforming sexual behavior, often of a pathological nature.

Sexual inadequacy: Inability or impaired ability to experience or give sexual gratification.

Shaping: Form of instrumental conditioning used in training animals, in which all responses that come close to the desired one are rewarded at first, then only the closest approximations, until the desired response is attained; also called successive approximation.

Sheltered workshops: Workshops where mentally retarded or otherwise handicapped individuals can engage in constructive work in the community.

"Shock" reaction: Transient personality decompensation in the face of sudden acute stress.

Shock therapy: Method of treating severe mental disturbances by inducing convulsions which are followed by a state of coma; usually induced by electricity.

Sibling: Term used to indicate the relationship between any two children of the same parents.

Sick role: Protected role provided by society via medical model for individual suffering from severe physical or mental disorder.

Simultaneous brightness contrast: Apparent change in gray to appear brighter (lighter) when seen next to black or darker when seen next to white.

Simultaneous hue contrast: Apparent change in hue of gray to take on the complementary hue of the color seen next to the gray.

Size constancy: Perceptual phenomenon by which we tend to perceive a known object as the same size regardless of its distance from us.

Situational stress reaction (acute): Superficial maladjustment to newly experienced life situations which are especially difficult or trying.

Situational orgasmic dysfunction: Inability of a women to have an orgasm with a particular person or in a particular situation.

Situational test: Test which measures performance in a simulated life situation.

Skinner box: Box containing a lever or other device which the animal must manipulate in order to obtain food or some other reward; used in experiments on operant conditioning.

Sleeper effect: An increase in the effect of a propaganda communication over a period of time, contrary to the normal expectation that the message would be forgotten; may occur when source of propaganda is discounted, since the discounting factor tends to be forgotten more rapidly than the message.

Social exchange: Model of interpersonal relationships based on the premise that such relationships are formed for mutual need gratification.

Social facilitation: Improvement of the performance of individuals by the mere presence of others.

Social perception: Awareness of group attitudes; requisite of a good leader.

Social stimulus value: The effect an individual has on others; includes his external appearance and his behavior toward others.

Social suggestion: Tendency to pay attention to what is pointed out by others, or to perceive an object in the same way others perceive it.

Social norms: Group standards concerning behaviors viewed as acceptable or unacceptable.

Social pathology: Abnormal patterns of social organization, attitudes, or behavior; undesirable social conditions which tend to produce individual pathology.

Social role: Behavior expected of individual occupying given position in group.

Social sanction: Punishment by group for violation of social norms.

"Social" self: The façade the individual displays to others as contrasted with his private self.

Social worker: Person in mental health field with a master's degree in social work (MSW) plus supervised training in clinical or social service agencies.

Sociocultural: Pertaining to board social conditions which influence the development and or behavior of individuals and groups.

Socioeconomic status: Position on social and economic scale in community; determined largely by income and occupational level.

Sociogenic: Having its roots in sociocultural conditions or causes.

Sociometric data: Measures of social acceptance and interaction used in studying intragroup relationships; sociometric choices are choices made by group members of those they like or would prefer for specified roles or activities.

Sociopathic disorder: Lack of social responsibility and inability to conform to prevailing social norms even when such norms are adaptive.

Sodium pentothal: Barbiturate drug sometimes used in psychotherapy to produce a state of relaxation and suggestibility.

Sodomy: Sexual intercourse via the anus.

Somatic: Pertaining to the body.

Sociotherapy: Process of modifying the patient's environment in such a way that he will stand a good chance of making a successful adjustment. Treatment of interpersonal aspects of the individual's life situation.

Somatic nervous system: Components of the nervons system which control the skeletal muscles; distinguished from the autonomic nervous system.

Somatic weakness: Special vulnerability of given organ systems to stress.

Somatosensory areas: Areas of cerebral cortex concerned with kinesthesis and the cutaneous senses; primary area lies just back of the fissure of Rolando and body surface is projected onto it; secondary area, just below, has the body projected on it less precisely and in reverse order.

Somatotype theory: A body-theory, proposed by Sheldon, relating physique to temperament and classifying individuals into three types: endomorph, mesomorph, and ectomorph.

Somesthesis: Body sensation, including kinesthetic and cutaneous sensations, controlled by the somatosensory areas of the brain.

Somnambulism: Sleepwalking.

Spasm: Intense involuntary, usually painful contraction of a spasticity. Marked hypertonicity or continual overcontraction of muscles, causing stiffness, awkwardness, and motor incoordination.

Spatial intelligence: Space visualization; ability to visualize the relationships of objects in space; a primary mental ability.

Specific nerve energies: Doctrine set forth by Johannes Miller which states that a sensory nerve will produce a certain type of experience no matter how it is stimulated.

Spectrum: The range of wavelengths; the visible spectrum goes from violet at the short-wave end to red at the long-wave end.

Speed of response: Criterion of learning based on num-sperm. Male gamete or germ cell.

Special vulnerability: Low tolerance for specific types of stress.

Sperm: Male gamete or germ cell.

Split-brain research: Research associated with split-brain surgery, which markedly impedes transmission of information from one cerebral hemisphere to the other.

Spinal reflex action: Simple stimulus-response behavior not ordinarily involving centers in the brain; can be studied by separating the spinal cord from higher centers or correlation.

Split brain: Brain in which the corpus callosum has been cut so that the two hemisphere are no longer connected;used in animal studies to learn more about brain function.

Spontaneous potentials: Rhythmic electrical oscillation which go continuously in the cerebral cortex; not evocated by specific sensory stimuli.

Spontaneous recovery. The return of a conditioned response following experimental extinction, after an interval of no stimulation.

Spontaneous recovery (remission): Recovery of a mental patient without treatment or with minimal treatment.

S-R psychologists: Psychologists who emphasize the role of stimulus-response (S-R) connections in learning. Also called associationists.

Spreading cortical depression: Reduction in electrical activity of the cerebral cortex induced by applying electrical potential to its surface through a hole bored in the skull.

Squint glasses: Glasses composed of prisms; used in studying color vision.

Stage of exhaustion: Third and final stage in the general-adaptation-syndrome, in which the organism is no longer able to resist continuing stress; may result in death.

Stage of resistance: Second stage of the general-adaptation-syndrome.

Standard deviation: A measure of variability; equal to the square root of the variance.

Standard error: A measure of how well a statistic represents a parameter; equal to the standard deviation of a sampling distribution.

Standard error of the mean: A measure of how well a sample mean represents a population mean; equal to the standard deviation of the sampling distribution of means.

Standard score: Score obtained by finding the difference between the raw score and the mean and dividing that difference by the standard deviation; useful in comparing scores on different tests.

Standardization: Process of obtaining norms, or standards, for comparing individual scores on a test; obtained by administering the test under standard conditions with standard instructions to a large group of persons who are representative of the individuals for whom the test is intended. Procedure for establishing the reliability startle reaction, or other group will appear, think, feel, or act.

Standard interview: Interview in which predetermined questions are asked in a set order.

Stereotype: Persistent and inappropriate repetition of phrases, gestures, or acts.

Stapes: The last of three hinged bones in the ear which transmit vibrations from the eardrum to the oval window; also called the stirrup.

Statistic: A number which represents a certain property of a series of measurements taken on a sample.

Statistical analysis: Method used to identify the component abilities involved in complex tasks and skills.

Statistical control: Technique of controlling variables statistical inference. Procedure of drawing general conclusions by studying samples.

Statistical significance: The degree to which the outcome of an experiment is contradictory to the null hypothesis; the probability of obtaining a given experimental outcome if the null hypothesis is correct.

Stimulation method: Method of determining which parts of the brain are related to muscular activity by stimulating areas of the brain and observing which, muscles move.

Stimulus: Energy given off by a stimulus object which, if strong enough, excites a receptor or group of receptors.

Stimulus generalization: Spread of a conditioned response to other objects similar to the original stimulus.

Stimulus objects: The parts of the environment that cause an individual, to react at any particular moment, or that are capable of making him react.

Stimulants: Drugs that tend to increase feelings of alertness, reduce feelings of fatigue, and enable individual to stay awake over sustained periods of time.

Stimulus generalization: The spread of a conditioned response to some stimulus similar to, but not identical with, the conditioned stimulus.

Stress: Unpleasant emotional upheaval which the individual experiences in response to frustration; any adverse condition such as extreme cold, heat, loud noise, etc.

Stressor: Anything injurious to the organism, either physically or psychologically.

Stress: Any adjustive demand that requires coping behavior on part of individual or group.

Stress-decompensation model: View of abnormal behavior which emphasizes progressive disorganization of behavior under excessive stress.

Stress interview: Interview of a subject under simulated stress conditions.

Stress tolerance (frustration tolerance): Nature, degree, and undergoing serious personality decompensation.

Structuralists: School of psychologists who studied conscious experience, conceived as made up of elementary mental states observable through introspection.

Stupor: Condition of lethargy and unresponsiveness, with partial or complete unconsciousness.

Stuttering: Speech disorder characterized by a blocking or repetition of initial sounds of words.

Subcortical structures: Structures of the brain below the cerebral cortex and above the midbrain.

Sublimation: Indirect expression of a need which cannot be satisfied directly, through acceptance of an alternate goal which provides a socially acceptable outlet of expression; usually refers specifically to indirect expressions of the sexual urge. Ego-defense mechanism by means of which frustrated sexual energy is partially channeled into substitutive activities.

Subliminal: Below the threshold; term applied to energy too weak to produce a response.

Substitution: Acceptance of substitute goals or satisfactions successive approximation. Expression of frustrated impulses indirectly but with no change in the conscious quality of the desire; often involves socially unacceptable activities.

Summation: Production of a response by a combination of stimuli that, singly, are too weak to produce a response temporal summation is accomplished through the repetition of a weak stimulus; spatial summation through the simultaneous stimulation of two or more adjacent points.

Superego: In psychoanalytic theory, that part of the personality which guards the ideas of right and wrong learned as a child; in constant conflict with the id; corresponds to the "conscience." Conscience; ethical or moral dimensions attitudes of personality.

Suicide: Taking one's own life.

Suppression: Conscious forcing of desires or thoughts out of consciousness; conscious inhibition of desires or impulses.

Surrogate: Substitute parental figure.

Survey method: Obtaining data from a selected group by means of questionnaires or interviews.

Symbol: An image; object, or activity that represents and can be substituted for somethingelse.

Symbolic rewards: Words or objects which cannot themselves satisfy biological drives but which come to be associated with primary rewards until they eventually acquire a reward value of their own.

Swinging: Mate swapping and other group sex practices.

Symbolism: Representation of one idea or object by another.

Sympathetic division: Division of the autonomic nervous system which is active in emergency conditions of extreme cold, violent effort, and emotions. Or division of the autonomic nervous system which is active in emergency conditions of extreme cold, violent effort or exercise, and states of fear or rage; fibers originate in spinal cord segments in middle of back.

Symptom: An observable manifestation of a physical or mental disorder.

Synapse: Association, without direct contact, between the end brushes of one neuron and the dendrites of another.

Synaptic knob: Rounded expansion at the end of each branch of the end brush of a neuron; comes very close to the next neuron and nerve impulse can "jump" across.

Synesthesia: Translation of sensory experience from one sensory mode to another, as in seeing colors when sounds are heard.

Systematic desensitization: Form of action therapy using the reciprocal inhibition technique; relaxation is induced while patient contemplates situations which produce anxiety; developed by Wolpe.

Syncope: Temporary loss of consciousness resulting from cerebral anemia.

Syndrome: Group or pattern of symptoms which occur together in a disorder and represent the typical picture of the disorder.

Syphilophobia: Morbid fear of syphilis.

System: An assemblage of interdependent parts, living or nonliving.

Systematic desensitization: A behavior therapy technique for eliminating maladaptive anxiety responses.

Ratio: A ratio similar to a critical ratio except that it takes into account the size of the sample; used in null hypothesis testing.

Tachycardia: Rapid pulse.

Tactual hallucinations: Hallucinations involving the sense of touch, such as feeling cockroaches crawling over one's body.

Tachistoscope: Apparatus which can project images or words onto a screen for a fraction of a second.

Tarantism: A mass psychosis or "dancing mania" which occurred occasionally in Italy and spain in the 17th century. Or a type of hysterical dancing occurring in epidemic form during the middle Ages.

Task-oriented reaction: Realistic rather than ego-defensive approach to stress.

Taraxein: A substance extracted from the blood of schizophrenic patients which, when injected into the blood of normal persons, will produce temporary psychotic symptoms.

Task-oriented dependency: Dependence on others for the performance of certain tasks; decreases and is discouraged as child learns to feed and clothe himself and perform other developmental tasks.

Taste buds: Clusters of receptors located on the tongue, responding to the four elemental qualities of taste, sweet, sour, salt, and bitter.

Tau effect: Phenomenon by which the timing of stimulation of points on the surface of the body can influence the perceived distance between them; similar phenomenon exsists in vision and hearing. If time between first and second stimulus is shouter than that between the second and third, the subject perceives the first two stimuli as closer together spatially than the second and third.

Tay-Sachs disease: Genetic disorder of lipoid metabolism usually resulting in death by age 3.

Telepathy: Communication from one person to another without use of any known sense organs.

Temporal lobe: Portion of cerebrum located in front of occipital lobe and separated from frontal and parietal lobes by the fissure of Sylvius.

Telephone theory: A frequency theory of hearing, according to which the basilar membrane plays the role of a telephone transmitter, realying impulses of various frequencies to the brain; unacceptable because a single nerve fiber cannot respond fast enough to handle frequencies greater than 1000 cycles per second.

Temperament factors: Traits of personality which describe the manner in which an individual characteristically operates.

Temporal lobe: Portion of the cerebrum separated from the frontal and parietal lobes by the fissure of Sylvius and lying just beneath the temples.

Tension: Condition arising out of the mobilization of psychobiological resources to meet a threat; physically, involves an increase in muscle tonus and other emergency changes; psychologically, is characterized by feelings if strain, uneasiness, and anxiety.

Tertiary prevention: Preventive techniques focusing on short-term hospitalization and intensive aftercare when an emotional breakdown has occurred. With aim of returning individual to his family and community setting as soon as possible.

Testes: Male reproductive glands or gonads (sex glands).

Testicular androgens: Male sex hormones produced by the testes; the major hormones responsible for the development of masculine characteristics during adolescence.

Testosterone: Male sex hormone.

Thalamus: Structure almost in the center of the brain; relay station for incoming sensory messages from all parts of the body. Responsible for sensations of pain and some diffuse, poorly localized sensations of pleasure or discomfort.

Theory: A logically organized set of principles propounded for the purpose of explaining a given group of phenomena.

Thinking: The manipulation or organization of elements of the environment by means of symbols rather than overt activity.

Therapeutic: Pertaining to treatment or healing.

Therapeutic community: The hospital environment used for therapeutic purposes.

Therapy: Treatment; application of various treatment techniques.

Theta wave: Brain wave having a frequency of only 5 to 7 cycles per second.

Threat: Real or imagined danger to individual.

Throughput: In cybernetics (as applied to man), activity within the nervous system which activates muscles to produce a response.

Thymus: An endocrine gland, most active in early life, which plays a role in developing immunity. Gland of uncertain function located in neck and upper thorax; usually atrophies in human adults.

Thyroids: Endocrine glands located in the neck which affect body metabolism, influence intelligence, and help control the rate of physical growth.

Thyroxin: Hormone secreted by the thyroids.

Tlc: Intermittent twitching or jerking, usually of facial muscles.

Timbre: Quality of sound determined by the complexity of the sound wave, that is, by the number of over-tones or partials which sound with the fundamental tone.

Tinnitus: Ringing in the ears.

Tone deafness: Inability to tell one note or pitch form another.

Token economy: Reinforcement technique often used in hospital or institutional settings in which individuals are rewarded for socially constructive behavior with tokens that can then be exchanged for desired objects or activities.

Tolerance: Physiological condition in which increased dosage of an addictive drug is needed to obtain effects previously produced by smaller dose.

Tonic: Pertaining to muscle tension or contraction; muscle tone.

Toxic: Poisonous.

Toxic deleria (psychoses): Severe disturbances in cerebral functions resulting from toxins.

Trait: Characteristic of individual which can be observed or measured.

Tranquilizer: Drug which calms and soothes the patient.

Trance: Sleep-like state in which the range of consciousness is limited and voluntary activities are suspended; a deep hypnotic state.

Tranquilizers: Drugs used for antipsychotic purposes and/or reduction of anxiety and tension.

Transactional analysis: Form of interpersonal therapy based on interaction of "child," "Adult." Ego states.

Transference: Process whereby client projects attitudes and emotions applicable to another significant person onto the therapist; emphasized in psychoanalytic therapy. Or process by which a patient in psychoanalytic therapy attaches to the therapist feelings formerly held toward some person who figured in an emotional conflict, often a parent or a lover.

Transitional cortex: A band of cortex running from the midline side of the frontal lobe across its underside and onto the temporal lobe; stimulation in this area produces visceral responses and vocalizations which are interpreted as emotional responses.

Translent situational disorder: Temporary mental disorder developing under conditions of overwhelming stress, as in military combat or civilian catastrophes.

Transsexualism: Identification of oneself with members of opposite sex, as opposed to acceptance of one's sexual identity.

Transavestism: Persistent desire to dress in clothing of the opposite sex, often accompanied by sexual excitement.

Trauma: Severe psychological or physiological stress resulting in injury or wound.

Traumatic: Pertaining to a wound or injury.

Traumatic neurosis: See "Shock" reaction.

Tremor: Repeated fine spastic movement.

Turner's syndrome: Form of mental retardation associated with sex chromosome anomaly.

Trial and error: Attempts to solve a problem by trying out alternative possibilities and discarding those that prove to be unsatisfactory.

Two–tailed test: A test of statistical significance in which the critical region lies at both extremes of the sampling distribution.

Two-way analysis of variance: Analysis of variance used in experiments in which there are two independent variables.

Two-way classification: Classification of each subject in an experiment according to two independent variables.

Uncertainty principle: Principle holding that measurements can never be absolutely accurate because an object or process may be altered by very process of being measured.

Unconditioned response (UCR): Response made to an unconditioned stimulus; often the case of salivation in reponse to food.

Unconditioned stimulus (USC): Stimulus which elicits a response in the absence of conditioning.

Ulcer: Open sore in mucosa lining of the stomach.

Unconscious: Lack of awareness; as used by Freud. Psychological material that has been repressed. Also loss of consciousness.

Unconscious motivation: Motivation for individual's behavior of which he is unaware.

Unconscious mental processes: Psychological processes or events which are below the level of consciousness (often as result of repression) but which exert an important influence on the individual's behavior; first postulated by Freud.

Undoing: Form of intellectualization in which the individual divests himself of painful feelings by making use of a cleansing ritual after some act which cases him to feel guilty; a defense mechanism.

Universe: The ultimate group to which an inference is to be made from data drawn from a representative sample; also called population.

Utricle: Sac-like chamber in the vestibule at the base of the semicircular canals of the ear, containing receptors which respond to the static force of gravity and to straight-line motion; important to our sense passive movement.

Underarousal: Inadequate physiologic response to a give stimulus.

Undoing: Ego-defense mechanism by means of which the individual performs activities designed to alone for his misdeeds, thereby, in a sense, "undoing" them.

Unsocialized aggressive reaction: Behavior disorder of childhood.

Vaginismus: An involuntary muscle spasm at the entrance to the vagian that prevents penetration and sexual intercourse.

Validity: Extent to which a measuring instrument actually measures what it purports to measure.

Values: Assumptions concerning good and bad, right and wrong.

Variable: A characteristic or property that may assume any one of a set of different qualities.

Variability: Spread or deviation; often used as means of determining how far above or below the average of his fellows an individual is in a given trait; the most common measure of variability is the standard deviation.

Variable interval schedule: Schedule by which reinforcement is given after differing lengths of time regardless of the number of correct responses made in between; leads to a relatively constant rate of response.

Variable ratio schedule: Schedule by which reinforcement is given after a variable number of responses; leads to a high and constant rate of responding.

Variance: A measure of variability which is computed by adding the square of the difference between each measurement and the mean, and dividing by the number of measurements; square of the standard deviation.

Vasomotor: Pertanining to the walls of the blood vessels.

Vegetative: Withdrawn or deterior to the point where the individual leads a passive vegetable-like existence.

Verbal learning: Any case of learning to respond to or with words.

Verbatim learning: Word for- word memorization.

Verbigeration: Prolonged and monotonous repetition of meaningless words and phrases.

Vertige: Dizziness.

Vicarious living: Attempt to evade efforts toward self-fulfillment by repressing one's own individuality and identifying with some hero or ideal.

Vicious circle: Chain reaction in which individual resorts to an unhealthy defensive reaction in trying to solve his problems, which only serves to complicated them and make them harder to solve.

Vigilance task: Task which requires the detection of specified changes in the environment over extended periods of times.

Virilism: Accentuation of masculine secondary sex characteristic, especially in a woman or young boy, caused by overactivity of the adrenal cortex.

Viscera: Internal organs.

Visceral: Pertaining to the internal organs; components of the nervous system which control the glands and the muscles of the internal organs.

Visual acuity: Sharpness of vision.

Visual area: Occipital lobe of the brain to which the optic nerves connect the two retinas.

Visual hallucinations: Hallucinations involving sense of sight.

Voyeurism: Achievement of sexual pleasure through clandestine "peeping," usually watching other persons disrobe and/or engage in sexual activities.

Volley theory: Auditory theory that nerve fibers operate in groups and that various fibers discharge their volley of impulses at different times, making it possible for bundle of fibers to reproduce high frequencies. Adequate for frequencies up to 5000, with a resonance (place theory being needed to explain higher frequencies the combination is known as the place volley theory.

Wassermann test: Serum test used in the diagnosis of syphilis.

Waxy flexibility: Condition in which a patient will maintain the position in which his limbs are placed for an unusually long period of time.

Wavelength: Linear distance from a point on one light wave or sound wave to the corresponding point on the next wave. Wavelength of light are the physical stimuli for sensations of hue; wavelengths of sound are the stimuli for sensations of pitch.

Weber's law: Law stating that the difference threshold or smallest noticeable difference in perceived intensity is a constant proportion of the original stimulus this law does not hold for extreme values.

Wernicke's center: Area on cortex of temporal lobe below the auditory area, extending backward and curving up around the end of the inability to understand spoken language.

Wisdom of the body: Ability to choose proper foods according to needs of the body; evidenced in infants but largely undermined by acquired tastes in abults.

Withdrawal reactions: Defense mechanisms involving physical flight or psychological withdrawal from the frustrating situation.

Within variance: A measurement of variation based on variance within samples, which is the result of random variation in relevant variables.

Wrong-way impulses: See Centrifugal impulses.

Withdrawal: Intellectual, emotional or physical retreat.

Withdrawal symptoms: Wide range of symptoms evidence by addicts when the drug on they are physiologically dependent is not available.

Word salad's: Jumbled or incoherent use of words by psychotic or disoriented individuals. Working through confronting and dealing with a problem situation until satisfactory adjustments are achieved and established.

Worry: Persistent concern about past behavior or about anticipated dangers in the present or future.

Index

B

C